Handbook of Drug Therapy

Handbook of Drug Therapy

Editor: Horace Dawson

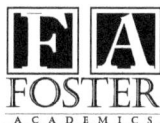

FA
FOSTER
ACADEMICS

www.fosteracademics.com

www.fosteracademics.com

FA FOSTER
ACADEMICS

Cataloging-in-Publication Data

Handbook of drug therapy / edited by Horace Dawson.
    p. cm.
Includes bibliographical references and index.
ISBN 978-1-63242-479-2
1. Chemotherapy. 2. Therapeutics. 3. Drugs. 4. Immunotherapy. I. Dawson, Horace.
RM262 .H36 2017
615.58--dc23

Foster Academics,
118-35 Queens Blvd., Suite 400,
Forest Hills, NY 11375, USA

ISBN 978-1-63242-479-2 (Hardback)

Contents

Preface

Drug therapy is defined as the cure and treatment of illness through drugs. Long-term consumption of drugs and drug treatment require careful monitoring and advice, as well as regulation of nutrition and a balanced diet. This book brings forth some of the most innovative concepts and elucidates the unexplored aspects of drug therapy. The various advancements in this field are glanced at and their applications as well as ramifications are looked at in detail. Those in search of information to further their knowledge will be greatly assisted by this text. This book will be very useful for students and researchers in the field of pharmaceuticals, pharmacology and medicinal chemistry.

The researches compiled throughout the book are authentic and of high quality, combining several disciplines and from very diverse regions from around the world. Drawing on the contributions of many researchers from diverse countries, the book's objective is to provide the readers with the latest achievements in the area of research. This book will surely be a source of knowledge to all interested and researching the field.

In the end, I would like to express my deep sense of gratitude to all the authors for meeting the set deadlines in completing and submitting their research chapters. I would also like to thank the publisher for the support offered to us throughout the course of the book. Finally, I extend my sincere thanks to my family for being a constant source of inspiration and encouragement.

Editor

Peritoneal Tumor Carcinomatosis: Pharmacological Targeting with Hyaluronan-Based Bioconjugates Overcomes Therapeutic Indications of Current Drugs

Isabella Monia Montagner[1], Anna Merlo[1], Gaia Zuccolotto[2], Davide Renier[3], Monica Campisi[3], Gianfranco Pasut[4], Paola Zanovello[1,5], Antonio Rosato[1,5]*

1 Veneto Institute of Oncology IOV - IRCCS, Padua, Italy, 2 Department of Medicine, University of Padua, Padua, Italy, 3 Fidia Farmaceutici S.p.A., Abano Terme, Italy, 4 Department of Pharmaceutical and Pharmacological Sciences, University of Padua, Padua, Italy, 5 Department of Surgery, Oncology and Gastroenterology, University of Padua, Padua, Italy

Abstract

Peritoneal carcinomatosis still lacks reliable therapeutic options. We aimed at testing a drug delivery strategy allowing a controlled release of cytotoxic molecules and selective targeting of tumor cells. We comparatively assessed the efficacy of a loco-regional intraperitoneal treatment in immunocompromised mice with bioconjugates formed by chemical linking of paclitaxel or SN-38 to hyaluronan, against three models of peritoneal carcinomatosis derived from human colorectal, gastric and esophageal tumor cell xenografts. *In vitro*, bioconjugates were selectively internalized through mechanisms largely dependent on interaction with the CD44 receptor and caveolin-mediated endocytosis, which led to accumulation of compounds into lysosomes of tumor cells. Moreover, they inhibited tumor growth comparably to free drugs. *In vivo*, efficacy of bioconjugates or free drugs against luciferase-transduced tumor cells was assessed by bioluminescence optical imaging, and by recording mice survival. The intraperitoneal administration of bioconjugates in tumor-bearing mice exerted overlapping or improved therapeutic efficacy compared with unconjugated drugs. Overall, drug conjugation to hyaluronan significantly improved the profiles of *in vivo* tolerability and widened the field of application of existing drugs, over their formal approval or current use. Therefore, this approach can be envisaged as a promising therapeutic strategy for loco-regional treatment of peritoneal carcinomatosis.

Editor: Irina V. Lebedeva, Columbia University, United States of America

Funding: This work was supported by Italian Association for Cancer Research (AIRC, IG-13121; and Special Program Molecular Clinical Oncology 5 per mille ID 10016 to AR). The funders had no role in study design, data collection and analysis, decision to publish, or preparation of the manuscript.

Competing Interests: The authors declare the affiliation of two co-authors (Dr. Davide Renier and Dr. Monica Campisi) to Fidia Farmaceutici S.p.A. company.

* Email: antonio.rosato@unipd.it

Introduction

Colorectal (CRC) and gastric cancers are the second and third most common causes of cancer-related death worldwide, respectively [1,2]. Both tumor histotypes frequently spread in the peritoneal cavity, thus causing peritoneal carcinomatosis (PC) even in the early phase of the disease [3–5]. Patients with peritoneally diffused disease have a poor prognosis, with median survival of just few months [3–5]. Esophageal carcinoma is the sixth most common cancer in the world, with a long-term survival rate of only 27–41% [6]. In the advanced stages, this type of carcinoma shows extensive peritoneal tumor spread [7].

Once established, PC can be essentially regarded as a terminal clinical condition that is poorly amenable to further chemotherapeutic aggression [8]. Nonetheless, the last years have witnessed new therapeutic treatments based on cytoreductive surgery combined with intraperitoneal chemotherapy under hyperthermic condition, to produce a loco-regional control of peritoneal metastasis and to improve long-term survival of patients [9,10].

This approach, however, requires the development of more efficient and less toxic chemotherapeutic agents [11].

Macromolecular drug delivery systems have been proposed as advanced approaches for improving antitumor treatments, especially with the aim of overcoming drug resistance, water insolubility, lack of selectivity and increasing tolerability [12]. Polymeric conjugates of chemotherapy agents are largely based on biocompatible polymers like dextran [13,14], synthetic poly(L-glutamic acid) polymers [15], polyanhydrides [16], N-(2-hydroxypropyl)methacrylamide copolymers [17,18], poly(ethyleneglycol) (PEG) [19,20] and hyaluronan (HA), as reviewed by Duncan *et al.* [12]. HA [21,22] is a linear polysaccharide that is ubiquitously distributed in the extracellular matrix, the synovial fluid of joints and the cartilage. By promoting cell motility, adhesion and proliferation, HA plays a pivotal role in biological processes as morphogenesis, wound repair, inflammation and cancer metastasis [23,24]. These phenomena rely on the interaction with several receptors, among which the most representative are CD44 [25,26], the receptor for hyaluronan-mediated cell motility

(RHAMM, CD168) [24], and HARE (HA receptor for endocytosis) [27]. Since CD44 and RHAMM are overexpressed in a wide variety of cancers, including colorectal [11], gastric [28] and esophageal carcinoma [29], hyaluronan-drug bioconjugates should present a markedly enhanced selectivity for cancerous cells. Therefore, such approach can be envisaged to achieve an enhanced targeting of tumor tissue, and to prolong the retention of drugs within the body, besides providing advantages in drug solubilization, stabilization, localization and controlled release. In this regard, HA has already been conjugated to different antineoplastic drugs, generating new compounds with promising antitumor effects toward a broad panel of tumor histotypes [11,21,30–32].

Here, we compared the therapeutic effectiveness of two bioconjugates derived from the chemical linking of paclitaxel [21] or SN-38 [11], the active metabolite of irinotecan, to HA against three models of human PC xenografts in immunocompromised mice. We show that they performed successfully after intraperitoneal administration, having a comparable or enhanced therapeutic efficacy profile respect to free drugs, thus supporting their testing in clinical trials.

Materials and Methods

Drugs

The hyaluronan-based paclitaxel (ONCOFID-P) [21] and SN-38 (ONCOFID-S) [11] bioconjugates have been previously described. The batch of ONCOFID-S used was characterized by a SN-38 loading of 9.4%. Paclitaxel (Taxol) was from Bristol-Myers Squibb Italia (Rome, Italy), while irinotecan (CPT-11) and SN-38 were purchased from Antibioticos (Rodano, Italy). When needed, bioconjugates were labeled with the fluorochrome BODIPY TR cadaverine (Invitrogen, San Giuliano Milanese, Italy), as previously described [33].

Tumor cell lines

The following human tumor cell lines were used: HCT-15 [34], HT-29 [35] and LoVo [36], colorectal adenocarcinoma; OE-33 [37], esophageal adenocarcinoma; KYSE-30 [38] and OE-21 [37], esophageal squamous carcinoma; MKN-45 [39], gastric adenocarcinoma. A CD44^{high} subpopulation of HCT-15 was isolated by immunomagnetic sorting, as previously reported [40]. Cells were grown in RPMI 1640 (EuroClone, Milan, Italy) supplemented with 10% (v/v) heat-inactivated fetal bovine serum (Gibco BRL, Paisley, UK), 2 mM L-glutamine (Gibco BRL), 10 mM HEPES (PAA Laboratories, Linz, Austria), 200 U/mL penicillin (Pharmacia & Upjohn, Milan, Italy), 200 U/mL streptomycin (Bristol-Myers Squibb Italia) and 1 mM sodium pyruvate (Lonza, Basel, Switzerland; not added in the case of MKN-45 cells), hereafter referred as to complete medium. Cell lines were maintained at 37°C in a humidified atmosphere containing 5% CO_2.

Cytotoxicity assay

The *in vitro* cytotoxicity of free drugs, ONCOFID-P, ONCOFID-S and fluorochrome-labeled bioconjugates was assessed against all cell lines using the ATPlite luminescence adenosine triphosphate (ATP) detection assay system (PerkinElmer, Zaventem, Belgium) [41], according to the manufacturer's instructions. Briefly, cells were resuspended in complete medium and seeded into 96-well flat-bottomed plates (8×10^3/well); the day after, different drug concentrations were added (final volume, 100 μL/well) for 72 hours. At day 4, 50 μL of lysis solution were added to each well followed by addition of 50 μL of substrate solution and

final counting of luminescence by the TopCount Microplate Counter (PerkinElmer). Within each experiment, determinations were performed in triplicate and experiments were repeated 5 times for each cell line. The percentage of cell survival was calculated by determining the counts per second (cps) values according to the formula: $[(cps_{tested} - cps_{blank})/(cps_{untreated\ control} - cps_{blank})] \times 100$, with cps_{blank} referring to the cps of wells that contained only medium and ATPlite solution. IC_{50} values were calculated from semi-logarithmic dose-response curves by linear interpolation.

Flow cytometry analysis

CD44 and CD168 (RHAMM) expression in all tumor cell lines was evaluated by flow cytometry, as previously reported [33]. Interaction of bioconjugates with tumor cells was evaluated by incubating 3×10^5 cell/sample in 1 mL of medium containing BODIPY-labeled ONCOFID-P (50 μg/mL in paclitaxel equivalents) or ONCOFID-S (50 μg/mL in SN-38 equivalents) at 37°C. At different time points thereafter (0.5, 1, 2, 5, 10, 15, 30 or 60 minutes), cells were harvested as previously described [21] and the fluorescence was compared with that of untreated cells. Where indicated, tumor cells were treated with BODIPY-labeled ONCOFID-P, and then with hyaluronidase (HA:hyaluronidase molar ratio of 25:1 w/w; Sigma-Aldrich) for 4 hours at 37°C in PBS to remove non-internalized conjugates, before flow cytometry analysis. To evaluate the role of CD44 receptor in the interaction of ONCOFID-P with cancer cell lines, cells were incubated with BODIPY-labeled bioconjugate for 30 minutes in the presence of an anti-CD44 blocking mAb (10 μg/ml, clone 5F12, Lifespan Biosciences, Seattle, WA).

Chemical inhibitors of endocytosis

To dissect the endocytosis pathway involved in cellular entry of bioconjugates, tumor cells were treated with different chemical inhibitors for 1 hour at 37°C in RPMI before drug exposure and hyaluronidase treatment, as reported above. The following inhibitors were used: amiloride (inhibitor of phagocytosis/micropinocytosis; 50 μM), chlorpromazine (inhibitor of clathrin-dependent endocytosis; 20 μg/ml), cytochalasin D (inhibitor of phagocytosis/micropinocytosis; 10 μg/ml), and filipin III (inhibitor of clathrin-independent, caveolin-mediated endocytosis; 10 μg/ml), all purchased from Sigma-Aldrich.

Confocal microscopy analysis

To assess cell internalization of bioconjugates by confocal microscopy, tumor cell lines were seeded on glass coverslips in 12-well tissue culture plates at the concentration of 5×10^5 cells/well. After 24 hours of culture, cells were incubated with BODIPY-labeled bioconjugates for 1 hour at 37°C, and then fixed for 20 minutes in 4% formaldehyde. Sample analysis was carried out with a Zeiss LSM 510 microscope (Carl Zeiss, Jena, Germany), using a long pass 560 nm filter. Lysosomal colocalization and microtubular visualization studies were carried out as previously described [40].

Assessment of Topoisomerase I activity by plasmid relaxation assay

Topoisomerase I (Topo I) was isolated from tumor cell lines by Qproteome Nuclear Protein Kit (Qiagen, Milan, Italy), after incubation of cells (5×10^6/sample) with ONCOFID-S (50 μg/mL in SN-38 equivalents), SN-38 (50 μg/mL) or complete medium (untreated cells) at 37°C for 1 hour. Enzyme activity was assessed using the Human Topo I Assay Kit for cell extracts (Inspiralis,

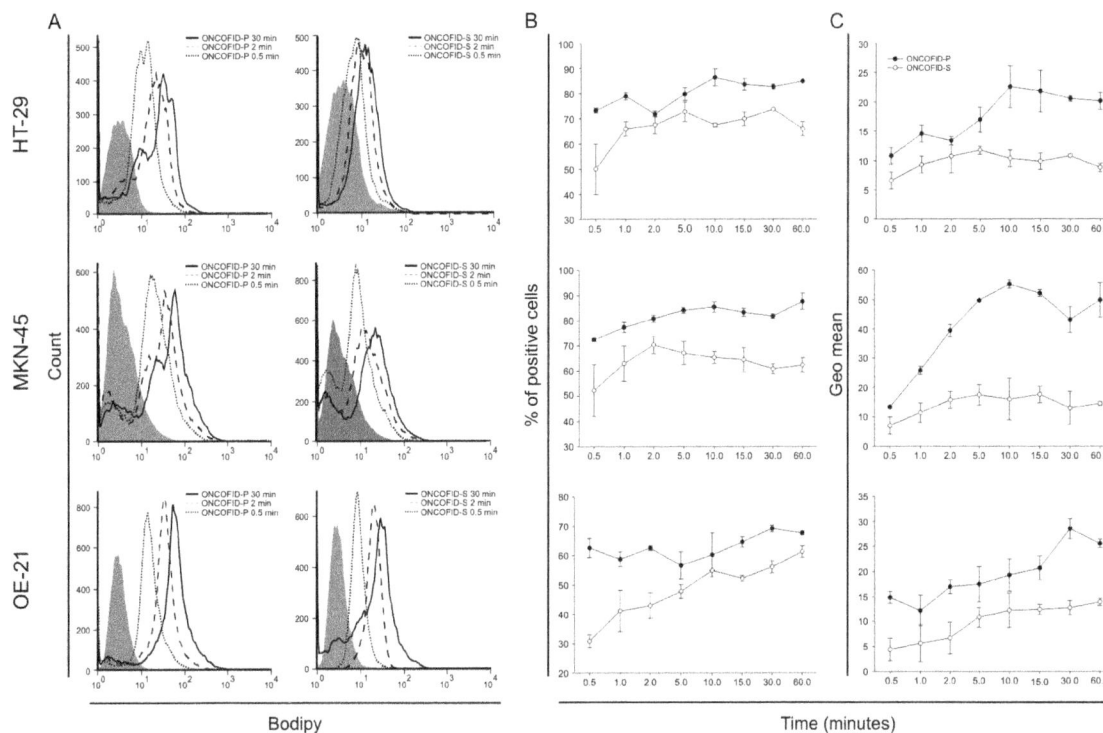

Figure 1. Interaction of bioconjugates with cancer cell lines. A, BODIPY-labeled ONCOFID-P (50 µg/mL in paclitaxel equivalents) or ONCOFID-S (50 µg/mL in SN-38 equivalents) were added to tumor cells and flow cytometry analysis was performed at different time points thereafter (0.5, 1, 2, 5, 10, 15, 30 or 60 minutes). Panels illustrate cytometry profiles at 3 representative time points. B, whole kinetics of interaction at all time points tested. C, kinetics of the fluorescence intensity (geo mean) detected on tumor cells at the same time points analysed as in B. Panels B and C report mean ± SD of 3 independent experiments.

Norwich, United Kingdom). Dilutions of cell extracts (1:5, 1:10, 1:50, 1:100 and 1:500) were incubated for 30 minutes at 37°C with the relaxation mix containing a supercoiled DNA substrate (pBR322). Reaction was stopped by adding an equal volume of chloroform/isoamyl alcohol (24:1). Samples were fractionated by 0.8% agarose gel electrophoresis, visualized by ethidium bromide staining and quantified by UV densitometry using the supercoiled and relaxed pBR322 plasmid as positive or negative control, respectively. Inhibition of Topo I activity was calculated as the ratio between the supercoiled fractions in treated cells and the positive control and expressed as percentage.

Mice

Six to eight week-old female severe combined immunodeficiency (SCID) mice were purchased from Charles River Laboratories (Calco, Italy), and housed in our Specific Pathogen Free (SPF) animal facility.

In vivo experiments and optical imaging

SCID mice were inoculated i.p. with 1×10^6 HT-29, MKN-45 or OE-21 tumor cells. Pharmacological treatments were started at day 7 from tumor injection and carried out according to a q7dx3 schedule (every 7 days for 3 doses). Each experiment comprised groups of animals (six mice/group) that received ONCOFID-P i.p. (40 mg/kg in paclitaxel equivalents), or ONCOFID-S i.p. (19.2 mg/kg in SN-38 equivalents), or paclitaxel i.p. (10 mg/kg), or CPT-11 i.p. (60 mg/kg), or paclitaxel i.v. (20 mg/kg) or CPT-11 i.v. (100 mg/kg). Injected tumor cells had been previously transduced with a lentiviral vector coding for the firefly luciferase reporter gene [42] to track tumor growth *in vivo*. Bioluminescence

(BLI) images were acquired at different time points after *in vivo* cell injection using the IVIS Lumina II Imaging System (PerkinElmer). Ten minutes before each imaging session, animals were anesthetized with isoflurane/oxygen and administered i.p. with 150 mg/kg of D-luciferin (PerkinElmer) in DPBS. A constant region of interest (ROI) was manually selected around the abdomen of animals and the signal intensity was measured as radiance (photon/sec) using the LivingImage software 3.2 (PerkinElmer). Tumor growth and response to therapy were monitored by BLI and by recording survival. Procedures involving animals and their care were in conformity with institutional guidelines (D.L. 116/92 and subsequent implementing circulars), and experimental protocols (project ID: 3/2012) were approved by the local Ethical Committee of Padua University (CEASA). During *in vivo* experiments, animals in all experimental groups were examined daily for a decrease in physical activity and other signs of disease or drug toxicity; severely ill animals were euthanized by carbon dioxide overdose.

Statistical analysis

Survival curves and probabilities were estimated using the Kaplan-Meier technique. A log-rank test for comparisons, an Anova test or a Mann-Whitney Rank Sum Test were used when required. Analysis of data were done using the MedCalc (version 12) and SigmaPlot (version 12.3) statistical packages.

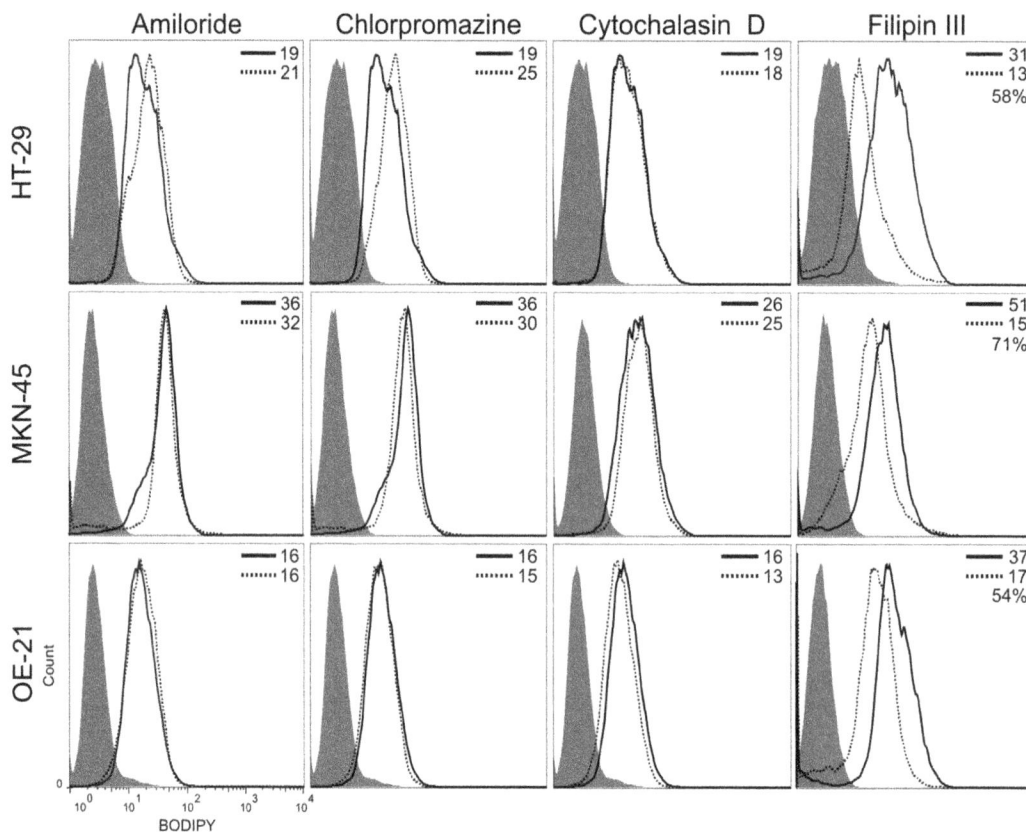

Figure 2. Endocytosis pathways involved in bioconjugate cell entry. HT-29, MKN-45 and OE-21 tumor cells were left untreated (solid line) or treated (dashed line) for 1 hour with selective chemical inhibitors of different pathways involved in endocytosis (amiloride, chlorpromazine, cytochalasin D and filipin III). Subsequently, cells were exposed for 30 minutes to ONCOFID-P and then treated with hyaluronidase for 4 hours, to be finally analyzed by flow cytometry. Data at the upper-right corner of each panel report the respective geo mean values, and the percentage of reduction induced by treatment.

Results

HA receptor expression on target cancer cell lines

CD44 and CD168 are regarded as important receptors for hyaluronan binding. To assess their expression on colorectal, esophageal and gastric tumor cell lines, flow cytometry analysis was carried out. Results showed that CD44 was intensely expressed on all cell lines examined but HCT-15, which disclosed a weak positivity (about 20% of population; Fig. S1, inset). This cell line was immunomagnetically sorted in two subpopulations expressing the relevant marker at high and low intensity (Fig. S1A), to be further analyzed and compared with the parental cell line for sensitivity to the conjugated drugs (see below). RHAMM expression was more erratic and exclusively intracellular (Fig. S1B), being membrane levels of the receptor almost undetectable (data not shown).

Analysis of interaction of bioconjugates with target cancer cell lines

To assess the direct interaction of ONCOFID-P and ONCO-FID-S with CD44 expressing target cells, bioconjugates were labeled with the BODIPY fluorophore, incubated with tumor lines and analyzed cytofluorimetrically at different time points. Results disclosed that the bioconjugates readily bound to target cancer cells in a time-dependent manner (Fig. 1A and B). Indeed, the percentage of positive cells was already sensibly high just after 30 seconds, and progressively increased over time along with

fluorescence intensity (Fig. 1C). To assess whether the fluorescent signal was simply due to a physical association to the cell membrane or truly reflected the internalized compound, the potentially non-internalized bioconjugates were removed by hyaluronidase treatment. For this and the following set of experiments, ONCOFID-P was selected as a prototype compound, since the critical moiety involved in cell interaction for both conjugates is represented by HA with the same MW and characteristics, and therefore results obtained with one can reliably apply also to the other bioconjugate. Results disclosed that such treatment slightly impacted the kinetics of physical binding between ONCOFID-P and tumor cells, as these latter readily became positive both in the presence or in the absence of hyaluronidase. On the other hand, removal of the membrane-bound labeled compound strongly reduced the fluorescence signal intensity and disclosed that a plateau was reached very rapidly, thus indicating that most of the bioconjugate was internalized in the first few minutes of interaction (Fig. S2).

Moreover, tumor cells were treated with a blocking anti-CD44 mAb to disclose the relevance of this receptor in the interaction of HA-conjugated drugs with target cells. While the fluorescent signal turned out to be strongly reduced, treatment with the blocking antibody did not completely abrogate the binding to the cells, thus suggesting a prominent but not exclusive role of CD44 in the uptake of the HA-conjugated compound ([24]; Fig. S3).

To dissect the different mechanisms of trafficking across the plasma membrane, tumor cells were treated with chemical agents

A

B

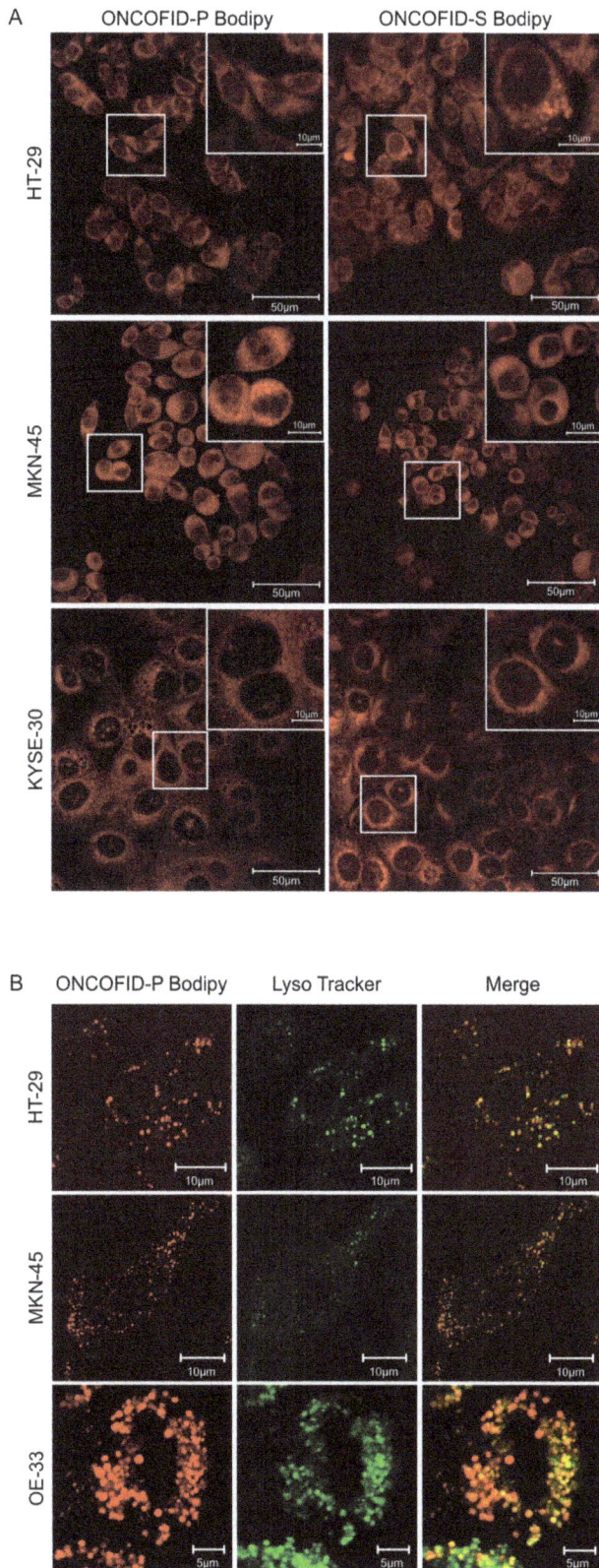

Figure 3. Confocal microscopy analysis and co-localization studies. A, accumulation of bioconjugates in HT-29, MKN-45 and KYSE-30. Cells were incubated with BODIPY-labeled ONCOFID-P (50 μg/mL in paclitaxel equivalents) or ONCOFID-S (50 μg/mL in SN-38 equivalents) for 1 hour, washed and fixed before analysis. B, co-localization analysis of bioconjugates in lysosomes. HT-29, MKN-45 and OE-33 cells were

treated with LysoTracker green, incubated with BODIPY-labeled compounds and finally analyzed by confocal microscopy. Left pictures show the fluorescence of the labeled bioconjugates (red) in single cells, while central pictures illustrate signals (green) from lysosomes. The merging of the 2 components is visible in right pictures. Lysosomes were occupied by bioconjugates by ~90% to 100%, as assessed by the Zeiss' profile software tool. Experiments were repeated at least twice with consistent results.

that selectively block specific endocytic pathways. Amiloride, chlorpromazine and cytochalasin D leaved the internalization of ONCOFID-P substantially unaffected, thus ruling out phagocytosis/micropinocytosis and clathrin-mediated endocytosis as mechanisms for cellular entry. Conversely, the treatment with filipin III strongly reduced the intensity of fluorescence signal (Fig. 2), thus indicating that a clathrin-independent, caveolin-mediated endocytic pathway represents the major mechanism of internalization for HA-conjugates, in agreement with previously published data [43]. Overall, these data suggest that the bioconjugates physically associate to the cells, to be subsequently sequestered and accumulated. Indeed, this latter aspect was formally demonstrated by confocal microscopy analysis (Fig. 3A), which disclosed a relevant cytoplasmic accumulation. Moreover, bioconjugates appeared undergoing a rapid compartmentalization into discrete subcellular sites that were strongly reminiscent of lysosomes, as a similar pattern of fluorescence was observed by labeling tumor cells with a green fluorescent lysosome tracker. In fact, fluorescence signals derived from cells treated with the labeled compounds and the lysosome tracker completely overlapped (Fig. 3B and data not shown), thus demonstrating that bioconjugates did actually accumulate into the lysosomal compartments. Fluorochrome labeling of compounds did not modify their biological activity, as the fluorescent bioconjugates fully retained the cytotoxic potential (Fig. S4 and data not shown).

Assessment of the mechanism of action of bioconjugates

Paclitaxel profoundly interferes with the intracellular microtubular mesh. To evaluate the effects of ONCOFID-P on the cytoskeleton architecture, target cell lines were incubated with the bioconjugate or the free drug, and stained with an anti-β-tubulin mAb to be finally imaged by confocal microscopy. Results showed that the bioconjugate led to the formation of tubulin bundles similar to those induced by treatment with free drug (Fig. 4A), thus suggesting that the paclitaxel released by ONCOFID-P fully retains the capacity of interfering with the microtubule polymerization dynamics.

After being produced from irinotecan, SN-38 blocks the activity of Topo I, a nuclear enzyme which makes single-strand cuts in DNA to favor relaxation before cell duplication. To assess the effects of ONCOFID-S or the free drug on Topo I activity, nuclear protein extracts from treated cells were incubated with a plasmid DNA and the ratio between the supercoiled and relaxed forms was visualized (Fig. 4B) and quantified (Fig. 4C) by gel electrophoresis. Both ONCOFID-S and SN-38 inhibited the enzyme activity, even though the free drug appeared more efficient in particular in the colorectal and esophageal histotypes. Nonetheless, results suggest that active SN-38 molecules are released by the bioconjugate and have access to the nucleus where they can block Topo I activity.

Evaluation of *in vitro* tumor growth inhibition activity of bioconjugates

To test ONCOFID-P and ONCOFID-S *in vitro* efficacy against target cancer lines, cells were incubated with escalating

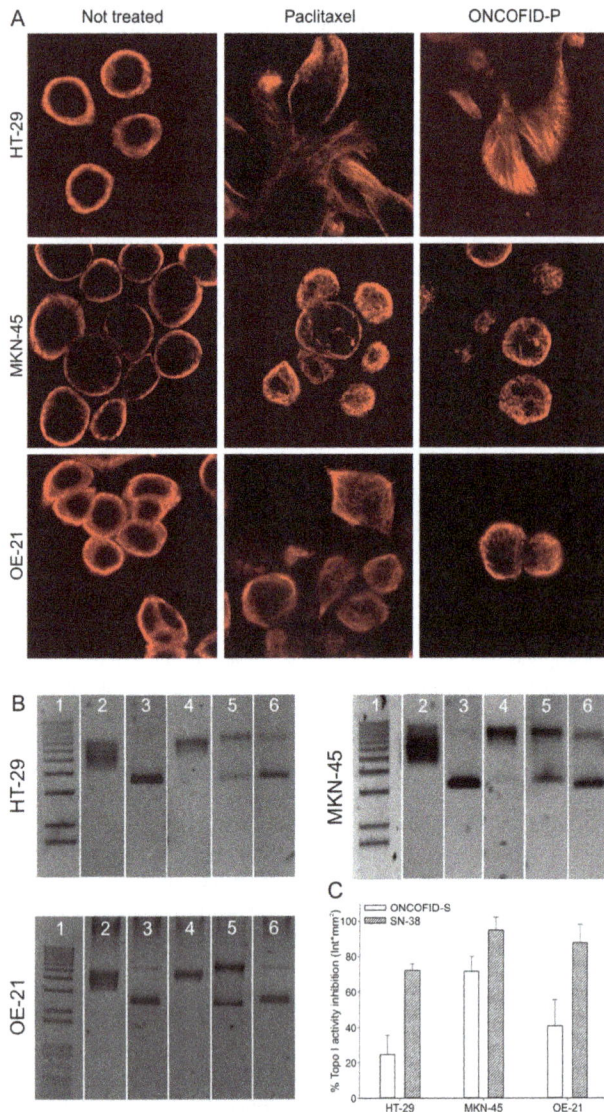

Figure 4. Assessment of bioconjugate mechanism of action. A, rearrangement of tumor cell microtubular architecture after drug treatment. HT-29, MKN-45 and OE-21 cells were treated with ONCOFID-P or free paclitaxel for 4 hours at 37°C. After treatment, cells were fixed, permeabilized, and stained with an anti-β-tubulin mAb and anti-mouse Ig Alexa 546-conjugated antiserum. Cells treated with free drug or bioconjugate disclosed the same interferences on the microtubular mesh. B, inhibition of Topo I activity after ONCOFID-S or SN-38 treatment in HT-29, MKN-45 and OE-21 cells. Gels show the supercoiled or relaxed forms of pBR322 plasmid after incubation with a 1:50 dilution of nuclear protein neat extracts obtained from tumor cells treated with conjugated or free drug for 4 hours. Lane 1, marker; lane 2, relaxed pBR322 plasmid (positive control); lane 3, supercoiled plasmid (negative control); lane 4, supercoiled plasmid in the presence of nuclear protein neat extract from drug-untreated cells; lane 5, supercoiled pBR322 admixed with nuclear protein neat extract from ONCOFID-S treated cells; lane 6, supercoiled pBR322 admixed with nuclear protein neat extract from SN-38-treated cells. C, quantification of the reactions shown in B. Figure reports mean ± SD of 3 independent experiments.

concentrations of bioconjugates and the resulting dose-dependent growth inhibition activity was compared to that exerted by the commercial free drugs. The antiproliferative activity of bioconjugates turned out to be comparable to that observed with the

unconjugated drugs (Table S1); as expected, the inhibitory activity of irinotecan was limited because such drug requires *in vivo* activation and conversion [44]. No toxic effects could be ascribed to HA (data not shown).

As CD44 appears critically involved in binding HA-conjugated drugs (Fig. S3 and [40]), we further addressed the role of CD44 in conjugate binding and activity by isolating two HCT-15 sublines expressing respectively high and low levels of the receptor, to test their sensitivity to bioconjugate cytotoxicity respect to the parental cell line. Using either ONCOFID-P or ONCOFID-S, almost a one-log differential susceptibility was observed between HCT-15 sublines (Fig. S5). The total cell population did not display a perfectly intermediate behaviour between CD44^{high} and CD44^{low} cells, likely due to a receptor expression very close to that of the CD44^{low} subline. As controls, both HCT-15 sublines and parental cells exhibited the same sensitivity to the unconjugated drugs (Fig. S5, left panels).

In vivo therapeutic activity of ONCOFID-P and ONCOFID-S

To test the therapeutic efficacy of bioconjugates in a PC context, models of diffuse carcinomatosis were set up for each tumor histotype under investigation by i.p. injection of MKN-45, HT-29 and OE-21 tumor cell lines. Pharmacological treatments were started at day 7 from tumor injection and carried out according to a q7dx3 schedule. In each experiment, groups of mice were injected with either ONCOFID-P or ONCOFID-S i.p., or the free drugs administered through the i.p. or i.v. routes for comparison. The low water solubility and high side toxicity precluded the use of free SN-38, which was then replaced by its precursor CPT-11, commonly used in the clinical setting. The therapeutic impact of the different approaches was assessed by luminescence, as the tumor cell lines tested had been previously transduced with a lentiviral vector coding for the firefly luciferase reporter gene to track tumor growth, and by recording survival.

As illustrated in Figure 5, ONCOFID-P loco-regional treatment brought about relevant therapeutic effects against all peritoneal carcinomatosis models, with a particular emphasis in gastric and esophageal cancers. When such results were compared to those obtained using the free drug given through different administration routes, it turned out that free paclitaxel given i.p. exhibited a modest efficacy, being less efficient against gastric and esophageal cancer but not colon carcinoma, and with a significant reduced activity compared to the conjugated form. On the other hand, the same free drug given i.v. was slightly more efficient in mediating antitumor effects, but not superior to ONCOFID-P (data not shown). Notably, a relevant tumor growth inhibition was also obtained with ONCOFID-S.

These results were partially confirmed by survival analysis (Fig. 6 and Table S2). Indeed, ONCOFID-P treatment significantly prolonged survival in all tumor models compared to controls, a result comparable to that obtained with the free drug irrespective of i.v. or i.p. administration. A notable exception was represented by OE-21 tumor-bearing mice, where the bioconjugate performed significantly better than the free drug. Similarly, ONCOFID-S exerted an important therapeutic activity against colon carcinoma and gastric, but not esophageal, peritoneal carcinomatosis, thus performing equally to the free CPT-11 drug administered either i.v. or i.p.

Discussion

Peritoneal carcinomatosis is a severe condition often representing the final and fatal evolution of tumors arising in the

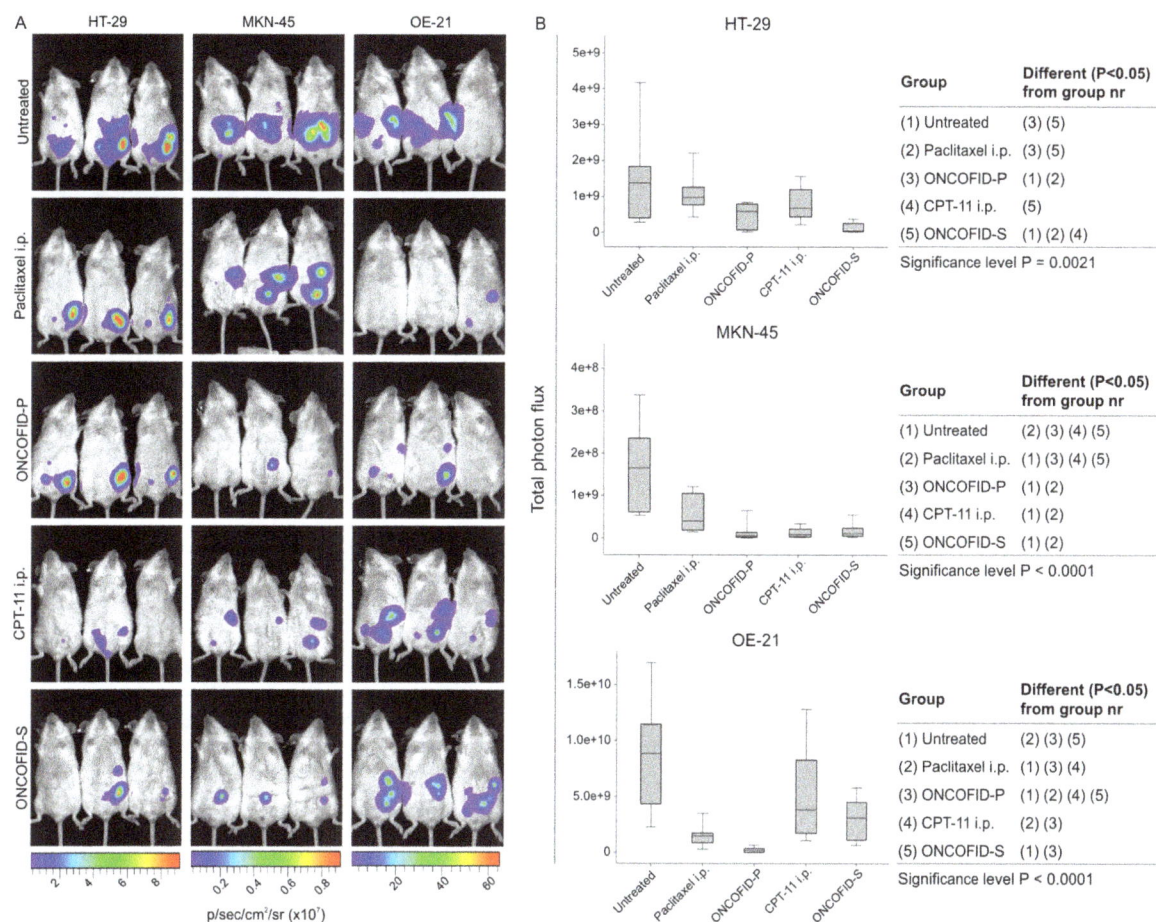

Figure 5. Assessment of *in vivo* tumor growth and response to therapy. A, bioluminescence imaging of pharmacologically treated or untreated mice with peritoneal carcinomatosis induced by luciferase-transduced tumors. Panels show three representative mice per group at one month after tumor injection. B, cumulative results. Each box plot reports mean ± SD of total photon emission from 6 mice per group at one month from peritoneal carcinomatosis induction. Statistical analysis (Kruskal-Wallis test) is reported in tables at the right of each panel.

gastrointestinal tract. However, the anatomical characteristics of the peritoneum make a loco-regional treatment an attractive and valid option to the systemic chemotherapy, which is widely used as support and palliative care. Indeed, in the last two decades cytoreductive surgery [45] followed by intraperitoneal chemotherapy (with or without associated hyperthermia) has increased the patients survival [46,47].

However, in addition to drug-related adverse effects (in particular, bone marrow suppression [45]), these procedures are invasive, impact negatively the quality of life of patients [48], are not well standardized and also require high degree of specialization, since related morbidity and mortality rates (ranging from 25 to 41% and from 0 to 8%, respectively [49]) are critically lower in centers of expertise [9]. Other concerns arise from the limited choice of pharmacological loco-regional treatments, which is primarily dictated by the histotype of the original tumor and is presently based on the off-label use of i.v. drug formulations characterized by unsatisfactory pharmacokinetics and pharmacodynamics properties [50]. To the best of our knowledge, to date only catumomaxomab obtained the FDA approval for malignant ascites treatment [50]. Thus, *ad hoc* drug delivery strategies are focused on achieving higher local concentration of the drugs with a higher retention time in the cavity, thus reducing systemic adverse effects and local toxicity. To this end, different formulations have been exploited involving microspheres, nanoparticles, liposomes, micelles, implants and injectable depots. Nonetheless, each approach presents some drawbacks regarding the retention time, tumor penetration capacity, induction of inflammatory reactions or technical difficulties, as recently reviewed [51].

In such context, the use of hyaluronan-based bioconjugates can potentially overcome these issues. Based on the promising results obtained with the loco-regional use of ONCOFID-P [21,33,40,52] and ONCOFID-S [11], we propose the administration of these bioconjugates for the treatment of peritoneal carcinomatosis. In addition to its well-known biocompatibility, hyaluronan was chosen because of its capability to selectively target tumor cells through the binding to CD44. This receptor is over-expressed in a wide variety of cancers, including tumor histotypes reported in this study [11,28,29].

Indeed, in addition to the results from competition experiments with anti-CD44 blocking mAb, the selectivity of these bioconjugates was confirmed by the fact that a $CD44^{low}$ human colon cancer subline disclosed a differential susceptibility to ONCOFID-P and to ONCOFID-S respect to the related $CD44^{high}$ counterpart. While conferring this selectivity, the chemical linking of paclitaxel and SN-38 to hyaluronan did not impact their biological effects, as demonstrated *in vitro* by the assessment of the microtubular structure alterations and the Topo I activity

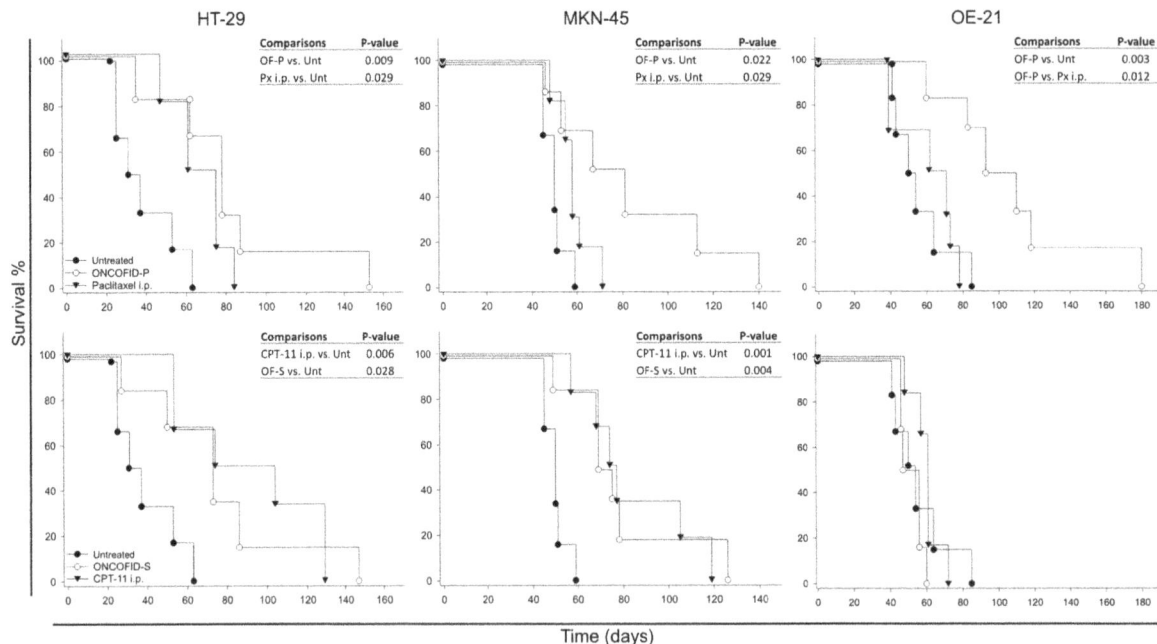

Figure 6. *In vivo* **therapeutic activity of bioconjugates.** Kaplan-Meier survival curves of mice with peritoneal carcinomatosis from HT-29, MKN-45 or OE-21 tumor cells. Animals were randomly assigned to an experimental group and drug treatment was initiated according to therapeutic schedule reported in Materials and Methods. All experimental groups were statistically compared each other, but only significant values are reported in each panel.

inhibition, respectively. This in turn reflects on biological activity *in vitro* and also *in vivo*, both shortly after the completion of the drug administration schedule (in terms of tumor growth as assessed by imaging), and long-term when considering survival. ONCO-FID-P significantly reduced the short-term tumor burden in all analysed histotypes respect to the free drug; similar results were obtained for ONCOFID-S. Interestingly, ONCOFID-P performed equally to ONCOFID-S in both colorectal and gastric carcinomatosis. In this regard, it should be noted that the conjugation with HA allows the successful employment of paclitaxel against colorectal carcinoma, an use that has not a FDA approval and consideration in the clinical setting.

In long-term analysis, ONCOFID-P improved therapeutic outcome of esophageal peritoneal carcinomatosis respect to the related free drugs; moreover, an increase in median survival could be also observed against MKN-45 model, while not reaching statistical significance. In all other cases, the bioconjugates displayed encouraging results fully overlapping those achieved by the related free drugs. Nonetheless, the conjugation with HA brings about relevant advantages. From a pharmacological point of view, it increases the water solubility of paclitaxel, thus eliminating the adverse effects related to the currently used solvent Cremophor EL (inflammatory and hypersensitivity reactions, massive leukocyte infiltration involving both the mesothelial lining and the underlying muscle abdominal wall [33], neurotoxicity [53] and the need for long infusion time [54]). In addition, the conjugation with HA allows the administration of the CPT-11 active metabolite SN-38, which is at least 100 fold more active *in vitro* than CPT-11 at equimolar concentrations, but whose use is precluded due to its intrinsic toxicity and extremely low water solubility [11]. Moreover, it has been demonstrated that the hyaluronan *per se* reduces postoperative and disease-related adhesions without impacting the metastatic potential of tumor cells [55]. From a clinical point of view, the therapeutic outcome is

achieved with negligible adverse effects. Indeed, we and others [33,11] previously reported that both bioconjugates did not induce any sign of local toxicity, when administered at the same or even superior amounts. In addition, ONCOFID-S does not cause myelotoxicity, thus potentially representing an attractive candidate for the treatment of UGTA1 genotype patients, which are predisposed to develop severe neutropenia related to CPT-11 [11]. The virtually absence of critical side effects and the specific tumor targeting allow the use of increased administration doses (a 4- and 3-times increase for ONCOFID-P *vs* paclitaxel i.p. and for ONCOFID-S *vs* CPT-11 i.p. in SN-38 equivalents, respectively).

Moreover, it is worth noting that our results are mainly obtained with drugs used for off-label indications, administered only anecdotally against the tumor histotypes under study. In particular, as for short-term tumor growth analysis, the treatment of colorectal carcinoma with ONCOFID-P improves mice survival at a comparable extent to ONCOFID-S, which carry the on-label, widely used CPT-11 metabolite.

In conclusion, these data corroborate previously successful results in the management of bladder and ovarian cancer, and envisage that the conjugation with HA can widen the use of existing drugs over their formal approval or current use, thus providing a strategy to potentially improve the loco-regional treatment of peritoneal carcinomatosis.

Supporting Information

Figure S1   CD44 and intracellular RHAMM expression in different tumor cell lines. A, viable cells were stained with a FITC-labeled anti-human CD44 mAb. B, fixed and permeabilized cells were stained with an anti-human CD168 mAb followed by an Alexa 546-conjugated anti-Ig mouse serum. In both panels A and B, insets show flow cytometry analysis of HCT-15 parental cell line.

Figure S2 Kinetics of interaction between ONCOFID-P and tumor cell lines, in the presence of hyaluronidase. BODIPY-labeled ONCOFID-P was added to tumor cells for different time points (0.5, 1, 2, 5, 10 and 15 minutes); after extensive washing, samples were added with hyaluronidase for 4 hours or left untreated, and flow cytometry analysis was finally performed. A, whole kinetics of interaction at all time points tested. B, kinetics of the fluorescence intensity (geo mean) detected on tumor cells at the same time points analyzed as in A. Panels A and B report mean ± SD of 3 independent experiments.

Figure S3 Blocking of the ONCOFID-P-receptor interaction by an anti-CD44 antibody. HT-29, MKN-45 and OE-21 tumor cells were incubated with BODIPY-labeled ONCOFID-P alone (solid line) or in the presence of an anti-CD44 blocking mAb (dashed line), and analyzed by flow cytometry. Data at the upper-right corner of each panel report the respective geo mean values and the percentage of reduction induced by anti-CD44 mAb blocking treatment.

Figure S4 BODIPY labeling does not alter ONCOFID-S activity. Representative tumor cell lines were incubated with escalating concentrations of unlabeled and BODIPY-labeled ONCOFID-S, and the resulting growth inhibition was evaluated by ATPlite assay. Unlabeled and labeled bioconjugates showed fully overlapping dose-response curves. The values of IC_{50} reported were calculated from these semi-logarithmic dose-response curves by linear interpolation.

Figure S5 Impact of differential CD44 expression on bioconjugate cytotoxic activity. The parental (HCT-15) and the selected CD44^{low} (HCT-15 CD44^{low}) and CD44^{high} (HCT-15 CD44^{high}) HCT-15 colorectal cell lines were incubated with escalating doses of paclitaxel (upper left panel), ONCOFID-P (upper right panel), SN-38 (lower left panel) and ONCOFID-S (lower right panel). The resulting growth inhibition was evaluated by ATPlite assay. Figure shows mean ± SD of three independent experiments. Extrapolated IC_{50} values are reported in pg/mL in free drug equivalents.

Table S1 IC_{50} values of free and HA-conjugated drugs. The values of the reported IC_{50} are the mean ± SE of five viability experiments carried out for each tumor cell line. For each experiment, the IC_{50} was calculated from each single semi-logarithmic dose-response curve by linear interpolation, and obtained values were then averaged. Values are reported in ng/mL and for each bioconjugate they are expressed in terms of free drug equivalents. No significant difference is evidenced between the activities of HA-bound and free drugs (Mann-Whitney Rank Sum Test).

Author Contributions

Conceived and designed the experiments: IMM PZ AR. Performed the experiments: IMM. Analyzed the data: IMM. Contributed reagents/materials/analysis tools: DR MC GP. Contributed to the writing of the manuscript: IMM AM GZ AR.

References

1. Walker AS, Zwintscher NP, Johnson EK, Maykel JA, Stojadinovic A, et al. (2014) Future directions for monitoring treatment response in colorectal cancer. J Cancer 5: 44–57.
2. Correa P (2013) Gastric cancer: Overview. Gastroenterol Clin North Am 42: 211–217.
3. Elias D, Quenet F, Goere D (2012) Current status and future directions in the treatment of peritoneal dissemination from colorectal carcinoma. Surg Oncol Clin N Am 21: 611–623.
4. Glockzin G, Piso P (2012) Current status and future directions in gastric cancer with peritoneal dissemination. Surg Oncol Clin N Am 21: 625–633.
5. Bozzetti F, Yu W, Baratti D, Kusamura S, Deraco M (2008) Locoregional treatment of peritoneal carcinomatosis from gastric cancer. J Surg Oncol 98: 273–276.
6. Schweigert M, Dubecz A, Stein HJ (2013) Oesophageal cancer–an overview. Nat Rev Gastroenterol Hepatol 10: 230–244.
7. Gros SJ, Dohrmann T, Rawnaq T, Kurschat N, Bouvet M, et al. (2010) Orthotopic fluorescent peritoneal carcinomatosis model of esophageal cancer. Anticancer Res 30: 3933–3938.
8. Coccolini F, Gheza F, Lotti M, Virzi S, Iusco D, et al. (2013) Peritoneal carcinomatosis. World J Gastroenterol 19: 6979–6994.
9. Brucher BL, Piso P, Verwaal V, Esquivel J, Derraco M, et al. (2012) Peritoneal carcinomatosis: Cytoreductive surgery and HIPEC–overview and basics. Cancer Invest 30: 209–224.
10. Konigsrainer I, Beckert S (2012) Cytoreductive surgery and hyperthermic intraperitoneal chemotherapy: Where are we? World J Gastroenterol 18: 5317–5320.
11. Serafino A, Zonfrillo M, Andreola F, Psaila R, Mercuri L, et al. (2011) CD44-targeting for antitumor drug delivery: A new SN-38-hyaluronan bioconjugate for locoregional treatment of peritoneal carcinomatosis. Curr Cancer Drug Targets 11: 572–585.
12. Duncan R, Vicent MJ (2013) Polymer therapeutics-prospects for 21st century: The end of the beginning. Adv Drug Deliv Rev 65: 60–70.
13. Varshosaz J (2012) Dextran conjugates in drug delivery. Expert Opin Drug Deliv 9: 509–523.
14. Sugahara S, Kajiki M, Kuriyama H, Kobayashi TR (2007) Complete regression of xenografted human carcinomas by a paclitaxel-carboxymethyl dextran conjugate (AZ10992). J Control Release 117: 40–50.
15. Northfelt DW, Allred JB, Liu H, Hobday TJ, Rodacker MW, et al. (2012) Phase 2 trial of paclitaxel polyglumex with capecitabine for metastatic breast cancer. Am J Clin Oncol.
16. Jain JP, Chitkara D, Kumar N (2008) Polyanhydrides as localized drug delivery carrier: An update. Expert Opin Drug Deliv 5: 889–907.
17. Nakamura H, Etrych T, Chytil P, Ohkubo M, Fang J, et al. (2014) Two step mechanisms of tumor selective delivery of N-(2-hydroxypropyl)methacrylamide copolymer conjugated with pirarubicin via an acid-cleavable linkage. J Control Release 174: 81–87.
18. Larson N, Yang J, Ray A, Cheney DL, Ghandehari H, et al. (2013) Biodegradable multiblock poly(N-2-hydroxypropyl)methacrylamide gemcitabine and paclitaxel conjugates for ovarian cancer cell combination treatment. Int J Pharm 454: 435–443.
19. Patnaik A, Papadopoulos KP, Tolcher AW, Beeram M, Urien S, et al. (2013) Phase I dose-escalation study of EZN-2208 (PEG-SN38), a novel conjugate of poly(ethylene) glycol and SN38, administered weekly in patients with advanced cancer. Cancer Chemother Pharmacol 71: 1499–1506.
20. Clementi C, Miller K, Mero A, Satchi-Fainaro R, Pasut G (2011) Dendritic poly(ethylene glycol) bearing paclitaxel and alendronate for targeting bone neoplasms. Mol Pharm 8: 1063–1072.
21. Rosato A, Banzato A, De Luca G, Renier D, Bettella F, et al. (2006) HYTAD1-p20: A new paclitaxel-hyaluronic acid hydrosoluble bioconjugate for treatment of superficial bladder cancer. Urol Oncol 24: 207–215.
22. Laurent TC, Fraser JR (1992) Hyaluronan. FASEB J 6: 2397–2404.
23. Liao YH, Jones SA, Forbes B, Martin GP, Brown MB (2005) Hyaluronan: Pharmaceutical characterization and drug delivery. Drug Deliv 12: 327–342.
24. Entwistle J, Hall CL, Turley EA (1996) HA receptors: Regulators of signalling to the cytoskeleton. J Cell Biochem 61: 569–577.
25. Isacke CM, Yarwood H (2002) The hyaluronan receptor, CD44. Int J Biochem Cell Biol 34: 718–721.
26. Aruffo A, Stamenkovic I, Melnick M, Underhill CB, Seed B (1990) CD44 is the principal cell surface receptor for hyaluronate. Cell 61: 1303–1313.
27. Zhou B, McGary CT, Weigel JA, Saxena A, Weigel PH (2003) Purification and molecular identification of the human hyaluronan receptor for endocytosis. Glycobiology 13: 339–349.
28. Takaishi S, Okumura T, Tu S, Wang SS, Shibata W, et al. (2009) Identification of gastric cancer stem cells using the cell surface marker CD44. Stem Cells 27: 1006–1020.

29. Zhao JS, Li WJ, Ge D, Zhang PJ, Li JJ, et al. (2011) Tumor initiating cells in esophageal squamous cell carcinomas express high levels of CD44. PLoS One 6: e21419.

30. Oommen OP, Garousi J, Sloff M, Varghese OP (2013) Tailored doxorubicin-hyaluronan conjugate as a potent anticancer glyco-drug: An alternative to prodrug approach. Macromol Biosci.

31. Sorbi C, Bergamin M, Bosi S, Dinon F, Aroulmoji V, et al. (2009) Synthesis of 6-O-methotrexylhyaluronan as a drug delivery system. Carbohydr Res 344: 91–97.

32. Dong Z, Zheng W, Xu Z, Yin Z (2013) Improved stability and tumor targeting of 5-fluorouracil by conjugation with hyaluronan. J Appl Polym Sci 130: 927–32.

33. Banzato A, Bobisse S, Rondina M, Renier D, Bettella F, et al. (2008) A paclitaxel-hyaluronan bioconjugate targeting ovarian cancer affords a potent in vivo therapeutic activity. Clin Cancer Res 14: 3598–3606.

34. Jaganathan SK, Supriyanto E, Mandal M (2013) Events associated with apoptotic effect of p-coumaric acid in HCT-15 colon cancer cells. World J Gastroenterol 19: 7726–7734.

35. Faryammanesh R, Lange T, Magbanua E, Haas S, Meyer C, et al. (2014) SDA, a DNA aptamer inhibiting E- and P-selectin mediated adhesion of cancer and leukemia cells, the first and pivotal step in transendothelial migration during metastasis formation. PLoS One 9: e93173.

36. Kumar SS, Price TJ, Mohyieldin O, Borg M, Townsend A, et al. (2014) KRAS G13D mutation and sensitivity to cetuximab or panitumumab in a colorectal cancer cell line model. Gastrointest Cancer Res 7: 23–26.

37. Smit JK, Faber H, Niemantsverdriet M, Baanstra M, Bussink J, et al. (2013) Prediction of response to radiotherapy in the treatment of esophageal cancer using stem cell markers. Radiother Oncol 107: 434–441.

38. Yuan Y, Chen H, Ma G, Cao X, Liu Z (2012) Reelin is involved in transforming growth factor-beta1-induced cell migration in esophageal carcinoma cells. PLoS One 7: e31802.

39. Aoyagi K, Kouhuji K, Miyagi M, Kizaki J, Isobe T, et al. (2013) Molecular targeting therapy using bevacizumab for peritoneal metastasis from gastric cancer. World J Crit Care Med 2: 48–55.

40. Montagner IM, Banzato A, Zuccolotto G, Renier D, Campisi M, et al. (2013) Paclitaxel-hyaluronan hydrosoluble bioconjugate: Mechanism of action in human bladder cancer cell lines. Urol Oncol 31: 1261–1269.

41. Crouch SP, Kozlowski R, Slater KJ, Fletcher J (1993) The use of ATP bioluminescence as a measure of cell proliferation and cytotoxicity. J Immunol Methods 160: 81–88.

42. Keyaerts M, Verschueren J, Bos TJ, Tchouate-Gainkam LO, Peleman C, et al. (2008) Dynamic bioluminescence imaging for quantitative tumour burden assessment using IV or IP administration of D: -Luciferin: Effect on intensity,

time kinetics and repeatability of photon emission. Eur J Nucl Med Mol Imaging 35: 999–1007.

43. Contreras-Ruiz L, de la Fuente M, Parraga JE, Lopez-Garcia A, Fernandez I, et al. (2011) Intracellular trafficking of hyaluronic acid-chitosan oligomer-based nanoparticles in cultured human ocular surface cells. Mol Vis 17: 279–290.

44. Dodds HM, Haaz MC, Riou JF, Robert J, Rivory LP (1998) Identification of a new metabolite of CPT-11 (irinotecan): Pharmacological properties and activation to SN-38. J Pharmacol Exp Ther 286: 578–583.

45. Al-Shammaa HA, Li Y, Yonemura Y (2008) Current status and future strategies of cytoreductive surgery plus intraperitoneal hyperthermic chemotherapy for peritoneal carcinomatosis. World J Gastroenterol 14: 1159–1166.

46. Elias D, Gilly F, Boutitie F, Quenet F, Bereder JM, et al. (2010) Peritoneal colorectal carcinomatosis treated with surgery and perioperative intraperitoneal chemotherapy: Retrospective analysis of 523 patients from a multicentric french study. J Clin Oncol 28: 63–68.

47. Gill RS, Al-Adra DP, Nagendran J, Campbell S, Shi X, et al. (2011) Treatment of gastric cancer with peritoneal carcinomatosis by cytoreductive surgery and HIPEC: A systematic review of survival, mortality, and morbidity. J Surg Oncol 104: 692–698.

48. Passot G, Bakrin N, Roux AS, Vaudoyer D, Gilly FN, et al. (2013) Quality of life after cytoreductive surgery plus hyperthermic intraperitoneal chemotherapy: A prospective study of 216 patients. Eur J Surg Oncol.

49. Glockzin G, Schlitt HJ, Piso P (2009) Peritoneal carcinomatosis: Patients selection, perioperative complications and quality of life related to cytoreductive surgery and hyperthermic intraperitoneal chemotherapy. World J Surg Oncol 7: 5-7819-7-5.

50. Lu Z, Wang J, Wientjes MG, Au JL (2010) Intraperitoneal therapy for peritoneal cancer. Future Oncol 6: 1625–1641.

51. De Smet L, Ceelen W, Remon JP, Vervaet C (2013) Optimization of drug delivery systems for intraperitoneal therapy to extend the residence time of the chemotherapeutic agent. ScientificWorldJournal 2013: 720858.

52. Bassi PF, Volpe A, D'Agostino D, Palermo G, Renier D, et al. (2011) Paclitaxel-hyaluronic acid for intravesical therapy of bacillus calmette-guerin refractory carcinoma in situ of the bladder: Results of a phase I study. J Urol 185: 445–449.

53. Authier N, Gillet JP, Fialip J, Eschalier A, Coudore F (2001) Assessment of neurotoxicity following repeated cremophor/ethanol injections in rats. Neurotox Res 3: 301–306.

54. Gelderblom H, Verweij J, Nooter K, Sparreboom A (2001) Cremophor EL: The drawbacks and advantages of vehicle selection for drug formulation. Eur - J Cancer 37: 1590–1598.

55. Pucciarelli S, Codello L, Rosato A, Del Bianco P, Vecchiato G, et al. (2003) Effect of antiadhesive agents on peritoneal carcinomatosis in an experimental model. Br J Surg 90: 66–71.

2

HIV Cure Strategies: How Good Must They Be to Improve on Current Antiretroviral Therapy?

Paul E. Sax[1,3]*, **Alexis Sypek**[5,7], **Bethany K. Berkowitz**[5,7], **Bethany L. Morris**[5,7], **Elena Losina**[2,3,5,7,8], **A. David Paltiel**[10], **Kathleen A. Kelly**[5,7], **George R. Seage III**[4], **Rochelle P. Walensky**[1,3,6,7], **Milton C. Weinstein**[4], **Joseph Eron**[11], **Kenneth A. Freedberg**[3,4,5,6,7,9]

1 Division of Infectious Diseases, Brigham and Women's Hospital, Boston, Massachusetts, United States of America, 2 Department of Orthopedic Surgery, Brigham and Women's Hospital, Boston, Massachusetts, United States of America, 3 Harvard University Center for AIDS Research, Harvard University, Boston, Massachusetts, United States of America, 4 Harvard School of Public Health, Harvard University, Boston, Massachusetts, United States of America, 5 Division of General Medicine, Department of Medicine, Massachusetts General Hospital, Boston, Massachusetts, United States of America, 6 Division of Infectious Diseases, Department of Medicine, Massachusetts General Hospital, Boston, Massachusetts, United States of America, 7 Medical Practice Evaluation Center, Department of Medicine, Massachusetts General Hospital, Boston, Massachusetts, United States of America, 8 Department of Biostatistics, Boston University School of Public Health, Boston, Massachusetts, United States of America, 9 Department of Epidemiology, Boston University School of Public Health, Boston, Massachusetts, United States of America, 10 Yale School of Public Health, New Haven, Connecticut, United States of America, 11 Division of Infectious Disease, School of Medicine, University of North Carolina at Chapel Hill, Chapel Hill, North Carolina, United States of America

Abstract

Background: We examined efficacy, toxicity, relapse, cost, and quality-of-life thresholds of hypothetical HIV cure interventions that would make them cost-effective compared to life-long antiretroviral therapy (ART).

Methods: We used a computer simulation model to assess three HIV cure strategies: Gene Therapy, Chemotherapy, and Stem Cell Transplantation (SCT), each compared to ART. Efficacy and cost parameters were varied widely in sensitivity analysis. Outcomes included quality-adjusted life expectancy, lifetime cost, and cost-effectiveness in dollars/quality-adjusted life year ($/QALY) gained. Strategies were deemed cost-effective with incremental cost-effectiveness ratios <$100,000/ QALY.

Results: For patients on ART, discounted quality-adjusted life expectancy was 16.4 years and lifetime costs were $591,400. Gene Therapy was cost-effective with efficacy of 10%, relapse rate 0.5%/month, and cost $54,000. Chemotherapy was cost-effective with efficacy of 88%, relapse rate 0.5%/month, and cost $12,400/month for 24 months. At $150,000/procedure, SCT was cost-effective with efficacy of 79% and relapse rate 0.5%/month. Moderate efficacy increases and cost reductions made Gene Therapy cost-saving, but substantial efficacy/cost changes were needed to make Chemotherapy or SCT cost-saving.

Conclusions: Depending on efficacy, relapse rate, and cost, cure strategies could be cost-effective compared to current ART and potentially cost-saving. These results may help provide performance targets for developing cure strategies for HIV.

Editor: Nicolas Sluis-Cremer, University of Pittsburgh, United States of America

Funding: This research was funded by the National Institute of Allergy and Infectious Diseases (http://www.niaid.nih.gov/Pages/default.aspx): R37 AI042006 (PS, AS, BB, BM, EL, ADP, KK, RW, MW, KF), AI051966 (GS), R01 AI093269 (RW, KF, ADP, MW), U01 AI 069472 (PS, EL, KF, RQ, ADP, AS, BB, BM, KK) (Partners/Harvard AIDS Clinical Trials Unit), U01 AI068636 (PS, EL, KF, RQ, ADP, AS, BB, BM, KK) (Central AIDS Clinical Trials Group), and UM1 AI 069423 (JE) (UNC Global Clinical Trials Unit). The funders had no role in study design, data collection and analysis, decision to publish, or preparation of the manuscript.

Competing Interests: Dr. Sax has served as a consultant to AbbVie, BMS, Gilead, GSK, Merck and Janssen, and has received grant support from BMS, Gilead, and GSK. Dr. Weinstein serves as a consultant to OptumInsight for work unrelated to the submitted research. Dr. Eron has served as a consultant to Abbvie, BMS, Gilead, GSK, Merck, Janssen and ViiV, and has received grant support from BMS, ViiV and Merck. All other authors report no conflicts of interest.

* Email: psax@partners.org

Introduction

Combination antiretroviral therapy (ART) durably controls HIV replication and halts progression of clinical HIV disease in the vast majority of patients who receive and continue treatment [1]. Projected survival for people with HIV is now estimated to be several decades. Some reports suggest that survival for people with HIV on successful therapy approaches that of those without infection if therapy is initiated early and HIV suppression is sustained [2].

Despite the remarkable success of treatment, ART nonetheless has many limitations. Although much less toxic than earlier regimens, current treatment still may be associated with cardio-vascular, renal, bone, and other complications [3,4]. The inflammation and immune activation that persist in many patients on suppressive ART may have long-term negative consequences [5]. Therapy in the US and Europe remains costly, and, because not curative, it must be continued indefinitely [6,7]. Successful ART also does not eliminate the stigma associated with HIV infection [8].

The first report of successful HIV cure after allogeneic stem cell transplant for acute leukemia demonstrated that eradicating HIV from an individual is viable [9]. While allogeneic transplant in the absence of usual indications carries substantial risk, cost, and post-transplant consequences of chronic immunosuppression, other strategies are being studied that could potentially cure HIV and be practically deployed [10–12]. In this analysis we aim to establish thresholds of efficacy, toxicity, durability, cost, and quality of life necessary for a cure strategy to compare favorably with current antiretroviral therapy in the United States.

Methods

Analytic Overview

To analyze the potential life expectancy and cost-effectiveness of HIV cure strategies under study, we utilized the Cost-Effectiveness of Preventing AIDS Complications (CEPAC) model, a Monte-Carlo microsimulation of HIV disease and treatment [13]. We completed a 'what if' analysis, in order to understand the possible role of HIV cure strategies as they are developed. Model outputs included life expectancy, quality-adjusted life expectancy, and lifetime costs (2012 USD), all discounted to present value at 3% annually [14]. Incremental cost-effectiveness ratios (ICERs) were calculated by comparing each hypothetical cure strategy to the standard of care, lifelong ART. We determined parameter thresholds at which potential cure strategies were either cost-effective, defined as ICERs <$100,000/quality-adjusted life year (QALY), or cost-saving compared to current ART [15].

Strategies Evaluated

We evaluated three hypothetical HIV cure strategies: a "low efficacy," "low risk" gene therapy approach (Gene Therapy); a "moderate efficacy," "moderate risk" chemotherapy approach (Chemotherapy); and a "high efficacy," "high risk" allogeneic stem cell transplant (SCT). Costs of these strategies would likely vary widely and are currently uncertain.

The Gene Therapy strategy was modeled after the use of zinc finger nucleases to modify the CCR5 receptor on the surface of CD4 cells [12]. Patients undergo pheresis, their cells are modified using zinc finger nucleases, and re-infused with the goal of establishing a CCR5-negative cell population that is resistant to HIV infection. Based on preliminary reports, this type of procedure would have lower risk and toxicity than Chemotherapy and SCT and, we assumed, lower likelihood of achieving cure [16–19]. Simulated patients were modeled to receive the benefit of cure one month after Gene Therapy, if effective. Input parameters for all strategies were varied widely in sensitivity analysis, as described below.

The Chemotherapy intervention was derived from both in vitro and in vivo experiments using histone deacetylase inhibitors (such as vorinostat) to stimulate and eliminate the HIV viral reservoir [10]. Simulated patients received ART combined with Chemo-therapy for 96 weeks, after which, if effective, they had the benefit of cure. There was increased cost and toxicity for the chemother-apy-based administration of vorinostat [17,20].

SCT had the highest assumed risk of mortality and toxicity, but was assumed the most effective. Simulated SCT patients received the benefit of cure in the first month after successful transplant.

The Cost-Effectiveness of Preventing AIDS Complications (CEPAC) Model

Simulations were performed using the CEPAC model, a widely-published, validated state-transition microsimulation of HIV disease [13]. HIV natural history is modeled as a series of monthly transitions between health states characterized by CD4 count and HIV RNA. Without treatment, patients' CD4 counts decline according to a viral load-dependent trajectory [21]. Patients are also subject to age- and sex-specific non-HIV-related mortality [22].

Once patients initiate ART, the probability of virologic suppression and subsequent CD4 count increases, with the greatest CD4 gain occurring in the first two months [23]. CD4 count gains are associated with reduced risk of developing opportunistic infections and HIV-related death. Patients' HIV RNA and CD4 counts are routinely monitored to detect treatment failure. Upon virologic rebound, patients switch to the next available ART regimen. Costs of HIV treatment and care are from the health system perspective and derived from HIV Research Network data and the Medicare fee schedule [24–27].

Cure Simulation

This analysis focused on patients who had received fully suppressive first-line ART for one year and were thereby eligible for a cure strategy, as is the case in planned or ongoing cure trials [28]. We maintained the CD4 benefit associated with virologic suppression for each cure strategy. With each cure regimen, patients faced strategy-specific probabilities of achieving cure as well as toxicity, quality of life (QOL) decrements and increases (associated with both toxicity and the regimen itself), and monthly probabilities of relapse. Additionally, patients accrued strategy-specific intervention costs. Cured patients were no longer subject to monthly probabilities of opportunistic infections and AIDS-related death, but were subject to monthly probabilities of relapse and subsequent return to ART. After cure, patients faced monthly probabilities of non-AIDS mortality and accrued monthly costs for routine care and continued HIV RNA monitoring for relapse. Patients who failed cure, or later relapsed after cure, resumed first-line ART, followed by additional ART regimens if virologic failure occurred later.

Model Inputs and Analysis

We used the CEPAC model itself to determine the distribution of CD4 counts in the eligible population by simulating a cohort of patients entering the model with the age, sex, and CD4 count distribution of HIV-infected patients in North America at care presentation. Patients were given a first-line ART regimen of efavirenz, tenofovir, and emtricitabine for one year [29]. Per current guidelines, all patients received ART, regardless of CD4 count [30]. Following one year on suppressive ART, patients became eligible for a cure intervention, beginning these cure strategies with mean CD4 count of 564/µl (SD 250/µl), based on this initialization.

Patients assigned to a cure intervention were subject to a strategy-specific probability of being cured (Table 1). All efficacies were hypothetical, since cure interventions do not currently exist. Cured patients had undetectable viremia for the duration of their lifetimes, unless they relapsed. We assumed relapse rates were highest during the first five years after a cure intervention (0.5%/

month); after five years the relapse rate was reduced by one half (0.25%/month). Relapse was detected through routine virologic monitoring. Both acute and chronic non-fatal toxicities resulted in a QOL decrement of 0.04, which lasted one month for acute non-fatal toxicities and until the patient failed the cure strategy for chronic toxicities [31]. Because the cohort was comprised only of patients virologically suppressed on first-line ART for one year, we assumed high rates of virologic re-suppression after a failed cure intervention. Those patients were also at risk for later virologic failure, at a rate of 0.13%/month [32]. Costs associated with each of the interventions and their associated toxicities were based on reported costs for similar procedures for other conditions (Table 1). In the base case, we assumed no additional QOL benefit related to achieving HIV cure compared to being on effective ART. In sensitivity analyses, we considered scenarios in which cured patients had an increase in their QOL from the base case. Any QOL benefit was suspended if the patient relapsed and re-initiated ART.

Gene Therapy was assumed to have an efficacy of 10.0% with no risk of fatal toxicity [16]. Patients incurred a 25.0% risk of acute, non-fatal toxicity (e.g., headache or oropharyngeal pain) lasting for one month [16]. While receiving Gene Therapy, patients incurred an immediate cost of $100,000, based on current estimates for gene therapies, plus $2,000 for continued ART (from weighted average of current drug prices) during the month they received Gene Therapy [20,33,34]. This intervention cost was based on ivacaftor, an oral cystic fibrosis medication that acts on the genetic mutation causing the disease [20].

Chemotherapy was assumed to have an efficacy of 20.0%, and 1.2% probability of fatal toxicity [17]. Patients incurred a 6.0% risk of acute non-fatal toxicity and 5.8% risk of chronic non-fatal toxicity [17,18]. Chemotherapy was modeled as a 96-week course (24 months) with monthly costs of $12,400; $2,000/month was included for maintenance ART [17]. At any point in the 96-weeks patients could fail ART and experience HIV virologic rebound. Patients who had not experienced ART failure during the 96 weeks could be cured at the end of that period (assumed efficacy 20.0%).

SCT was assumed to have an efficacy of 70.0%, with 5.0% mortality from the procedure [35]. Patients had a 47.3% probability of acute graft-versus-host disease and 37.2% probability of chronic graft-versus-host-disease [19]. The initial cost of the transplant was assumed to be $150,000 with monthly costs of $1,000 for six months for immunosuppressive medications [36,37].

Sensitivity Analysis

Because the focus of this analysis was on strategies under research and development, we conducted extensive sensitivity analysis on all cure parameters to identify those most important in changing the main conclusions. For each cure strategy and parameter, we determined thresholds at which the strategy would become cost-effective at a threshold of $100,000/QALY, as well as become cost-saving compared to ART. For sensitivity analyses involving relapse rates, early ($\leq$5 years) and late (>5 years) relapse rates were varied together. Recognizing the impact a cure might have on patients' well-being (physical, emotional, and social), we

Table 1. Parameter inputs for a model-based analysis of potential HIV cure strategies.

Variable: Base Case (Range)	Gene Therapy	Chemotherapy	Stem Cell Transplant	References
Cohort Characteristics				
CD4 count, mean cells/µl (SD)	564 (250)	564 (250)	564 (250)	See Methods[a]
Age, mean years (SD)	44 (12)	44 (12)	44 (12)	[29]
Percent male	84	84	84	[29]
Cure Characteristics				
Efficacy (%)	10.0 (10.0–90.0)	20.0 (10.0–90.0)	70.0 (10.0–90.0)	Assumptions
Monthly relapse rate (%), early/late	0.50/0.25 (0.0–2.0)	0.50/0.25 (0.0–2.0)	0.50/0.25 (0.0–2.0)	Assumptions
Initial cost ($)	100,000 (50,000–200,000)	12,400/month[b] (6,200–24,800)	150,000 (75,000–300,000)	Assumptions based on [20,33,34,36]/[20]/[36]
Additional cost ($, while on cure regimen only)	2,000/month[c]	2,000/month[c]	1,000/month[d] (for 6 months)	[20,34]/[20,34]/[37]
Fatal Toxicity				
Probability (%)	0.0	1.2	5.0	Assumption based on [16]/[17]/[35]
Cost ($)	–	63,110	63,110	Derived from [24,25,27,46]
Acute Non-fatal Toxicity				
Probability (%)	25.0	6.0	47.3	Assumption based on Ivacaftor package insert [16]/[18]/[19]
Cost ($)	50	3,100	18,700	[25]/[47]/Derived from [48]
Chronic Non-fatal Toxicity				
Probability (%)	0.0	5.8	37.2	Assumption based on [16]/[18]}/[19]
Cost ($)	–	1,040	1,900	[49]/Derived from [50]

SD: standard deviation; **QOL:** quality-of-life.
[a]Determined through initialization run of simulated cohort; [b]For 24 months based on vorinostat; [c]For monthly antiretroviral therapy, derived from weighted averages of current therapies until gene- or chemo-therapy is complete; [d]For immunosuppressive agents, including methotrexate with tacrolimus.

also conducted sensitivity analysis on health-related QOL, both prior to and following HIV cure. Due to the major toxicity, including fatal toxicity, involved in SCT, we focused the QOL sensitivity analysis on the Gene Therapy and Chemotherapy strategies.

Ethics Statement

This study was reviewed and approved by the Partners Heath Care Human Research Committee (Protocol 2000P001927), Boston, Massachusetts, USA, as it was determined to meet the criteria for exemption from human studies. A waiver for written informed consent from participants was not necessary because only secondary data were used in this study and no human subjects were involved. Secondary patient data that serve as our model inputs were anonymized and de-identified prior to analysis.

Results

Base Case Scenarios

The standard of care (lifelong ART) had a discounted projected life expectancy of 19.0 years (16.4 QALYs) and discounted lifetime cost of $591,400. Undiscounted life expectancy with standard of care was 32.3 years, compared to 32.8, 32.3, and 32.6 years, for Gene Therapy, Chemotherapy, and SCT under the base case set of assumptions. Gene Therapy (10% efficacy) resulted in a discounted life expectancy of 19.3 years (16.6 QALYs) and increased discounted lifetime costs to $658,700, for an ICER of $330,600/QALY gained compared to continued ART. Chemotherapy (20% efficacy) led to a discounted life expectancy of 19.0 years (16.4 QALYs) and discounted lifetime cost of $807,300, and was more expensive and less effective than ART. SCT resulted in a discounted life expectancy of 19.0 years (16.3 QALYs) and increased costs to $607,400; it was also more expensive and less effective than ART (Table 2).

One-way Sensitivity Analyses

With efficacy increased to 22% and other inputs remaining the same, Gene Therapy had an ICER <$100,000/QALY, and at an efficacy of 34% became cost-saving, relative to ART (Table 3). With a reduced cost of $54,000, Gene Therapy achieved an ICER<$100,000/QALY gained even at 10% efficacy; it was cost-saving at $34,000. Chemotherapy was not cost-effective unless efficacy increased to 88% and was not cost-saving at any efficacy. Varying any other single parameter within reasonable limits did not result in Chemotherapy reaching thresholds for cost-effectiveness or cost savings (Table 3). The efficacy threshold for SCT was 79% to achieve cost-effectiveness and 80% to achieve cost savings. Reducing fatal toxicity to 3.0% from 5.0% also led to SCT becoming cost-effective (Table 3).

Multiway Sensitivity Analyses

With no relapse risk, Gene Therapy was cost-saving with efficacy of at least 30%. With increasing relapse rates, higher efficacy was required to achieve cost savings. At a decreased cost of $50,000, Gene Therapy became cost-effective at the base case values for relapse and efficacy and cost-saving with lower relapse rates or higher efficacies (Figure 1). At increased cost of $200,000, the intervention was not cost-effective compared to standard of care ART for almost all combinations of input parameters (Figure 1).

For Chemotherapy, at the base case cost and relapse rate of greater than 0.5%/month, the intervention was never cost-effective (Figure 2). With no relapse risk, the intervention was not cost-effective at efficacies of 20–50% but was cost-saving at efficacies above 60%. If the cost was halved ($6,200/month), Chemotherapy was cost-saving at substantially lower efficacies and higher relapse rates than in the base case. For example, at this decreased cost, Chemotherapy was cost-saving with relapse rate of 0.5%/month with efficacy 60%. If the cost of Chemotherapy was doubled to $24,800/month, it was not cost-effective with any combination of efficacy (20–90%) and relapse rate (0.0–2.0%). The window for cost-effectiveness was narrow; with most parameter combinations, Chemotherapy was either cost-saving or not cost-effective.

In most sensitivity analyses, SCT was not cost-effective. In selected cases where the cost was extremely low or efficacy very high, SCT became cost-saving (Figure 3). For one parameter combination, SCT was less effective and less expensive than ART, but it was not cost-effective because the ICER of ART was < $100,000/QALY compared to SCT. If the cost of SCT was halved ($75,000), the combinations where the intervention was cost-saving remained roughly the same, but several scenarios that were not cost-effective in the base case became less expensive and less effective than ART.

With an efficacy of 10% for Gene Therapy, improving QOL to a utility of 1.00 (i.e., the equivalent of perfect health) after successful cure would be insufficient to achieve an ICER < $100,000/QALY gained. With efficacy of 20%, however, an ICER <$100,000/QALY gained could be achieved if patient utility following cure increased from 0.85 to 0.88, or the equivalent of facing a 3% decreased risk of death every year. For efficacies of 30% or more, the Gene Therapy strategy would always be cost-effective, regardless of whether the cure had any impact on QOL. At the base-case QOL utility of 0.85, Chemotherapy was not cost-effective at any efficacy below 60%, even with the maximum QOL improvement. At an efficacy of 60% for Chemotherapy, cost-effectiveness could be achieved if patient utility following cure increased from 0.85 to 0.97. If the baseline QOL utility while living with HIV were 0.50, Chemotherapy would not reach the

Table 2. Base case results of an analysis of hypothetical HIV cure strategies*.

Strategy	Discounted Life Years (Undiscounted)	Discounted QALYs	Cost ($)	Incremental Cost-effectiveness compared to standard of care ($/QALY)
Standard of care ART	19.0 (32.3)	16.4	591,400	–
Gene Therapy	19.3 (32.8)	16.6	658,700	330,600
Chemotherapy	19.0 (32.3)	16.4	807,300	Dominated
Stem Cell Transplant	19.0 (32.6)	16.3	607,400	Dominated

*Based on assumptions for efficacy, durability, toxicity, and cost in Methods and Table 1. Life expectancy, QALYs, and costs all discounted at 3%/year. **ART:** antiretroviral therapy; **QALY:** Quality-adjusted life year; **Dominated:** Less effective and more costly than the standard of care ART strategy.

Table 3. Threshold which key parameters would need to reach for each type of HIV cure strategy to be cost-effective (ICER< $100,000/QALY gained) or cost-saving.

Parameter	Base case value	ICER<$100,000/QALY gained	Cost-saving
Gene Therapy (base case ICER: $330,600/QALY gained)			
Efficacy (%)	10	22	34
Fatal Toxicity (%)	0.0	None	None
Monthly relapse rate (%), early (late)	0.5/0.25	None	None
Intervention cost ($)	100,000, one-time	54,000, one-time	34,000, one-time
Chemotherapy (base case ICER: Dominated)			
Efficacy (%)	20	88	None
Fatal Toxicity (%)	1.2	None	None
Monthly relapse rate (%), early (late)	0.5/0.25	None	None
Intervention cost ($)	12,400/month, for 24 months	*	*
Stem Cell Transplant (base case ICER: Dominated)			
Efficacy (%)	70	79	80
Fatal Toxicity (%)	5.0	3.0	None
Monthly relapse rate (%), early (late)	0.5/0.25	None	0.25/0.125
Intervention cost ($)	150,000, one-time	*	*

ICER: incremental cost-effectiveness ratio; **QALY:** quality-adjusted life year; **QOL:** quality of life; **Dominated:** strategy was less effective and more expensive than current ART.
*Cost reductions led to the strategy being less effective and less expensive than current ART. One could calculate an ICER for ART compared to Chemotherapy or Stem Cell Transplant, but it is not clinically plausible that these strategies would be used if they resulted in worse outcomes than standard of care with ART, even if they saved money by avoiding the costs of lifelong ART.

cost-effectiveness threshold of <$100,000/QALY at cure efficacies below 40%. At cure efficacy of 40%, Chemotherapy would achieve an ICER below $100,000/QALY gained with improvement in QOL utility to 0.88. If we used ICER thresholds below $150,000 or $200,000 per QALY gained to define cost-effectiveness, there were no appreciable changes in results [15].

Discussion

With intense pre-clinical investigation underway towards finding a cure for HIV, we sought to evaluate the cost-effectiveness of three potential HIV cure approaches, each compared to standard of care ART. We used a variety of assumptions,

anchored in published data on gene-targeted therapy, chemotherapy, and stem cell transplant for diseases other than HIV. By doing extensive sensitivity analyses on efficacy, toxicity, relapse rates, and cost, we defined a range of benchmarks that might justify the adoption of a cure strategy, and identified combinations of parameters under which these could potentially be cost-effective or cost-saving. For a Gene Therapy approach, modest increases in efficacy (above 10%) or moderate decreases in cost (below $100,000), led to this strategy being cost-saving compared to ART. For Chemotherapy and SCT, the inventions became cost-saving with very high efficacies and low relapse rates.

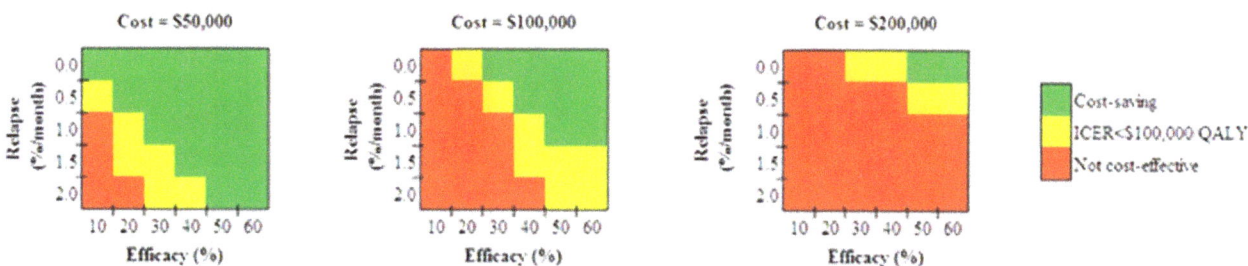

Figure 1. Gene Therapy compared to standard of care ART. The figure depicts the cost-effectiveness of Gene Therapy compared to standard of care ART as a function of the three influential parameters identified via the one-way sensitivity analysis in Table 3: cost, relapse rate, and efficacy. In each panel, the horizontal axis denotes efficacy while the vertical axis denotes the relapse rate. Inside each panel, the shading denotes the resultant cost-effectiveness finding, ranging from cost-saving (green), through cost-effective (with an ICER<$100,000/QALY, yellow), to not cost-effective (≥ $100,000/QALY or more expensive and less effective than ART, red). **ART:** antiretroviral therapy; **ICER:** incremental cost-effectiveness ration; **QALY:** quality-adjusted life year.

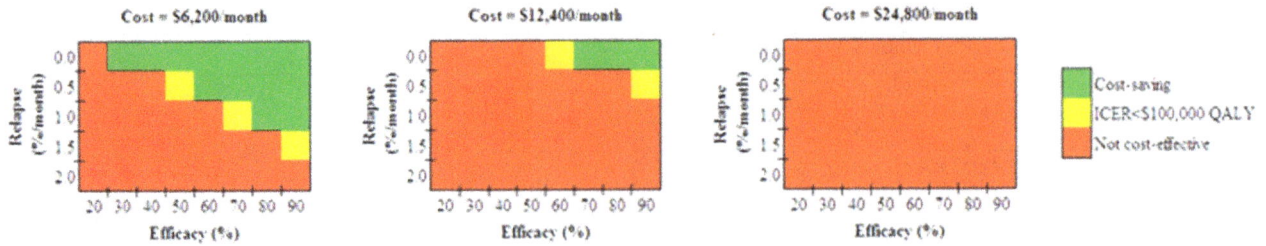

Figure 2. Chemotherapy compared to standard of care ART. The figure depicts the cost-effectiveness of Chemotherapy compared to standard of care ART as a function of the three influential parameters identified via the one-way sensitivity analysis in Table 3: cost, relapse rate, and efficacy. In each panel, the horizontal axis denotes efficacy while the vertical axis denotes the relapse rate. Inside each panel, the shading denotes the resultant cost-effectiveness finding, ranging from cost-saving (green), through cost-effective (with an ICER<$100,000/QALY, yellow), to not cost-effective (≥$100,000/QALY or more expensive and less effective than ART, red). **ART:** antiretroviral therapy; **ICER:** incremental cost-effectiveness ration; **QALY:** quality-adjusted life year.

We found that changes in efficacy, relapse rates, and/or cost rapidly moved the strategies from being worse than ART to being cost-saving – that is, to being both equally or more effective and less costly. The range in which any strategy would be cost-effective but not cost-saving is narrow (Figures 1–3, yellow area). High initial costs of cure strategies could be justified, and would save money, if (and essentially only if) the strategy eliminates the lifetime cost of ART. For example, with an initial cost of $100,000 and an efficacy of 34%, the Gene Therapy strategy is cost-saving compared to ART, even if all other assumptions remain the same. In such a scenario, identification of conditions that could theoretically increase the likelihood of cure – such as ART started during acute infection, or heterozygosity of the CCR5delta32 gene – would make a cure strategy even more attractive [38]. Alternatively a substantial decrease in the cost of lifelong ART would make these interventions less cost-effective.

It is possible that combination approaches to cure may be needed to improve efficacy [39]. These would, nonetheless, each have some combination of efficacy, toxicity, and cost. The value in terms of cost-effectiveness, compared to ART, can be inferred from those combinations as shown in Figures 1–3. Further, some lower-risk interventions, such as zinc finger nucleases, could also have higher efficacy than other interventions. If so, then they would both be more effective and less costly, and thus 'dominant' from a cost-effectiveness perspective, compared to those other interventions, such as HDAC inhibitors.

No published studies to date have examined the cost-effectiveness of hypothetical HIV cure strategies in comparison to ART. Similar model-based analyses have, however, been done for other previously unproven strategies in HIV, including therapeutic and preventive HIV vaccines and pre-exposure prophylaxis (PrEP) [40–42]. These analyses have been used to design subsequent vaccine and PrEP research. In the case of PrEP, modeled results before proven efficacy closely matched the outcome of some later trials [43].

At present, strategies to cure HIV have only progressed to the proof of concept stage. Given this early stage, current complexity, anticipated cost, and possible risks, a cure strategy will not be ready for implementation anytime soon. However, this analysis suggests that potential HIV cure strategies must be moderately effective and have low toxicity and low relapse rates to compare favorably to standard of care ART. The optimal cost threshold for such strategies will depend on both the likelihood of durable cure (initial efficacy and subsequent relapse rate) and the cost of ART. As initial efforts at cure are developed, this work can help investigators determine the efficacy and toxicity targets which would make the strategies attractive. Further, if any cure strategies are proven effective, the results of this analysis can help inform policymakers as to their appropriate role. This issue has recently been highlighted by the high efficacy and cost of new HCV cures [44].

From a societal and quality-of-life perspective, with a base case utility of 0.85 for patients doing well on ART, improvements in

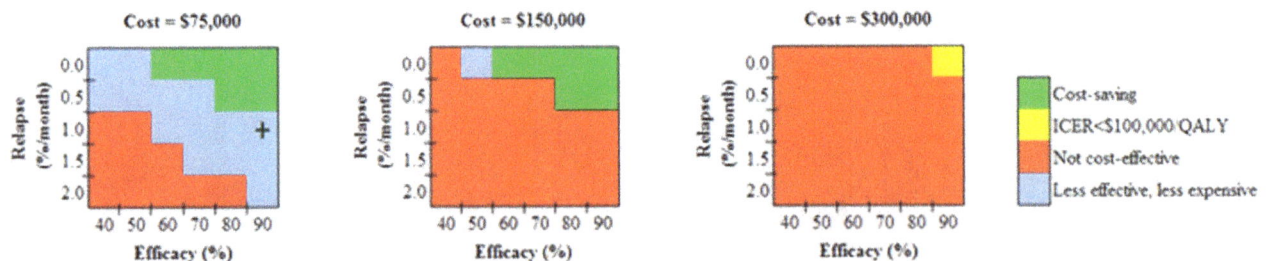

Figure 3. Stem Cell Transplantation compared to standard of care ART. The figure depicts the cost-effectiveness of Stem Cell Transplantation compared to standard of care ART as a function of the three influential parameters identified via the one-way sensitivity analysis in Table 3: cost, relapse rate, and efficacy. In each panel, the horizontal axis denotes efficacy while the vertical axis denotes the relapse rate. Inside each panel, the shading denotes the resultant cost-effectiveness finding, ranging from cost-saving (green), through cost-effective (with an ICER<$100,000/QALY, yellow), to not cost-effective (≥$100,000/QALY or more expensive and less effective than ART, red). Instances where the intervention is both less expensive and less effective than ART are denoted in blue, but most were not cost-effective because the ICER of ART was <$100,000/QALY compared to SCT. The plus sign indicates a strategy that had an ICER for ART compared to SCT >$100,000/QALY gained. **ART:** antiretroviral therapy; **ICER:** incremental cost-effectiveness ration; **QALY:** quality-adjusted life year.

quality of life after cure do not have a major impact on cost-effectiveness. However, many might argue that there is an important psychological, social, and emotional distinction to be drawn between curing HIV and controlling it via therapy.

Our study has several limitations. The most important is that HIV cure interventions do not yet exist, so model parameters such as efficacy, mortality, cost, and relapse rates were assumed using specific data wherever possible and then varied widely. The effect of cure strategies on the incidence and severity of "non-HIV" complications, such as malignancies, heart disease, and other chronic non-communicable diseases was not included; one might anticipate either an increase or decrease in these complications, based on the strategy employed. If non-AIDS events are driven primarily by HIV-mediated immune activation and inflammation, then curing HIV would presumably ameliorate these processes. In addition, adverse effects of antiretroviral drugs would also be eliminated. By contrast, some of the treatments proposed for HIV cure may themselves increase risks of non-AIDS events. For example, some are analogous to cancer chemotherapy, and such treatments may increase the risk of secondary malignancies; radiation used for stem cell transplant could also raise cardiovascular risk; and alteration in stem cells could also increase the long-term risk of cancers. The demographics of the suppressed patients eligible for cure interventions were based on the demographics of the population presenting to care in the United States and may not be completely representative of those who achieve suppression after one year. Since we modeled only patients virologically suppressed after a year, this represents the most adherent subset of patients. If cure strategies were utilized in a broader group of patients, such as those with early infection, the strategies might be more or less effective and cost-effective compared to ART, depending on the requirements of the particular cure strategy. Gene therapy may require stem cell modification to achieve cure, which could increase the risk of rare but substantial toxicity of cancer induction; this risk was not included. Although we did include relapse rates – indicating a later chance of HIV viral rebound after initial cure – we did not include the possibility of re-infection among cured patients, which has been documented after successful HCV cure [45]. Adding this possibility would make any cure strategy less attractive. Increased use of newer, more effective branded therapies, however, may keep the costs of ART in their current range [20].

In summary, the key determinants of the cost-effectiveness of HIV cure strategies, compared to current antiretroviral therapy, are initial efficacy, toxicity, relapse rate, and cost. Potential cure strategies must have moderate efficacy, low toxicity, and relatively low risk of relapse to be cost-effective and, in combination, would likely be cost-saving.

Author Contributions

Conceived and designed the experiments: PES AS BKB BLM EL ADP KAK GRS RPW MCW JE KAF. Analyzed the data: PES AS BKB BLM EL ADP KAK GRS RPW MCW JE KAF. Contributed to the writing of the manuscript: PES AS BKB BLM EL ADP KAK GRS RPW MCW JE KAF. Performed model analyses: AS BKB BLM KAK.

References

1. Moore RD, Bartlett JG (2011) Dramatic decline in the HIV-1 RNA level over calendar time in a large urban HIV practice. Clin Infect Dis 53: 600–604.
2. Rodger AJ, Lodwick R, Schechter M, Deeks S, Amin J, et al. (2013) Mortality in well controlled HIV in the continuous antiretroviral therapy arms of the SMART and ESPRIT trials compared with the general population. AIDS 27: 973–979.
3. Sabin CA, Worm SW, Weber R, Reiss P, El-Sadr W, et al. (2008) Use of nucleoside reverse transcriptase inhibitors and risk of myocardial infarction in HIV-infected patients enrolled in the D:A:D study: a multi-cohort collaboration. Lancet 371: 1417–1426.
4. Martin A, Bloch M, Amin J, Baker D, Cooper DA, et al. (2009) Simplification of antiretroviral therapy with tenofovir-emtricitabine or abacavir-Lamivudine: a randomized, 96-week trial. Clin Infect Dis 49: 1591–1601.
5. Lederman MM, Funderburg NT, Sekaly RP, Klatt NR, Hunt PW (2013) Residual immune dysregulation syndrome in treated HIV infection. Advances in immunology 119: 51–83.
6. Farnham PG, Gopalappa C, Sansom SL, Hutchinson AB, Brooks JT, et al. (2013) Updates of lifetime costs of care and quality-of-life estimates for HIV-infected persons in the United States: late versus early diagnosis and entry into care. J Acquir Immune Defic Syndr 64: 183–189.
7. Finzi D, Hermankova M, Pierson T, Carruth LM, Buck C, et al. (1997) Identification of a reservoir for HIV-1 in patients on highly active antiretroviral therapy. Science 278: 1295–1300.
8. Andrinopoulos K, Clum G, Murphy DA, Harper G, Perez L, et al. (2011) Health related quality of life and psychosocial correlates among HIV-infected adolescent and young adult women in the US. AIDS Educ Prev 23: 367–381.
9. Allers K, Hutter G, Hofmann J, Loddenkemper C, Rieger K, et al. (2011) Evidence for the cure of HIV infection by CCR5Delta32/Delta32 stem cell transplantation. Blood 117: 2791–2799.
10. Archin NM, Liberty AL, Kashuba AD, Choudhary SK, Kuruc JD, et al. (2012) Administration of vorinostat disrupts HIV-1 latency in patients on antiretroviral therapy. Nature 487: 482–485.
11. Margolis DM, Hazuda DJ (2013) Combined approaches for HIV cure. Curr Opin HIV AIDS 8: 230–235.
12. Tebas P, Stein D, Tang WW, Frank I, Wang SQ, et al. (2014) Gene editing of CCR5 in autologous CD4 T cells of persons infected with HIV. N Engl J Med 370: 901–910.
13. Walensky RP, Sax PE, Nakamura YM, Weinstein MC, Pei PP, et al. (2013) Economic savings versus health losses: the cost-effectiveness of generic antiretroviral therapy in the United States. Ann Intern Med 158: 84–92.
14. Siegel JE, Weinstein MC, Russell LB, Gold MR (1996) Recommendations for reporting cost-effectiveness analyses. Panel on Cost-Effectiveness in Health and Medicine. JAMA 276: 1339–1341.
15. Ubel PA, Hirth RA, Chernew ME, Fendrick AM (2003) What is the price of life and why doesn't it increase at the rate of inflation? Arch Intern Med 163: 1637–1641.
16. Vertex Pharmaceuticals Incorporated (2012) Kalydeco (ivacaftor) package insert. Available: http://pi.vrtx.com/files/uspi_ivacaftor.pdf. Accessed 18 August 2014.
17. Merck Sharp & Dohme Corp. (2006) Zolinza (vorinostat) [package insert]. Available: http://www.merck.com/product/usa/pi_circulars/z/zolinza/zolinza_pi.pdf. Accessed 18 August 2014.
18. Kavanaugh SM, White LA, Kolesar JM (2010) Vorinostat: A novel therapy for the treatment of cutaneous T-cell lymphoma. Am J Health Syst Pharm 67: 793–797.
19. Stamatovic D, Balint B, Tukic L, Elez M, Tarabar O, et al. (2011) Impact of stem cell source on allogeneic stem cell transplantation outcome in hematological malignancies. Vojnosanit Pregl 68: 1026–1032.
20. RED BOOK Online (2013) Product Information for antiretroviral drug prices, Kalydeco, Zolinza, and Tivicay. Micromedex 2.0, Truven Health Analytics.
21. Mellors JW, Muñoz A, Giorgi JV, Margolick JB, Tassoni CJ, et al. (1997) Plasma viral load and CD4+ lymphocytes as prognostic markers of HIV-1 infection. Ann Intern Med 126: 946–954.
22. United Nations, Department of Economic and Social Affairs and Population Division (2009) World Population Prospects: The 2008 Revision, Highlights, Working Paper No. ESA/P/WP.210 Available: http://www.un.org/esa/population/publications/wpp2008/wpp2008_highlights.pdf. Accessed 10 June 2013.
23. Pozniak AL, Gallant JE, DeJesus E, Arribas JR, Gazzard B, et al. (2006) Tenofovir disoproxil fumarate, emtricitabine, and efavirenz versus fixed-dose zidovudine/lamivudine and efavirenz in antiretroviral-naive patients: virologic, immunologic, and morphologic changes-a 96-week analysis. J Acquir Immune Defic Syndr 43: 535–540.
24. Centers for Medicare and Medicaid Services (2012) Clinical Diagnostic Laboratory Fee Schedule 2012. Available: https://www.cms.gov/Medicare/Medicare-Fee-for-Service-Payment/ClinicalLabFeeSched/clinlab.htm. Accessed 18 August 2014.
25. Centers for Medicare and Medicaid Services (2012) Medicare Physician Fee Schedule 2012. Available: http://www.cms.gov/apps/physician-fee-schedule/overview.aspx. Accessed 20 January 2014.
26. University HealthSystems Consortium (2008) CDP Online Report. Available: www.uhc.edu. Accessed 28 January 2014.
27. Bozzette SA, Berry SH, Duan N, Frankel MR, Leibowitz AA, et al. (1998) The care of HIV-infected adults in the United States. HIV Cost and Services Utilization Study Consortium. N Engl J Med 339: 1897–1904.
28. Mellors J, McMahon D (2014) Evaluating the safety and efficacy of single-dose romidepsin in combination with antiretroviral therapy in HIV-infected adults

with suppressed viral load. NCT01933594. Available: http://clinicaltrials.gov/ct2/show/NCT01933594?term=romidepsin+hiv&rank=1. Accessed 23 Janaury 2014.

29. Althoff KN, Gange SJ, Klein MB, Brooks JT, Hogg RS, et al. (2010) Late presentation for human immunodeficiency virus care in the United States and Canada. Clin Infect Dis 50: 1512–1520.

30. Panel on Antiretroviral Guidelines for Adults and Adolescents (2013) Guidelines for the prevention and treatment of opportunistic infections in HIV-infected adults and adolescents: recommendations from the Centers for Disease Control and Prevention, the National Institutes of Health, and the HIV Medicine Association of the Infectious Diseases Society of America. Department of Health and Human Services. Available: http://aidsinfo.nih.gov/contentfiles/lvguidelines/adult_oi.pdf. Accessed 18 August 2014.

31. Pepper PV, Owens DK (2002) Cost-effectiveness of the pneumococcal vaccine in healthy younger adults. Med Decis Making 22: S45–57.

32. Messou E, Chaix ML, Gabillard D, Minga A, Losina E, et al. (2011) Association between medication possession ratio, virologic failure and drug resistance in HIV-1-infected adults on antiretroviral therapy in Côte d'Ivoire. J Acquir Immune Defic Syndr 56: 356–364.

33. Dotinga R (2010) Gene therapy for HIV inches forward. Available: http://health.usnews.com/health-news/managing-your-healthcare/genetics/articles/2010/06/16/gene-therapy-for-hiv-inches-forward. Accessed 7 May 2014.

34. US Department of Health and Human Services (2005) Medicaid drug price comparisons: average manufacturer price to published prices. Available: http://oig.hhs.gov/oei/reports/oei-05-05-00240.pdf. Accessed 16 January 2014.

35. Shenoy S (2011) Hematopoietic stem cell transplantation for sickle cell disease: current practice and emerging trends. Hematology Am Soc Hematol Educ Program 2011: 273–279.

36. National Bone Marrow Transplant Link (2010) Bone marrow/stem cell transplant frequently asked questions. Available: http://nbmtlink.org/resources_support/faq/faq_question8.html. Accessed 18 August 2014.

37. Kasiske BL, Cohen D, Lucey MR, Neylan JF (2000) Payment for immunosuppression after organ transplantation. American Society of Transplantation. JAMA 283: 2445–2450.

38. Saez-Cirion A, Bacchus C, Hocqueloux L, Avettand-Fenoel V, Girault I, et al. (2013) Post-treatment HIV-1 controllers with a long-term virological remission after the interruption of early initiated antiretroviral therapy ANRS VISCONTI Study. PLoS Pathog 9: e1003211.

39. Lewin SR (2014) Finding a Cure for HIV: Much Work to Do. Ann Intern Med 161: 368–369.

40. Paltiel AD, Freedberg KA, Scott CA, Schackman BR, Losina E, et al. (2009) HIV preexposure prophylaxis in the United States: impact on lifetime infection risk, clinical outcomes, and cost-effectiveness. Clin Infect Dis 48: 806–815.

41. Leelahavarong P, Teerawattananon Y, Werayingyong P, Akaleephan C, Premsri N, et al. (2011) Is a HIV vaccine a viable option and at what price? An economic evaluation of adding HIV vaccination into existing prevention programs in Thailand. BMC Public Health 11: 534.

42. Walensky RP, Paltiel AD, Goldie SJ, Gandhi RT, Weinstein MC, et al. (2004) A therapeutic HIV vaccine: how good is good enough? Vaccine 22: 4044–4053.

43. Grant RM, Lama JR, Anderson PL, McMahan V, Liu AY, et al. (2010) Preexposure chemoprophylaxis for HIV prevention in men who have sex with men. N Engl J Med 363: 2587–2599.

44. Petta S, Cabibbo G, Enea M, Macaluso FS, Plaia A, et al. (2014) Cost-effectiveness of sofosbuvir-based triple therapy for untreated patients with genotype 1 chronic hepatitis C. Hepatology 59: 1692–1705.

45. Lambers FA, Prins M, Thomas X, Molenkamp R, Kwa D, et al. (2011) Alarming incidence of hepatitis C virus re-infection after treatment of sexually acquired acute hepatitis C virus infection in HIV-infected MSM. AIDS 25: F21–27.

46. Gebo KA, Moore RD, Fleishman JA (2003) The HIV Research Network: a unique opportunity for real time clinical utilization analysis in HIV. Hopkins HIV Rep 15: 5–6.

47. Havrilesky LJ, Pokrzywinski R, Revicki D, Higgins RV, Nycum LR, et al. (2012) Cost-effectiveness of combination versus sequential docetaxel and carboplatin for the treatment of platinum-sensitive, recurrent ovarian cancer. Cancer 118: 386–391.

48. Dignan FL, Potter MN, Ethell ME, Taylor M, Lewis L, et al. (2013) High readmission rates are associated with a significant economic burden and poor outcome in patients with grade III/IV acute GvHD. Clin Transplant 27: E56–63.

49. Elting LS, Cantor SB, Martin CG, Hamblin L, Kurtin D, et al. (2003) Cost of chemotherapy-induced thrombocytopenia among patients with lymphoma or solid tumors. Cancer 97: 1541–1550.

50. Crespo C, Perez-Simon JA, Rodriguez JM, Sierra J, Brosa M (2012) Development of a population-based cost-effectiveness model of chronic graft-versus-host disease in Spain. Clin Ther 34: 1774–1787.

3

Azathioprine versus Beta Interferons for Relapsing-Remitting Multiple Sclerosis: A Multicentre Randomized Non-Inferiority Trial

Luca Massacesi[1,2]*, **Irene Tramacere**[3], **Salvatore Amoroso**[4], **Mario A. Battaglia**[5], **Maria Donata Benedetti**[6], **Graziella Filippini**[3], **Loredana La Mantia**[7], **Anna Repice**[2], **Alessandra Solari**[3], **Gioacchino Tedeschi**[8], **Clara Milanese**[3]

1 Dipartimento di Neuroscienze, Psicologia, Farmaco e Salute del Bambino Università di Firenze, Firenze, Italy, 2 Neurologia 2, Azienda Ospedaliero-Universitaria Careggi, Firenze, Italy, 3 Fondazione IRCCS Istituto Neurologico Carlo Besta, Milano, Italy, 4 Dipartimento di Neuroscienze, Sezione di Farmacologia, Università Politecnica delle Marche, Ancona, Italy, 5 Associazione Italiana Sclerosi Multipla (AISM), Fondazione Italiana Sclerosi Multipla (FISM), Genova, Italy, 6 Dipartimento Universitario di Neurologia, Azienda Ospedaliera Universitaria Integrata di Verona, Verona, Italy, 7 Unità di Neurologia - Multiple Sclerosis Center, I.R.C.C.S. Santa Maria Nascente Fondazione Don Gnocchi, Milano, Italy, 8 Clinica Neurologica, Università di Napoli, Napoli, Italy

Abstract

For almost three decades in many countries azathioprine has been used to treat relapsing-remitting multiple sclerosis. However its efficacy was usually considered marginal and following approval of β interferons for this indication it was no longer recommended as first line treatment, even if presently no conclusive direct β interferon-azathioprine comparison exists. To compare azathioprine efficacy versus the currently available β interferons in relapsing-remitting multiple sclerosis, a multicenter, randomized, controlled, single-blinded, non-inferiority trial was conducted in 30 Italian multiple sclerosis centers. Eligible patients (relapsing-remitting course; ≥ 2 relapses in the last 2 years) were randomly assigned to azathioprine or β interferons. The primary outcome was annualized relapse rate ratio (RR) over 2 years. Key secondary outcome was number of new brain MRI lesions. Patients (n = 150) were randomized in 2 groups (77 azathioprine, 73 β interferons). At 2 years, clinical evaluation was completed in 127 patients (62 azathioprine, 65 β interferons). Annualized relapse rate was 0.26 (95% Confidence Interval, CI, 0.19–0.37) in the azathioprine and 0.39 (95% CI 0.30–0.51) in the interferon group. Non-inferiority analysis showed that azathioprine was at least as effective as β interferons (relapse $RR_{AZA/IFN}$ 0.67, one-sided 95% CI 0.96; p<0.01). MRI outcomes were analyzed in 97 patients (50 azathioprine and 47 β interferons). Annualized new T2 lesion rate was 0.76 (95% CI 0.61–0.95) in the azathioprine and 0.69 (95% CI 0.54–0.88) in the interferon group. Treatment discontinuations due to adverse events were higher (20.3% vs. 7.8%, p = 0.03) in the azathioprine than in the interferon group, and concentrated within the first months of treatment, whereas in the interferon group discontinuations occurred mainly during the second year. The results of this study indicate that efficacy of azathioprine is not inferior to that of β interferons for patients with relapsing-remitting multiple sclerosis. Considering also the convenience of the oral administration, and the low cost for health service providers, azathioprine may represent an alternative to interferon treatment, while the different side effect profiles of both medications have to be taken into account.

Trial Registration: EudraCT 2006-004937-13

Editor: Klemens Ruprecht, Charite - Universitätsmedizin Berlin, Germany

Funding: The present study was funded by AIFA (Agenzia Italiana del Farmaco, www.agenziafarmaco.gov.it). The funder had no role in study design, data collection and analysis, decision to publish, or preparation of the manuscript.

Competing Interests: Dr. Solari, Dr. Massacesi and Dr. Tedeschi have read the journal's policy and have the following conflicts: Dr. Solari was a board member for Novartis, Biogenidec and Merck Serono, and has received speaker honoraria from Sanofi-Aventis. Dr. Massacesi has received reimbursements for meeting participation or educational grants from Biogen-Idec, Merk-Serono, Sanofi-Aventis and Novartis. In addition, he is a member of the Scientific Advisory Group Neurology of the European Medicine Agency (EMA) and of the Italian Medicine Agency (Agenzia Italiana del Farmaco, AIFA) Advisory Committee on Neurology, but the opinions included in this paper do not involve this activity. Dr. Tedeschi has received reimbursements for meeting participation or educational grants from Biogen-Idec, Merk-Serono, Sanofi-Aventis and Novartis. In addition, he was a member of the Italian Medicine Agency (Agenzia Italiana del Farmaco, AIFA) Advisory Committee on Neurology, but the opinions included in this paper do not involve this activity. All the other authors have declared that no competing interests exist.

* Email: massacesi@unifi.it

Introduction

For almost three decades azathioprine (AZA) has been used in many countries to treat relapsing-remitting multiple sclerosis (MS) based on placebo controlled randomized clinical trials (RCTs) [1–4]. Efficacy however was usually considered marginal [5,6], and following approval of β interferons (IFNs) AZA was no longer recommended as first-line therapy [7]. Lack of MRI evaluation, methodological weaknesses and the low power of the trials may have fostered perception of the poor efficacy of AZA, whereas consistently efficacious and safe IFN trials in MS [8–11] have made IFN a drug of choice for this indication [7]. However, meta-analyses [12–14], new comparative RCTs [15,16], and MRI results [17,18] suggest a similar effect size of AZA in relapsing-remitting MS. Presently no conclusive direct IFN-AZA comparison exists. This paper documents an independent multicenter RCT evaluating the non-inferiority of the efficacy of AZA vs. IFNs on clinical and MRI measures of disease activity in relapsing-remitting MS.

Materials and Methods

The protocol for this trial and supporting CONSORT checklist are available as supporting information; see Protocol S1, Amendment S1, and Checklist S1.

Ethics statement

This study was approved by ethics committees in the coordinating center (Careggi University Hospital, Ethic Committee, Florence) and in each of the participating centers (**Fondazione IRCCS Istituto Neurologico Carlo Besta**, Milano; **Clinica Neurologica**, Novara; **Università "La Sapienza"**, Roma; **Policlinico "G. Rodolico" Azienda Ospedaliero-Universitaria**, Catania; **Clinica Neurologica 2**, Genova; **Azienda Ospedaliera Universitaria Integrata**, Verona; **Ospedale Clinicizzato "Colle Dall'Ara"**, Chieti; **Università di Sassari**, Sassari; **Università di Napoli**, Napoli; **Ospedale S. Antonio**, Padova; **Ospedale Civile S. Agostino-Estense**, Modena; **Ospedale Santa Maria**, Reggio Emilia; **Policlinico Universitario Mater Domini**, Catanzaro; **Ospedale S. Gerardo**, Monza; **Azienda Ospedaliero-Universitaria S. Anna**, Ferrara; **Ospedali Riuniti**, Ancona; **Istituto S. Raffaele "G. Giglio"**, Cefalù; **Azienda Ospedaliero San Giovanni Battista**, **Università di Torino**, Torino; **Ospedale Sacro Cuore**, Negrar; **Ospedale Santa Chiara**, Trento; **Ospedale Regionale**, Bolzano; **Azienda Ospedaliero-Universitaria Senese, Policlinico "Le Scotte"**, Siena; **Ospedale "Misericordia e Dolce"**, Prato; **Università degli Studi di Pisa**, Pisa; **Policlinico "G. Martino"**, Messina; **Università degli Studi di Palermo**, Palermo; **Università Cattolica, Policlinico Gemelli**, Roma; **Dipartimento Neuroriabilitativo ASL CN1**, Cuneo; **Luigi Gonzaga Hospital**, Orbassano Ethics Committees), adhered to Good Clinical Practice (GCP) guidelines and Declaration of Helsinki. The original trial was registered in 2006 in the EudraCT register (EUDRACT n.: 2006-004937-13) at a time that was prior to being accepted as a registry that fulfills the requirements by the International Committee of Medical Journal Editors (ICMJE) (http://www.icmje.org/faq_clinical.html). Since this registry was only considered to fulfill the requirements by the ICMJE since June 2011 and was not publicly available for several years after it was established, this precluded fulfilment of the requirements outlined by the ICMJE. We confirm that all ongoing and future trials are now registered.

Study design and patients

Designed as a multicenter, randomized, single-blinded, phase III clinical trial, the study assesses non-inferiority of AZA efficacy vs. IFNs over two years. Patients were recruited between February 2007 and March 2009 in 30 MS centers throughout Italy. Inclusion criteria were: age, 18–55 years; relapsing-remitting MS [19]; at least two clinical relapses in the preceding two years; a baseline Expanded Disability Status Scale (EDSS) [20] score from 1.0 to 5.5; effective female contraception and a signed informed

consent. Exclusion criteria were: clinical relapses or steroid therapy 30 days prior to study entry; immunomodulatory or immunosuppressive treatments in the preceding year; concomitant diseases precluding IFN or AZA treatment; pregnancy or breastfeeding; cognitive decline preventing informed consent; pathological conditions interfering with MS evolution; non-steroidal anti-inflammatory drugs (NSAID) allergy or intolerance to AZA or IFNs.

The study was an independent academic initiative supported by the Italian Medicine Agency (Agenzia Italiana del Farmaco, AIFA) through a competitive Grant following a public call aimed to support independent Clinical Trials.

Randomization and blinding

Patients were selected for AZA or IFNs using a computer generated central randomization list (1:1 ratio), in blocks of four and stratified by disability score (EDSS≤3.5 or >3.5). Patients were assessed by an unblinded treating and a blinded examining neurologist at their centers. Brain MRI images were centrally analyzed by two blinded independent experts at the Image Analysis Centre of the University of Florence (Italy).

Interventions

Treatment was prescribed free of charge by treating neurologists and self-administered within one month after screening and one week after randomization.

Standard treatment. The IFN-treated patients were either administered 250 µg of IFNβ-1b subcutaneously on alternate days (Betaferon), 30 µg of IFNβ-1a IM, weekly (Avonex); 22/44 µg of subcutaneous IFNβ-1a thrice weekly (Rebif). The type of IFNβ (Betaferon, Avonex or Rebif) was selected by the treating neurologist. The standard dose was titrated over the first four weeks.

Experimental treatment. The AZA-treated patients were given an oral target dose of 3 mg/kg/day, individually adjusted to their differential white cell counts. The initial 50 mg/day dose was subsequently titrated for the first six to eight weeks, increasing 50 mg every fortnight to the target dose.

Treatment adjustment and discontinuation criteria. For all medications, treatment adjustment criteria included: reaching grade two for adverse events (AEs) of Common Toxicity Criteria (CTC) [21], including n<800/µl lymphocyte count and n<3000/µl white blood cells. For AZA in case of grade two AEs, a 25/50 mg dose reduction was required. When the AE occurred during dose titration the higher dose was not prescribed. Returning to the target dose after reduction or increasing dose during titration was allowed for AEs occurring only once, otherwise the low dose was maintained. The treatment monitoring, including hemato-chemical tests (erythrocytes, hemoglobin, leukocytes with differential count, platelets, ALT, AST, GGT, ALP, and bilirubin), were performed quarterly. These tests were performed every fortnight during the first two months of treatment (one month for the IFNs) and when a grade two AE occurred. Treatment was discontinued for grade two AEs persistent at two subsequent controls after dose reduction. Other withdrawal criteria were: a grade three AE or AEs considered intolerable by patients or treating neurologists; treatment failure (i.e., more relapses during the study than in the previous two years, or an equal number of relapses and increase of at least one EDSS point confirmed after six months, or shift to a secondary progressive course); pregnancy; and consent withdrawal.

Co-interventions. Symptomatic treatments were allowed and 1 g of I.V. methylprednisolone was given for three-five days for relapses, as prescribed by the treating neurologist.

Procedures

The treating neurologist oversaw the overall medical management of patients, including drug prescription and self-administration instruction, scheduled (quarterly) and unscheduled (i.e., at the onset of new symptoms or complications) follow-up visits where he/she recorded symptoms, blood test results, clinical AEs and their management, and any treatment decision, including discontinuation. The examining neurologist was responsible for the neurological examination and EDSS scoring at scheduled (every six months) and unscheduled visits, that were requested by the treating neurologist to confirm relapses. These included the onset of new neurological symptom(s), or worsening of pre-existing ones from MS, determining worsening of at least one point in one or more functional system or at least 0.5 EDSS points. A new symptom was considered part of a new relapse if it lasted at least 48 hours with no fever, and if reported at least 30 days from the end of a previous relapse. To discontinue treatment a final visit was planned within 30 days from the last dose.

A Contract Research Organization (CRO) visited all centers before enrolment and every four months thereafter.

Outcomes

Clinical efficacy. The primary outcome was annualized relapse rate ratio (RR) over two years. Secondary clinical outcomes were: a) annualized relapse rate during the first and second year; b) proportion of patients with 0, 1, and ≥2 relapses during the first and second year; c) proportion of patients with corticosteroid-treated relapses; d) time to first relapse after randomization; e) proportion of patients with no confirmed disability progression, i.e., without an increase of at least one EDSS point confirmed after at least six months over two years; f) mean EDSS change from baseline to the end of follow-up; g) number of treatment failures; h) mean change of the MSQOL-54 scale [22] over two years.

Brain MRI. Brain lesions were evaluated through MRI scans performed over 30 days prior to treatment (baseline) and at two years (study completion). In the MRI study participated 23 Centers, all identified prior to the beginning of the study. The primary MRI outcome was the number of new T2 brain lesions, defined as new or enlarging lesions on T2-weighted scans. Secondary outcomes were: a) proportion of patients with 0, 1–2, ≥3 new T2 brain lesions; b) combined new and enhancing lesions (CE); c) mean and median Gadolinium contrast enhancing (Gd+) lesions on T1-weighted scans; d) proportion of patients with 0, 1–2, ≥3 Gd+ lesions. New lesion numbers were evaluated through dedicated software packages (Analyze 10.0), comparing each scan obtained at study completion with the corresponding baseline scan [see Methods S1 in File S1 for details].

Safety. Data was collected on: 1) AEs and serious AEs (SAEs); 2) patients with any AE; 3) patient withdrawal after any AE; 4) severity of any AE and their correlation with treatments as judged by the treating neurologist. Frequency and severity of AEs were actively assessed every three months or upon patient request. Severity was graded using the National Cancer Institute Common Terminology Criteria for AE [21]. SAE notification was sent to a specifically appointed Pharmacological Surveillance Unit (PSU).

Non-inferiority margin, power and sample size

Non-inferiority margin. To compare treatment relapse rates, a non-inferiority margin (M) was calculated following published guidelines [23–25], as a fraction of the mean effect of IFNs vs. placebo ($E_{IFNvsPlacebo}$) on the same outcome measure in previous trials with the same inclusion criteria and follow-up period [8,9,11]. By next expressing the $E_{IFNvsPlacebo}$ as a relapse

rate ratio, M was expressed as 50% of the excess to 1.0 of this rate ratio. Given the historical $E_{IFNvsPlacebo}$ of 1.46 (= 2.55/1.75, corresponding to the relapse rate reduction through IFN treatment), M = 1.23 was therefore selected [8,9]. The annualized new T2 lesion rate over two years was chosen as the primary MRI outcome, as this was the main MRI outcome available in the pivotal trial aimed at establishing the efficacy of IFNβ-1b vs. placebo and whose inclusion criteria and follow-up length were identical [8,11], thereby enabling precise evaluation of the $E_{IFNvsPlacebo}$ on new T2 lesion rates, as their ratio was 2.67 (= 6.4/2.4). Based on these data, a non-inferiority margin of M = 1.84 was established *a priori*, as 50% of the excess to 1.0 of the 2.67 historical ratio.

Power and sample size. Sample size was calculated to verify the non-inferiority of AZA against IFNs. With a power of 80%, α of 5% and under the hypothesis of no difference between the means of relapse rates (new T2 lesion rates for MRI), with an expected loss of 20% at follow-up, 360 patients (175/treatment arm) for relapse, and 192 patients (96/treatment arm) for MRI were needed. However, the sample size of the study was undermined by the revision of the Italian National Health System reimbursement criteria, that occurred during the recruitment period and allowed IFN therapy from the first MS attack, thus overcoming the required presence of at least two relapses during the previous two years, which was one of the inclusion criteria of this study. This change remarkably reduced the number of eligible patients and the recruitment slowed to such a low rate that the Steering Committee of the study judged the planned sample size not feasible any more. For this reason a protocol amendment, approved by the Independent Data and Safety Management Committee (IDSMC) and by the Ethic Committee of the Coordinating Center, recommended a 150 patient recruitment ceiling, accepting a power of 60–65% for relapses, and 80% for MRI outcome, under the hypothesis of no differences between the means of relapse/new T2 lesion rates [see Protocol S1 and Amendment S1 for details]. It is worth to note that the request of amendment was submitted by the Steering Committee exclusively on the basis of the observed accrual rate, when no data or codes were available.

Statistical analyses

Baseline characteristics. Baseline clinical and demographic characteristics were analyzed using χ^2 test for categorical, and t-test (or Mann-Whitney test in the absence of Normal distribution) for continuous variables.

Clinical outcome measures. AZA efficacy was judged non-inferior to IFNs if the upper limit (U_L) of the one-sided 95% confidence interval (95% CI) of the annualized relapse $RR_{AZA/IFN}$ over two years, calculated by Poisson regression, was <M = 1.23. Secondary outcomes were analyzed using χ^2 test with one degree of freedom for rate comparison (based on Poisson regression); χ^2 test with two degrees of freedom for number of relapsed patients; Kaplan-Meier curves, log-rank test and Cox proportional-hazards model for time to first relapse; Fisher's exact test for patients with no confirmed disability progression; and t-test for EDSS and MSQOL-54 score changes. For the annualized relapse rate, sensitivity analyses were performed adjusting for baseline covariates (number of relapses during the previous two years, baseline EDSS score, and disease duration from onset of symptoms), and excluding Avonex treated patients. An additional sensitivity analysis was performed to include in the analysis patients lost to follow-up, using two multiple imputation methods (monotone logistic regression and fully conditional specification [FCS] logistic regression method) [26–28], taking the randomized treatment as

the covariate (i.e., incorporating possible different uncertainty due to different dropout rates between the two randomized treatment groups). All analyses were performed in the intention to treat (ITT) and per-protocol (PP, i.e. after excluding noncompliant patients and drop-outs) populations. In the analyses based on relapse rates and on proportion of patients with relapses or disability progression, patients lost to follow-up were excluded.

Brain lesions. AZAs were judged non-inferior to IFNs if the U_L of the one-sided 95% CI of the annualized new T2 lesion rate ratio over two years, calculated by Poisson regression, was $<M = 1.84$. Secondary outcomes were analyzed through χ^2 test with one degree of freedom for rate comparison (based on Poisson regression); χ^2 test with two degrees of freedom for number of patients with lesions; and Mann-Whitney test for Gd+ lesion number. All analyses were performed in the ITT and PP populations.

Adverse Events. AEs were analyzed as rates, in terms of patients with AEs and overall number of AEs, using χ^2 test based on Poisson regression for rate comparison, and χ^2 test for categorical variable comparison for discontinued interventions after AEs, AE severity and correlation of AE with treatment. SAEs were described reporting their postulated correlation with treatment and any consequent discontinuation.

Data were reported following the CONSORT guidelines [29].

Results

Characteristics of participants

Figure 1 presents patient allocation and follow-up. Of the 150 randomized patients 77 and 73 were AZA- and IFN-assigned respectively. In the IFN group, 26 (36%) were assigned to Avonex, 5 (7%) to Betaferon, 35 (48%) to Rebif 22, and 7 (10%) to Rebif 44. Of the 150 patients screened at baseline, 127 completed the ITT follow-up: 62 (81%) in the AZA group, and 65 (89%) in the IFN group (overall 85%). Eight patients, initially randomized to AZA, refused consent and received IFN (out of these, four were lost to follow up). Including losses to follow up, treatment discontinuations were respectively 30 in the AZA group (39%; with the patients who refused to begin the treatment, n = 8) and 19 in the IFN group (26%). The majority of the discontinuations under AZA occurred in the first year (n = 26; 87%) whereas those under IFN occurred in the second year (n = 12; 63%). The discontinuations were 22 (32%) and 18 (25%) respectively, if only patients who began the treatments are included in the analysis of pharmacological compliance.

Fourteen (47%) of 30 treatment discontinuations in the AZA group and 6 (32%) of 19 discontinuations in the IFN group were due to AEs; 2 (7%) of 30 patients in the AZA group and 3 (16%) of 19 patients in the IFN group discontinued for lack of efficacy. Demographic, clinical characteristics and MRI findings at baseline were highly comparable in both groups (Table 1), even considering the ITT (n = 127), the PP (n = 101), and the MRI (n = 97) populations who completed follow-up [data not shown]. Baseline characteristics were comparable even separately considering patients enrolled during the first and second year of recruitment [data not shown].

Efficacy - clinical outcomes

From the primary efficacy analysis, AZA emerges as significantly non-inferior to IFN (Fig. 2), as the upper limit (U_L) of the one-sided 95% CI for the annualized relapse $RR_{AZA/IFN}$ was 0.96, i.e., below the non-inferiority margin M (= 1.23; p<0.01). This U_L is also significantly (p = 0.03) below a more stringent non-inferiority margin M1 = 1.0, corresponding to 100% of the effect

of IFNs vs. placebo. The U_L of the one-sided 99% CI for the $RR_{AZA/IFN}$ (i.e., 1.12), corresponding to the 75% of the IFN effect vs. placebo, was also significantly below the non-inferiority margin of M = 1.23 (p<0.01). The annualized relapse rates observed over two years among the AZA and the IFN treated subjects were 0.26 and 0.39, respectively (p = 0.07, adjusted p = 0.06; Table 2). The corresponding $RR_{AZA/IFN}$ was 0.67 (95% CI, 0.43–1.03) based on the 127 patients who completed follow-up, 0.67 (95% CI, 0.40–1.12) based on 150 randomized patients and using the monotone logistic regression multiple imputation method, and 0.69 (95% CI, 0.43–1.10) using the FCS logistic regression multiple imputation method [data not shown]. Adjusted analysis gave similar results (Table 2), confirming the robustness of the findings. In addition, comparable results were obtained in a sensitivity analysis excluding the Avonex treated patients (the annualized relapse rate over two years among Betaferon or Rebif treated patients was 0.37, with a corresponding $RR_{AZA/IFN}$ of 0.70, 95% CI, 0.43–1.15) [data not shown]. No significant difference was noted between AZA and IFN in the proportion of patients with 0, 1, 2, $\geq$3 relapses over two years and separately in the first or the second year, the proportion of patients with corticosteroid-treated relapses, and the proportion of patients with no confirmed disability progression over two years. (Table 2). There were six treatment failures in the AZA group and five in the IFN group. For QOL, no difference was observed between the treatments, for both physical and mental-QOL (p = 0.94 and 0.93, respectively) [data not shown]. Figure 3 shows Kaplan-Meier curves of the time to first relapse: no significant difference was observed in terms of log-rank (p = 0.11) or Cox proportional-hazards model results, with a hazard ratio of 0.66 (95% CI, 0.40–1.10). Similar results were obtained in sensitivity analyses excluding Avonex treated patients (log-rank p = 0.15) [data not shown]. The analyses performed in the PP population yielded similar findings [data not shown].

Efficacy - MRI outcomes

Of the 122 patients given baseline MRI (61 per group), 97 completed the ITT follow-up: 50 (82%) in the AZA group, and 47 (77%) in the IFN group. The ratio of annualized new T2 lesion rates of AZA vs. IFNs was 1.10 (Fig. 4). The corresponding U_L of the 95% one-sided CI was 1.45, below the non-inferiority margin M = 1.84, indicating an AZA vs. IFN effect equivalent to at least 73% of the IFNs vs. placebo effect. Moreover, the U_L of the one-sided 99% CI for the new T2 lesion $RR_{AZA/IFN}$ (i.e., 1.63) was also significantly below the non-inferiority margin of M = 1.84 (p< 0.01). Table 3 summarizes the MRI outcomes: no significant difference was noted between AZA and IFNs for new T2, new CE, and Gd+ lesions. The annualized new T2 lesion rate was 0.69 (95% CI, 0.54–0.88) in the IFN and 0.76 (95% CI, 0.61–0.95) in the AZA patients (p = 0.75). Adjustments for inflammatory activity at baseline, expressed by the Gd+ lesion number confirmed these findings. Analyses performed in the PP population (81 patients: 40 in the AZA and 41 in the IFN group) confirmed these results [data not shown].

Safety comparison

The rate of patients with at least one AE was not different between the two groups (p = 0.28), however the rate of AEs was higher in the AZA group (p<0.01) (Table 4). The most frequently reported AEs were flu-like symptoms, more frequent in IFNs (p< 0.01), nausea/vomiting and abnormal blood count more frequent in AZA-treated patients (p<0.01). AE-related discontinued interventions were more frequent among AZA (20.3%) than IFN (7.8%) patients (p = 0.03). SAEs and other AEs are described in Tables S1 and S2 in File S1.

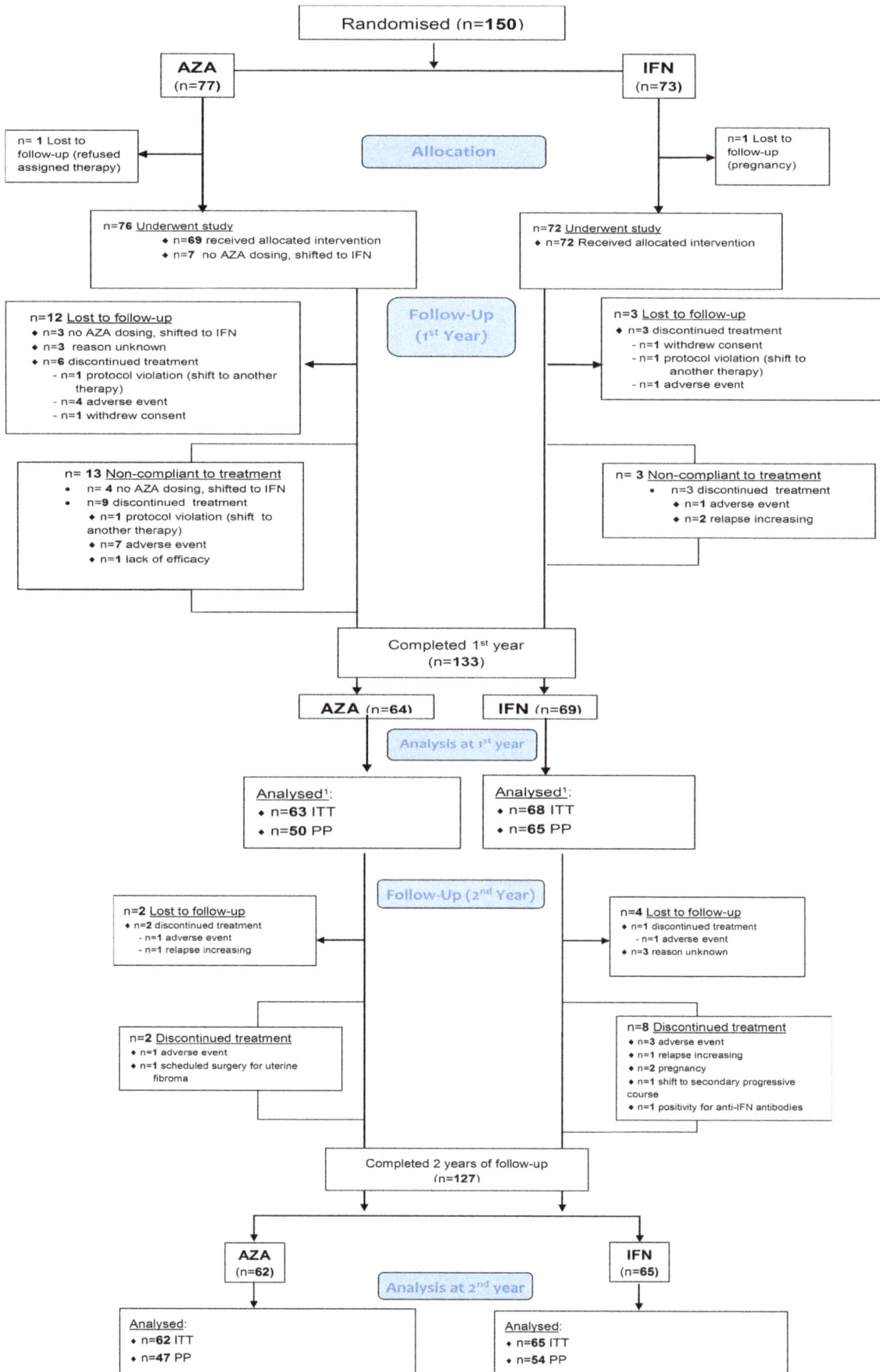

Randomised (n=**150**)

AZA
(n=**77**)

IFN
(n=**73**)

n= **1** Lost to
follow-up (refused
assigned therapy)

Allocation

n=1 Lost to
follow-up
(pregnancy)

n=76 Underwent study
 • n=**69** received allocated intervention
 • n=**7** no AZA dosing, shifted to IFN

n=72 Underwent study
 • n=**72** Received allocated intervention

n=**12** Lost to follow-up
 • n=3 no AZA dosing, shifted to IFN
 • n=3 reason unknown
 • n=6 discontinued treatment
   - n=1 protocol violation (shift to another
     therapy)
   - n=4 adverse event
   - n=1 withdrew consent

Follow-Up
(1st Year)

n=**3** Lost to follow-up
 • n=3 discontinued treatment
   - n=1 withdrew consent
   - n=1 protocol violation (shift to
     another therapy)
   - n=1 adverse event

n= **13** Non-compliant to treatment
 • n=4 no AZA dosing, shifted to IFN
 • n=9 discontinued treatment
   • n=1 protocol violation (shift to
     another therapy)
   • n=7 adverse event
   • n=1 lack of efficacy

n= **3** Non-compliant to treatment
 • n=3 discontinued treatment
   • n=1 adverse event
   • n=2 relapse increasing

Completed 1st year
(n=**133**)

AZA (n=64)

IFN (n=69)

Analysis at 1st year

Analysed[1]:
 • n=**63** ITT
 • n=**50** PP

Analysed[1]:
 • n=**68** ITT
 • n=**65** PP

n=2 Lost to follow-up
 • n=2 discontinued treatment
   - n=1 adverse event
   - n=1 relapse increasing

Follow-Up (2nd Year)

n=4 Lost to follow-up
 • n=1 discontinued treatment
   - n=1 adverse event
 • n=3 reason unknown

n=2 Discontinued treatment
 • n=1 adverse event
 • n=1 scheduled surgery for uterine
   fibroma

n=8 Discontinued treatment
 • n=3 adverse event
 • n=1 relapse increasing
 • n=2 pregnancy
 • n=1 shift to secondary progressive
   course
 • n=1 positivity for anti-IFN antibodies

Completed 2 years of follow-up
(n=**127**)

AZA
(n=**62**)

IFN
(n=**65**)

Analysis at 2nd year

Analysed:
 • n=**62** ITT
 • n=**47** PP

Analysed:
 • n=**65** ITT
 • n=**54** PP

Figure 1. Flow-chart: patient allocation and follow-up. Abbreviations: AZA, azathioprine; IFN, interferon; ITT, intention to treat; PP, per-protocol. [1]One missing CRF at month 12.

Discussion

Principal findings

This study directly compared AZA and IFN efficacy on clinical and MRI outcomes in relapsing-remitting MS patients. The results indicated that AZA was non-inferior to IFNs in reducing relapses and new brain lesions over two years. The effect size on the primary end point (annualized relapse rate ratio) was 0.67, with the upper CIs indicating that in the worst case scenario efficacy of AZA vs. placebo can be estimated as at least 100% (95% CI) or as

Table 1. Baseline characteristics of the patients.

Characteristic	AZA (N = 77)	IFN (N = 73)	p-value[1]
Demographic characteristics			
Female – No. (%)	49 (63.6%)	50 (68.5%)	p = 0.53
Age - Years			
Mean ± SD	38.1±8.9	36.6±8.8	p = 0.31
Median (range)	37.9 (21.3–56.5)	37.6 (19.1–58.8)	
Clinical characteristics			
Duration of disease from onset of symptoms - Years			
Mean ± SD	6.8±7.1	5.7±5.5	
Median (range)	3.4 (0.5–25.3)	3.4 (0.3–24.8)	p = 0.53
Relapses in previous 2 years			
Mean ± SD	2.38±0.78	2.41±0.89	
Median (range)	2 (0–5)	2 (0–6)	p = 0.91
No. patients with relapses in previous 2 years - No. (%)			
0–1[2]	3 (3.9%)	2 (2.7%)	
2	48 (62.3%)	47 (64.4%)	p = 0.91
≥3	26 (33.8%)	24 (32.9%)	
No. patients with previous histories of … - No. (%)			
AZA treatment	1 (1.3%)	1 (1.4%)	p = 0.95
IFN treatment	4 (5.2%)	3 (4.1%)	
EDSS score[3]			
Mean ± SD	1.9±0.9	1.9±0.9	
Median (range)	1.5 (1.0–5.5)	1.5 (0.0–5.0)	p = 0.86
Patients with concomitant diseases – No. (%)[4]	5 (6.9%)	4 (5.8%)	p = 0.80
	AZA (N = 61)	**IFN (N = 61)**	**p-value[1]**
MRI findings			
Gd+ lesion number			
Mean ± SD	1.64±3.85	2.32±4.53	
Median (range)	0 (0–24)	1 (0–20)	p = 0.38
No. patients with Gd+ lesions - No. (%)			
0	32 (52.5%)	27 (44.3%)	
1–2	20 (32.8%)	23 (37.7%)	p = 0.36
≥3	9 (14.8%)	11 (18.0%)	
T2 lesion load (FLAIR sequences; mm³)			
Mean ± SD	15,284±16,466	10,283±11,696	p = 0.16
Median (range)	9,197 (338–73,226)	7,205 (326–61,025)	

Abbreviations: AZA, azathioprine; EDSS, Expanded Disability Status Scale; IFN, interferon; SD, standard deviation.
[1]P-values for AZA vs. IFN comparison were obtained through: χ^2 test with one or two degrees of freedom for sex, number of patients with previous histories of AZA/IFN treatment, number of patients with relapses with concomitant disease and with Gd+ lesions; t-test for age; Mann-Whitney test for duration of disease, number of relapses, EDSS score, number of Gd+ lesions and T2 lesion load.
[2]Protocol violations.
[3]Scores on the EDSS range from 0 to 10, with higher scores indicating greater degree of disability.
[4]The sum does not add up to the total because of some missing values.

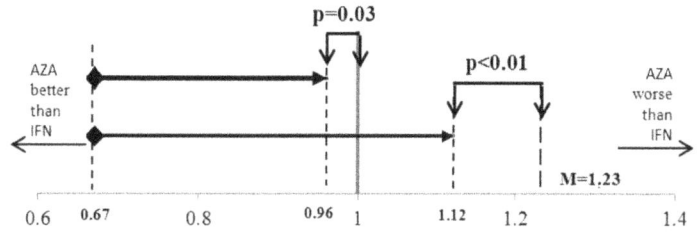

	AZA (n=62)	IFN (n=65)	Rate Ratio (RR_AZAvsIFN)
relapses/PY (rate)	33/126 (0.26)	52/132 (0.39)	0.67

Figure 2. Primary clinical outcome over 2 years: non-inferiority of effect of AZA vs. IFN, represented as annualized relapse rate ratio (RR_AZA/IFN) compared with the pre-established non-inferiority margin M (= 1.23) and with a margin M_1 = 1.0. One-sided 99% CI of the 0.67 ratio (upper-limit, $U_L = 1.12$), represents an effect of AZA vs. IFNs equivalent to at least 75% of the effect of IFNs vs. Placebo. One-sided 95% CI of the same ratio ($U_L = 0.96$), represents an effect of AZA vs. IFNs equivalent to at least 100% of the effect of IFNs vs. Placebo. Abbreviations: AZA, azathioprine; IFN, interferon; PY, person-years; RR, rate ratio.

at least 75% (99% CI) of that of IFNs, according to the CIs level selected. The effect size on new brain lesions (the main secondary outcome measure) was 1.1 with the upper CI levels (95%) indicating that in the worst case scenario efficacy of AZA vs. placebo could be estimated as at least 73% of that of the IFNs. The direct comparison of AZA and IFN efficacy therefore indicated a similar effect size, in reducing both relapses and new brain lesions. Both treatments were similarly efficacious in time to the first relapse, in slowing disability accumulation, and in the other secondary clinical and MRI outcome measures examined. Both medications showed better efficacy in the second year, probably for a delay in fully exerting their activity during the first months of treatment, at least in part determined by the initial dose titration. The observed lag of efficacy was similar for both treatments.

Similar efficacy of AZA and IFNs was observed both in the ITT and in the PP analysis and in the different sensitivity analyses performed. As in this study the comparator treatment included all the IFNs as a group, a sensitivity analysis excluding Avonex treated patients (probably the less efficacious of the IFNs [30]) confirmed the results of the main analysis.

AZA was compared to all the IFNs as a group because a centralized choice of one specific IFN could have raised allegation of conflict of interests, as in this academically driven independent study the medications were prescribed and charged to the NHS. In addition, under these experimental conditions, a centralized selection of a specific IFN could have reduced and distorted patient accrual in the participating centers.

The remarkable internal consistency between clinical and MRI data, between the ITT and the PP analysis and among the different sensitivity analyses, supported the robustness of the results. It must be pointed out that consistency between ITT and PP analysis is a critical requirement for reliability of non-inferiority studies [23–25].

The present study strengthens previous results of AZA vs. placebo [1–4] or vs. IFN [14–16], and expands previous available data as for the first time MRI was included as an outcome of AZA efficacy, thus allowing contemporary assessment of relapses and brain lesions accumulation. The previous MRI studies [17–18] indeed were informative for supporting the hypothesis of AZA efficacy on brain lesions, but were not aimed to assess clinical

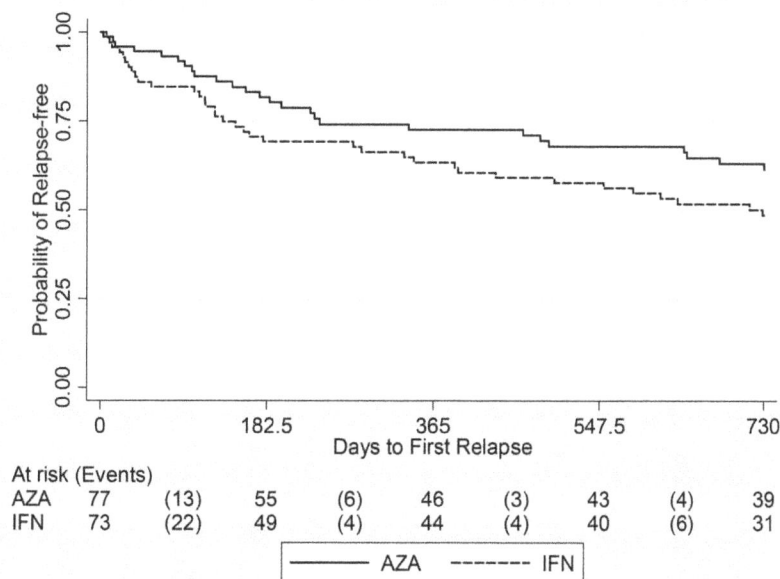

Figure 3. Time to first relapse. Beneath the plot patients at risk and number of events (in brackets) by treatment were reported for each interval of 6 months. Abbreviations: AZA, azathioprine; IFN, interferon.

Table 2. Secondary clinical outcomes.

Outcome	1st Year			2nd Year			Overall (2 years of follow-up)		
	AZA (N=63)	IFN (N=68)	p-value[1]	AZA (N=62)	IFN (N=65)	p-value[1]	AZA (N=62)	IFN (N=65)	p-value[1]
Relapses									
Annualised relapse rate (95% CI)	0.37 (0.25–0.56)	0.47 (0.34–0.67)	p=0.37	0.18 (0.10–0.32)	0.29 (0.18–0.45)	p=0.19	0.26 (0.19–0.37)	0.39 (0.30–0.51)	p=0.07
Adjusted annualised relapse rate (95% CI)[2]	-	-	-	-	-	-	0.27 (0.19–0.38)	0.41 (0.31–0.54)	p=0.06
No. of patients with relapse - No. (%)									
0	45 (71.4%)	44 (64.7%)	p=0.63	52 (83.9%)	49 (75.4%)	p=0.42	39 (62.9%)	31 (47.7%)	p=0.22
1	14 (22.2%)	17 (25.0%)		9 (14.5%)	13 (20.0%)		15 (24.2%)	23 (35.4%)	
≥2	4 (6.4%)	7 (10.3%)		1 (1.6%)	3 (4.6%)		8 (12.9%)	11 (16.9%)	
No. of patients with relapses treated with corticosteroids – No. (%)									
0	-	-	-	-	-	-	40 (64.5%)	34 (52.3%)	p=0.22
1	-	-	-	-	-	-	16 (25.8%)	22 (33.9%)	
≥2	-	-	-	-	-	-	6 (9.7%)	9 (13.9%)	
Disability[3]									
Patients with no confirmed disability progression - % (95% CI)[4]	-	-	-	-	-	-	98.2 (91.5–99.9)	92.0 (81.8–97.4)	p=0.19
Change from baseline in EDSS score – Mean (95% CI)[5]	-	-	-	-	-	-	−0.08 (−0.31; 0.16)	0.22 (−0.03; 0.47)	p=0.08

Abbreviations: AZA, azathioprine; IFN, interferon.
[1] P-values for AZA vs. IFN comparison were obtained through χ^2 test with one degree of freedom for rate comparison, χ^2 test with two degrees of freedom for number of patients with relapses, Fisher's exact test for patients with no confirmed disability progression, and t-test for change in EDSS score.
[2] The analyses were adjusted for number of relapses during the previous two years, baseline EDSS score, and duration of disease from symptom onset.
[3] The analyses were based on 56 AZA and 50 IFN patients respectively, because of some missing values.
[4] A confirmed disability progression was defined as an increase of no less than one point of the EDSS score confirmed at least after six months; 95% CI were estimated through the exact method. All the patients, with the exception of two (who did not report a disability progression), had a baseline EDSS score between 1 and 5.
[5] Adjusted for baseline EDSS score.

	AZA (n=50)	IFN (n=47)	Rate Ratio (RR$_{AZAvsIFN}$)
lesions/PY (rate)	76/100 (0.76)	65/94 (0.69)	1.10

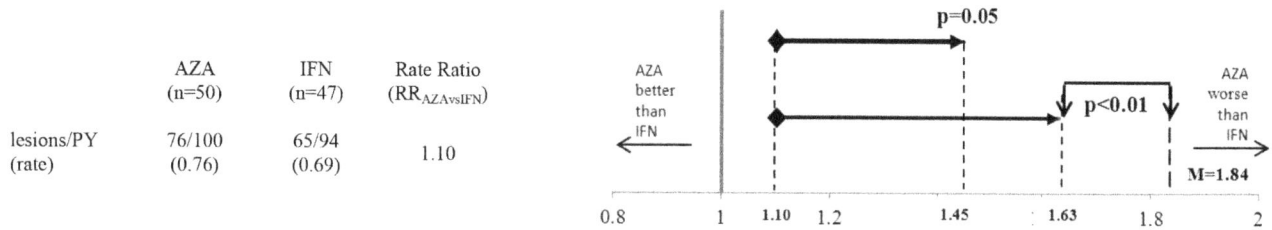

Figure 4. Non-inferiority of the effect AZA vs. IFN on new T2 lesions over 2 years. One-sided 99% CI (upper-limit, U$_L$ = 1.63), and one-sided 95% CI (U$_L$ = 1.45), of the effect of AZA vs. IFNs as for annualized new T2 lesion rate ratio (RR$_{AZA/IFN}$), compared with the pre-established non-inferiority margin (M = 1.84), representing an effect of AZA vs. IFNs equivalent to the 73% of the effect of IFNs vs placebo. Abbreviations: AZA, azathioprine; IFN, interferon; PY, person-years; RR, rate ratio.

outcomes and were based on retrospective or open label designs [17–18].

It must be noted that the results of the present study were obtained administering AZA at the target dose of 3 mg/Kg/day, adjusted according to leuko/lymphocyte count. This approach was similar to that of the trials that also showed the most remarkable reduction in relapse rates induced by AZA [2–4,15], suggesting that appropriate dosage represents an important variable administering this treatment.

No unknown AEs occurred. Overall similar numbers of patients developed at least one AE. Leuko/lymphopenia in the AZA group was not associated with a higher incidence of infections and should be considered part of the desired mechanism of action. However, treatment discontinuations after AEs were significantly higher in the AZA group, mainly occurring during the first months of treatment. Most of the discontinuations for IFNs were in the

second year, confirming already known different temporal AE profile of each treatment.

Strengths and weaknesses of the study

The main limit of the study was probably the sample size, which resulted smaller than planned. This was due to difficulties in recruiting and retaining patients in the trial, particularly following the change in the Italian NHS reimbursement criteria that occurred during the recruitment period. Indeed, rational basis of a direct comparison and randomization between an old generic medication and a new approved drug were sometimes hard to explain both to neurologists and patients and contributed to these difficulties.

However, the sample size affected only the initial power estimate based on the conservative hypothesis of no difference between the means of the relapse rates. Indeed, the data obtained during the study, showing a difference favoring AZA, allowed a

Table 3. MRI outcomes. New brain lesions.

Outcome	Overall (2 years of follow-up)		
	AZA (N = 50)	IFN (N = 47)	p-value[1]
New T2 lesions			
Annualised new T2 lesion rate (95% CI)	0.76 (0.61–0.95)	0.69 (0.54–0.88)	p = 0.75
No. of patients with new T2 lesions - No. (%)			
0	27 (54.0%)	21 (45.0%)	
1–2	11 (22.0%)	18 (38.0%)	p = 0.41
≥3	12 (24.0%)	8 (17.0%)	
New Combined Unique (CE) lesions			
Annualised new CE lesion rate (95% CI)	0.78 (0.63–0.98)	0.70 (0.55–0.90)	p = 0.53
Gd+ lesions			
Gd+ lesion number			
Mean ± SD	0.20±0.50	0.40±1.35	
Median (range)	0 (0–2)	0 (0–5)	p = 0.52
No. patients with Gd+ lesions - No. (%)			
0	41 (84.0%)	43 (91.5%)	
1–2	8 (16.0%)	1 (2.0%)	p = 0.39
≥3	0 (0.0%)	3(6.5%)	
Missing data	1	0	

Abbreviations: AZA, azathioprine; IFN, interferon.
[1]P-values for AZA vs. IFN comparison were obtained through χ^2 test with one degree of freedom for rate comparison, χ^2 test with two degrees of freedom for number of patients with lesions, and Mann-Whitney test for Gd+ lesion number.

Table 4. Adverse Events.

Event	AZA	IFN	p-value[1]
	($N_{patients}=69$, $N_{events}=308$, PY = 108)	($N_{patients}=77$, $N_{events}=241$, PY = 136)	
All AEs[2]			
Patients – No./PY and rate (95%CI)	65/108	68/136	p = 0.28
	0.60 (0.47–0.77)	0.50 (0.40–0.64)	
AEs - No./PY and rate (95%CI)	308/108	241/136	p<0.01
	2.85 (2.54–3.19)	1.77 (1.56–2.01)	
Most frequently reported AEs[2]			
Influenza-like illness			
Patients – No./PY and rate (95%CI)	3/108	39/136	p<0.01
	0.03 (0.01–0.08)	0.29 (0.20–0.39)	
AEs - No./PY and rate (95%CI)	3/108	41/136	p<0.01
	0.03 (0.01–0.08)	0.30 (0.22–0.41)	
Fever			
Patients – No./PY and rate (95%CI)	2/108	19/136	p<0.01
	0.02 (0.00–0.07)	0.14 (0.08–0.22)	
AEs - No./PY and rate (95%CI)	2/108	20/136	p = 0.01
	0.02 (0.00–0.07)	0.15 (0.09–0.23)	
Local allergic reaction			
Patients – No./PY and rate (95%CI)	0/108	13/136	-
		0.10 (0.05–0.16)	
AEs - No./PY and rate (95%CI)	0/108	14/136	-
		0.10 (0.06–0.17)	
Systemic allergic reaction			
Patients – No./PY and rate (95%CI)	3/108	0/136	-
	0.03 (0.01–0.08)		
AEs - No./PY and rate (95%CI)	3/108	0/136	-
	0.03 (0.01–0.08)		
Nausea/vomiting			
Patients – No./PY and rate (95%CI)	30/108	1/136	p<0.01
	0.28 (0.19–0.40)	0.01 (0.00–0.04)	
AEs - No./PY and rate (95%CI)	35/108	1/136	p<0.01
	0.32 (0.23–0.45)	0.01 (0.00–0.04)	
Abnormal blood count			
Patients – No./PY and rate (95%CI)	46/108	24/136	p<0.01
	0.43 (0.31–0.57)	0.18 (0.11–0.26)	
AEs - No./PY and rate (95%CI)	106/108	39/136	p<0.01
	0.98 (0.80–1.19)	0.29 (0.20–0.39)	
Other abnormal blood tests[3]			
Patients – No./PY and rate (95%CI)	24/108	37/136	p = 0.44
	0.22 (0.14–0.33)	0.27 (0.19–0.37)	
AEs - No./PY and rate (95%CI)	46/108	54/136	p = 0.72
	0.43 (0.31–0.57)	0.40 (0.30–0.52)	
Other AE			
Patients – No./PY and rate (95%CI)	51/108	47/136	p = 0.12
	0.47 (0.35–0.62)	0.35 (0.25–0.46)	
AEs - No./PY and rate (95%CI)	70/108	54/136	p<0.01
	0.65 (0.51–0.82)	0.40 (0.30–0.52)	
Discontinued interventions due to AEs			
No. of patients with discontinued interventions due to AEs (%)	14 (20.3%)	6 (7.8%)	p = 0.03

Table 4. Cont.

Event	AZA	IFN	p-value[1]
	($N_{patients} = 69$, $N_{events} = 308$, PY = 108)	($N_{patients} = 77$, $N_{events} = 241$, PY = 136)	
Seriousness of AE[5]			
No. of events (%)[4]			
Minor/Moderate	291 (96.0%)	236 (98.3%)	p = 0.12
Major/Serious	12 (4.0%)	4 (1.7%)	
Correlation with study treatment			
No. of events (%)[4]			
Non-correlated/Unlikely	63 (20.7%)	49 (20.4%)	p = 0.95
Possible/Likely	242 (79.3%)	191 (79.6%)	

Abbreviations: AZA, azathioprine; IFN, interferon; PY, person-years.
[1]P-values for AZA vs. IFN comparison were obtained through χ^2 test with one degree of freedom for rate comparison, discontinued interventions due to adverse events, seriousness of adverse event, and correlation of event with treatment.
[2]All 95% CI were estimated using the exact method.
[3]Liver enzymes, thyroid function and bilirubin level.
[4]The sum does not add up to the total because of some missing values.
[5]Seriousness judged by the treating neurologist. SAEs classified according to the National Cancer Institute Common Terminology Criteria for AE [21] are reported in Table S1 in File S1.

power sufficient to establish non-inferiority at statistically robust levels of significance. Moreover, as documented by Schulz and Grimes [31] trials with low sample size might be acceptable if investigators use methodological rigor to eliminate bias and properly report to avoid misinterpretation.

Another possible limitation could be related to patient knowledge of the treatment. Indeed, out of the patients who refused the assigned treatment, all had been randomized to AZA. As this occurred before the first dose of AZA was administered, it was necessarily due to a different perception by the patients of this therapy with respect to the IFNs, which were specifically approved for MS. Successfully blinding of patients seemed unrealistic given the profoundly different side effects of AZA and IFNs of which the patients had been informed in detail. Indeed, analysis of blinding in previous studies revealed a strong tendency to treatment awareness in patients receiving IFNs [10,32].

Dropout rates was another possible issue in this study. Although the overall number of patients who withdrew the study was only 15%, a higher number of patients were lost to follow up in the AZA than in the IFN group, mainly during the first year. As this event may have diluted true differences between treatments, sensitivity analyses, based on two multiple imputation methods, were performed and no difference in the $RR_{AZA/IFN}$ estimate was observed, thus confirming the results obtained in the analysis of patients who completed the follow-up.

Finally, the different number of treatment discontinuations observed between the two groups (i.e., 39% of patients on AZA and 26% on IFN) could have impacted the study effect size. However, if only patients who began the treatment according to the study protocol are considered, a similar number of patients discontinued (32% on AZA and 25% on IFNs), suggesting similar compliance of the two medications over two years. The clear difference was that treatment interruptions were more frequent in the first year in the AZA group and in the second year in the IFN group.

Implications for clinical practice

The present study was the first independent RCT that directly compared efficacy of a generic medication (AZA) to a drug specifically approved for MS (IFN) using a non-inferiority design. The authors believe that the results of this study are robust, clinically meaningful and relevant for clinical practice, supporting AZA as a rational and effective alternative to IFNs in relapsing-remitting MS, particularly considering the convenience of oral administration and the cost, lower than the other available treatments. Nevertheless, the different side effect profiles of both medications have to be taken into account.

Supporting Information

Checklist S1   CONSORT checklist.

Protocol S1   Trial protocol.

Amendment S1   Amendment to the protocol.

File S1   Methods S1, Outcomes. Brain MRI: Scan acquisition specifications. **Table S1**, Serious Adverse Events (SAEs). **Table S2**, AEs – subtypes.

Acknowledgments

The authors wish to thank: The Italian Medicines Agency (Agenzia Italiana del Farmaco, AIFA) for the financial support; the Interdipartimental Center for Magnetic Resonance Imaging of University of Florence for the support in the MRI analysis; Paul Bowerbank for his help in reviewing the English of the manuscript.
Group information
The Multicenter Azathioprine Interferon-ß Non-Inferiority (M.A.I.N.) Trial Group and investigators are as follows: *Steering committee:* L Massacesi (Dipartimento di Neuroscienze, Psicologia, Farmaco e Salute del Bambino Università di Firenze, Italy; Neurologia 2, Azienda Ospedaliero-Universitaria Careggi, Firenze, Italy.), G Filippini, C Milanese, A Solari (Fondazione IRCCS Istituto Neurologico Carlo Besta, Milano), L La Mantia (Unità di Neurologia - Multiple Sclerosis Center, I.R.C.C.S. Santa Maria Nascente Fondazione Don Gnocchi, Milano), MD Benedetti (Dipartimento Universitario di Neurologia, Azienda Ospedaliera Universitaria Integrata, Verona), S Amoroso (Dipartimento di Neuroscienze,

Sezione di Farmacologia, Università Politecnica delle Marche, Ancona), G Mancardi (Dipartimento Neuroscienze, Università di Genova, Genova), D Orrico (Divisione di Neurologia, Ospedale Civile Santa Chiara, Trento), G Tedeschi (Clinica Neurologica, Università di Napoli), M Battaglia (AISM, FISM, Genova), MG Valsecchi (Centro di Biostatistica per l'Epidemiologia Clinica, Università Milano-Bicocca, Monza). *Study coordinators* C Milanese, L Massacesi. *Randomization centre* A Solari. *Data Coordination and Analysis:* G Filippini, I Tramacere (Fondazione IRCCS Istituto Neurologico Carlo Besta, Milano). *Image Analysis Centre:* L Massacesi, L Vuolo (Dipartimento di Neuroscienze, Azienda Ospedaliero-Universitaria Careggi, Firenze). *Independent data safety management committee (IDSMC)* G Tognoni (Istituto Mario Negri, Milano), R D'Alessandro (Clinica Neurologica, Università di Bologna), L Provinciali (Clinica Neurologica, Ospedali Riuniti, Ancona). *Pharmacologic surveillance Unit* S Amoroso (Dipartimento di Neuroscienze, Sezione di Farmacologia, Università Politecnica delle Marche, Ancona). *Study sites and hospitals (PI = Principal investigator)* **Dipartimento di Neuroscienze, Psicologia, Farmaco e Salute del Bambino Università di Firenze** and Neurologia 2, Azienda Ospedaliero-Universitaria Careggi, Firenze; L Massacesi (PI), A Repice, A Barilaro, L Vuolo. **Fondazione IRCCS Istituto Neurologico Carlo Besta, Milano**; C Milanese (PI), P Confalonieri. **Unità di Neurologia - Multiple Sclerosis Center, I.R.C.C.S. Santa Maria Nascente Fondazione Don Gnocchi, Milano**; L La Mantia. **Clinica Neurologica, Novara**; M Leone (PI), S Ruggerone, P Naldi. **Dipartimento di Scienze Neurologiche "La Sapienza", Roma**; C Pozzilli (PI), F De Angelis. **Policlinico "G. Rodolico", Azienda Ospedaliero-Universitaria, Catania**; F Patti (PI), S Messina. **Dipartimento di Neuroscienze, Clinica Neurologica 2, Genova**; G Mancardi (PI), E Capello. **Dipartimento Universitario di Neurologia, Azienda Ospedaliera Universitaria Integrata, Verona**; MD Benedetti (PI), A Gajofatto. **Centro Sclerosi Multipla, Clinica Neurologica, Ospedale Clinicizzato "Colle Dall'Ara", Chieti**; A Lugaresi (PI), G De Luca. **Clinica Neurologica, Università di Sassari**; G Rosati (PI), M Pugliatti. **Clinica Neurologica, Università di Napoli**; G Tedeschi (PI), S. Bonavita. **UO Neurologia, Ospedale S. Antonio, Padova**; B Tavolato (PI). **Dipartimento di Neuroscienze, Clinica Neurologica, Modena**; P Sola (PI). **Ospedale Santa Maria, Reggio Emilia**; L Motti (PI). **Clinica Neurologica, Policlinico Universitario Mater Domini, Catanzaro**; A Quattrone (PI). **Clinica Neurologica, Ospedale S. Gerardo, Monza**; M Frigo (PI). **Clinica Neurologica, Azienda Ospedaliero-Universitaria S. Anna, Ferrara**; MR Tola (PI). **Clinica Neurologica, Ospedali Riuniti, Ancona**; M Danni (PI). **UO Neurologia, Istituto S. Raffaele "G. Giglio", Cefalù**; L Grimaldi (PI). **Dipartimento di Neuroscienze, Azienda Ospedaliero San Giovanni Battista, Università di Torino, Torino**; P Cavalla (PI). **UO Neurologia, Ospedale Sacro Cuore, Negrar**; F Marchioretto (PI), M Pellegrini. **Divisione Neurologia, Ospedale Santa Chiara, Trento**; D Orrico (PI). **Divisione di Neurologia, Ospedale Regionale, Bolzano**; R Schoenhuber (PI). **Azienda Ospedaliero-Universitaria Senese, Policlinico "Le Scotte", Siena**; M Ulivelli (PI). **UO Neurologia, Ospedale "Misericordia e Dolce", Prato**; M Falcini (PI). **Dipartimento di Neuroscienze, Sezione di Neurologia, Pisa**; A Iudice (PI). **UOC Neurologia, Policlinico "G. Martino", Messina**; C Messina (PI). **Dipartimento di Neuroscienze, Clinica Neurologica, Palermo**; G Savettieri (PI). **Dipartimento di Neuroscienze, Università Cattolica, Policlinico Gemelli, Roma**; AP Batocchi (PI). **Dipartimento Neuroriabilitativo ASL CN1, Cuneo**; F Perla (PI). **Ospedale S. Luigi Gonzagal, Orbassano**; A Bertolotto (PI).

Author Contributions

Conceived and designed the experiments: LM CM MDB LL GF AS. Performed the experiments: LM CM MDB GT. Analyzed the data: IT AR. Wrote the paper: GF IT LM. Critical revision of the manuscript for important intellectual content: SA MDB LL AS GT CM. Obtained funding: LM CM. Administrative, technical, and material support: MAB AR. Study supervision: LM CM.

References

1. The British, Dutch MSATG. (1988) Double-masked trial of azathioprine in multiple sclerosis. british and dutch multiple sclerosis azathioprine trial group. Lancet 2: 179–183.

2. Ellison GW, Myers LW, Mickey MR, Graves MC, Tourtellotte WW, et al. (1989) A placebo-controlled, randomized, double-masked, variable dosage, clinical trial of azathioprine with and without methylprednisolone in multiple sclerosis. Neurology 39: 1018–1026.

3. Goodkin DE, Bailly RC, Teetzen ML, Hertsgaard D, Beatty WW. (1991) The efficacy of azathioprine in relapsing-remitting multiple sclerosis. Neurology 41: 20–25.

4. Milanese C, La Mantia L, Salmaggi A, Eoli M. (1993) A double blind study on azathioprine efficacy in multiple sclerosis: Final report. J Neurol 240: 295–298.

5. Clegg A, Bryant J, Milne R. (2000) Disease-modifying drugs for multiple sclerosis: A rapid and systematic review. Health Technol Assess 4: i–iv, 1–101.

6. Yudkin PL, Ellison GW, Ghezzi A, Goodkin DE, Hughes RA, et al. (1991) Overview of azathioprine treatment in multiple sclerosis. Lancet 338: 1051–1055.

7. Goodin DS, Frohman EM, Garmany GP, Jr, Halper J, Likosky WH, et al. (2002) Disease modifying therapies in multiple sclerosis: Report of the therapeutics and technology assessment subcommittee of the American Academy of Neurology and the MS council for clinical practice guidelines. Neurology 58: 169–178.

8. IFNB MSG. (1993) Interferon beta-1b is effective in relapsing-remitting multiple sclerosis. I. clinical results of a multicenter, randomized, double-blind, placebo-controlled trial. the IFNB multiple sclerosis study group. Neurology 43: 655–661.

9. PRISMS. (1998) Randomised double-blind placebo-controlled study of interferon beta-1a in relapsing/remitting multiple sclerosis. PRISMS (prevention of relapses and disability by interferon beta-1a subcutaneously in multiple sclerosis) study group. Lancet 352: 1498–1504.

10. Jacobs LD, Cookfair DL, Rudick RA, Herndon RM, Richert JR, et al. (1996) Intramuscular interferon beta-1a for disease progression in relapsing multiple sclerosis. the multiple sclerosis collaborative research group (MSCRG). Ann Neurol 39: 285–294.

11. Paty DW, Li DK. (1993) Interferon beta-1b is effective in relapsing-remitting multiple sclerosis. II. MRI analysis results of a multicenter, randomized, double-blind, placebo-controlled trial. UBC MS/MRI study group and the IFNB multiple sclerosis study group. Neurology 43: 662–667.

12. Casetta I, Iuliano G, Filippini G. (2007) Azathioprine for multiple sclerosis. Cochrane Database Syst Rev (4): CD003982.

13. Filippini G, Munari L, Incorvaia B, Ebers GC, Polman C, et al. (2003) Interferons in relapsing remitting multiple sclerosis: A systematic review. Lancet 361: 545–552.

14. Palace J, Rothwell P. (1997) New treatments and azathioprine in multiple sclerosis. Lancet 350: 261.

15. Etemadifar M, Janghorbani M, Shaygannejad V. (2007) Comparison of interferon beta products and azathioprine in the treatment of relapsing-remitting multiple sclerosis. J Neurol 254: 1723–1728.

16. Milanese C, La Mantia L, Salmaggi A, Caputo D. (2001) Azathioprine and interferon beta-1b treatment in relapsing-remitting multiple sclerosis. J Neurol Neurosurg Psychiatry 70: 413–414.

17. Cavazzuti M, Merelli E, Tassone G, Mavilla L. (1997) Lesion load quantification in serial MR of early relapsing multiple sclerosis patients in azathioprine treatment. A retrospective study. Eur Neurol 38: 284–290.

18. Massacesi L, Parigi A, Barilaro A, Repice AM, Pellicano G, et al. (2005) Efficacy of azathioprine on multiple sclerosis new brain lesions evaluated using magnetic resonance imaging. Arch Neurol 62: 1843–1847.

19. McDonald WI, Compston A, Edan G, Goodkin D, Hartung HP, et al. (2001) Recommended diagnostic criteria for multiple sclerosis: Guidelines from the international panel on the diagnosis of multiple sclerosis. Ann Neurol 50: 121–127.

20. Kurtzke JF. (1983) Rating neurologic impairment in multiple sclerosis: An expanded disability status scale (EDSS). Neurology 33: 1444–1452.

21. CTC (2003). Cancer therapy evaluation program, common terminology criteria for adverse event, version 3.0, DCTD, NCI, NIH, DHHS.

22. Solari A, Filippini G, Mendozzi L, Ghezzi A, Cifani S, et al. (1999) Validation of Italian multiple sclerosis quality of life 54 questionnaire. J Neurol Neurosurg Psychiatry 67: 158–162.

23. Committee for medicinal product for human use (CHMP) (2005). Guideline on the choise of the non-inferiority margin. doc. ref. EMEA/CPMP/EWP/2158/99.

24. Piaggio G, Elbourne DR, Altman DG, Pocock SJ, Evans SJ, et al. (2006) Reporting of noninferiority and equivalence randomized trials: An extension of the CONSORT statement. JAMA 295: 1152–1160.

25. Sackett DL. (2004) Superiority trials, noninferiority trials, and prisoners of the 2-sided null hypothesis. ACP J Club 140: A11.

26. Rubin DB. (1987) Multiple imputation for nonresponse in surveys. New York: John Wiley & Sons.

27. Brand JPL. (1999) Development, implementation and evaluation of multiple imputation strategies for the statistical analysis of incomplete data sets, ph.D. thesis, erasmus university, rotterdam.

28. van Buuren S, Boshuizen HC, Knook DL. (1999) Multiple imputation of missing blood pressure covariates in survival analysis. Stat Med 18: 681–694.

29. Piaggio G, Elbourne DR, Pocock SJ, Evans SJ, Altman DG; CONSORT Group. (2012) Reporting of noninferiority and equivalence randomized trials: extension of the CONSORT 2010 statement. JAMA 308:2594–2604.

30. Filippini G, Del Giovane C, Vacchi L, D'Amico R, Di Pietrantonj C, et al. (2013) Immunomodulators and immunosuppressants for multiple sclerosis: A network meta-analysis. Cochrane Database Syst Rev 6: CD008933.

31. Schulz KF, Grimes DA. (2005) Sample size calculations in randomised trials: Mandatory and mystical. Lancet 365: 1348–1353.

32. The IFNB Multiple Sclerosis Study Group and The University of British Columbia MS/MRI Analysis Group. (1995) Interferon beta-1b in the treatment of multiple sclerosis: Final outcome of the randomized controlled trial. Neurology 45: 1277–1285.

4

Adoptive Immunotherapy of Cytokine-Induced Killer Cell Therapy in the Treatment of Non-Small Cell Lung Cancer

Min Wang[1][⅁][¶], Jun-Xia Cao[1][⅁][¶], Jian-Hong Pan[2], Yi-Shan Liu[1], Bei-Lei Xu[1], Duo Li[1], Xiao-Yan Zhang[1], Jun-Li Li[1], Jin-Long Liu[1], Hai-Bo Wang[1], Zheng-Xu Wang[1]*

1 Biotherapy Center, General Hospital of Beijing Military Command, Beijing, China, 2 Department of Biostatistics, Peking University Clinical Research Institute, Peking University Health Science Center, Beijing, China

Abstract

Aim: The aim of this study was to systemically evaluate the therapeutic efficacy of cytokine-induced killer (CIK) cells for the treatment of non-small cell lung cancer.

Materials and Methods: A computerized search of randomized controlled trials for CIK cell-based therapy was performed. The overall survival, clinical response rate, immunological assessment and side effects were evaluated.

Results: Overall, 17 randomized controlled trials of non-small cell lung cancer (NSCLC) with a total of 1172 patients were included in the present analysis. Our study showed that the CIK cell therapy significantly improved the objective response rate and overall survival compared to the non-CIK cell-treated group. After CIK combined therapy, we observed substantially increased percentages of $CD3^+$, $CD4^+$, $CD4^+CD8^+$, $CD3^+CD56^+$ and NK cells, whereas significant decreases were noted in the percentage of $CD8^+$ and regulatory T cell (Treg) subgroups. A significant increase in Ag-NORs was observed in the CIK-treated patient group ($p = 0.00001$), whereas carcinoembryonic antigen (CEA) was more likely to be reduced to a normal level after CIK treatment ($p = 0.0008$). Of the possible major side effects, only the incidence of fever in the CIK group was significantly higher compared to the group that received chemotherapy alone.

Conclusion: The CIK cell combined therapy demonstrated significant superiority in the overall survival, clinical response rate, and T lymphocytes responses and did not present any evidence of major adverse events in patients with NSCLC.

Editor: Nupur Gangopadhyay, University of Pittsburgh, United States of America

Funding: This research work was supported by the National Natural Science Foundation of China (No. 31171427 and 30971651 to Zheng-Xu Wang), Beijing Municipal Science & Technology Project; Clinical characteristics and Application Research of Capital (No. Z121107001012136 to Zheng-Xu Wang) and the Postdoctoral Foundation of China (No. 20060400775 to Jun-Xia Cao). Zheng-Xu Wang designed the research; Jun-Xia Cao is one of the people who performed the research and wrote the paper. The funders had no role in study design, data collection and analysis, decision to publish, or preparation of the manuscript.

Competing Interests: The authors have declared that no competing interests exist.

* Email: zhxwang18@hotmail.com

⅁ These authors contributed equally to this work.

¶ These authors are co-first authors on this work.

Introduction

Lung cancer is the leading cause of cancer-related mortality worldwide [1]. According to the 2012 Chinese cancer registration annual report, more than 3 million new cases of lung cancer will be diagnosed every year, and the approximately 2.7 million deaths from lung cancer will account for 13% of allmortalities. There is no doubt that the incidence and mortality of lung cancer are far too prevalent [2]. In patients with advanced lung disease, 1-year survival rates are typically 35%, and 2-year survival rates were shown to approach 15%-20% in recent studies [3]. At best, the 5-year overall survival rate of localized cancer is 15.9%, and only half of extended-stage patients have a 3.7% chance of surviving 5 years [4]. Most NSCLC patients have locally advanced or metastatic cancer at stage IIIB-IV at the time of diagnosis, leaving only palliative therapeutic options. Based on the existing clinical data, chemotherapy appears to have limited benefits and disappointed prognoses [5].

The novel approach of adoptive cell immunotherapy relies on an ex vivo expansion of the autologous tumor-specific effector cells before their reinfusion into the host [6]. Since the development of this immunotherapy, a number of immunological effector cells have been employed to treat cancer and eliminate residual tumor cells after surgery, such as CIK cells, lymphokine-activated killer cells (LAKs), tumor-infiltrating lymphocytes (TILs), natural killer cells (NKs), and cytotoxic T lymphocyte cells (CTLs) [7,8]. Among them, LAKs, which are a mixture of lymphokine-activated $CD3^+$ T lymphocytes and $CD3^-CD56^+CD16^+$ NK cells, were cultured with recombinant interleukin-2 (rIL-2) for 3 days, and CTLs were isolated from a patient's own tissues, including peripheral blood mononuclear cells (PBMCs), TILs, draining lymph nodes, or PBMCs after vaccination with irradiated autologous tumor cells (ATCs) [7,8]. After adoptive cell immunotherapy made great strides due to the efforts of several generations of researchers, CIK cells were found to possess greater proliferative and cytolytic capacities than NK or LAK cells. CIK cells are MHC-unrestricted cytotoxic lymphocytes that can be generated in vitro from PBMCs and cultured with the addition of IFN-γ, IL-2 and CD3 monoclonal antibody (CD3mAb). Anti-tumor cytotoxic activity is represented by surface markers for both T cells (TCR-α/β, CD3) and NKT cells (CD3$^+$CD56$^+$) [9].

The first clinical trial using CIK cell therapy for cancer patients was reported in 1999 [10]. Soon afterward, a growing number of clinical trials have suggested that CIK therapy yields highly compelling objective clinical responses in several solid carcinomas compared to other immunological effectors. A pooled analysis of 792 patients with solid carcinomas indicated that treatment with CIK cells is associated with a significant prolonging of the mean survival time and disease control rate [11]. Recently, both chinese clinical trials with 563 patients and international registered clinical trials with 426 cases of CIK cell therapy provided evidence for a broad clinical application based on a positive evaluation of the immunological and clinical responses [12,13]. Some systematic reviews have analyzed CIK cell therapy and shown it to be safe and efficient to treat renal cell carcinoma, hepatocellular carcinoma, and colon cancer [14–16]. Furthermore, CIK cell therapy has been perceived to have significant survival benefits in a few NSCLC clinical trials [17–22]. These studies showed that the immunotherapy of cancers with CIK cells may improve immunological and clinical responses, promote the quality of life (QoL) of cancer patients, and extend their life spans under certain conditions. However, there is no systematic review to assess the therapeutic efficacy of CIK cell therapies combined with chemotherapy in NSCLC; therefore, we performed a systematic meta-analysis of CIK cell therapy with randomized controlled trials on NSCLC. Our large-scale CIK cell immunotherapy clinical trials systematically analyzed the clinical efficiency and safety considering the overall survival, clinical response, immunological assessments and side effects.

Methods

Study design, search strategy and eligibility criteria

The relevant studies were identified by searching PubMed, the Cochrane Center Register of Controlled Trials, Science Direct, Embase, and China National Knowledge Infrastructure for randomized controlled trials (RCT) in the most recent decades. The search strategy included the keywords 'non-small-cell lung cancer,' 'adoptive immunotherapy,' and 'cytokine induced killer cells' adoptive immunotherapy arms with no adjuvant treatment in NSCLC patients except those who had undergone the same chemotherapy compared with control arms. In addition, we manually searched a website of clinical trials for ongoing trials. We searched keywords 'non-small-cell lung cancer' and 'cytokine induced killer cells' on the website http://www.clinicaltrials.gov/. The registered clinical trials with publication citations are displayed at the bottom of the Full Text View tab of a study record, under the More Information heading. Reference lists of previously published trials and relevant review articles were examined for other eligible trials. No language restriction was applied. Review papers and postgraduate theses were also examined for published results. Furthermore, we performed manual searches in reference lists and conference proceedings of the American Society of Clinical Oncology (ASCO) annual

meetings and the European Cancer Conference (ECCO). We excluded abstracts that were never subsequently published as full papers and studies on animals and cell lines.

Data selection criteria

Data extraction was independently conducted by two reviewers (Min Wang and Jun-Xia Cao) using a standardized approach. Disagreement was adjudicated by a third reviewer (Zheng-Xu Wang) after referring back to the original publications. The selection criteria were as follows: (1) English language studies on human clinical trials with patients at all stages of NSCLC were included; (2) RCT with CIK cell-based immunotherapy combined with chemotherapy versus chemotherapy alone for the treatment of NSCLC were included; (3) all trials approved by the local ethical committee and in which all patients signed a study-specific consent form prior to study entry were included; (4) case studies, review articles, and studies involving fewer than 10 patients were excluded; (5) uncontrolled metabolic disease, inadequate hepatic function, renal dysfunction, neurological disorders and other infectious diseases were excluded from the study; and (6) blood samples receiving any chemotherapy or radiotherapy within one month before treatment were excluded.

The overall quality of each included paper was evaluated by the Jadad scale [23]. A few of the major criteria were employed as a grading scheme: (1) randomization; (2) allocation concealment; (3) blinding; (4) lost to follow up; (5) ITT (intention to treat); and (6) baseline. We also used a funnel plot to evaluate the publication bias.

Definition of outcome measures

The primary clinical endpoints in RCT for cancer therapies employed the measures of median survival time (MST) and progression-free survival (PFS). The time to progression (TTP) may not consider those patients who die from other causes but is often used as equivalent to PFS. The secondary endpoints were the clinical response rate, including the objective response rate (ORR) and disease control rate (DCR). The ORR was defined as the sum of the partial rates (PRs) and complete response rates (CRs), and the DCR was defined as the sum of the stable disease (SD), PR and CR, according to the World Health Organization criteria. The side effects and toxicity were graded according to the National Cancer Institute Common Toxicity Criteria. The data were either obtained directly from the articles or calculated using the graphed data in articles using Photoshop and a software graph digitizer scout.

Statistical analysis

The analysis was performed using Review Manager Version 5.0 (Nordic Cochran Centre, Copenhagen, Denmark). Heterogeneity was assessed to determine which model should be used. To assess the statistical heterogeneity between the studies, the Cochran Q-test was performed using a predefined significance threshold of 0.1. The treatment effects are reflected by odds ratios (ORs), which were obtained using a method reported by Mantel and Haenszel. To evaluate whether the results of the studies were homogeneous, Cochran's Q test was performed. We also calculated the quantity I^2, which describes the percentage of variation across studies that is due to heterogeneity rather than chance. The OR was obtained using a fixed-effect model with no statistically significant heterogeneity; otherwise, a random-effects model was employed. P-values <0.05 were considered statistically significant. All reported P-values were two-sided.

Results

Selection of the trials

The data searches yielded 167 references, 91 of which were considered ineligible for different reasons (44 non-CIK immuno-therapy, 19 multiple cancer analyses, 18 reviews, and 10 animal models). The remaining 76 articles were further evaluated, and 59 trials were excluded due to language, lack of an RCT, and insufficient data. The final 17 articles were included in the meta-analysis with RCTs of CIK cell-based therapy for the treatment of NSCLC (Figure 1, also see the checklist S1).

The quality assessment of the 17 studies is summarized in Table 1. We also used a funnel plot to evaluate the publication bias. In our analysis, overall survival, clinical response rate, and side effects suffered low published bias. However, immunological assessment and T cell subgroups observed a high published bias (Figure 2), which demonstrated that the node of the vertical line does not meet the horizontal one at the midpoint by analysis with Review Manager Version 5.0.

Characteristics of CIK cell-based therapy

The characteristics of the 17 trials are listed in Table 2. Our selected 17 trials with a total of 1172 NSCLC patients in stage I-IV were included in the present analysis, and 90% of them included metastatic or locally advanced NSCLC. The enrolled ages were between 28 and 82 years of age, with a median age greater than 50.

In all 17 trials, the control arm was chemotherapy or cyberknife alone, whereas the treatment arm was chemotherapy or cyberknife combined with CIK cell therapy. In each trial, all of the patients in the CIK group were treated identically to those in the chemotherapy group in terms of chemotherapy doses and cycles. In all 17 trials of the treatment arm, most of the patients were treated with CIK cells plus DC immunotherapy combined with chemotherapy, although patients in four of the trials were injected with CIK cells combined with chemotherapy [6,30,38,39]. Most of the CIK groups used DCs without pulse, i.e., the DCs were only induced to become mature before co-culture with CIK cells. In 4 out of 17 studies, the DCs were injected while being pulsed with lung cancer antigens or tumor lysate [17,22,33,37]. Some of the necessary cytokines were supplied in a culture of CIK, IL-2, IFN-γ, and CD3mAb in a variety of culture media. The patients received cell infusions of 1×10^9 to 2×10^{12} cells per course, mostly at a 10^9 order of magnitude. Most of the treatments with repeated CIK cell infusions were administered for at least 2 weeks, and some of them lasted over 1 month. The injected route for immunotherapy was mainly intravenous for CIK cells and via subcutaneous injection for DCs (File S1 and File S2).

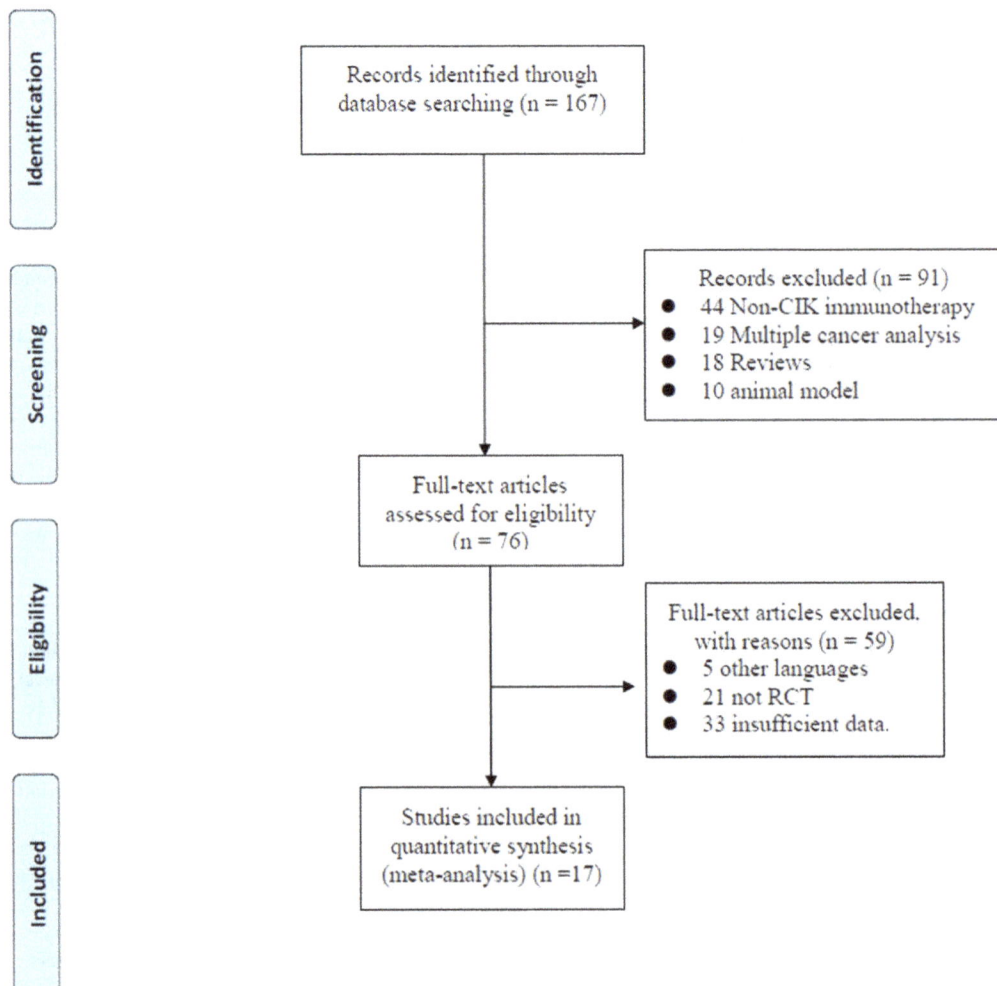

Figure 1. Flow diagram of the study selection process.

Table 1. Jadad Scale for the 17 randomized controlled studies.

Included studies	Randomization	Allocation concealment	Blinding	Lost to follow up	ITT analysis	Baseline	Quality grading
Li 2009 [17]	Yes	Unclear	Unclear	No	Yes	Similar	B
Li 2012 [30]	Yes	Unclear	Unclear	No	Yes	Similar	B
Mo 2010 [18]	Yes	Unclear	Unclear	Yes	Unclear	Unclear	C
Peng 2012 [19]	Yes	Unclear	Unclear	No	Yes	Similar	B
Sheng 2011 [20]	Yes	Unclear	Unclear	No	Yes	Similar	B
Shi 2012 [21]	Yes	Unclear	Unclear	No	Yes	Similar	B
Wang 2013 [39]	Yes	Unclear	Unclear	Yes	Yes	Similar	B
Wu 2008 [6]	Yes	Unclear	Unclear	No	Yes	Similar	B
Xu 2010 [31]	Yes	Unclear	Unclear	No	Yes	Similar	B
Xu 2011 [32]	Yes	Unclear	Unclear	No	Yes	Similar	B
Yang 2013 [33]	Yes	Unclear	Unclear	No	Yes	Similar	B
You 2012 [34]	Yes	Unclear	Unclear	Yes	Yes	Unclear	B
Yuan 2011 [35]	Yes	Unclear	Unclear	Yes	Yes	Unclear	C
Zhang 2012 [36]	Yes	Unclear	Unclear	No	Yes	Similar	B
Zheng 2012 [38]	Yes	Unclear	Unclear	No	Yes	Similar	B
Zhong 2008 [37]	Yes	Unclear	Unclear	No	Yes	Similar	B
Zhong 2011 [22]	Yes	Unclear	No	No	Yes	Similar	B

ITT: intention-to-treat. A: adequate, with correct procedure; B: unclear, without a description of the methods; C: inadequate procedures, methods, or information.
Each criterion was graded as follows: Yes, adequate, with correct procedure; Unclear, without a description of the methods; No, inadequate procedures, methods, or information. Each involved study was graded as follows: A, studies with a low risk of bias and which were scored as grade of A for all items; B, studies with a moderate risk of bias, with one or more grades of B; and C, studies with a high risk of bias, with one or more grades of C.

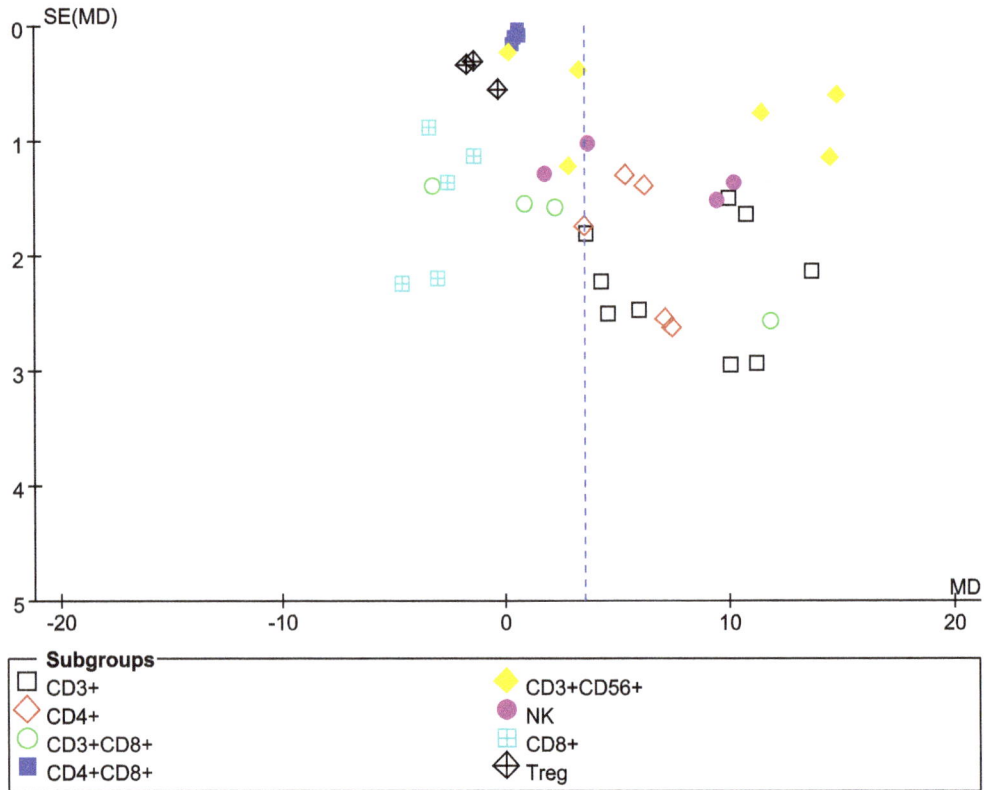

Figure 2. Funnel plot to evaluate the publication bias of T-cell subgroups. The analysis was performed using Review Manager Version 5.0.

Survival

The patients in the CIK group had significantly prolonged MST compared with those in the non-CIK group (95%CI −7.45 to −0.66, $p = 0.02$) (Table 3). The results of the pooled analysis showed that the CIK arm significantly extended overall survival at the end of follow-up, compared with the non-CIK group (Table 4). Three subgroups of patients of the CIK cell-based therapy group at 1-year survival, 2-year survival, and 3-year survival presented significant survival benefits compared to the patients in the non-CIK group (OR 0.64, 95%CI 0.46–0.91, $p = 0.01$; OR 0.36, 95%CI 0.22–0.59, $p<0.0001$; OR 0.37, 95%CI 0.20–0.70, $p = 0.002$, respectively), which was consistent with the overall survival (OR 0.50, 95%CI 0.39–0.64, $p<0.0001$). Based on the results of our analysis, the short-term survival subgroup showed a significant difference at the 1-year and 2-year survivals. The 1-year survival for the 282 patients in the CIK group was 56%, whereas a slightly lower 1-year survival rate was found for the non-CIK group (45% of 278 patients). A significant difference was also demonstrated in the 2-year survival group, which was 43.22% for 236 patients in the CIK group and 27.47% of 233 patients without the CIK cell treatment. The long-term survival rates in the CIK group showed a slight decrease compared with the short-term survival rate; however, a significant difference in the long-term survival rates was found compared to the non-CIK group ($p = 0.002$).

Concerning the median PFS, the CIK group did not produce any significant improvement compared with the corresponding control groups (95%CI −13.27 to 3.89, $p = 0.28$), whereas the median TTP clearly prolonged the median time to disease progression in the CIK group (95%CI −2.70 to −0.47, $p = 0.005$) (Table 3).

Response rate

The CIK cell-based therapy group showed favorable results when subjected to both analysis of the ORR (OR 0.58, 95%CI 0.44–0.78, $p = 0.00003$) and the DCR (OR 0.41, 95%CI 0.29–0.58, $p<0.0001$), compared with the corresponding control arms. With no significant heterogeneity, a fixed-effect model was used in the ORR and DCR analyses (Table 4). Cochran's Q test resulted in a statistically significant P-value, and the corresponding quantity for I^2 was 0% for both groups, indicating that there was no evidence of heterogeneity among the individual studies.

Immunological assessment of T-cell subgroups

When heterogeneity was observed in the T-cell subgroups, a random-effects model was applied for the overall and subgroup analysis of T-cell immunological assessments (Table 5). The results demonstrated a substantially increased ratio of CD3$^+$ (MD 8.21, 95%CI 5.79–10.64, $p<0.00001$), CD4$^+$ (MD 5.59, 95%CI 4.10–7.07, $p<0.00001$), CD4$^+$CD8$^+$ (MD 0.49, 95%CI 0.37–0.61, $p<0.00001$), CD3$^+$CD56$^+$ (MD 7.80, 95%CI 2.61–12.98, $p = 0.003$) and NK cells (CD3$^-$CD16$^+$CD56$^+$) (MD 6.21, 95%CI 2.25–10.17, $p = 0.002$), whereas the ratio of CD3$^+$CD8$^+$ (MD 2.55, 95%CI −2.46 to 7.56, $p = 0.32$) generated no statistical improvement after CIK treatment. In addition, the pooled analysis showed a significant decrease in the percentage of CD8$^+$ (MD −2.75, 95%CI −3.88 to −1.63, $p<0.00001$) and Treg (CD4$^+$CD25$^+$CD127$^-$) (MD −1.26, 95%CI −1.94 to −0.58,

Table 2. Clinical information from the eligible trials in the meta-analysis.

Trials	Age	No. of pts	Operative method	Tumor Stage	CIK regimens	CIK culture	DC modification
Li 2009 [17]	40–80; (M61)	42;42	Chemo; Chemo+DC-CIK	I-IIIA	1.3×10^9/course, 4 treatments at intervals of a month	X-Vivo 20, IL-1α, IL-2, IFN-γ, CD3	ATL (100 µg/ml)
Li 2012 [30]	UK	37; 37	Chemo; Chemo+ CIK	III-IV	13×10^9/course, twice in a cycle, at least 3 cycles	X-Vivo 20,IL-1α, IL-2, IFN-γ, CD3	NO DC
Mo 2010 [18]	39–77; (M60)	20;21	Chemo; Chemo+ DC-CIK	IV	2–6×10^6/course, 6 times every second day	RPMI1640, IL-1α, IL-2, IFN-γ, CD3mAb	NI-DC
Peng 2012 [19]	65–79; (M71)	23; 24	Chemo; Chemo+ DC-CIK	III-IV	1×10^{10}–2×10^{12}/course, 2–3 times a week, 7 days intervals for 4 cycles	CM, IL-1α, IL-2, IFN-γ, CD3	NI-DC
Sheng 2011 [20]	35–65; (M54)	33; 32	Chemo; Chemo+ DC-CIK	III-IV	5×10^9/course, 4 treatments in a week for 2 weeks	RPMI1640, IL-1α, IL-2, IFN-γ, CD3	NI-DC
Shi 2012 [21]	UK	30; 30	Chemo; Chemo+ DC-CIK	III-IV	5 times every second day	RPMI1640, IL-1, IL-2, CD3	NI-DC
Wang 2013 [39]	UK	11; 11	CK; CK+ CIK	AS	2×10^{10}/course, 2 courses in 2 months	UK	No DC
Wu 2008 [6]	38–78; (M60)	30; 29	Chemo; Chemo+ CIK	III-IV	1×10^9/course, 5 times every second day	RPMI1640, IL-1α, IL-2, IFN-γ, CD3	No DC
Xu 2010 [31]	47–75; (M59.6)	40; 38	Chemo; Chemo+ DC-CIK	III-IV	1.6×10^9/course, 2 times a week in next following 4–5 weeks	RPMI1640, IL-2, IFN-γ, CD3	NI-DC
Xu 2011 [32]	45–73; (M59)	40; 45	Chemo; Chemo+ DC-CIK	III	1.3×10^9/course, 2 times a week in 5–6 weeks	RPMI1640, IL-2, IFN-γ, CD3	NI-DC
Yang 2012 [33]	28–82; (M63.5)	61; 61	Chemo; Chemo + DC-CIK	III-IV	1.2×10^9/course, 30day intervals for 4 cycles	X-vivo 20, IFN-γ,IL-1α,IL-2,CD3McAb	ATL (100 µg/ml)
You 2012 [34]	M 52	50; 55	Chemo; Chemo+ DC-CIK	III-IV	5×10^9/course, 4 times a cycle, 2–6 cycles	RPMI1640, IL-1α, IL-2, IFN-γ, CD3mAb	NI-DC
Yuan 2011 [35]	M 66	32; 32	Chemo; Chemo+ DC-CIK	AS	4 times a cycle	Unknown	NI-DC
Zhang 2012 [36]	35–72; (M57)	50; 50	Chemo; Chemo+ DC-CIK	III-IV	28day intervals for 2 cycles	GT-T551,IL-2, IFN-γ, CD3	NI-DC
Zheng 2012 [38]	M 59	36; 36	γK; γK +CIK	III	1×10^{10}/course, 1 month intervals for 2 cycles	RPMI1640, IL-1α, IL-2,IFN-γ, CD3mAb	No DC
Zhong 2008 [37]	M 53.6	44; 22	Chemo; Chemo+ DC-CIK	IB	2 times in 4 days	UK	CEA PI-DC
Zhong 2011 [22]	40–65	14; 14	Chemo; Chemo+ DC-CIK	IIIB- IV	1–1.7×10^9/course,30day intervals for 4 cycles	CM, IFN-γ, IL-2,CD3McAb	CEA, PI-DC (10 µg/ml)

M: median; UK: unknown; AS: advanced stage; Chemo: chemotherapy; CK: cyberknife; γK: γ-knife; NI-DC: non-impulsed DC; ATL: Autologous tumor lysate; PI-DC: peptide impulse DC; Pts: Patients. The selective data include the authors' names, year of publication, trial period, sample size per arm, regimen used, median or mean age of patients, cell preparation, CIK-based therapy treatment and information pertaining to the study design.

Table 3. Comparison of MTTP, MST, and MPFS between the non-CIK and CIK groups.

Event	No. of Trials [Ref]	No. of pts Non-CIK	CIK	Mean Difference	95% CI	P value	Heterogeneity (I²)
MTTP	4 [6,21,31,36]	97	100	−1.59	−2.70 to −0.47	0.005	0%
MST	4 [6,31,32,37]	154	134	−4.06	−7.45to −0.66	0.02	0%
MPFS	3 [21,30,37]	161	139	−4.69	−13.27to 3.89	0.28	56%

MTTP: median time to progression; MST: median survival time; MPFS: median progression-free survival; Pts: patients; 95%CI: 95% confidence interval; significant difference: P value <0.05.

Table 4. Comparison of OS, ORR and DCR between the non-CIK and CIK groups.

Event	No. of Trials [Ref]	No. pts of Non-CIK	CIK	Odds Ratio (OR)95% CI		P value	Heterogeneity (I²)
1 yr OS	8 [6,18,19,22,31,32,33,36]	278	282	0.64	0.46 to 0.91	0.01	0%
2 yr OS	6 [6,17,18,31–33]	233	236	0.36	0.22 to 0.59	<0.0001	0%
3 yrOS	4 [17,20,31,37]	154	136	0.37	0.20 to 0.70	0.002	13%
ORR	11 [6,18–20,31–36,38]	401	410	0.58	0.44 to 0.78	0.0003	0%
DCR	10 [6,18–20,31–34,36,38]	369	378	0.41	0.29 to 0.58	<0.00001	0%

Forest plot comparing the 1-, 2- and 3-year OS between the non-CIK and CIK groups.OR, odds ratio; OS, overall survival. Due to the low heterogeneity detected, the fixed-effect model was used in this OS meta-analysis. Comparison of the ORR and the DCR between the non-CIK group and CIK group. OR, odds ratio; ORR, objective response rate; DCR, disease control rate. Due to the lack of heterogeneity, the fixed-effect model was used. OS: overall survival; ORR: objective response rate; DCR: disease control rate.

Table 5. Comparison of $CD3^+$, $CD4^+$, $CD3^+CD8^+$, $CD4^+CD8^+$, $CD3^+CD56^+$, NK, $CD8^+$ and Treg before CIK treatment and after CIK therapy.

Event	No. of Trials [Ref]	No. of pts Before-CIK CIK	Mean Difference	95% CI	P value	Heterogeneity (I^2)
CD3+	9 [6,17,20,21,31–33,35,36]	359	8.21	5.79 to 10.64	<0.00001	67%
CD4+	5 [6,21,31,32,35]	174	5.59	4.10 to 7.07	<0.0001	0%
CD3+CD8+	4 [17,18,33,36]	174	2.55	-2.46 to 7.56	0.32	89%
CD4+CD8+	4 [6,31,32,35]	144	0.49	0.37 to 0.61	<0.00001	53%
CD3+CD56+	6 [6,18,19,30,36,38]	222	7.80	2.61 to 12.98	0.003	99%
NK	4 [6,21,32,36]	154	6.21	2.25 to 10.17	0.002	90%
CD8+	5 [6,21,31,32,35]	174	-2.75	-3.88 to -1.63	<0.00001	0%
Treg	3 [17,33,36]	153	-1.26	-1.94 to -0.58	0.0003	58%

Forest plot for the comparison of T-cell subgroups, before and after treatment with the CIK cell-based therapy. The random-effects meta-analysis model was used in this analysis.

$p = 0.0003$) subgroups after treatment with CIK cell-based therapy.

Immunological assessment of Ag-NORs and CEA expression

Due to the limited data presented in the published papers, only some of the immunological assessments, e.g., Ag-NORs (argyrophilic nucleolar organizer regions), and NSCLC tumor markers, e.g., CEA, were subjected to analysis. Heterogeneity was observed, and a random-effects model was therefore applied for the analysis of the subgroups and the overall analysis. The analysis showed that the CIK group significantly improved the patients' T lymphocyte immune activity, showing better Ag-NORs (MD -0.71, 95%CI -0.94 to -0.47, $p = 0.00001$) compared with the non-CIK therapy group (Table 6). The CEA expression level in the analysis was based on two trials [38,39]. The plasma CEA was markedly decreased in the CIK group compared to the non-CIK group (MD 3.96, 95%CI 1.64–6.28, $p = 0.0008$) (Table 6).

Toxicity and adverse reactions

The patients in the CIK group observed fewer severe side effects from chemotherapy, such as fewer cases of grade III and IV leucopenia, gastrointestinal adverse reactions, anemia and liver dysfunction (Figure 3). Without significant heterogeneity, a fixed-effect model (Mantel-Haenszel method) was used for the side effect analysis.

After CIK cell transfusion, most of the patients developed a slight fever, between 37.5 and 39 degrees, but the patients recovered within a few days without severe side effects. Four types of serious chemotherapy side effects could lead to toxic reactions in both groups of patients. The pooled analysis showed that the adverse effects of gastrointestinal adverse reactions (OR 1.77, 95%CI 1.20–2.59, $p = 0.004$) and anemia (OR 2.80, 95%CI 1.37–5.73, $p = 0.005$) generated a significant difference, with fewer episodes in the CIK group. Leucopenia and liver dysfunction were observed less frequently in the patients receiving the CIK treatment, but neither set of data displayed a significant difference compared with the non-CIK group (OR 1.59, 95% CI 0.93–2.72, $p = 0.09$; OR 1.11, 95%CI 0.60–2.06, $p = 0.73$).

Discussion

Immunotherapy has benefited from an increased understanding of tumor immunology and genetics. A number of studies have confirmed that immunotherapy is a safe and feasible treatment option for cancer patients [12–16]. Therefore, conventional therapy combined with adoptive cell immunotherapy is associated with a favorable prognosis compared to chemotherapy alone [18]. Our analysis was designed to elucidate the effects of CIK cell therapy on improving the therapeutic efficacy and safe treatment of NSCLC patients based on a variety of evaluation indexes, including clinical survival outcomes, clinical response rates, immunophenotypes and adverse effects.

In our study, 17 trials were selected for the analysis of the culture of CIK cells and treatment regimens. Most of the trials collected 50–100 ml of autologous peripheral blood and separated the mononuclear cells for further induction. Some of the necessary cytokines were supplied to the cultures of CIK cells, such as IL-2, IFN-γ, and CD3mAb, in 1640 or serum-free medium. Based on our study, most of the treatments with repetitive infusions of 1×10^9 to 2×10^{12} CIK cells were administered for at least 2 weeks on every second day for a minimum of two treatment cycles. However, the different doses and cycles of CIK cell transfusions may lead to different outcomes and immune responses.

Table 6. Comparison of the immunological assessment of Ag-NORs and CEA expression between the CIK and non-CIK group.

Event	No. of Trials [Ref]	No. of pts Non-CIK	CIK	Mean Difference	95% CI	P value	Heterogeneity (I^2)
Ag-NORs	2 [20,38]	69	68	−0.71	−0.94 to −0.47	0.00001	33%
CEA	2 [38,39]	47	47	3.96	1.64–6.28	0.0008	0%

Summary of the significant points in the Ag-NORs and CEA expression level between the CIK group and the non-CIK group with meta-analysis. The random-effects model was used for the calculations. Ag-NORs: argyrophilic nucleolar organizer regions; CEA: carcinoembryonic antigen; Pts: patients; 95%CI: 95% confidence interval; significant difference: P value <0.05.

In the present study, the CIK cell-based therapy group was associated with favorable results based on an evaluation of both the overall survival and clinical responses (Table 4). The 1-year survival (OR 0.64, 95%CI 0.46–0.91, $p = 0.01$), 2-year survival (OR 0.36, 95%CI 0.22–0.59, $p<0.0001$), and 3-year survival (OR 0.37, 95%CI 0.20–0.70, $p = 0.002$) showed significantly prolonged durations in the CIK cell therapy group. A favorable DCR and ORR were also observed in patients receiving CIK cell therapy ($p<0.0001$). The MTTP and MST also showed significant improvements in the CIK group ($p = 0.005$, $p = 0.02$). CIK cells, which are also known as NKT cells, exhibit both the cytotoxicity activities of T-lymphocytes and the restrictive tumor-killing activity by non-MHC of NK cells, among which the main effectors are $CD3^+CD56^+$ cells [7]. In total, 4 of 17 trials used DCs pulsed with lung cancer antigens or tumor lysate, whereas 9 trials used mature DCs co-cultured with CIK cells (Table 2). DCs possess antigen-presenting activities on the extracellular surface and are able to activate the proliferation of T cells and CIK cells. Therefore, considering the poor immunogenicity of NSCLC, CIK infusion with an immunoadjuvant or tumor-specific antigen pulsed DCs boosted the immune responses [24]. Therefore, CIK cell-based therapy even acting through completely different mechanisms for fighting cancer cells, can lead to an improvement in the clinical objective responses based on the assessment of traditional RECIST criteria [40].

The human immune response against cancer cells is mainly dependent on cellular immunity. Previous studies have found that the numerical ratios of T-lymphocyte subsets in the peripheral blood are disordered in tumor patients [17]. In the present study, we observed a substantially increased percentage of $CD3^+$ and $CD4^+$ ($p<0.001$), the ratio of $CD4^+CD8^+$ and $CD3^+CD56^+$ ($p<0.001$) and NK cells ($p = 0.002$), but a significant decrease in the percentage of the $CD8^+$ ($p<0.001$) and Treg ($p = 0.0003$) subgroups after DC-CIK treatment by meta-analysis. Many studies have demonstrated that CIK cells possess strong cytotoxicity against a variety of T-lymphocyte populations, among which $CD3^+CD56^+$ is mainly responsible for the MHC unrestricted antitumor activity [8]. In addition, the number of $CD4^+$ and $CD8^+$ T-cells plays an important role in affecting clinical outcomes in NSCLC. The activation of $CD4^+$ T cells contributes to the secretion of immune regulatory cytokines, including IL-2, IL-12, and IFN-γ, which in turn facilitate an elevation in the cytolytic $CD8^+$ T cell responses, thereby inducing tumor cell death [25]. The activation of $CD4^+$ T cells also enhances the killing activity of NK cells and the phagocytic activity of macrophages, triggering a humoral immune response that leads to antibody production, thus $CD4^+$ and $CD8^+$ have a synergistic relationship in immune responses. Our meta-analysis demonstrated that $CD3^+$, $CD4^+$, $CD4^+CD8^+$, $CD3^+CD56^+$ and NK cells were increased after DC-CIK treatment, therefore suggesting the improvement of immune function after immunotherapy in the NSCLC patients.

In addition, we should note that $CD8^+$ T cells were not significantly increased after the immunotherapy, which also showed the varied immunophenotypes compared with the results of other T-cell assessments by the CIK treatment in different solid carcinomas [11–13]. Naïve $CD4^+$ T lymphocytes undergo cell differentiation in the presence of antigen, co-stimulatory molecules and cytokines, and these cells can be divided into several major groups: Th1, Th2 and Treg cells [26]. Th1 helper cells are the host immunity effectors against intracellular bacteria and protozoa. These are triggered by IL-12, IL-2 and the effector cytokine IFN-γ. The main effector cells of Th1 immunity are macrophages, CD8 T cells, IgG B cells, and CD4 T cells. Th2 helper cells are the host immunity effectors against multicellular helminthes [26]. The

Study or Subgroup	Non-CIK Events	Total	CIK Events	Total	Weight	Odds Ratio M-H, Fixed, 95% CI	Odds Ratio M-H, Fixed, 95% CI
4.1.1 Leucopenia							
Xu 2010	32	40	31	38	5.5%	0.90 [0.29, 2.79]	
Xu 2011	33	40	36	45	5.2%	1.18 [0.39, 3.52]	
Zheng 2012	28	36	20	36	3.9%	2.80 [1.01, 7.80]	
Zhong 2008	10	44	4	22	3.6%	1.32 [0.36, 4.82]	
Zhong 2011	13	14	10	14	0.6%	5.20 [0.50, 54.05]	
Subtotal (95% CI)		**174**		**155**	**18.8%**	**1.59 [0.93, 2.72]**	
Total events	116		101				
Heterogeneity: Chi² = 3.49, df = 4 (P = 0.48); I² = 0%							
Test for overall effect: Z = 1.70 (P = 0.09)							
4.1.2 Gastrointestinal adverse reaction							
Peng 2012	5	23	2	24	1.3%	3.06 [0.53, 17.66]	
Xu 2010	30	40	29	38	6.5%	0.93 [0.33, 2.62]	
Xu 2011	32	40	37	45	6.1%	0.86 [0.29, 2.57]	
You 2012	15	50	13	55	7.5%	1.38 [0.58, 3.30]	
Zhang 2012	27	50	16	50	6.4%	2.49 [1.11, 5.63]	
Zheng 2012	19	36	10	36	4.1%	2.91 [1.09, 7.74]	
Zhong 2008	6	44	2	22	2.0%	1.58 [0.29, 8.55]	
Zhong 2011	13	14	9	14	0.6%	7.22 [0.72, 72.70]	
Subtotal (95% CI)		**297**		**284**	**34.5%**	**1.77 [1.20, 2.59]**	
Total events	147		118				
Heterogeneity: Chi² = 6.93, df = 7 (P = 0.44); I² = 0%							
Test for overall effect: Z = 2.90 (P = 0.004)							
4.1.3 Anemia							
Zhang 2012	36	50	22	50	5.4%	3.27 [1.42, 7.52]	
Zhong 2008	1	44	0	22	0.6%	1.55 [0.06, 39.65]	
Zhong 2011	6	14	4	14	2.0%	1.88 [0.39, 9.01]	
Subtotal (95% CI)		**108**		**86**	**7.9%**	**2.80 [1.37, 5.73]**	
Total events	43		26				
Heterogeneity: Chi² = 0.51, df = 2 (P = 0.77); I² = 0%							
Test for overall effect: Z = 2.81 (P = 0.005)							
4.1.4 Liver dysfunction							
You 2012	26	50	20	55	8.0%	1.90 [0.87, 4.14]	
Zhang 2012	4	50	3	50	2.4%	1.36 [0.29, 6.43]	
Zhong 2011	1	14	8	14	6.5%	0.06 [0.01, 0.57]	
Subtotal (95% CI)		**114**		**119**	**16.8%**	**1.11 [0.60, 2.06]**	
Total events	31		31				
Heterogeneity: Chi² = 8.25, df = 2 (P = 0.02); I² = 76%							
Test for overall effect: Z = 0.34 (P = 0.73)							
4.1.5 No-infection fever							
Peng 2012	0	23	7	24	6.3%	0.05 [0.00, 0.93]	
Shi 2012	0	30	4	30	3.9%	0.10 [0.00, 1.88]	
Zhong 2008	0	44	4	22	5.1%	0.05 [0.00, 0.90]	
Zhong 2011	3	14	10	14	6.8%	0.11 [0.02, 0.61]	
Subtotal (95% CI)		**111**		**90**	**22.1%**	**0.08 [0.02, 0.26]**	
Total events	3		25				
Heterogeneity: Chi² = 0.39, df = 3 (P = 0.94); I² = 0%							
Test for overall effect: Z = 4.15 (P < 0.0001)							
Total (95% CI)		**804**		**734**	**100.0%**	**1.33 [1.05, 1.70]**	
Total events	340		301				
Heterogeneity: Chi² = 46.08, df = 22 (P = 0.002); I² = 52%							
Test for overall effect: Z = 2.33 (P = 0.02)							
Test for subgroup differences: Not applicable							

0.02   0.1   1   10   50
Favours CIK   Favours Non-CIK

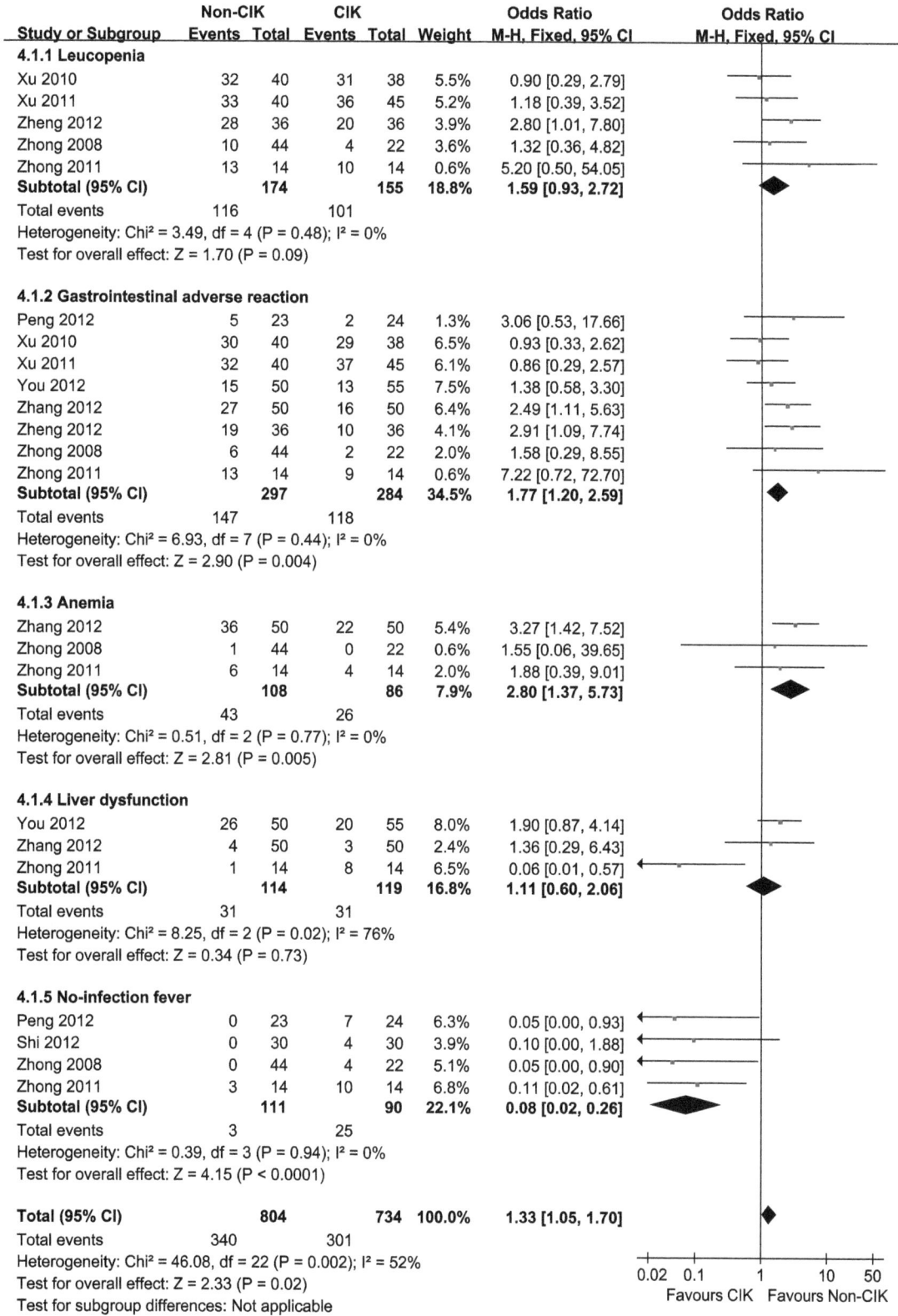

Figure 3. Forest plot comparing the toxicity and no treatment-related side effects between the CIK group and the non-CIK group.
Some serious adverse effects were observed significantly less frequently in the CIK group. Due to the lack of heterogeneity, the fixed-effect model was used.

main effector cells are eosinophils, basophils, and mast cells, as well as IgE B cells and IL-4/IL-5 CD4 T cells [27]. T regulatory cells express FoxP3 and produce TGF-β and $CD4^+CD25^+CD127^-$ T subgroups to suppress immune responses against Th1 and Th2. In addition, tumor cells also express high levels of $CD4^+CD25^+$ Treg cells, which help direct immunosuppressive cytokines to the tumor microenvironment [28], so the decrease of the Treg cell may be helpful to remove the immunosuppressive effect for NSCLC patients, and our results also demonstrated a lower number of Treg cells. Higher proportions of Treg and proliferating $CD8^+$ T cells were both associated with poor survival in malignancies lung cancer [41], suggesting that DC-CIK immunotherapy may play a role in enhancing the immune function of NSCLC patients.

Immunotherapy exerts its effect on the cellular immune response and requires time for immune cytokines to change the tumor burden or survival time. In our present study, we also evaluated T lymphocyte immune activity by Ag-NORs *in vivo* and the NSCLC tumor marker CEA. The significant increase in Ag-NORs ($p = 0.00001$) and the reduction in the CEA content ($p = 0.0008$) observed in the CIK group contributed to the prevention of short-term recurrence and improvement of clinical responses. We also analyzed clinical survival outcomes, clinical response rates, immunophenotypes and tumor markers, and we hypothesized that the CIK cells fight with tumor cells in several different ways, including direct cellular interactions (Fas/FasL pathway, granzyme B), the secretion of cytokines (IFN-γ, TNF-α, IL-2) and antibodies, and immune response regulations (T-lymphocyte variations) [29]. In all, our meta-analysis evaluated a variety of T-cell subgroups, and the differences in the cytokines used for immunotherapy, and we found that the results were consistent with the clinical therapeutic outcomes, such as the overall survival and clinical response.

In our analysis, CIK cell-based therapy yielded a disappointing result in non-infective fever (P<0.0001), and no other major side effect was observed. The pooled analysis showed that the adverse effects of gastrointestinal adverse reactions ($p = 0.004$) and anemia ($p = 0.005$) generated significant differences with fewer episodes in the CIK group. Thus, CIK cell immunotherapy with chemotherapy has proven to be a feasible and effective method for the treatment of NSCLC without severe side effects.

Limitation of the study

The 17 trials included in this meta-analysis were selected with an RCT to improve statistical reliability. To avoid bias in the identification and selection of trials, we minimized the possibility of overlooking published papers to the greatest extent. Although we selected using RCT as much as possible, there are some major criteria that did not receive a good grade under the Jadad scale, such as allocation concealment and intention-to-treat, meaning our study may have a moderate risk of bias. We also used a funnel plot to evaluate the publication bias. In our analysis, overall survival, clinical response rate, and side effects suffered low published bias; however, immunological assessment and T cell subgroups observed a high published bias. Therefore, there are some limitations to our study. First, CIK cell-based therapy is a greater concern for Chinese scholars; therefore, all 17 selected trials were from Asia, because there is a global lack of any multinational large-sample multicenter clinic research regarding CIK cell therapy for NSCLC. Second, some of the papers had to be excluded due to the lack of a control arm during the experimental design; however, some of the papers produced even better prognosis after the CIK treatment. Third, our analyzed data were selected from published papers rather than drawn first-hand

from patient records, potentially causing an overestimation of the analytical results. Therefore, only the enrollment of a larger sample could minimize this bias. However, various crucial issues for CIK cell-based immunotherapy need to be conquered before it can be approved as a standard treatment for NSCLC tumors due to several obstacles. First, the different dosage and treatment regimens of CIK cell transfusions may lead to different outcomes and immune responses. Second, although most of our selected papers focused on therapeutic outcomes based on chemotherapy RECIST criteria, due to the different tumor killing mechanisms, a novel immune-related response criterion (irRC) should also be used for the assessment of immunotherapy clinical activities [40]. Third, due to the poor immunogenicity of NSCLC, optimizing DC modifications combined with CIK cell infusion may contribute to more favorable clinical outcomes in NSCLC patients.

Taken together, the CIK-combined therapy for NSCLC presented a significantly prolonged overall survival, an improved clinical response rate, a strengthened immune system, and low rates of adverse side effects. The CIK therapy is more concerned with reducing the tumor burden stage than curing cancer. The CIK adoptive immune therapy showed potential regarding improved clinical outcomes, and there is increasing evidence that the CIK therapy treatment of NSCLC evokes specific humoral and cellular antitumor immune responses. However, the timing of the immunotherapy, dosage, regimens and efficient tumor antigens still require further research.

Conclusion

In total, 17 randomized controlled trials of NSCLC with 1172 patients were included in the present analysis. Combined CIK cell therapy for the treatment of NSCLC demonstrated significant superiority in terms of overall survival and objective response compared with the non-CIK group. The T-lymphocyte subgroups also seemed to favorably affect the immune system after chemotherapy. The data also indicated that CIK therapy relieves the side effects of chemotherapy without causing any additional major side effects aside from non-infective fever. This analysis supports a further larger-scale meta-analysis for the evaluation of the efficacy of CIK adoptive cell therapy for the treatment of NSCLC in the future.

Acknowledgments

This research work was supported by the National Natural Science Foundation of China (No. 31171427 and 30971651 to Zheng-Xu Wang), Beijing Municipal Science and Technology Project for Clinical Characteristics and Application Research of Capital (No. Z121107001012136 to Zheng-Xu Wang); the National Natural Science Foundation of China (No. 30700974 to Jun-Xia Cao) and the Postdoctoral Foundation of China (No. 20060400775 to Jun-Xia Cao).

Author Contributions

Conceived and designed the experiments: ZXW. Performed the experiments: MW JXC. Analyzed the data: MW JXC BLX XYZ J. Li J. Liu HBW. Contributed reagents/materials/analysis tools: JHP YSL DL. Wrote the paper: MW JXC.

References

1. Parkin DM, Bray F, Ferlay J, Pisani P (2005) Global cancer statistics. CA Cancer J Clin 55: 74–108.
2. Chen WQ, Zheng RS, Zhang SW, Zhao P, Li GG, et al. (2013) Chinese cancer registration annual report: National cancer registration center of lung cancer. Chin J Cancer Res 25(1): 10–21.
3. Arango BA, Castrellon AB, Santos ES, Raez LE (2009) Second-line therapy for non-small-cell lung cancer. Clin Lung Cancer 10(2): 91–98.
4. National Institutes of Health (2012) Cancer of the Lung and Bronchus-SEER Stat Facts Sheet. http://seer.cancer.gov/statfacts/htm/lungb.html.
5. Jiang J, Liang X, Zhou X, Huang R, Chu Z, et al. (2013) Non-platinum doublets were as effective as platinum-based doublets for chemotherapy-naïve advanced non-small-cell lung cancer in the era of third-generation agents. J Cancer Res Clin Oncol 139(1): 25–38.
6. Wu C, Jiang J, Shi L, Xu N (2008) Prospective study of chemotherapy in combination with cytokine-induced killer cells in patients suffering from advanced non-small cell lung cancer. Anticancer Res 28(6B): 3997–4002.
7. Choi D, Kim TG, Sung YC (2012) The past, present, and future of adoptive T cell therapy. Immune Netw 12(4): 139–147.
8. Sangiolo D (2011) Cytokine induced killer cells as promising immunotherapy for solid tumors. J Cancer 2: 363–368.
9. Rutella S, Iudicone P, Bonanno G, Fioravanti D, Procoli A, et al. (2012) Adoptive immunotherapy with cytokine-induced killer cells is generated with a new good manufacturing practice-grade protocol. Cytotherapy 14(7): 841–850.
10. Schmidt-Wolf IG, Finke S, Trojaneck B, Denkena A, Lefterova P, et al. (1999) Phase I clinical study applying autologous immunological effector cells transfected with the interleukin-2 gene in patients with metastatic renal cancer, colorectal cancer and lymphoma. Br J Cancer 81: 1009–1016.
11. Ma Y, Zhang Z, Tang L, Xu YC, Xie ZM, et al. (2012) Cytokine-induced killer cells in the treatment of patients with solid carcinomas: a systematic review and pooled analysis. Cytotherapy 14(4): 483–493.
12. Hontscha C, Borck Y, Zhou H, Messmer D, Schmidt-Wolf IG (2011) Clinical trials on CIK cells: first report of the international registry on CIK cells (IRCC). J Cancer Res Clin Oncol 137(2): 305–310.
13. Li XD, Xu B, Wu J, Ji M, Xu BH, et al. (2012) Review of Chinese clinical trials on CIK cell treatment for malignancies. Clin Transl Oncol 14(2): 102–108.
14. Jäkel CE, Hauser S, Rogenhofer S, Müller SC, Brossart P, et al. (2012) Clinical studies applying cytokine induced killer cells for the treatment of renal cell carcinoma. Clin Dev Immunol 2012: 473245.
15. Ma Y, Xu YC, Tang L, Zhang Z, Wang J, et al. (2011) Cytokine-induced killer (CIK) cell therapy for patients with hepatocellular carcinoma: efficacy and safety. Exp Hematol Oncol 1(1): 11.
16. Wang ZX, Cao JX, Liu ZP, Cui YX, Li CY, et al. (2014) Combination of chemotherapy and immunotherapy for colon cancer in China: A meta-analysis. World J Gastroenterol 20(4): 1095–1106.
17. Li H, Wang C, Yu J, Cao S, Wei F, et al. (2009) Dendritic cell-activated cytokine-induced killer cells enhance the anti-tumor effect of chemotherapy on non-small cell lung cancer in patients after surgery. Cytotherapy 11(8): 1076–1083.
18. Mo C, Gao J, Wang J, Huang Y, Wu X, et al. (2005) Clinical efficacy of DC-activated and cytokine-induced killer cells combined with chemotherapy in treatment of advanced lung cancer. Chinese J Cancer Biotherapy 17(4): 419–423. doi: 10. 3872/j. issn. 1007-385X. 2010. 04. 011.
19. Peng D, Li J, Yuan J, Liu Y, Yu W, et al. (2012) Efficacy and safety of autologous DC and CIK cells cominedPemetrexed in the treatment of elderly patients with non-small cell lung cancer. Chinese J Immunol 28(7): 648–652. doi: 10.3969/j.issn.1000-484X.2012. 07.017.
20. Sheng CH, Bao F, Xu S, Chang CY (2011) Clinical research on chemotherapy combined with dendritic cell-cytokine induced killer cells for non-small cell lung cancer. Journal of Practical Oncology 26(5): 503–506.
21. Shi SB, Ma TH, Li CH, Tang XY (2011) Effect of maintenance therapy with dendritic cells: cytokine-induced killer cells in patients with advanced non-small cell lung cancer. Tumori 98(3): 314–319.
22. Zhong R, Teng J, Han B, Zhong H (2011) Dendritic cells combining with cytokine-induced killer cells synergize chemotherapy in patients with late-stage non-small cell lung cancer. Cancer Immunol Immunother 60(10): 1497–1502.
23. Jadad AR, Moore RA, Carroll D, Jenkinson C, Reynolds DJ, et al. (1996) Assessing the quality of reports of randomized clinical trials: Is blinding necessary? Control Clin Trials 17: 1–12.
24. Shepherd FA, Douillard JY, Blumenschein GR Jr (2011) Immunotherapy for non-small cell lung cancer: novel approaches to improve patient outcome. J Thorac Oncol 6(10): 1763–1773.
25. Arens R, Schoenberger SP (2010) Plasticity in programming of effector and memory CD8 T-cell formation. Immunological Reviews 235: 190–205.
26. Mucida D, Cheroutre H (2010) The many face-lifts of CD4 T helper cells. Advances in Immunology 107: 139–152.
27. Neurath MF, Finotto S, Glimcher LH (2002) The role of Th1/Th2 polarization in mucosal immunity. Nature Medicine 8: 567–573.
28. Gallimore A, Godkin A (2008) Regulatory T cells and tumor immunity observations in mice and men. Immunology 123: 157–163.
29. Yu J, Zhang W, Jiang H, Li H, Cao S, et al. (2008) CD4+T cells in CIKs (CD4+ CIKs) reversed resistance to fas-mediated apoptosis through CD40/CD40L ligation rather than IFN-gamma stimulation. Cancer Biother Radio pharm 23(3): 342–354.
30. Li R, Wang C, Liu L, Du C, Cao S, et al. (2012) Autologous cytokine-induced killer cell immunotherapy in lung cancer: a phase II clinical study. Cancer Immunol Immunother 61(11): 2125–2133.
31. Xu Y, Xu D, Zhang N, Chen F, Liu J (2011) Observation of Chemotherapy Combined with Cytokine-induced Killer Cells and Dendritic Cells in Patients with the Advanced Non-Small Cell Lung Cancer. Prac J Cancer 25(2): 163–166.
32. Xu Y, Xu D, Zhang N, Chen F, Zhang G, et al. (2011) Effection of NP concurrent chemotherapy radiotherapy and sequential adoptive immunity cell for locally advanced non-small cell lung cancer. Chinese J Cancer Prev Treat 18(13): 1032–1035.
33. Yang L, Ren B, Li H, Yu J, Cao S, et al. (2013) Enhanced antitumor effects of DC-activated CIKs to chemotherapy treatment in a single cohort of advanced non-small-cell lung cancer patients. Cancer Immunol Immunother 62(1): 65–73.
34. You Z, Su X, Liu Y (2012) Observation on Clinical Efficacy of DC-CIK Biotherapy Auxiliary Interventional Chemotherapy on Central Non-Small-Cell Lung Carcinoma. Anti-tumor Phar 2(3): 193–196. doi: 10.3969/j.issn.2095-1264.2012.03.010.
35. Yuan J, Peng D, Li J (2011) Clinical effects of administering dendritic cells and cytokine induced killer cells combined with chemotherapy in the treatment of advanced non-small cell lung cancer. J Clin Pulmonary Med 16(12): 1910–1911.
36. Zhang J, Mao G, Han Y, Yang X, Feng H, et al. (2012) The clinical effects of DC-CIK cells combined with chemotherapy in the treatment of advanced NSCLC. Chin Ger J Clin Oncol 11(2): 67–71.
37. Zhong R, Han B, Zhong H, Gong L, Sha H, et al. (2008) Dendritic cells immunotherapy combined with chemotherapy inhibits postoperative recurrence and metastasis in stage IB of NSCLC after radical surgery. China Oncol 18(10): 760–764.
38. Zheng FC, Zhang XY, Feng HZ, Chen J, Sun Y, et al. (2012) Clinical Study of Stereotactic Conformal Body γ-knife Combined with Adoptive Immunotherapy (Dendritic Cell and Cytokine-induced Killer Cell) in the Treatment for Advanced Non-small Cell Lung Cancer. Journal of Chinese Oncology 18(11): 815–818.
39. Wang YY, Wang YS, Liu T, Yang K, Yang GQ, et al. (2013) Efficacy study of Cyber Knife stereotactic radio surgery combined with CIK cell immunotherapy for advanced refractory lung cancer. Exp Ther Med 5(2): 453–456.
40. Wolchok JD, Hoos A, O'Day S, Weber JS, Hamid O, et al. (2009) Guidelines for the evaluation of immune therapy activity in solid tumors: immune-related response criteria. Clin Cancer Res 15: 7412–7420.
41. McCoy MJ, Nowak AK, van der Most RG, Dick IM, Lake RA (2013) Peripheral CD8(+) T cell proliferation is prognostic for patients with advanced thoracic malignancies. Cancer Immunol Immunother 62(3): 529–539.

5

Iron Overload and Apoptosis of HL-1 Cardiomyocytes: Effects of Calcium Channel Blockade

Mei-pian Chen[1], Z. Ioav Cabantchik[2], Shing Chan[1], Godfrey Chi-fung Chan[1]*, Yiu-fai Cheung[1]*

1 Department of Pediatrics and Adolescent Medicine, The University of Hong Kong, Hong Kong, China, 2 Department of Biological Chemistry, Alexander Silberman Institute of Life Sciences, Hebrew University of Jerusalem, Safra Campus at Givat Ram, Jerusalem, Israel

Abstract

Background: Iron overload cardiomyopathy that prevails in some forms of hemosiderosis is caused by excessive deposition of iron into the heart tissue and ensuing damage caused by a raise in labile cell iron. The underlying mechanisms of iron uptake into cardiomyocytes in iron overload condition are still under investigation. Both L-type calcium channels (LTCC) and T-type calcium channels (TTCC) have been proposed to be the main portals of non-transferrinic iron into heart cells, but controversies remain. Here, we investigated the roles of LTCC and TTCC as mediators of cardiac iron overload and cellular damage by using specific Calcium channel blockers as potential suppressors of labile Fe(II) and Fe(III) ingress in cultured cardiomyocytes and ensuing apoptosis.

Methods: Fe(II) and Fe(III) uptake was assessed by exposing HL-1 cardiomyocytes to iron sources and quantitative real-time fluorescence imaging of cytosolic labile iron with the fluorescent iron sensor calcein while iron-induced apoptosis was quantitatively measured by flow cytometry analysis with Annexin V. The role of calcium channels as routes of iron uptake was assessed by cell pretreatment with specific blockers of LTCC and TTCC.

Results: Iron entered HL-1 cardiomyocytes in a time- and dose-dependent manner and induced cardiac apoptosis via mitochondria-mediated caspase-3 dependent pathways. Blockade of LTCC but not of TTCC demonstrably inhibited the uptake of ferric but not of ferrous iron. However, neither channel blocker conferred cardiomyocytes with protection from iron-induced apoptosis.

Conclusion: Our study implicates LTCC as major mediators of Fe(III) uptake into cardiomyocytes exposed to ferric salts but not necessarily as contributors to ensuing apoptosis. Thus, to the extent that apoptosis can be considered a biological indicator of damage, the etiopathology of cardiosiderotic damage that accompanies some forms of hemosiderosis would seem to be unrelated to LTCC or TTCC, but rather to other routes of iron ingress present in heart cells.

Editor: Alexander G. Obukhov, Indiana University School of Medicine, United States of America

Funding: This work was supported by Children's Thalassemia Foundation and Edward Sai Kim Hotung Pediatric Education and Research Fund (http://www.thalassaemia.org.hk). The funders had no role in study design, data collection and analysis, decision to publish, or preparation of the manuscript.

Competing Interests: The authors have declared that no competing interests exist.

* Email: gcfchan@hku.hk (GCFC); xfcheung@hku.hk (YFC)

Introduction

As an essential element for almost all living organisms, iron serves as a critical component in different metabolic processes including oxygen transport and storage, DNA, RNA and protein synthesis, and electron transport [1]. Tight regulation of iron concentrations is required for maintenance of cellular function, while excessive iron leads to generation of oxidative stress by increasing production of reactive oxygen species [2–4]. Of the different organs, the heart is particularly vulnerable to iron toxicity [5].

Iron overload cardiomyopathy (IOC) is well documented in patients with β-thalassemia major and is an important cause of morbidity and mortality [6–9]. Clinical manifestations include systolic and diastolic ventricular dysfunction, cardiac arrhythmias, and end-stage cardiomyopathy [5,8,10,11]. However, the mechanisms of iron-induced subclinical cardiac dysfunction and end-stage cardiomyopathy remain unclear. Progressive loss of cardio-myocytes, albeit at a low level, through apoptosis is believed to contribute to the remodeling process and ventricular dysfunction in heart failure [12–17]. There is, however, a paucity of data on the phenomenon of cardiomyocyte apoptosis and the pathway involved in the setting of iron overload.

Under physiologic condition, iron uptake into cardiomyocytes is mediated through transferrin-transferrin receptor-mediated endocytosis with negative feedback regulatory mechanisms [18]. However, under iron overloading conditions, transferrin becomes saturated and excess plasma iron will present as non-transferrin-bound iron (NTBI), which contributes to the intracellular labile iron pool and the generation of reactive oxygen species [9]. Reported mechanisms of NTBI entry into cardiomyocytes are nonetheless controversial [19]. While some studies have proposed L-type calcium channels (LTCC) to be a major pathway for NTBI entry [20–22], others suggest that T-type calcium channel (TTCC) may be the alternative portal of entry [23,24]. However, direct evidence for possible protective effects of calcium channel blockers against iron-induced cardiomyocyte apoptosis is lacking.

Using HL-1 cardiomyocytes, a spontaneously contracting cardiomyocyte cell line that expresses both LTCC and TTCC molecularly and functionally [25–27], together with the real-time technique tracing cellular iron uptake and flow cytometry, we explored (i) the phenomenon of and mechanisms involved in cardiomyocyte apoptosis induced by iron overload, (ii) the effects of LTCC and TTCC blockers on Fe(II) and Fe(III) entry into cardiomyocytes, and (iii) the potential protective effect on iron-induced cardiomyocyte apoptosis by calcium channel blockade.

Materials and Methods

Cell culture

HL-1 cardiomyocytes were kindly provided by Prof. W.C. Claycomb (Louisiana State University Health Science Center, New Orleans, LA, USA) who created the cell line [25]. HL-1 cells were established from the AT-1 mouse atrial cardiomyocyte tumor, and can be serially passaged while maintaining contractile phenotype. The cells were grown in culture vessels pre-coated with 0.02% gelatin (Difco, Fisher Scientific, Suwanee, GA, USA) - 5 μg/ml fibronectin (Sigma, St Louis, MO, USA) solution at 37°C in a humidified 5% CO_2 incubator, maintained in Claycomb Medium (SAFC Biosciences, Sigma) supplemented with 10% fetal bovine serum (Sigma), 0.1 mM norepinephrine (Sigma), 2 mM L-glutamine (Invitrogen, Life Technologies, Grand Island, NY, USA) and penicillin/streptomycin (100 U/ml:100 μg/ml) (Invitrogen). The medium was changed approximately 5 days per week.

Iron treatment and calcium channel blockade

For calcein green-acetomethoxy (CALG-AM) fluorescent assay, HL-1 cells were seeded at 6×10^4 cells/well in gelatin-fibronectin coated 96-well black CulturPlate (PerkinElmer, Waltham, Massachusetts, USA). Cells reached around 90% confluence after 24 hr culture. L-type calcium channel blockers including amlodipine (Cipla, India) and verapamil (Abbott, Ludwigshafen, Germany) and TTCC blocker, efonidipine (Sigma), were loaded at 0.1, 1, 10, 100 μM in assay buffer, which consisted of HEPES-buffered saline, pH 7.4 (HBS) supplemented with 0.5 mM probenecid (Sigma), 30 min before iron challenge, and the concentrations were maintained during the assay. $FeCl_3$ was loaded at 150, 300, 600 μM with and without 1 mM ascorbic acid in assay buffer, which has been indicated to represent Fe(II) and Fe(III) respectively [24,28,29]. Controls (with and without ascorbate) was defined as the conditions without calcium channel blockers and iron.

For flow cytometric assay, HL-1 cells were seeded at a density of 1.5×10^5 cells/ml in gelatin-fibronectin coated plates. After 24 hr incubation, culture medium was changed into norepinephrine-free medium containing 2% fetal bovine serum, 2 mM L-glutamine and penicillin/streptomycin (100 U/ml:100 μg/ml), and also 150, 300, 600 μM $FeCl_3$ with and without 1 mM ascorbic acid for test groups. Calcium channel blockers were pre-loaded at 1 μM 60 min before iron challenge without media change before treatment endpoint. For treatments with iron chelator deferiprone (Apotex, Toronto, Canada), 10 or 100 μM deferiprone was loaded 20 min after iron loading. Blank controls (with and without ascorbate) was defined as the conditions without calcium channel blockers, chelator and iron loading. After 72 hr of incubation, cells in the control group had confluency at around 90%, while cells in iron treatment groups had less. Cells were gently detached by 0.05% Trypsin-EDTA (Invitrogen) for flow cytometric assays.

CALG-AM fluorescent assay

To trace iron transport in live HL-1 cells, CALG-AM fluorescent assay was used [30]. Non-fluorescent CALG-AM is converted to green-fluorescent calcein once diffuses into live cells, going through acetoxymethyl ester hydrolysis by intracellular esterases. Cells were exposed to 0.25 μM CALG-AM (Molecular Probes, Life Technologies, Grand Island, NY, USA) at 37°C for 30 min in Claycomb Medium containing 10 mM Na-HEPES (Sigma). Cells were then rinsed with HBS, followed by the perfusion of assay buffer, HBS supplemented with 0.5 mM probenecid, which prevented leakage of anionic fluorescent probes from cells. Calcium channel blockers and ascorbic acid were added simultaneously under the conditions mentioned. Fluorescent intensity was measured using fluorescent plate reader Fusion (Packard, Perkin Elmer Life Sciences, Boston, MA, USA) at excitation/emission wavelength 485 nm/520 nm. Local average reading at 10 min after assay buffer loading was set as initial fluorescence level. $FeCl_3$ was loaded at 20 min after the first plate reading (Figure 1A). Calcein was quenched by intracellular labile iron, and hence, the fluorescence intensity was inversely proportional to the level of labile intracellular iron. Iron entry was terminated by adding 100 μM impermeant chelator diethylene-triamine-pentaacetic acid (DTPA) at 115 min after assay buffer loading. Identification of intracellular labile iron was verified by 100 μM permeant iron chelator deferasirox (Exjade, ICL670) at 136 min after assay buffer loading to reverse the calcein-Fe quenching. Control was defined as treatments without addition of calcium channel blockers, iron, DTPA and ICL670. Experiments were performed in triplicate. Each reading at any given time was normalized to the local initial fluorescence level.

Annexin V/PI assay

Fluorescein isothiocyanate (FITC) Annexin V Apoptosis Detection Kit (Becton Dickinson, Franklin Lakes, NJ, USA) was used according to manufacturer's instructions. Briefly, cells from cultures were collected and washed with cold PBS and then resuspended in annexin V binding buffer. After staining with annexin V-FITC and PI for 15 min at room temperature in the dark, cells suspended in annexin V binding buffer were tested by LSR II flow cytometer (Becton Dickinson). For each measurement, at least 10,000 cells were counted. Flow data were analyzed by FlowJo 8.8.4 (Tree Star). Only single cell events were gated out for analysis.

Activated caspase-3 assay

FITC Active Caspase-3 Apoptosis Kit (Becton Dickinson) was used according to manufacturer's instructions. Briefly, cells from culture were collected and washed with cold PBS, then fixed and permeabilized in BD Cytofix/Cytoperm solution for 20 min on ice. After washing with BD Perm/Wash buffer, cells were stained with FITC-conjugated anti- active caspase-3 antibody for 30 min at room temperature. With further wash with Perm/Wash buffer, cells suspended in Perm/Wash buffer were tested by LSR II flow cytometer. Flow cytometry was performed as aforementioned.

JC-1 assay

The mitochondrial membrane potential (Δψ) of HL-1 cardiomyocytes was evaluated by Flow Cytometry Mitochondrial Membrane Potential Detection Kit (Becton Dickinson). JC-1 (5,5′,6,6′-tetrachloro-1,1′,3,3′-tetraethylbenzimidazolcarbocyanine iodide) is a fluorochrome widely used to evaluate the status of Δψ. Mitochondria with normal Δψ increases JC-1 uptake, which leads to the formation of JC-1 aggregates that emit red

A

B

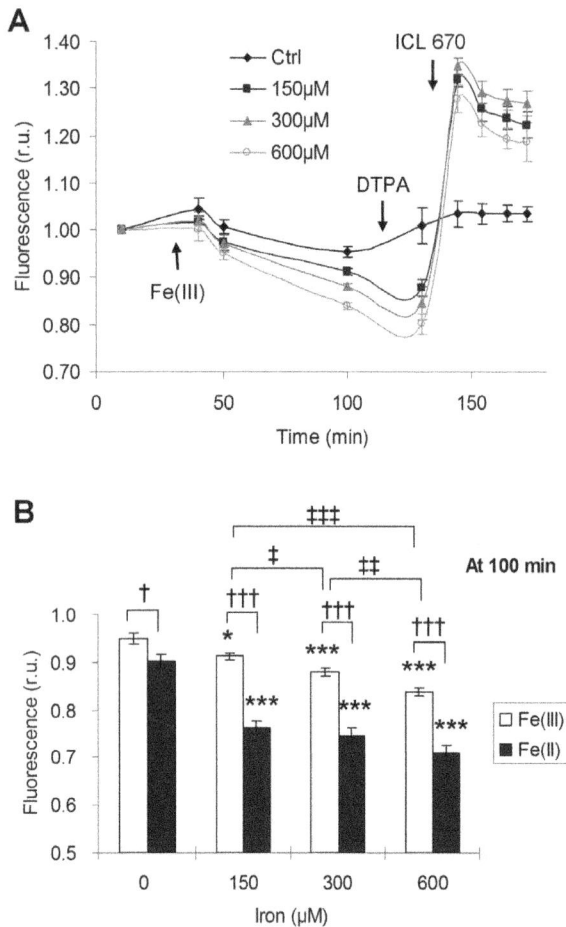

Figure 1. Exogenous iron entered cardiomyocytes in a time- and dose- dependent manner. (A) Fe(III) uptake by live HL-1 cells treated at 3 indicated doses, detected by CALG-AM fluorescent assay. Fluorescence intensity was carried out by fluorescent plate reader Fusion. Local average reading at 10 min was set as initial fluorescence level. Each reading at any given time was normalized to the local initial fluorescence level. FeCl₃ was load at 30 min. Impermeant chelator DTPA was loaded at 115 min; permeant iron chelator ICL 670 was loaded at 136 min. Control was defined as treatment without addition of iron, DTPA and ICL670. **(B)** Fe(III) and Fe(II) uptake at 100 min of the assessment time point indicated in (A), i.e. 70 min after iron loading. FeCl₃ loaded with ascorbate represented Fe(II) treatment. Both controls with and without ascorbate were shown. *, †, ‡, $p < 0.05$; **, ††, ‡‡, $p < 0.01$; ***, †††, ‡‡‡, $p < 0.001$; * versus respective controls. The results represented as mean ± SEM of five independent triplicate experiments.

fluorescence at 590 nm. In depolarized mitochondria, low concentration of JC-1 inside would stay at monomer form, emitting green fluorescence maximally at 527 nm. The staining protocol followed manufacturer's instructions. Briefly, cells were collected and incubated in JC-1 solution for 15 min at 37°C in CO_2 incubator. After subsequent washes with Assay Buffer, cells were resuspended in Assay Buffer for flow cytometry by LSR II as aforementioned.

Statistical analysis

Data are presented as mean ± SEM. Statistical analysis was performed using one-way analysis of variance (ANOVA) with post test for multiple comparisons, and unpaired t test for comparisons of two groups by GraphPad Instat 3 (GraphPad Software, Inc.,

San Diego, CA, USA). A $p < 0.05$ was regarded as statistically significant.

Results

Exogenous iron entered cardiomyocytes in a time- and dose- dependent manner

To detect intracellular labile iron, iron influx was visualized in real time by tracking the gradual decrease of fluorescence signals in the live HL-1 cardiomyocytes. Within the detection period from 10 to 70 min after iron loading (Figure 1A), we observed iron entering HL-1 cells in a time-dependent manner. With elimination of extracellular iron by addition of the impermeable chelator DTPA, the subsequent addition of permeable chelator ICL670 restored the calcein fluorescence quenched by labile iron significantly, confirming that CALG-AM assay could assess intracellular iron in HL-1 cardiomyocytes effectively.

Based on the difference of uptake rate at 70 min after iron challenge with or without ascorbate, Fe(II) was found to be significantly more permeable than Fe(III) ($p < 0.001$) (Figure 1B). Fe(III) showed a dose-dependent acquisition at 150, 300, 600 μM loading. In contrast, Fe(II) achieved a near plateau loading at 150 μM (Figure 1B).

Iron loading induced cardiomyocyte apoptosis

Annexin V/Propidium Iodide (PI) flow cytometric assay was used to quantify the amount of apoptosis. Cells positive for annexin V but negative for PI represented those undergoing early apoptosis, while cells stained positive for both annexin V and PI represented the population undergoing late apoptosis or necrosis [31,32]. By quantifying the percentage of total annexin V positive cells (lower and upper right quadrant in the representative flow cytometry charts as shown in Figure 2A), we found a dose-dependent increase in apoptotic cell population when HL-1 cells were treated with FeCl₃ with or without ascorbic acid for 72 hr (Figure 2A) (pH of each condition changed within 7.4–7.8). Such increase in apoptosis was noted in cells treated with concentrations of FeCl₃ at ≥300 μM ($p < 0.001$). At the concentration of 600 μM, Fe(II) induced significantly more apoptosis than Fe(III) ($p < 0.01$).

To further define the underlying apoptotic mechanism of iron overload on HL-1 cardiomyocytes, caspase-3 activity and mitochondrial membrane potential change were also assessed. In line with the findings of annexin V/PI assay, iron overload induced a dose-dependent activation of caspase-3 (Figure 2B) and alteration of mitochondrial membrane potential (Figure 2C), which suggested an involvement of the intrinsic apoptotic pathway.

High-dose LTCC but not TTCC ameliorated Fe(III) entry under condition of iron load

The potential roles of LTCC and TTCC for iron entry into HL-1 cardiomyocytes were evaluated using CALG-AM fluorescent assay, with treatments with LTCC blockers, amlodipine and verapamil, and TTCC blocker, efonidipine, at 30 min prior to iron loading. The blockade effects for Fe(III) (Figure 3A) and Fe(II) (Figure 3B) treated at 150, 300, 600 μM were assessed at logarithmic increments of calcium channel blocker concentrations from 0.1 to 100 μM. The time point of assay was at 70 min after iron loading, which was approximately 100 min after administration of different calcium channel blockers. Fluorescent signal changes were normalized to respective negative controls of each treatment arm.

Compared with the increase in iron entry into cells under Fe(III) treatment alone with decreased fluorescent signals, pretreatment with 10 to 100 μM of amlodipine and verapamil significantly

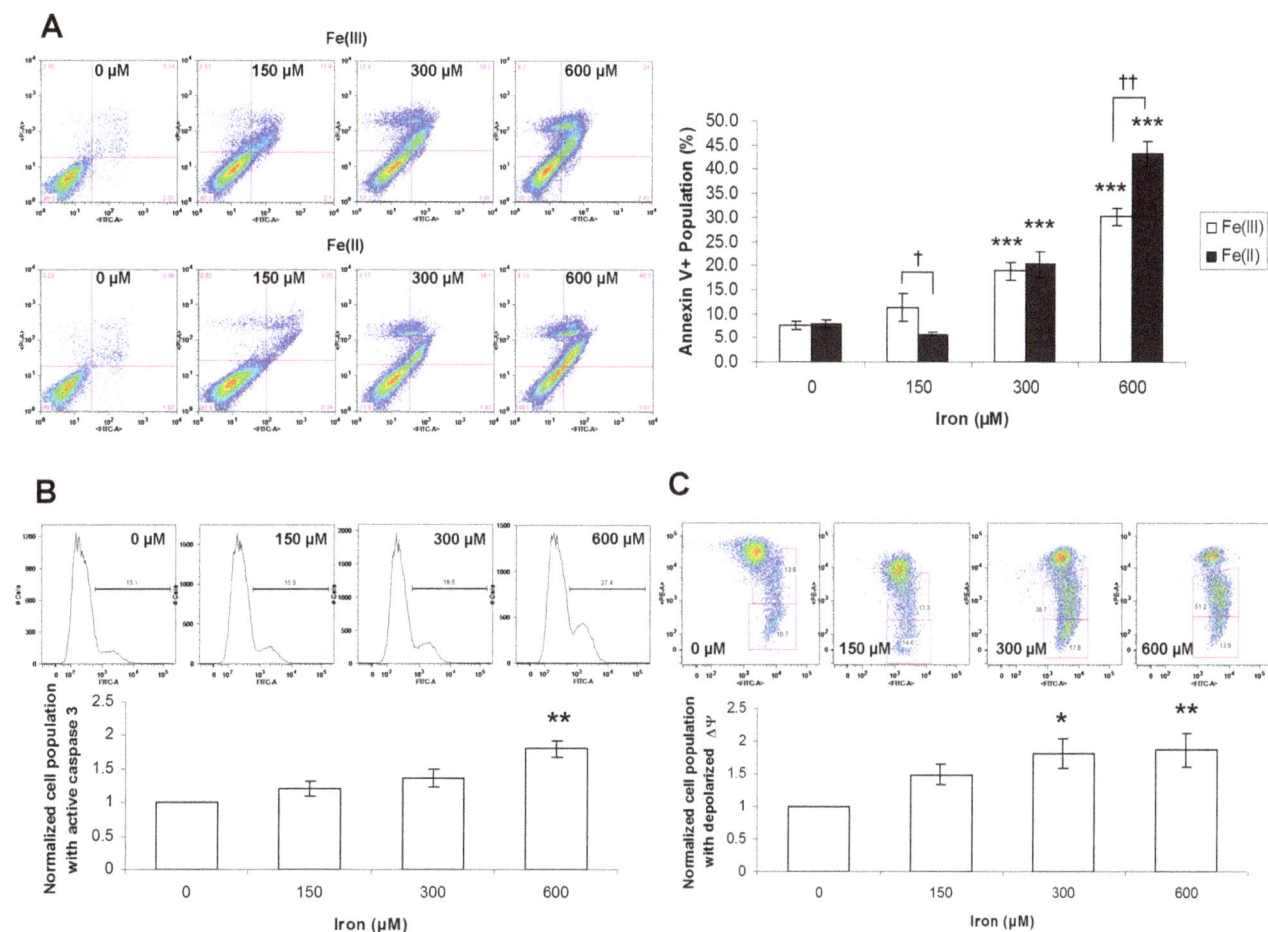

Figure 2. Iron overload induced cardiomyocyte apoptosis. HL-1 cells were treated with Fe(III) and Fe(II) for 72 hr, followed by **(A)** annexin V/PI flow cytometry assay, **(B)** active caspse-3 flow cytometry assay, and **(C)** JC-1 flow cytometry assay. *, †, $p<0.05$; **, ††, $p<0.01$; ***$p<0.001$; * versus respective controls. The results represented as mean ± SEM of five to six independent experiments.

increased normalized fluorescent signals (Figure 3A). The effect was more pronounced with 300 μM and 600 μM than 150 μM of Fe(III) load. These findings suggested blockade of Fe(III) entry by both LTCC blockers. However, efonidipine did not exert significant blocking effect on iron entry in Fe(III) overload.

Trend of LTCC and TTCC blockade of Fe(II) entry

With regard to Fe(II) loading condition, increased trends of fluorescent signals were observed with increased LTCC and TTCC blockade (Figure 3B). However, statistical significance was only found with pretreatment using 100 μM amlodipine.

Calcium channel blockers could not salvage cardiomyocytes from iron-induced apoptosis

To further explore whether calcium channel blockade could reduce HL-1 cardiomyocyte apoptosis induced by iron overload, annexin V/PI assay was performed on HL-1 cells loaded with Fe(III) and Fe(II) at different concentrations, with pretreatment of LTCC and TTCC blockers at a concentration of 1 μM. There was no significant decrease in apoptotic cell population, whether loaded with Fe(III) (Figure 4A) or Fe(II) (Figure 4B).

The findings suggested that calcium channel blockers at this concentration had no protective effects on HL-1 cells against iron-induced apoptosis. However, at the doses of 10 μM or 100 μM,

amlodipine or verapamil, which showed significant iron blockade effect on HL-1 cells (Figure 3), appeared to have high cellular toxicity (Figure 5A). Pretreatment of TTCC blockers in iron treated HL-1 cells led to similar or even worse effects.

By contrast, the commonly-used iron chelator deferiprone induced less toxic effect under non-iron overloaded condition (Figure 5A) and further showed protective effect on iron-induced apoptosis of cardiomyocytes (Figure 5B).

Discussion

The present study shows that i) iron induces apoptosis of HL-1 cardiomyocytes via the mitochondria-mediated caspase-3 dependent pathway, ii) blockade of LTCC but not TTCC prevented Fe(III) but not Fe(II) entry under iron overload condition and iii) blockade of neither LTCC nor TTCC could salvage the cultured cardiomyocytes from iron overload induced apoptosis.

Iron-induced cardiomyocyte apoptosis

The levels of plasma NTBI in thalassemia patients under iron overload are variable, with an estimation suggested to be 0-25 μM [33]. For the proof of principle, comparable iron concentrations as previously reported were used in the current *in vitro* study [24,34]. The apoptotic effect of iron overload on HL-1 cells and its involvement of mitochondria-dependent pathway were suggested

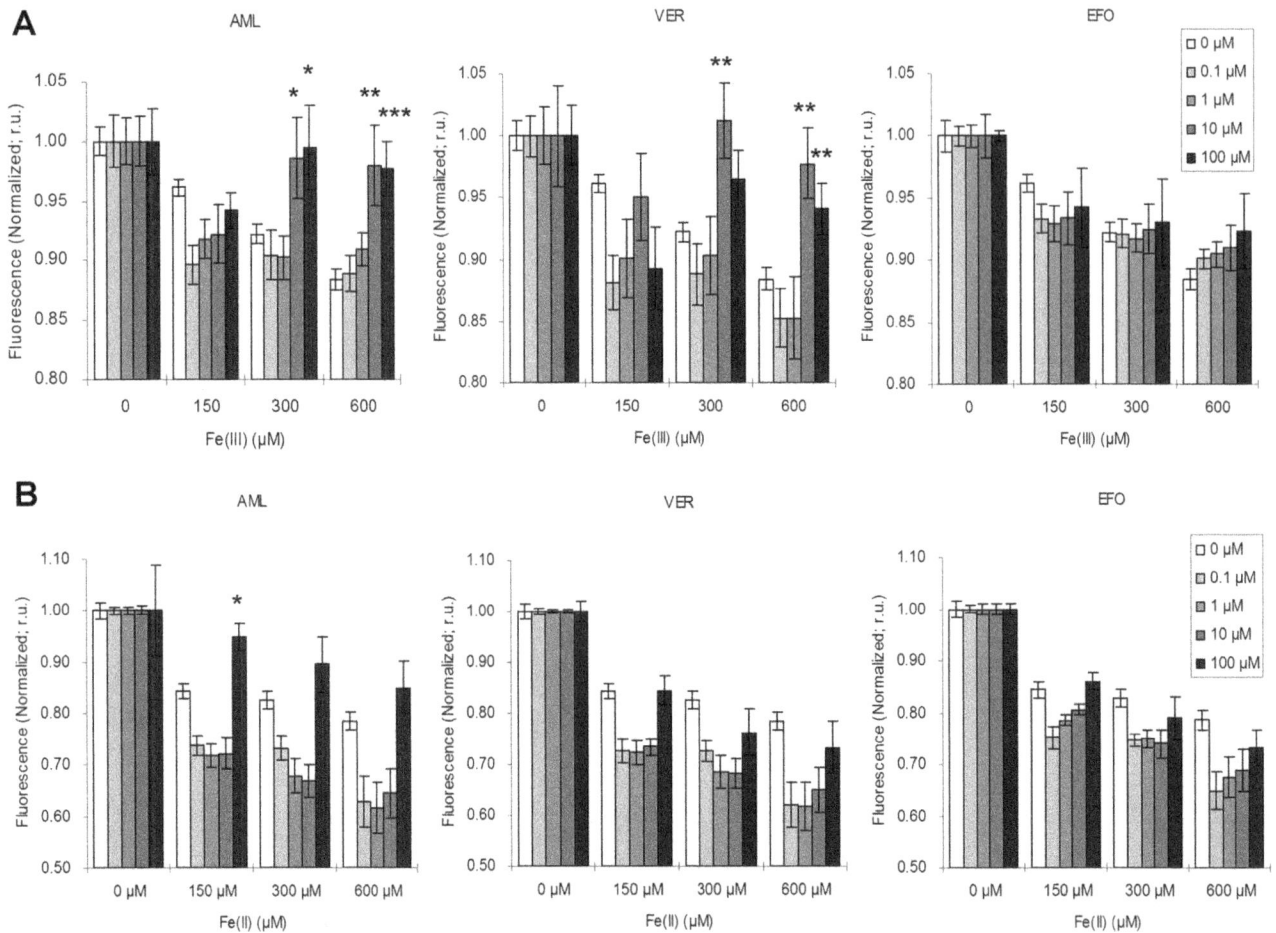

Figure 3. Iron blockade effects of LTCC and TTCC blockers on iron-overloaded cardiomyocytes. In this CALG-AM fluorescent assay, HL-1 cells were pretreated with LTCC blockers, amlodipine (AML) and verapamil (VER), and TTCC blocker, efonidipine (EFO), at logarithmic scale from 0.1 to 100 μM. 3 indicated doses of Fe(III) (**A**) and Fe(II) (**B**) were loaded 30 min after blocker treatment. Fluorescence readings were at 70 min after iron loading. Fluorescence signal changes were normalized to respective negative controls of each treatment arm. $*p<0.05$; $**p<0.01$; $***p<0.001$. The results represented as mean ± SEM of four independent triplicate experiments.

by the findings of increase in phosphatidylserine exposure, increased caspase-3 activity, and a dose-dependent drop on mitochondrial membrane potential in iron-overloaded HL-1 cells. Our results are in agreement with the *in vivo* studies suggesting the cardiac apoptotic effect of iron overload on mice [20] and gerbils [35] as revealed by increased nucleic DNA fragmentation and caspase activity. Although other study suggesting the necrotic effect of iron overload on cardiomyocytes [36], more evidences will be of interest to the further mechanism behind, including the postulated cross link between apoptosis and necrosis in series or parallel [37], as well as the differences among experimental models.

Fe(II) and Fe(III) entry into cardiomyocytes

As both redox states of iron have been shown to form cardiac iron deposit [28], our study explored both ferric and ferrous irons. The results agree with those reported previously regarding the more permeative nature of ferrous iron, which is maintained with ascorbate as a reducing agent [24], as evaluated by kinetic parameters [28,38]. Previous studies have implicated either the LTCC or TTCC as the main candidate for NTBI entry into cardiomyocytes. The controversies have in part been related to different models and methods used.

The effect of LTCC blockade on iron entry

Calcium channels play an important role in myocardial contractility and remain open for long duration (>400 ms) in each contraction cycle [39]. Except for the primary transport of Ca^{2+}, LTCC also facilitate transport for many other divalent cations including Fe^{2+}, Co^{2+} and Zn^{2+} [22,40,41]. Previous studies suggest that LTCC is the major portal for iron uptake into cardiomyocytes in IOC [20–22]. For a further mechanism, we assessed the role of LTCC in iron-overloaded cardiomyocytes by the real-time approach.

Our results showed significant reduction of ferric iron ingress by both LTCC blockers at higher doses of iron treatment, 300 μM and 600 μM, but not at lower dose of iron at 150 μM. This phenomenon implicated the classic concept of iron delivery through transferrin at lower dose of iron treatment [9], while confirming the blockade effect from LTCC blockers toward excessive iron, Fe(III) from this result, uptake into cardiomyocytes [20–22]. It is worth noting, however, that LTCC blockers displayed their iron blockade effect only at concentrations of 10 and 100 μM, higher than the therapeutic serum levels of 0.1 to 1 μM [42,43]. Hence, the clinical translation of the use of LTCC blockers to prevent iron-induced cardiotoxicity remains uncertain.

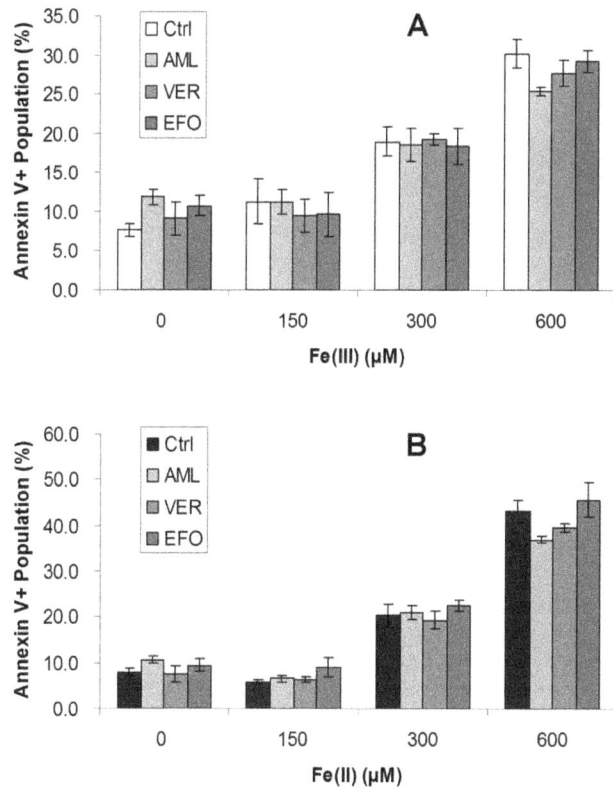

Figure 4. Calcium channel blockers could not salvage HL-1 cells from iron overload induced apoptosis. HL-1 cells were pretreated with LTCC blockers AML or VER, and TTCC blocker EFO for 1 hr, followed by Fe(III) (**A**) and Fe(II) (**B**) loading for 72 hr. Controls were defined as treatments without blockers. Apoptosis was determined by annexin V/PI flow cytometry assay. Total annexin V positive cell portion was counted. The results represented as mean ± SEM of three independent experiments.

Figure 5. Cellular toxicity of LTCC blockers and the comparison with deferiprone. (A) Apoptotic effects of 10 or 100 µM AML, VER and deferiprone on HL-1 cells for 72 hr were assessed by annexin V/PI flow cytometry assay. (B) HL-1 cells were challenged with 300 µM Fe(III) or Fe(II), followed by treatments of 10 or 100 µM deferiprone 20 min after iron loading. Apoptosis was determined after 72 hr incubation by annexin V/PI assay. Data were shown as total annexin V positive cell portion with normalization to respective negative controls. * $p<0.05$; ** $p<0.01$. The results represented as mean ± SEM of three independent experiments, except 100 µM AML and VER (n = 1).

It is widely recognized that the promiscuous property of LTCC for the transport of other metals is limited to divalent, but not trivalent cations [22,40,41,44]. Interestingly, our data indicated a significant reduction of Fe(III) uptake, but only a trend to reduce Fe(II) uptake, at the presence of LTCC blockers. Together with evidence that a reduction of Fe(III) is required for NTBI uptake into cardiomyocytes [22,28], it raised the possibility that LTCC blockers achieve the effect on NTBI blockade not by stopping Fe(II) entry directly but through alternative mechanism. Recent studies provide an alternative explanation on the role of LTCC in NTBI entry. LTCC has been shown to contribute to the activation of endocytotic machinery in neuronal cells [45]. Interestingly, endocytosis has also been demonstrated to be a possible pathway for macromolecule-associated NTBI uptake into various cell types including cardiomyocytes [38,46]. As LTCC blockade interferes calcium-induced endocytosis, a subsequent interruption of Fe(III) uptake via such pathway can be a possible speculation.

The effect of TTCC blockade on iron entry

With abundant expression in embryonic cardiomyocytes, and subsequent suppression shortly after birth [47], TTCC has been shown to reappear in murine hearts with pathological abnormalities including hypertrophy [48], myocardial infarction [49] and also thalassemia [23,24]. Using efonidipine, the TTCC blocker, Kumfu et al. shows effective blockade of iron uptake both *in vitro*

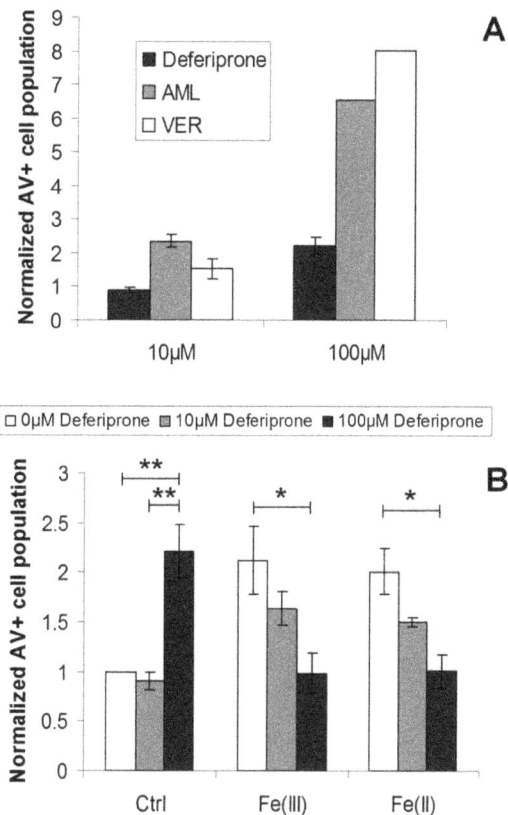

and *in vivo* using the thalassemic mice model, together with the protection effects as assessed *in vivo*, while LTCC blockers appeared inferior [23,24]. However, in our present experimental model, with pretreatment of efonidipine, uptake of neither Fe(II) nor Fe(III) was significantly decreased in iron-overloaded HL-1 cardiomyocytes, implicating an insignificant role of TTCC in HL-1 cells for excessive iron uptake.

Differences in study models

The mechanisms and portal of iron entry into cardiomyocytes under iron overload condition have been controversial, in part being related to differences in experiment approaches, types of iron load models, and the nature of cardiomyocytes explored. In the present study, immortalized HL-1 atrial myocytes were used, which have the advantages of being the only cardiomyocyte cell line currently available that continuously divides and spontaneously contracts while retaining a differentiated adult cardiac phenotype [25,26]. Apart from the superior cardiac properties and cell purity compared with isolated primary cardiomyocytes, HL-1 cells express, from molecular and functional regards, both LTCC and TTCC *in vitro* [27]. In addition, atrial myocytes may provide a model for the study of cardiac iron toxicity, given that atrial dilation and dysfunction have been reported to be earlier markers than depressed ventricular function of cardiac iron toxicity in patients with thalassemia major [50].

LTCC blockade and cardiomyocyte apoptosis

For the therapy of IOC, protection of iron overload induced cardiac apoptosis is apparently crucial beyond the maintenance of regular iron metabolism. Such protection effect was presented in our *in vitro* study by deferiprone, the effective iron chelator commonly used in current clinical practice [51]. However, in our assessment, none of the calcium channel blockers showed significant protection effect on iron overload induced apoptosis, though LTCC blockers, in particular amlodipine, presented slight protection at $600\ \mu M$ of ferric or ferrous iron challenge. This result is to a certain extent contrary to the previous finding that amlodipine and verapamil attenuate cardiac apoptosis in iron-overloaded mice evaluated by TUNEL assay [20]. One possible explanation is that NTBI initiates apoptosis of cardiomyocyte prior to its entry through cell membrane; and for the *in vivo* model, apart from the effect on NTBI blockade, it cannot rule out the possible contribution from the impacts of LTCC blockers on other physiological conditions which subsequently reduce such iron induced apoptosis. Furthermore, the different susceptibility to iron overload between atrial and ventricular cardiomyocytes should also be taken into consideration [52]. Despite the demonstrable ability of LTCC blockers to inhibit iron ingress into the cytosol of cardiomycytes, their apparent failure to protect them from apoptosis might be due to various properties associated with iron traffic within cells, particularly between cytosol and into mitochondria. As shown earlier [38,53,54], a major fraction of exogenously added iron can access mitochondria, by mechanism that seemingly by-pass the labile iron pool, which is sensed by the calcein probe, and it can even be refractory to some intracellular chelators [38]. While those features would imply that LTCC might provide a path for NTBI entry into cardiomyocytes, they also indicate that such paths might not be relevant for trafficking iron across cytosol to mitochondria, particularly in the pathophysiological context. Consequently, although the prevention of iron ingress into cardiomyocytes was observed in treatment with LTCC blockers at higher doses, due to their toxicity, at least shown *in vitro*, further studies would be of importance for their protective roles in iron-overloaded cardiomyocytes, and also for a better understanding of the etiology of IOC.

Clinical implications

Apoptosis is rare in normal human heart. In all reported cases, including those in failing hearts, apoptosis levels are substantially lower than 1% as revealed by TUNEL assay [55]. Due to the poor regenerative capacity of cardiomyocytes, a constant, albeit low, level of apoptosis can have serious consequence. Apart from limited studies showing the potential anti-apoptotic effect of deferasirox [35] and taurine [4] in myocardium of iron-overloaded murine model, little is known about the anti-apoptotic approach for iron overload. Further studies on the mechanism of iron induced apoptosis would provide novel targets for advanced therapy against IOC.

Limitations

Several limitations to this study warrant discussion. Firstly, the findings of the present *in vitro* study may reflect perhaps a relatively acute effect of iron load on cardiomyocytes. Ideally, the experimental protocols should be extended to longer duration with

lower iron levels. However, given the technical constraints including the confounding influence of cell proliferation with prolonged culture on fluorescent assay of iron entry and the need for medium change with alteration in iron concentrations, we have elected to adopt the current methodology. With regard to animal studies, previous works have been done on mouse [20,24] and gerbil [35], which mimic the effect of chronic iron overload better, although results remained controversial. Secondly, we have not assessed the effects of calcium channel blockade on cellular beating in the present study. Calcium channel blockade may reduce beating rate or cause cessation of cardiomyocyte contraction *in vitro* [56,57]. Nonetheless, LTCC and TTCC have been shown to remain functional in HL-1 cells without apparent contraction [27,58]. The effect of cardiomyocytes beating rate on iron uptake, however, requires further studies for its clarification. Thirdly, although HL-1 cells are the only cardiomyocyte cell line that retains contractile phenotype with differentiated cardiac characteristics [25,26], they are established from AT-1 mouse atrial cardiomyocyte tumor lineage. The different electrical properties, including calcium kinetics, between atrial and ventricular myocytes [52] may potentially lead to differences in response to iron overload between HL-1 cells and ventricular cardiomyocytes merit further studies. With advances in the induced pluripotent stem cell technology, the use of human ventricular cardiomyocytes may be a better model to study the effects of iron cardiotoxicity. Finally, we have not assessed the detailed pro-apoptotic signaling pathways in the present study. In mesenchymal stem cells [59,60], hepatocytes [61], neuroblastoma cells [62] and gerbil [63], p38 and JNK are activated under iron overload conditions. This would undoubtedly be important when designing future studies.

Conclusions

In summary, our current study illustrated the patterns of iron entry in HL-1 atrial myocytes under ferric or ferrous iron overload condition. The blockade of LTCC but not TTCC was identified to prevent labile ferric iron entry. The uptake of ferrous iron probably involves other mechanism. As expected, iron overload was shown to induce cardiac apoptosis via mitochondria-mediated caspase-3 dependent pathways. However, LTCC blockers have very limited protective effect toward iron induced apoptosis. Our study provided a better understanding to the role of LTCC and TTCC on NTBI uptake into cardiomyocytes, contributing to the conceptual framework in the development of advanced therapeutic strategy for IOC in combination with the current chelation therapy.

Acknowledgments

We thank Prof. William C. Claycomb (Louisiana State University Health Science Center, LA, USA) for HL-1 cardiomyocytes, and Dr. Wing Keung Chan (St. Jude Children's Research Hospital, TN, USA) for technical advice on experiments and data analysis. We also thank Prof. George J. Kontoghiorghes (Postgraduate Research Institute, Limassol,Cyprus) for comment on iron chelation experiment.

Author Contributions

Conceived and designed the experiments: MPC GCFC YFC. Performed the experiments: MPC. Analyzed the data: MPC GCFC YFC. Contributed reagents/materials/analysis tools: MPC ZIC SC. Wrote the paper: MPC ZIC GCFC YFC.

References

1. Lieu PT, Heiskala M, Peterson PA, Yang Y (2001) The roles of iron in health and disease. Mol Aspects Med 22: 1–87.

2. Esposito BP, Breuer W, Sirankapracha P, Pootrakul P, Hershko C, et al. (2003) Labile plasma iron in iron overload: redox activity and susceptibility to chelation. Blood 102: 2670–2677.

3. Hershko CM, Link GM, Konijn AM, Cabantchik ZI (2005) Iron chelation therapy. Curr Hematol Rep 4: 110–116.

4. Oudit GY, Trivieri MG, Khaper N, Husain T, Wilson GJ, et al. (2004) Taurine supplementation reduces oxidative stress and improves cardiovascular function in an iron-overload murine model. Circulation 109: 1877–1885.

5. Gujja P, Rosing DR, Tripodi DJ, Shizukuda Y (2010) Iron overload cardiomyopathy: better understanding of an increasing disorder. J Am Coll Cardiol 56: 1001–1012.

6. Kremastinos DT, Tiniakos G, Theodorakis GN, Katritsis DG, Toutouzas PK (1995) Myocarditis in beta-thalassemia major. A cause of heart failure. Circulation 91: 66–71.

7. Kremastinos DT, Flevari P, Spyropoulou M, Vrettou H, Tsiapras D, et al. (1999) Association of heart failure in homozygous beta-thalassemia with the major histocompatibility complex. Circulation 100: 2074–2078.

8. Muhlestein JB (2000) Cardiac abnormalities in hemochromatosis. In: Barton JC, Edwards CQ, editors. Hemochromatosis: genetics, pathophysiology, diagnosis, and treatment Cambridge University Press. pp. 297–310.

9. Murphy CJ, Oudit GY (2010) Iron-overload cardiomyopathy: pathophysiology, diagnosis, and treatment. J Card Fail 16: 888–900.

10. Olivieri NF, Nathan DG, MacMillan JH, Wayne AS, Liu PP, et al. (1994) Survival in medically treated patients with homozygous beta-thalassemia. N Engl J Med 331: 574–578.

11. Horwitz LD, Rosenthal EA (1999) Iron-mediated cardiovascular injury. Vasc Med 4: 93–99.

12. Narula J, Haider N, Virmani R, DiSalvo TG, Kolodgie FD, et al. (1996) Apoptosis in myocytes in end-stage heart failure. N Engl J Med 335: 1182–1189.

13. Olivetti G, Abbi R, Quaini F, Kajstura J, Cheng W, et al. (1997) Apoptosis in the failing human heart. N Engl J Med 336: 1131–1141.

14. Kang PM, Izumo S (2000) Apoptosis and heart failure: A critical review of the literature. Circ Res 86: 1107–1113.

15. Wencker D, Chandra M, Nguyen K, Miao W, Garantziotis S, et al. (2003) A mechanistic role for cardiac myocyte apoptosis in heart failure. J Clin Invest 111: 1497–1504.

16. Foo RS, Mani K, Kitsis RN (2005) Death begets failure in the heart. J Clin Invest 115: 565–571.

17. Lee Y, Gustafsson AB (2009) Role of apoptosis in cardiovascular disease. Apoptosis 14: 536–548.

18. Hentze MW, Muckenthaler MU, Andrews NC (2004) Balancing acts: molecular control of mammalian iron metabolism. Cell 117: 285–297.

19. Chattipakorn N, Kumfu S, Fucharoen S, Chattipakorn S (2011) Calcium channels and iron uptake into the heart. World J Cardiol 3: 215–218.

20. Oudit GY, Sun H, Trivieri MG, Koch SE, Dawood F, et al. (2003) L-type Ca2+ channels provide a major pathway for iron entry into cardiomyocytes in iron-overload cardiomyopathy. Nat Med 9: 1187–1194.

21. Oudit GY, Trivieri MG, Khaper N, Liu PP, Backx PH (2006) Role of L-type Ca2+ channels in iron transport and iron-overload cardiomyopathy. J Mol Med (Berl) 84: 349–364.

22. Tsushima RG, Wickenden AD, Bouchard RA, Oudit GY, Liu PP, et al. (1999) Modulation of iron uptake in heart by L-type Ca2+ channel modifiers: possible implications in iron overload. Circ Res 84: 1302–1309.

23. Kumfu S, Chattipakorn S, Chinda K, Fucharoen S, Chattipakorn N (2012) T-type calcium channel blockade improves survival and cardiovascular function in thalassemic mice. Eur J Haematol 88: 535–548.

24. Kumfu S, Chattipakorn S, Srichairatanakool S, Settakorn J, Fucharoen S, et al. (2011) T-type calcium channel as a portal of iron uptake into cardiomyocytes of beta-thalassemic mice. Eur J Haematol 86: 156–166.

25. Claycomb WC, Lanson NA Jr, Stallworth BS, Egeland DB, Delcarpio JB, et al. (1998) HL-1 cells: a cardiac muscle cell line that contracts and retains phenotypic characteristics of the adult cardiomyocyte. Proc Natl Acad Sci U S A 95: 2979–2984.

26. White SM, Constantin PE, Claycomb WC (2004) Cardiac physiology at the cellular level: use of cultured HL-1 cardiomyocytes for studies of cardiac muscle cell structure and function. Am J Physiol Heart Circ Physiol 286: H823–829.

27. Xia M, Salata JJ, Figueroa DJ, Lawlor AM, Liang HA, et al. (2004) Functional expression of L- and T-type Ca2+ channels in murine HL-1 cells. J Mol Cell Cardiol 36: 111–119.

28. Parkes JG, Olivieri NF, Templeton DM (1997) Characterization of Fe2+ and Fe3+ transport by iron-loaded cardiac myocytes. Toxicology 117: 141–151.

29. Randell EW, Parkes JG, Olivieri NF, Templeton DM (1994) Uptake of non-transferrin-bound iron by both reductive and nonreductive processes is modulated by intracellular iron. J Biol Chem 269: 16046–16053.

30. Glickstein H, El RB, Shvartsman M, Cabantchik ZI (2005) Intracellular labile iron pools as direct targets of iron chelators: a fluorescence study of chelator action in living cells. Blood 106: 3242–3250.

31. Lecoeur H, Melki MT, Saidi H, Gougeon ML (2008) Analysis of apoptotic pathways by multiparametric flow cytometry: application to HIV infection. Methods Enzymol 442: 51–82.

32. Oancea M, Mazumder S, Crosby ME, Almasan A (2006) Apoptosis assays. Methods Mol Med 129: 279–290.

33. Kontoghiorghes GJ (2006) Iron mobilization from transferrin and non-transferrin-bound-iron by deferiprone. Implications in the treatment of thalassaemia, anemia of chronic disease, cancer and other conditions. Hemoglobin 30: 183–200.

34. Nday CM, Malollari G, Petanidis S, Salifoglou A (2012) In vitro neurotoxic Fe(III) and Fe(III)-chelator activities in rat hippocampal cultures. From neurotoxicity to neuroprotection prospects. J Inorg Biochem 117: 342–350.

35. Wang Y, Wu M, Al-Rousan R, Liu H, Fannin J, et al. (2011) Iron-induced cardiac damage: role of apoptosis and deferasirox intervention. J Pharmacol Exp Ther 336: 56–63.

36. Munoz JP, Chiong M, Garcia L, Troncoso R, Toro B, et al. (2010) Iron induces protection and necrosis in cultured cardiomyocytes: Role of reactive oxygen species and nitric oxide. Free Radic Biol Med 48: 526–534.

37. Whelan RS, Kaplinskiy V, Kitsis RN (2010) Cell death in the pathogenesis of heart disease: mechanisms and significance. Annu Rev Physiol 72: 19–44.

38. Shvartsman M, Kikkeri R, Shanzer A, Cabantchik ZI (2007) Non-transferrin-bound iron reaches mitochondria by a chelator-inaccessible mechanism: biological and clinical implications. Am J Physiol Cell Physiol 293: C1383–1394.

39. Catterall WA, Striessnig J (1992) Receptor sites for Ca2+ channel antagonists. Trends Pharmacol Sci 13: 256–262.

40. Winegar BD, Kelly R, Lansman JB (1991) Block of current through single calcium channels by Fe, Co, and Ni. Location of the transition metal binding site in the pore. J Gen Physiol 97: 351–367.

41. Atar D, Backx PH, Appel MM, Gao WD, Marban E (1995) Excitation-transcription coupling mediated by zinc influx through voltage-dependent calcium channels. J Biol Chem 270: 2473–2477.

42. Hamann SR, Blouin RA, McAllister RG Jr (1984) Clinical pharmacokinetics of verapamil. Clin Pharmacokinet 9: 26–41.

43. Mak IT, Weglicki WB (1990) Comparative antioxidant activities of propranolol, nifedipine, verapamil, and diltiazem against sarcolemmal membrane lipid peroxidation. Circ Res 66: 1449–1452.

44. Lansman JB, Hess P, Tsien RW (1986) Blockade of current through single calcium channels by Cd2+, Mg2+, and Ca2+. Voltage and concentration dependence of calcium entry into the pore. J Gen Physiol 88: 321–347.

45. Rosa JM, Nanclares C, Orozco A, Colmena I, de Pascual R, et al. (2012) Regulation by L-Type Calcium Channels of Endocytosis: An Overview. J Mol Neurosci.

46. Sohn YS, Ghoti H, Breuer W, Rachmilewitz E, Attar S, et al. (2012) The role of endocytic pathways in cellular uptake of plasma non-transferrin iron. Haematologica 97: 670–678.

47. Yasui K, Niwa N, Takemura H, Opthof T, Muto T, et al. (2005) Pathophysiological significance of T-type Ca2+ channels: expression of T-type Ca2+ channels in fetal and diseased heart. J Pharmacol Sci 99: 205–210.

48. Martinez ML, Heredia MP, Delgado C (1999) Expression of T-type Ca(2+) channels in ventricular cells from hypertrophied rat hearts. J Mol Cell Cardiol 31: 1617–1625.

49. Huang B, Qin D, Deng L, Boutjdir M, Nabil ES (2000) Reexpression of T-type Ca2+ channel gene and current in post-infarction remodeled rat left ventricle. Cardiovasc Res 46: 442–449.

50. Li W, Coates T, Wood JC (2008) Atrial dysfunction as a marker of iron cardiotoxicity in thalassemia major. Haematologica 93: 311–312.

51. Kolnagou A, Kleanthous M, Kontoghiorghes GJ (2011) Efficacy, compliance and toxicity factors are affecting the rate of normalization of body iron stores in thalassemia patients using the deferiprone and deferoxamine combination therapy. Hemoglobin 35: 186–198.

52. Grandi E, Pandit SV, Voigt N, Workman AJ, Dobrev D, et al. (2011) Human atrial action potential and Ca2+ model: sinus rhythm and chronic atrial fibrillation. Circ Res 109: 1055–1066.

53. Shvartsman M, Fibach E, Cabantchik ZI (2010) Transferrin-iron routing to the cytosol and mitochondria as studied by live and real-time fluorescence. Biochem J 429: 185–193.

54. Shvartsman M, Ioav Cabantchik Z (2012) Intracellular iron trafficking: role of cytosolic ligands. Biometals 25: 711–723.

55. Chiong M, Wang ZV, Pedrozo Z, Cao DJ, Troncoso R, et al. (2011) Cardiomyocyte death: mechanisms and translational implications. Cell Death Dis 2: e244.

56. Wang T, Hu N, Cao J, Wu J, Su K, et al. (2013) A cardiomyocyte-based biosensor for antiarrhythmic drug evaluation by simultaneously monitoring cell growth and beating. Biosens Bioelectron 49: 9–13.

57. Jonsson MK, Wang QD, Becker B (2011) Impedance-based detection of beating rhythm and proarrhythmic effects of compounds on stem cell-derived cardiomyocytes. Assay Drug Dev Technol 9: 589–599.

58. Rao F, Deng CY, Wu SL, Xiao DZ, Huang W, et al. (2013) Mechanism of macrophage migration inhibitory factor-induced decrease of T-type Ca(2+) channel current in atrium-derived cells. Exp Physiol 98: 172–182.

59. Lu WY, Zhao MF, Chai X, Meng JX, Zhao N, et al. (2013) [Reactive oxygen species mediate the injury and deficient hematopoietic supportive capacity of umbilical cord derived mesenchymal stem cells induced by iron overload]. Zhonghua Yi Xue Za Zhi 93: 930–934.

60. Lu WY, Zhao MF, Sajin R, Zhao N, Xie F, et al. (2013) [Effect and mechanism of iron-catalyzed oxidative stress on mesenchymal stem cells]. Zhongguo Yi Xue Ke Xue Yuan Xue Bao 35: 6–12.

61. Dai J, Huang C, Wu J, Yang C, Frenkel K, et al. (2004) Iron-induced interleukin-6 gene expression: possible mediation through the extracellular signal-regulated kinase and p38 mitogen-activated protein kinase pathways. Toxicology 203: 199–209.

62. Salvador GA, Oteiza PI (2011) Iron overload triggers redox-sensitive signals in human IMR-32 neuroblastoma cells. Neurotoxicology 32: 75–82.

63. Al-Rousan RM, Paturi S, Laurino JP, Kakarla SK, Gutta AK, et al. (2009) Deferasirox removes cardiac iron and attenuates oxidative stress in the iron-overloaded gerbil. Am J Hematol 84: 565–570.

6

Comparison of Immunity in Mice Cured of Primary/Metastatic Growth of EMT6 or 4THM Breast Cancer by Chemotherapy or Immunotherapy

Reginald M. Gorczynski[1,2]*, Zhiqi Chen[1], Nuray Erin[3], Ismat Khatri[1], Anna Podnos[1]

1 University Health Network, Toronto General Hospital, Toronto, Canada, 2 Department of Immunology, Faculty of Medicine, University of Toronto, and Institute of Medical Science, University of Toronto, Toronto, Ontario, Canada, 3 Department of Medical Pharmacology, Akdeniz University, School of Medicine, Antalya, Turkey

Abstract

Purpose: We have compared cure from local/metastatic tumor growth in BALB/c mice receiving EMT6 or the poorly immunogenic, highly metastatic 4THM, breast cancer cells following manipulation of immunosuppressive CD200:CD200R interactions or conventional chemotherapy.

Methods: We reported previously that EMT6 tumors are cured in CD200R1KO mice following surgical resection and immunization with irradiated EMT6 cells and CpG oligodeoxynucleotide (CpG), while wild-type (WT) animals developed pulmonary and liver metastases within 30 days of surgery. We report growth and metastasis of both EMT6 and a highly metastatic 4THM tumor in WT mice receiving iv infusions of Fab anti-CD200R1 along with CpG/tumor cell immunization. Metastasis was followed both macroscopically (lung/liver nodules) and microscopically by cloning tumor cells at limiting dilution in vitro from draining lymph nodes (DLN) harvested at surgery. We compared these results with local/metastatic tumor growth in mice receiving 4 courses of combination treatment with anti-VEGF and paclitaxel.

Results: In WT mice receiving Fab anti-CD200R, no tumor cells are detectable following immunotherapy, and CD4+ cells produced increased TNFα/IL-2/IFNγ on stimulation with EMT6 in vitro. No long-term cure was seen following surgery/immunotherapy of 4THM, with both microscopic (tumors in DLN at limiting dilution) and macroscopic metastases present within 14 d of surgery. Chemotherapy attenuated growth/metastases in 4THM tumor-bearers and produced a decline in lung/liver metastases, with no detectable DLN metastases in EMT6 tumor-bearing mice-these latter mice nevertheless showed no significantly increased cytokine production after restimulation with EMT6 in vitro. EMT6 mice receiving immunotherapy were resistant to subsequent re-challenge with EMT6 tumor cells, but not those receiving curative chemotherapy. Anti-CD4 treatment caused tumor recurrence after immunotherapy, but produced no apparent effect in either EMT6 or 4THM tumor bearers after chemotherapy treatment.

Conclusion: Immunotherapy, but not chemotherapy, enhances CD4[+] immunity and affords long-term control of breast cancer growth and resistance to new tumor foci.

Editor: Fabrizio Mattei, Istituto Superiore di Sanità, Italy

Funding: Supported by a grant (RG-11) to RMG from the Canadian Cancer Society (www.cancer.ca). The funders had no role in study design, data collection and analysis, decision to publish, or preparation of the manuscript.

Competing Interests: The authors have declared that no competing interests exist.

* Email: rgorczynski@uhnres.utoronto.ca

Introduction

The immunoregulatory molecule CD200 has been reported to regulate growth of human solid tumors [1,2] and hematological tumors [3–5]. Using a transplantable EMT6 mouse breast cancer line CD200 expression, by tumor cells or host, increased local tumor growth and metastasis to DLN [6,7], which was abolished by neutralizing antibody to CD200, or following growth in mice lacking the primary inhibitory receptor for CD200 (CD200R1KO mice). In contrast to these observations, growth of the highly metastatic 4THM breast tumor (derived from a 4T1 parent line) was increased in CD200R1KO mice, with somewhat diminished

growth in CD200[tg] animals [8].Surgical resection in CD200R1KO EMT6 tumor-bearing mice, followed by immunization with CpG as adjuvant, cured CD200R1KO mice of breast cancer recurrence in the absence of lung/liver metastases, and of micro metastases (defined by limiting dilution cloning in vitro) in DLN [9].

Multiple factors both intrinsic to tumor cells themselves and host associated elements are implicated in tumor metastasis [10–14]. Many such factors are associated with altering trafficking of either host inflammatory-type cells to the local tumor environment where they can facilitate metastasis through a variety of mechanisms [15–17], including regulation of host resistance mechanisms [18–21]. Metastatic tumor cells are known to undergo changes in gene expression profile leading to increased cancer stem cell- like properties and the ability to survive, establish and grow in a foreign environment [22–24]. Like CD200, an inhibitory member of the B7 family of T cell co stimulation, expression of another such molecule, B7× (B7-H4) has been reported to influence metastasis using 4T1 tumor cells and B7KO mice [25]. B7KO mice with 4T1 tumors, like CD200R1KO with EMT6, showed enhanced survival and a memory response to tumor re-challenge, which was correlated with decreased infiltration of immunosuppressive cells, including tumor-associated neutrophils, macrophages, and regulatory T cells, into tumor-bearing metastatic lung tissue [25]. CD200R1KO mice showed increased growth of 4THM tumors [24].

The studies below compared protection seen in surgically treated/immunized EMT6 or 4THM tumor injected WT mice with/without manipulation of CD200:CD200R interactions using Fab anti-CD200R, with attenuation of disease after surgical resection followed by chemotherapy.

Materials and Methods [9]

Ethics approval and animal use guidelines

This study was carried out in strict accordance with the recommendations of the Canadian council for Animal Care (CCAC). The protocol was approved by the Committee on the Ethical use of Animals for experimentation at the University Health Network (Permit Number:AUP.1.5). All surgery was performed under sodium pentobarbital anesthesia, and all efforts were made to minimize suffering.

Mice

CD200KO and CD200R1 knockout mice are described elsewhere [9]. WT BALB/c mice were from Jax Labs. All mice were housed 5/cage in an accredited facility at UHN. Female mice were used at 8 wk of age.

Monoclonal antibodies, and CpG deoxyoligonucleotide for adjuvant use, are described elsewhere [6,9,26]

Rabbit Fab anti-CD200R1 antibody was prepared using a commercial kit (Pierce Protein Products, Rockford, IL, USA) and rabbit IgG isolated by Cedarlane Labs (Hornby, Ontario, Canada), following immunization of rabbits with 500 μg mouse CD200R1 emulsified in Freund's Adjuvant. In independent studies (not shown) this antibody (1:1000 dilution) inhibited binding (FACS analysis) of FITC-labeled mouse CD200 to Hek cells transduced to over-express murine CD200R1.

EMT6 breast tumor cells, induction of tumor growth in BALB/c mice, and limiting dilution cultures to establish frequency of metastasis to draining lymph nodes (DLN) were as described earlier [9,26]

4THM tumors, a highly metastatic variant of 4T1, were derived by Erin et al as reported elsewhere [24].

Surgical resection and immunotherapy/chemotherapy of tumor-bearing mice [9]

Mice receiving 5×10^5 EMT6 or 1×10^5 4THM tumor cells injected into the mammary fat pad in 100 μl PBS underwent surgical resection 14–16 d later. For immunotherapy, mice received intraperitoneal immunization with 3×10^6 EMT6 (or 4THM) tumor cells (irradiated with 2500Rads) mixed with 100 ug CpG ODN (see above) in 100 μl PBS, emulsified with an equal volume of Incomplete Freund's adjuvant, 2 days after surgery. Mice treated with chemotherapy post surgical resection, received 4 injections of paclitaxil intraperitoneally in 0.15 ml PBS (Taxol: 10 mg/Kg), beginning on the day of surgery, and at 21 day intervals thereafter. In addition, beginning on the day following surgery, and at 14 day intervals for a total of 6 injections, the same mice also received anti-VEGF (30 mg/Kg) iv in 0.3 ml PBS.

All animals were monitored ×3/week for weight loss and general health and sacrificed at the times indicated in individual experiments (>10% weight loss), with visible tumor colonies in the lung/liver enumerated. DLN cell suspensions were prepared from individual mice and cloned under limiting dilution in 96-well flat-bottomed microtitre plates to assess tumor colony formation [7]. Important variables measured were time post treatment to sacrifice, and tumor growth-note that aggressive uncontrolled tumor growth in some groups in individual experiments led to certain groups being sacrificed before others (see text).

Preparation of cells and cytotoxicity, proliferation and cytokine assays: see [9,26]

In brief, 5×10^6 splenocytes from mice treated as described in the text were stimulated in vitro in triplicate with 2×10^5 irradiated (2500Rads) tumor cells in 2 ml αMEM with 10% fetal calf serum. 100 μl aliquots of supernatants were assayed at 48 hr for various cytokines using commercial kits (BioLegend, San Diego, USA). Cells were harvested from cultures at 6 d, washed ×2, and incubated for 18 hr with 1×10^3 ^{3}HTdR-labelled tumor target cells at varying effector:target ratios to determine direct anti-tumor cytotoxicity.

Statistics

Cloneable tumor cell frequency was determined as before [6]. Within experiments, comparison between groups used ANOVA, with subsequent paired Student's t-tests as indicated.

Results

Surgical resection followed by immunization along with Fab anti-CD200R, or chemotherapy alone, prevents metastasis of EMT6, but not 4THM, in BALB/c mice

Surgical resection of a primary tumor in CD200R1KO mice followed by immunization prevented macroscopic lung/liver metastases enumerated at 90 d post tumor inoculation, compared with surgery alone [9]. As shown in Figure 1 (data pooled from 2 independent studies) no protection was seen in wild type (WT) mice Figure 1, panel a), but WT mice were cured if given Fab anti-CD200R following surgery/immunization (panel b). Note that aggressive tumor growth led to WT control mice having to be sacrificed within 18 d or 21 d of surgery (panels a/b), unlike immunotherapy-treated mice receiving anti-CD200R (panel b) where mice were able to be followed for ≥90 d post surgery. When mice in this latter group were sacrificed earlier (18–21 d post surgery) again no lung/liver colonies were observed (not shown, but note no colonies at 90 d). Both CD200R1KO and WT mice showed no evidence of macroscopic metastases following chemotherapy instead of immunotherapy post surgery (Figure 1, panels c/d respectively). Again note that addition of chemotherapy treatment allowed mice to be monitored for tumor metastases (90 d post surgery) much longer than non-chemotherapy controls (21 and 18 d in panels c, d respectively-however, in studies where chemotherapy mice were deliberately sacrificed early, no metastases were observed on days 18/21 (not shown-but note data for 90 d). In mice receiving 4THM tumors, attenuation of lung/liver metastasis was achieved using surgery+chemotherapy, but not by surgery followed by immunotherapy (see Figure 1, panels e and f respectively). Failure of immunotherapy to protect from 4THM tumors again led to these mice (panel e) being sacrificed much earlier (10 d post surgery) than with EMT6 mice (panels a–d) or 4THM mice receiving chemotherapy (panel f). Once again, in studies where chemotherapy-treated 4THM injected mice were sacrificed at 10 d post surgery, no metastases were seen (not shown-but seen marked attenuation of metastases even at 90 d in panel f).

DLN cell suspensions of mice sacrificed at the times shown in Figure 1 were cultured under limiting dilution conditions with cultures monitored over a 21-day period for colony growth, to enumerate the frequency of tumor cells in the initial DLN samples (Figure 2: panel a shows data for EMT6 tumors, panel b for 4THM) [7]. Data to the far left in each panel show the frequency of tumor cells cloned from DLN of mice sacrificed on the day of

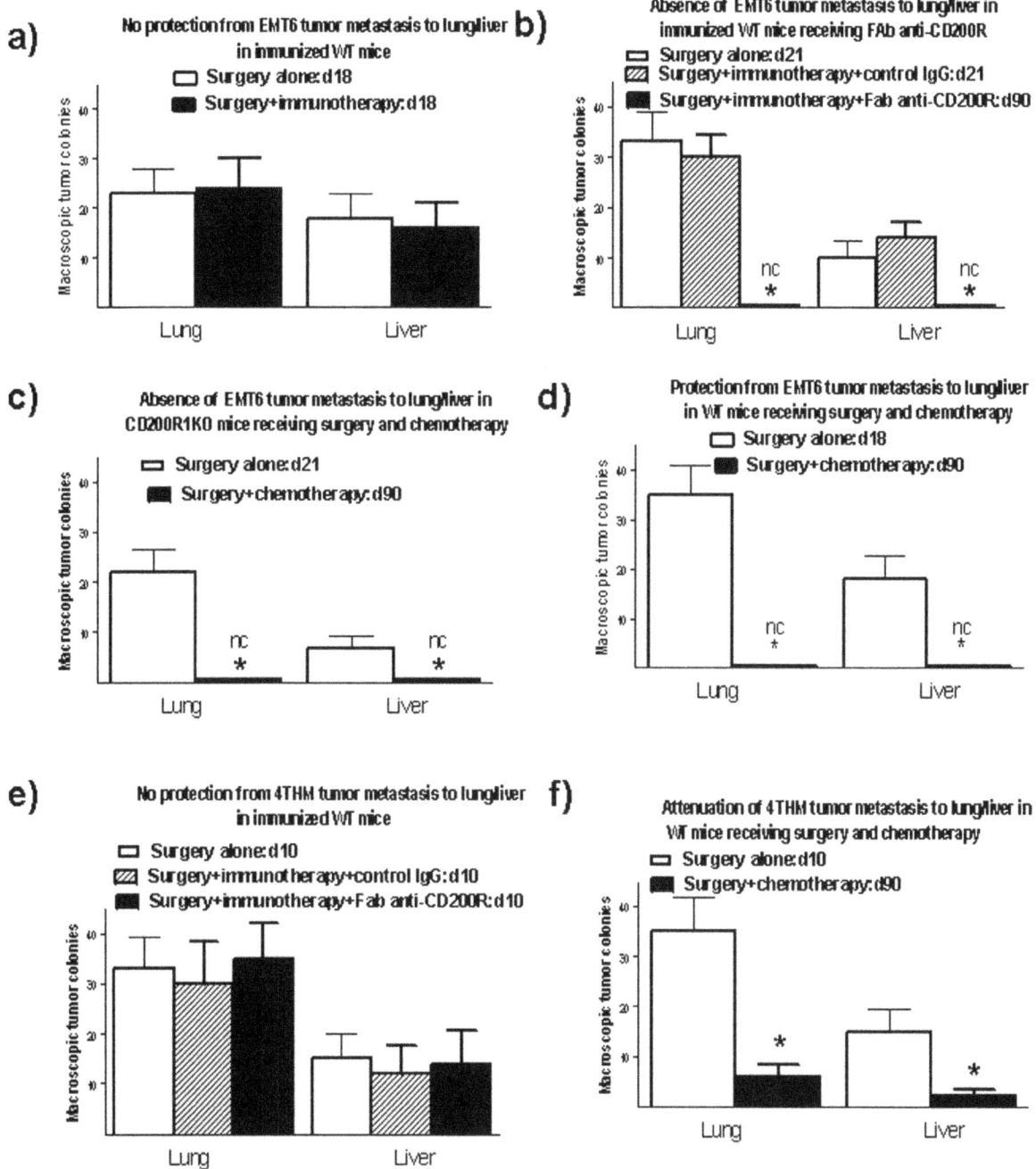

Figure 1. Comparison of lung and liver metastases of tumor cells in WT BALB/c mice receiving EMT6 or 4THM tumor cells and subsequently treated with surgical resection and chemotherapy/immunotherapy (see)Methods. 4 mice were used per group, with mice sacrificed at the times show post surgery (number above histogram bars) to measure macroscopic tumor metastases in the lung/liver. All data represent arithmetic means (±SD) for each group. nc indicates no metastatic colonies detected; *, p<0.05 relative to similar group receiving either immunotherapy or chemotherapy.

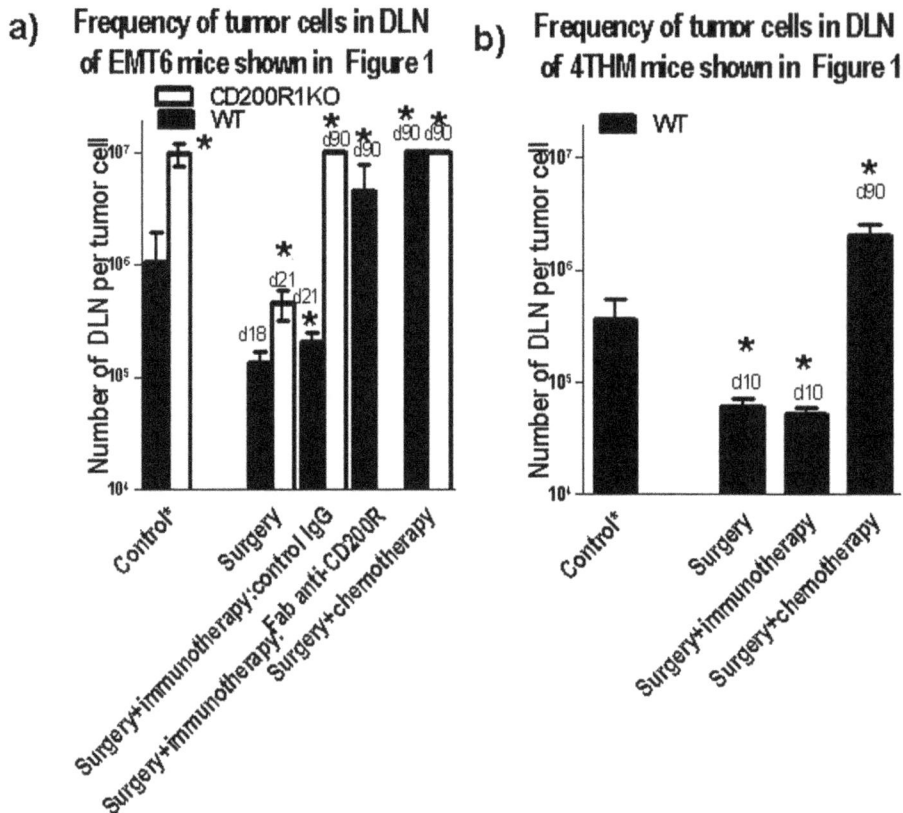

Figure 2. Attenuation of outgrowth of tumor from DLN of mice shown in Figure 1 as assessed by limiting dilution frequency (see Methods). DLN cells from separate mice were also cloned alone at the time of surgery (data to far left of each panel-control*). All frequencies were calculated based on the input numbers of cells from DLN of control mice only. *, $p<0.05$ compared with control* mice

tumor resection. Cells in all clones were stained (~100% positive) with anti-BTAK (anti-tumor) antibody (data not shown-see [7]).

The frequency of tumor cells cloned from DLN of both WT and CD200R1KO EMT6-injected mice treated only by surgical resection increased over 18–21 d post resection, relative to the frequency seen in DLN at the time of surgical resection (panel a). Surgical resection followed by immunotherapy and control IgG led to little decrease in the DLN tumor frequency in WT mice sacrificed at 21 d post surgery. Fab anti-CD200R along with surgery/immunization resulted in a marked decrease (>7x) in tumor cells cloned from DLN of WT mice (d90). In similarly treated CD200R1KO mice no tumor cells were detected (detection limits in assay ~1 in 1×10^7) at 90 d post surgery. No detectable tumor cells could be cloned from DLN of either WT or CD200R1KO mice 90 d post surgery if animals received chemotherapy following surgical resection (data to far right in Figure 2a). In 4THM tumor-bearers (panel b), sacrifice of mice 10 d after surgery with either no additional treatment, or immunotherapy (CpG+ irradiated 4THM), indicated an increase (~8x) in frequency of cloned tumor cells in DLN compared with the numbers present at the time of surgery. Surgery followed by chemotherapy decreased the number of cloned tumor cells at d90 (far right in Figure 2b).

In separate studies (not shown), no WT or CD200R1KO mice survived following treatment with surgery and anti-VEGF alone, and survival with paclitaxil as the sole chemotherapeutic agent was ≤50% of that seen using the combination shown, in both CD200R1KO and WT mice with each tumor used. Combined surgery and chemotherapy "cured" WT mice of EMT6 tumor

growth, as defined by an absence of macroscopic metastases at 300 d post surgery, and undetectable tumor cells cloned from DLN of mice at this time (limits of detection ~1 in 2×10^7 DLN cells)-see also [9]. All 4THM mice treated in this fashion died before110days post surgery (data not shown).

Absence of cells attenuating ability to clone tumor from DLN of mice receiving chemotherapy

Figure S1 investigated whether DLN of either immunotherapy- or chemotherapy-treated WT mice contained populations of cells which non-specifically attenuated growth of tumor cells, leading to inaccurate estimation of tumor cell frequency in limiting dilution [9]. Groups of 5WT mice were treated as in Figure 1 with EMT6 or 4THM tumor cells, followed by surgical resection and combined chemotherapy with anti-VEGF and paclitaxil. Mice were sacrificed 90 days post surgery. DLN cells from WT mice receiving either EMT6 or 4THM tumor cells 14d earlier (WT* in Figure S1) were cultured under limiting dilution conditions (from 2×10^3 to 1×10^5 cells/well) alone, or with a five-fold excess of DLN cells from the 90d chemotherapy-treated mice (from 1×10^4 to 5×10^5). Cells from these WT or CD200R1KO mice were also cloned alone. All tumor cells frequencies were subsequently calculated based on the input numbers of control cells only. Data shown in this Figure are pooled from 3 separate studies.

The frequency of detected tumor cells in the mice at 90 d post combined surgery/chemotherapy was below the limits of detection in this assay (see data to far right in each of the EMT6/4THM groups of Figure S1). Addition of a 5-fold excess of cells from the

DLN of these populations **did not** alter the measured frequency of cloneable tumor cells from DLN of WT* mice sacrificed at 14 d post tumor injection.

CD4$^+$ cells in immunotherapy-treated, but not in chemotherapy-treated mice, are responsible for decreased metastasis

Protection (in CD200KO or CD200R1KO mice) was not related to a direct immune response from recipient mice to CD200 expressed on tumor cells themselves [9,25]. CD200/CD200R is not expressed on 4THM tumors, and thus an immune response to such tumor-bearing epitopes could not explain the differences observed above. Immunotherapy of EMT6 tumor growth was abolished by infusion of anti-CD4 mAb [9]. To investigate whether an active CD4-dependent immune process was implicated in protection afforded by (surgery + chemotherapy) we performed the following study.

Groups of 30 WT mice received EMT6 or 4THM cells into the mammary fat pad, followed by surgical resection. 5 mice/group received no further treatment. Two subgroups of 15 mice each then received either combination chemotherapy, or immunotherapy with irradiated tumor cells, CpG and Fab anti-CD00R. 10 d after immunotherapy/chemotherapy was initiated 5mice/group began a course of anti-CD4mAb or control IgG injections (3 injections of 75 µg in 300 µlPBS at 72 hr intervals iv). Mice were monitored for overall health, with sacrifice of all mice when there was evidence of respiratory distress and/or weight loss (10%) in any individual. Note that in the case of 4THM mice not receiving chemotherapy, this necessitated sacrifice at 10 d post surgery, while for EMT6 control mice, or EMT6 mice receiving immunotherapy and anti-CD4 treatment, this necessitated sacrifice at18, 26 d post surgery respectively (see also text to Figure 1 above). All surviving mice were terminated at 90 d post surgery, and macroscopic liver/lung metastases determined, along with frequency of tumor cells in DLN (see Figure 2). In addition (see Figure S2), splenocytes from individual mice were stimulated in vitro with irradiated tumor cells for 6 d, with cytokine production measured (48 hr) and CTL assayed at 6 days, as described in the Methods. Data for 1 of 3 such studies are shown in Figure 3.

Macroscopically visible metastases in lung/liver (Figure 3a), along with increased frequency of tumor cells cloned from DLN (Figure 3b), was seen in EMT6 tumor injected mice receiving immunotherapy and anti-CD4 relative to mice receiving control Ig (see also [9])-as noted in Figure 1, where other immunotherapy-treated (but no anti-CD4) EMT6 groups were sacrificed at d18/26 (not 90 d as shown) there were, as expected, no metastases seen. Also as noted in Figure 1, immunotherapy afforded no protection from 4THM growth, regardless of subsequent anti-CD4 treatment, and these mice had to be sacrificed early in the study (10 d post surgery, by comparison to chemotherapy-treated mice, sacrificed at 90 d post surgery). In contrast to these data, following both EMT6 and 4THM tumor injection, the protection from macroscopic (lung/liver) and microscopic (DLN) metastases afforded by chemotherapy was apparently resistant to anti-CD4mAb therapy (Figure 3a/b). In separate studies (not shown) no affect was seen after infusion of anti-CD8 mAb into chemotherapy treated mice either. These in vivo studies need to be seen in the context of data from Figure S2, showing elevated cytotoxicity (CD4$^+$-dependent) only using splenocytes from immunotherapy-treated EMT6 tumor-injected mice (panel b), while in turn CD4$^+$ cells from these same mice produced increased cytokines (TNFα, IL-2 and IFNγ) relative to mice receiving surgery alone. Note that in the cytotoxicity assay used in Figure

S2b, killing itself was a function of CD8$^+$ cells in all groups (data not shown).

Resistance to implantation of fresh EMT6, but not 4THM, tumor in immunotherapy-treated EMT6-injected mice, but not in chemotherapy-treated EMT6/4THM-injected mice

The data in Figure 3 show that cure of both EMT6- and 4THM-injected mice of macroscopic and microscopic (DLN) tumor metastases following surgical resection and chemotherapy is resistant to anti-CD4 treatment, unlike mice cured of EMT6 tumor following surgery and immunotherapy. We next investigated resistance to fresh tumor implants of the same or different tumor in mice cured following immunotherapy/chemotherapy.

Groups of mice receiving EMT6/4THM tumors underwent surgical resection, followed by either chemotherapy (for all of 15 4THM- and 15 EMT6-injected mice) or immunotherapy (15 EMT6- injected mice). 90 d post surgical resection, with all animals free of obvious tumor growth and gaining weight, 5 mice/group, and 5 fresh mice, received either 5×10^5 EMT6 or 1×10^5 4THM tumors in the contralateral mammary fat pad to that used previously. Primary tumor growth was followed daily for all mice, and animals sacrificed 20 d later, with DLN harvested to assess tumor cells by limiting dilution. Data in Figure 4 show results (1 of 2 studies) for this experiment. None of the mice not receiving further tumor inoculation developed overt tumor recurrence in this time-data not shown to retain clarity.

Figure 4a shows that mice which undergo surgical eradication of EMT6, followed by immunotherapy, are refractory to re-challenge with EMT6 as monitored over 20 d by either visible tumor (panel a) or microscopic DLN metastases (panel b). There was no such protection seen if re-challenge was with 4THM tumor cells. Growth of either EMT6 or 4THM in mice receiving EMT6 followed by surgery/chemotherapy was equivalent to that seen in naive mice. Mice receiving primary injections with 4THM, and subsequently treated with chemotherapy, showed no resistance to re-challenge with either EMT6 or 4THM (Figure 4b). These data were mirrored by analysis of tumor cells frequencies in DLN of treated/re-challenged mice (Figure 4c). Only EMT6 tumor bearers cured by immunotherapy showed decreased DLN micro-metastasis after re-challenge with EMT6, but not 4THM, tumors. Note however, that in these mice (and mice cured of 4THM and re-challenged with EMT6) we cannot discern whether tumor cells measured were of EMT6 or 4THM origin.

Further evidence suggesting that immunotherapy, but not chemotherapy, treatment of EMT6-injected mice resulted in protective immunity to re-challenge with the same tumor came from studies using splenocytes pooled from 4mice/group 90 d post either surgical resection of primary tumors followed by either chemotherapy or immunotherapy. 50×10^6 of these cells were infused iv into fresh mice initially receiving 5×10^5 EMT6, or 1×10^5 4THM, tumor cells (Figure 5) 15 d earlier, and surgically removed 1 d before spleen cell transfer. Lung tumor colonies were enumerated in all groups at 15 days after surgery (14 d after spleen cell transfer), and DLN used to estimate tumor cell frequency by limiting dilution. Data for 1 of 2 studies are shown in Figure 5.

In this independent assay, protection from metastatic tumor colony growth, either macroscopic (to lung) or microscopic (DLN metastases assayed by limiting dilution), was afforded only by transfer of splenocytes from mice cured of EMT6 by surgical resection and immunotherapy, and not from mice cured by chemotherapy. Furthermore, no protection from growth of 4THM tumors was observed.

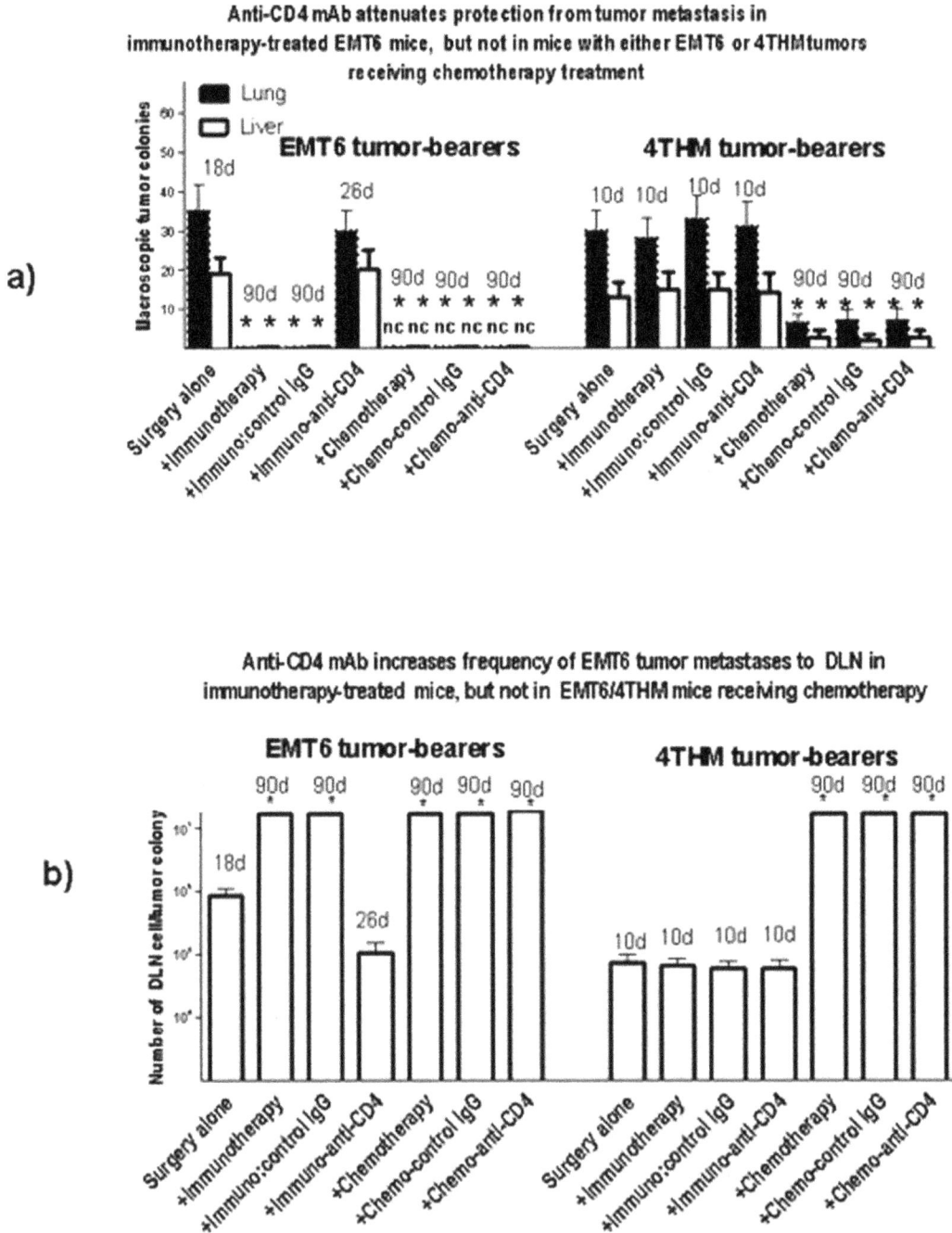

Figure 3. Effect of anti-CD4 mAb on lung/liver (panel a) or DLN (panel b) metastases in mice receiving EMT6 or 4THM tumor cells and treatment as in Figure 1. 5 mice were used per group for sacrifice at the time post surgery points shown (numbers above histogram bars). Data show means for macroscopic tumor colonies/group; nc = no visible tumor colonies. * indicates p<0.05, compared with control treated with surgery alone;

Discussion

Breast cancer cells are thought to be continuously monitored by host resistance mechanisms (immunosurveillance [27]), as evidenced by linkage of MHC expression (Class I) with breast cancer growth [28–30], as well as analysis of the role of other immune parameters on disease incidence/progression [31–34]. Included amongst such studies are several reporting on the possible importance of regulation of inflammation by T lymphocytes

[35–37]. Consistent with these concepts, lymphocyte infiltration into breast tumors is correlated with improved overall survival [38], and peripheral blood of breast cancer patients show evidence at both the cellular and humoral level of immunity to antigens (MUC-1 and Her-2/neu) associated with human breast cancer [39,40]. This in turn is reflected in the moderate success seen using Her-2/neu peptides, and other antigenic moieties, as a cancer vaccine [41,42]. While there remains controversy concerning whether development of CD4 or CD8 immunity will best predict

Specific host resistance to fresh EMT6 reinjection in mice cured of EMT6, but not 4THM, tumors by immuno- but not chemo-therapy

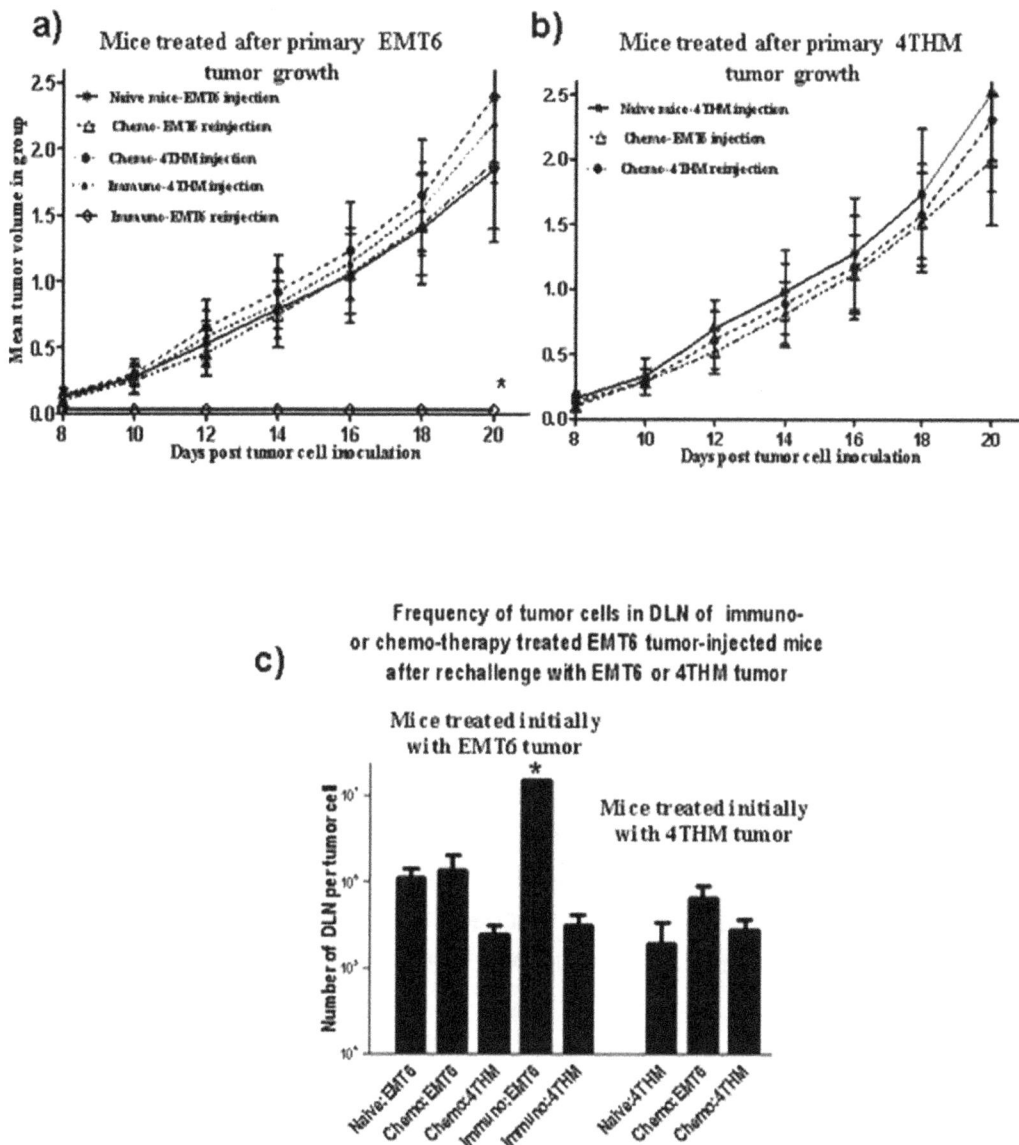

Figure 4. Specific protection from re-challenge with EMT6, but not 4THM, assaying either local tumor growth (panel a) or DLN metastases (panel c) in mice treated 90 d earlier by surgical tumor resection and immunotherapy. Naïve mice had had no previous EMT6 or 4THM tumor implants. All mice were sacrificed at 20 d post re-challenge. Data represent means for group. No protection was seen in mice initially treated with 4THM tumors before treatment/re-challenge (panel b). *, $p < 0.05$ compared with equivalent fresh control mice.

host-resistance [43,44], there is also concern that vaccination may augment induction of Tregs to block effective tumor immunity [45,46]. Compounding the complexity of understanding the role of immunotherapy in breast cancer treatment is the potential effect of concomitant chemotherapy on the immune system of the tumor host. Conventional cyclophosphamide-methotrexate-5-fluorouracil (CMF) chemotherapy decreases both NK cell activity [47]. In contrast, in studies of taxane-based chemotherapy in 30 women with advanced breast cancer, increased NK and LAK cell activity and increased IL-6, GM-CSF, and IFNγ levels with decreased IL-1 and TNFα levels were reported in cancer patients following chemotherapy, and correlated with clinical responses [48].

Similarly, cyclophosphamide which is known to suppress T reg cells, has been incorporated into some vaccine *HER2/neu* vaccine trials [39].

Anti-CD200 mAb protects mice from micro-metastasis of EMT6 to DLN, while EMT6 over-expressing a CD200 transgene, or growing in CD200[tg] hosts, grew more aggressively and metastasized at higher frequency [7]. CD200RKO mice were more resistant both to primary and metastatic growth of tumor [25]. In CD200R1KO mice cured (tumor-free for >300 d) by surgical tumor resection and immunotherapy, CD4[+] cells, rather than effector CD8[+] cells, were critical for protection [9]. Growth and metastasis of a highly aggressive metastatic variant (4THM) of

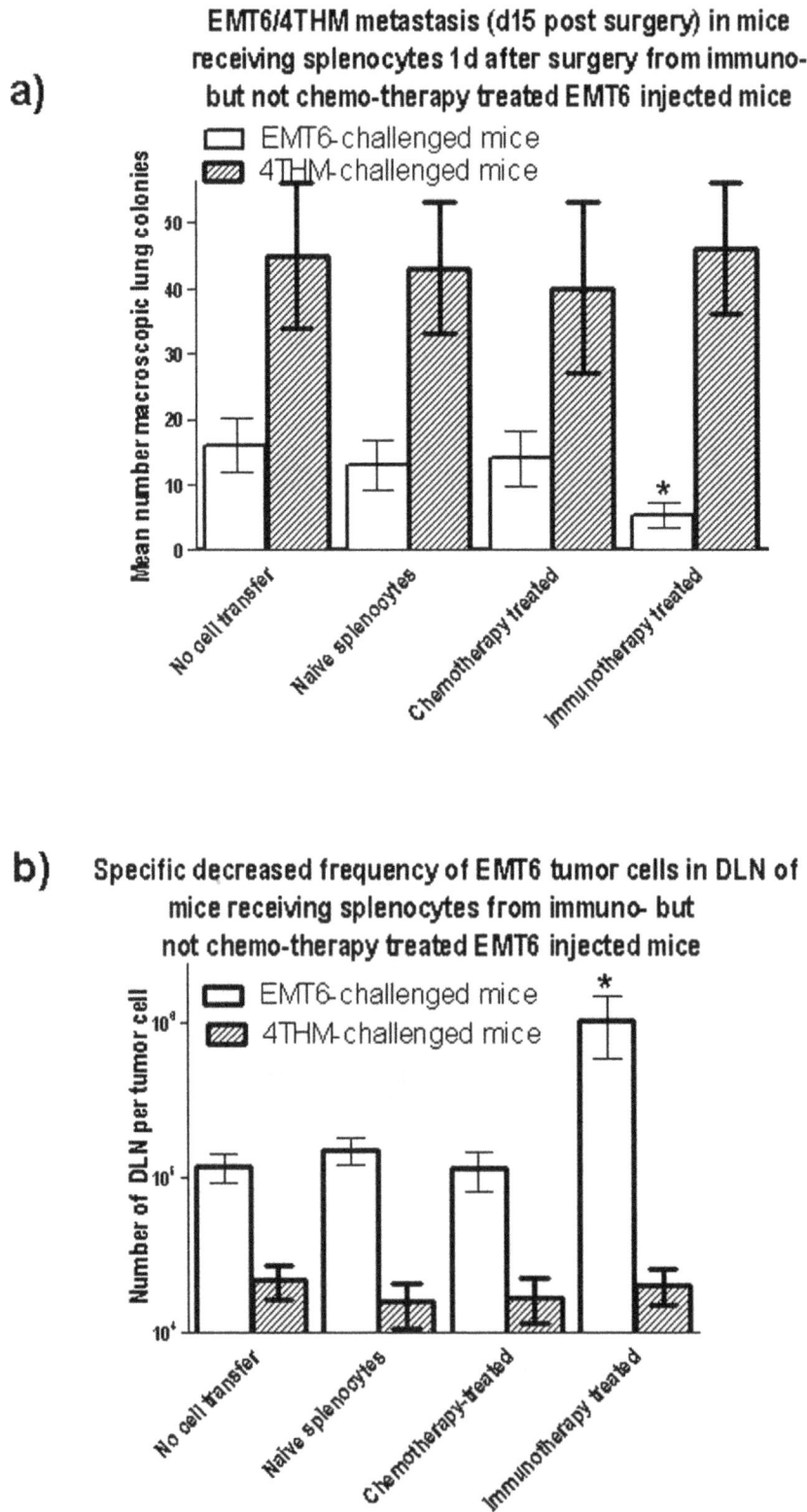

Figure 5. Adoptive transfer of splenocytes from immune- but not chemo-therapy treated mice receiving EMT6 tumors can decrease lung (panel a) and DLN (panel b) metastases in mice which had previously received EMT6 but not 4THM tumors. The tumors in the latter mice were surgically removed 1 d before spleen transfer, and all mice sacrificed 14 d after spleen cell transfer. Data show means (±SD). *, p< 0.01 relative to control (no cell transfer).

the breast tumor 4T1 was reported to be refractory to attenuation of CD200:CD200R interactions in CD200R1KO mice [8].

The current studies have extended our understanding of host resistance to EMT6 tumors using WT mice as tumor recipients, and, following surgical resection of tumor, by augmenting immunization with tumor cells (with CpG as adjuvant) with infusion of Fab anti-CD200R to block CD200:CD200R interactions. We compared this treatment with a more conventional approach using surgery followed by chemotherapy with anti-VEGF and paclitaxel, and compared results with EMT6 and the less immunogenic tumor, 4THM. 4THM mice were not effectively treated with immunotherapy, as was evident from the different times at which mice were sacrificed to measure tumor metastases endpoints in Figures 1–3. In contrast, chemotherapy was effective for both EMT6 and 4THM tumors, allowing us to study mice up to 90 d post surgery (Figures 1–3). Data in Figures 3–5, show that: (i) cure following chemotherapy in both tumor models is not abolished by anti-CD4 treatment, unlike cure of EMT6 tumors by immunotherapy (Figure 3-see also [9]). Immunotherapy in the EMT6 tumor model led to increased induction of direct killing (by CD8$^+$ effector cells) using splenocytes from treated mice, along with increased cytokine production in vitro-both effects were attenuated in mice receiving anti-CD4 treatment in vivo (Figure S2). (ii) following chemotherapy, mice initially cured of either 4THM or EMT6 tumors were not resistant to re-challenge with the same tumor, though immunotherapy of EMT6 tumors afforded resistance to re-challenge with the same tumor, but not with 4THM (Figure 4); and finally, (iii) only splenocytes from immuno- but not chemo-therapy treated EMT6 mice, could adoptively transfer protection from macroscopic/microscopic metastases to surgically treated WT mice (Figure 5) previously injected with the same tumor. Again no protection was afforded against 4THM tumors. Thus we were able to induce a tumor-protective immune response in WT mice with EMT6 tumors, but not mice with the more aggressive 4THM tumors. Additional features differentiating host inflammatory responses to EMT6 and 4THM have been described elsewhere by Erin et al (8). Given that the sensitivity of detection of metastases from DLN in our limiting dilution assay is ~1:10^7 cells, and that anti-CD4 treatment of immunotherapy-treated EMT6 tumor injected mice reveals increased metastases in mice otherwise "cured" of disease, we speculate that such mice may harbor quiescent tumor cells, whose growth is held in check by mechanisms which are CD4-dependent.

The nature of the resistant mechanism(s) in mice undergoing chemotherapy in the regimen prescribed is not yet clear. Preliminary data show a difference in intra-tumoral cytokine profiles in such animals, and a difference in phenotype of cells infiltrating the re-challenged EMT6 tumor in WT mice compared with those infiltrating a primary tumor challenge, with increased CD4$^+$ cells. This in itself is of interest given the data of Figure S2a, showing a CD4$^+$-dependent augmented cytokine production

(TNFα, IL-2 and IFNγ) in mice receiving immunotherapy, but not chemotherapy. Infusion of exogenous soluble CD200 into mice undergoing chemotherapy treatment did not attenuate cure or increase metastasis (RMG-unpublished), confirming the independence of this protection from an effect mediated by CD200:CD200R interactions, which is clearly implicated in the immunotherapy described. Our data suggest that optimal treatment of breast cancer should take into consideration the importance in "trade-off" between cancer cell sterilization by immunosuppressive drug treatment and the potential benefit of enhancing immune resistance by manipulation of co-inhibitory (CD200) pathways.

Supporting Information

Figure S1 DLN cell from (surgery+chemotherapy) treated WT mice do not antagonize outgrowth of tumor clones from DLN of WT mice sacrificed 14d post EMT6/4THM tumor cell injection. DLN cells from 5/group WT mice were harvested at 90 d post tumor resection and chemotherapy treatment (see Figures 1 and 2), and from separate groups of WT mice 14 d post EMT6/4THM injection-WT* in Figure). Cells from the latter were cultured under limiting dilution conditions (from 2×10^3 to 1×10^5 cells/well) alone, or with a 5-fold excess of cells from the 90 d treated mice. DLN cells from the latter were also cloned alone (data to far left in each subgroup in the Figure). All tumor cell frequencies cloned were calculated based on the input numbers of cells from DLN of WT* only.

Figure S2 Cytokine production (panel a) and CD8$^+$-dependent antigen specific lyses of ^{3}HTdR tumor target cells (panel b), using splenocytes from mice described in Figure 3. Control mice in each panel received no tumor cells-in this case only data are pooled for groups stimulated with either EMT6 or 4THM cells. Other mice shown were injected with EMT6 (left side of each panel) or 4THM tumor (right side of each panel), and received surgery alone, or followed by chemotherapy/immunotherapy. For all these studies splenocytes were harvested at 90 d post surgery, or earlier as necessary for groups where tumor growth was not controlled (see Figure 3), and re-stimulated in vitro with the same tumor cells (EMT6 or 4THM). Data show mean (±SD) for triplicate cultures, with a minimum of 4 individual spleen cells assayed/group. * p<0.05 compared with a surgery-only control group.

Author Contributions

Conceived and designed the experiments: RMG. Performed the experiments: RMG ZC IK AP. Analyzed the data: RMG NE IK. Contributed reagents/materials/analysis tools: RMG IK. Wrote the paper: RMG.

References

1. Petermann KB, Rozenberg GI, Zedek D (2007) CD200 is induced by ERK and is a potential therapeutic target in melanoma. J Clin Invest 117: 3922–3929.
2. Siva A, Xin H, Qin F, Oltean D, Bowdish KS, et al. (2008) Immune modulation by melanoma and ovarian tumor cells through expression of the immunosuppressive molecule CD200 Cancer Immunol Immunotherapy 57: 987–996.
3. Moreaux J, Veyrune JL, Reme T, DeVos J, Klein B (2008) CD200: A putative therapeutic target in cancer. Biochem Biophys Res Commun 366: 117–122.
4. McWhirter JR, KretzRommel A, Saven A (2006) Antibodies selected from combinatorial libraries block a tumor antigen that plays a key role in immunomodulation. Proc Nat Acad Sci Usa 103: 1041–1046.
5. Tonks A (2007) CD200 as a prognostic factor in acute myeloid leukemia. Leukemia 21: 566–571

6. Gorczynski RM, Chen Z, Diao J (2010) Breast cancer cell CD200 expression regulates immune response to EMT6 tumor cells in mice. Breast Cancer Res Treat 123: 405–415.
7. Gorczynski RM, Clark DA, Erin N, Khatri I (2011) Role of CD200 in regulation of metastasis of EMT6 tumor cells in mice. Breast Cancer Res Treatment 130: 49–60.
8. Erin N, Podnos A, Tanriover G, Duymus O, Cote E, Khatri I, et al. (2014) Bidirectional effect of CD200 on breast cancer development and metastasis, with ultimate outcome determined by tumor aggressiveness and a cancer-induced inflammatory response Oncogene: in press

9. Gorczynski RM, Chen Z, Khatri I, Podnos A, Yu K (2013) Cure of metastatic growth of EMT6 tumor cells in mice following manipulation of CD200:CD200R signaling. Breast Cancer Res Treatment 142: 271–282.

10. Pandit TS, Kennette W, MacKenzie L (2009) Lymphatic metastasis of breast cancer cells is associated with differential gene expression profiles that predict cancer stem cell- like properties and the ability to survive, establish and grow in a foreign environment. Int J Oncol 35: 297–308.

11. Pfeffer U, Romeo F, Noonan DM, Albini A (2009) Prediction of breast cancer metastasis by genomic profiling: where do we stand? Clin Exp Metastas 26: 547–558.

12. Pollard JW (2008) Macrophages define the invasive microenvironment in breast cancer. J Leukocyte Biol 84: 623–630.

13. Olkhanud PB, Baatar D, Bodogai M (2009) Breast Cancer Lung Metastasis Requires Expression of Chemokine Receptor CCR4 and Regulatory T Cells. Cancer Res 69: 5996–6004.

14. Lu X, Kang YB (2009) Chemokine (C-C Motif) Ligand 2 Engages CCR2(+) Stromal Cells of Monocytic Origin to Promote Breast Cancer Metastasis to Lung and Bone. J Biol Chem 284: 29087–29096.

15. Liang ZX, Yoon YH, Votaw J, Goodman MM, Williams L, et al. (2005) Silencing of CXCR4 blocks breast cancer metastasis. Cancer Res 65: 967–971.

16. Takahashi M, Miyazaki H, Furihata M (2009) Chemokine CCL2/MCP-1 negatively regulates metastasis in a highly bone marrow-metastatic mouse breast cancer model. Clin Exp Metastas 26: 817–828.

17. Ma XR, Norsworthy K, Kundu N (2009) CXCR3 expression is associated with poor survival in breast cancer and promotes metastasis in a murine model. Mol Cancer Ther 8: 490–498.

18. Huang B, Pan PY, Li QS (2006) Gr-1(+)CD115(+) immature myeloid suppressor cells mediate the development of tumor-induced T regulatory cells and T-cell anergy in tumor-bearing host. Cancer Res 66: 1123–1131.

19. Yang L, Debusk LM, Fukuda K (2004) Expansion of myeloid immune suppressor GR1+CD11b+ cells in tumor-bearing host directly promotes tumor angiogenesis. Cancer Cell 6: 409–421.

20. Qin FXF (2009) Dynamic Behavior and Function of Foxp3(+) Regulatory T Cells in Tumor Bearing Host. Cell Mol Immunol 6: 3–13.

21. Yang L, Huang JH, Ren XB (2008) Abrogation of TGF beta signaling in mammary carcinomas recruits Gr- 1+CD11b+ myeloid cells that promote metastasis. Cancer Cell 13: 23–35.

22. Pandit TS, Kennette W, MacKenzie L, Zhang GH, AlKatib W, et al. (2009) Lymphatic metastasis of breast cancer cells is associated with differential gene expression profiles that predict cancer stem cell- like properties and the ability to survive, establish and grow in a foreign environment. Int J Oncol. 35: 297–308.

23. Pakala SB, Rayala SK, Wang R, Ohshiro K, Mudvari P, et al. (2013) MTA1 Promotes STAT3 Transcription and Pulmonary Metastasis in Breast Cancer. Cancer Res. 73: 3761–3770

24. Erin N, Zhao W, Bylander J, Chase G, Clawson G (2006) Capsaicin-induced inactivation of sensory neurons promotes a more aggressive gene expression phenotype in breast cancer cells. Breast Cancer Res Treat 99: 351–364.

25. Abadi YM, Jeon H, Ohaegbulam KC, Scandiuzzi L, Ghosh K, et al. (2013) Host B7x Promotes Pulmonary Metastasis of Breast Cancer. J Immunol 190: 3806–3814

26. Podnos A, Clark DA, Erin N, Yu K, Gorczynski RM (2012) Further evidence for a role of tumor CD200 expression in breast cancer metastasis: decreased metastasis in CD200R1KO mice or using CD200-silenced EMT6. Breast Cancer Res Treatment 136: 117–127.

27. Standish LJ, Sweet ESND, Novack J, Wenner CA, Bridge C, et al. (2008) Breast Cancer and the Immune System. J Soc Integr Oncol. 6: 158–168.

28. Chaudhuri S, Cariappa A, Tang M (2000) Genetic susceptibility to breast cancer: HLA DQB*03032 and HLA DRB1*11 may represent protective alleles. Proc Natl Acad Sci USA 97: 11451–11454.

29. Marincola FM, Jaffee EM, Hicklin DJ (2000) Escape of human solid tumors from T-cell recognition: molecular mechanisms and functional significance. Adv Immunol 74: 181–273.

30. Camploi M, Changg CC, OLdford SA (2004) HLA antigen changes in malignant tumors of mammary epithelial origin: molecular mechanisms and clinical implications. Breast Dis 2004: 105–125.

31. Hamilton G, Reiner A, Teleky B (1988) Natural killer cell activities of patients with breast cancer against different target cells. J Cancer Res Clin Oncol. 114: 191–196.

32. Jarnicki AG, Lysaght J, Todryk S, Mills KH (2006) Suppression of antitumor immunity by IL-10 and TGF-beta-producing T cells infiltrating the growing tumor: influence of tumor environment on the induction of CD4+ and CD8+ regulatory T cells. J Immunol. 177: 896–904.

33. Ramsey-Goldman R, Mattai SA, Schilling E (1998) Increased risk of malignancy in patients with systemic lupus erythematosus. J Investig Med. 46: 217–222.

34. Calogero RA, Cordero F, Forni G, Cavallo F (2007) Inflammation and breast cancer. Inflammatory component of mammary carcino-genesis in ErbB2 transgenic mice. Breast Cancer Res. 9: 211–212.

35. Denardo DG, Coussens LM (2007) Inflammation and breast cancer. Balancing immune response: crosstalk between adaptive and innate immune cells during breast cancer progression. Breast Cancer Res. 9: 212–213.

36. Tan TT, Coussens LM (2007) Humoral immunity, inflammation and cancer. Curr Opin Immunol. 19: 209–216.

37. Einav U, Tabach Y, Getz G (2005) Gene expression analysis reveals a strong signature of an interferon-induced pathway in childhood lymphoblastic leukemia as well as in breast and ovarian cancer. Oncogene. 24: 6367–6375.

38. Menard S, Tomasic G, Casalini P (1997) Lymphoid infiltration as a prognostic variable for early onset breast carcinomas. Clin Cancer Res 3: 817–819.

39. Disis ML, Calenoff E, McLaughlin G (1994) Existent T cell and antibody immunity to Her-2/neu protein in patients with breast cancer. Cancer Res 54: 16–20.

40. Jerome KR, Domenech N, Finn OJ (1993) Tumor-specific cytotoxic T cell clones from patients with breast and pancreatic adenocarcinoma recognize EBV-immortalized B cells transfected with polymorphic epithelial mucin complementary DNA. J Immunol 151: 1654–1662.

41. Baxevanis CN, Sotiriadou NN, Gritzapis AD (2006) Immunogenic HER-2/neu peptides as tumor vaccines. Cancer Immunol Immunother 55: 85–95.

42. Anderson KS (2009) Tumor vaccines for Breast Cancer. Cancer Invest 27: 361–368.

43. Assudani DP, Horton RBV, Mathieu MG, McArdle SEB, Rees RC (2007) The role of CD4(+) T cell help in cancer immunity and the formulation of novel cancer vaccines. Cancer Immunol Immunother 56: 70–80.

44. Beyer M, Karbach J, Mallmann MR (2009) Cancer Vaccine Enhanced, Non-Tumor-Reactive CD8(+) T Cells Exhibit a Distinct Molecular Program Associated with "Division Arrest Anergy". Cancer Res 69: 4346–4354.

45. Zhou G, Drake CG, Levitsky HI (2006) Amplification of tumor-specific regulatory T cells following therapeutic cancer vaccines. Blood 107: 628–636.

46. Duraiswamy J, Kaluza KM, Freeman GJ, Coukos G (2013) Dual Blockade of PD-1 and CTLA-4 Combined with Tumor Vaccine Effectively Restores T-Cell Rejection Function in Tumors. Cancer Research 73: 3591–3603.

47. Tichatschek E, Zielinski CC, Muller C (1988) Long-term influence of adjuvant therapy on natural killer cell activity in breast cancer. Cancer Immunol Immunother. 27: 278–282.

48. Tsavaris N, Kosmas C, Vadiaka M (2002) Immune changes in patients with advanced breast cancer undergoing chemotherapy with taxanes. Br J Cancer. 87: 21–27.

7

A Polymeric Prodrug of 5-Fluorouracil-1-Acetic Acid Using a Multi-Hydroxyl Polyethylene Glycol Derivative as the Drug Carrier

Man Li[◗], **Zhen Liang**[◗], **Xun Sun, Tao Gong*, Zhirong Zhang***

Key Laboratory of Drug Targeting and Drug Delivery Systems, Ministry of Education, West China School of Pharmacy, Sichuan University, Chengdu, Sichuan, PR China

Abstract

Purpose: Macromolecular prodrugs obtained by covalently conjugating small molecular drugs with polymeric carriers were proven to accomplish controlled and sustained release of the therapeutic agents *in vitro* and *in vivo*. Polyethylene glycol (PEG) has been extensively used due to its low toxicity, low immunogenicity and high biocompatibility. However, for linear PEG macromolecules, the number of available hydroxyl groups for drug coupling does not change with the length of polymeric chain, which limits the application of PEG for drug conjugation purposes. To increase the drug loading and prolong the retention time of 5-fluorouracil (5-Fu), a macromolecular prodrug of 5-Fu, 5-fluorouracil-1 acid-PAE derivative (5-FA-PAE) was synthesized and tested for the antitumor activity *in vivo*.

Methods: PEG with a molecular weight of 38 kDa was selected to synthesize the *multi-hydroxyl polyethylene glycol* derivative (PAE) through an addition reaction. 5-fluorouracil-1 acetic acid (5-FA), a 5-Fu derivative was coupled with PEG derivatives via ester bond to form a macromolecular prodrug, 5-FA-PAE. The *in vitro* drug release, pharmacokinetics, *in vivo* distribution and antitumor effect of the prodrug were investigated, respectively.

Results: The PEG-based prodrug obtained in this study possessed an exceedingly high 5-FA loading efficiency of 10.58%, much higher than the maximum drug loading efficiency of unmodified PEG with the same molecular weight, which was 0.98% theoretically. Furthermore, 5-FA-PAE exhibited suitable sustained release in tumors.

Conclusion: This study provides a new approach for the development of the delivery to tumors of anticancer agents with PEG derivatives.

Editor: Ronald Hancock, Laval University Cancer Research Centre, Canada

Funding: The authors acknowledge the financial support from the National Natural Science Foundation of China (no. 30873167) and the National Basic Research Program of China (973 program, No: 2013CB932504). The funders had no role in study design, data collection and analysis, decision to publish, or preparation of the manuscript.

Competing Interests: The authors have declared that no competing interests exist.

* Email: gongtaoy@126.com (TG); zrzzl@vip.sina.com (ZZ)

◗ These authors contributed equally to this work.

Introduction

Cancer is one of the most life-threatening diseases worldwide, which seriously endangers human health and survival [1,2]. Surgery, radiotherapy, chemical medication, biological immunization therapies are the major treatment strategies, among which chemotherapy plays an important role in the treatment of cancer [3–9]. Regarding chemotherapies, 5-fluorouracil (5-Fu) is one of the most widely used antimetabolites in clinic [10], which shows significant inhibitory effect against a broad spectrum of solid tumors [11–13]. Traditional chemotherapies such as 5-Fu are cytotoxic agents that inhibit rapidly proliferating cancer cells. Due to its low specificity, side effects such as myelosuppression, mucositis, dermatitis and diarrhea are commonly observed during the clinical application of 5-Fu [14–16]. Additionally, 5-Fu has a very short half life of about 20 minutes and is rapidly eliminated after administration. The irregular oral absorption and the low bioavailability often results in poor clinical therapeutic outcome [17–19].

To address the aforementioned problems, researchers have tried various methods to improve the efficacy and to reduce the toxicity of 5-Fu, including modification of the chemical structure, formulation strategies and novel delivery systems. Several small molecular prodrugs of 5-Fu were developed, such as 5-fluoro-2'-deoxyuridine, 1-(2-tetrahydrofuryl)-5-fluorouracil and 3, 5-dioctanoyl 5-fluoro-2-deoxyuridine [20–22]. Various delivery systems have been developed for the targeted delivery of 5-Fu [23]. Menei *et al* developed biodegradable microspheres to obtain sustained delivery of 5-Fu for the treatment of glioblastoma [24]. Liposomes have been used as a sustained delivery system for 5-Fu [25]. In recent years, macromolecular carrier/delivery systems have been studied extensively. Macromolecular prodrugs obtained by combining small molecular drugs with polymeric carriers could slowly release the therapeutic agents *in vivo* with an improved half-life [26–31]. Moreover, the enhanced permeability and retention (EPR) effect may contribute to the accumulation of macromolecular prodrugs within the solid tumor, which would lead to a tumor-targeted drug delivery and reduced toxicity to normal tissues [32–34]. Moreover, the EPR effect has been regarded as the "golden rule" in the design of antitumor drugs. Based on the EPR effect, numerous tumor-targeted drug delivery systems were developed using macromolecules such as albumin (65 kDa), transferrin (90 kDa), IgG (immunoglobulin, 150 kDa), α2-macroglobulin (240 kDa) and ovomucoid of chicken eggwhite (29 kDa, highly glycosylated protein), and some have entered clinical trials [35].

In addition to the aforementioned macromolecular materials, polyethylene glycol (PEG) has become a material of great interests due to its low toxicity, low immunogenicity and high biocompatibility [36–38]. The molecular weight of PEG used in forming macromolecular prodrugs would impact the *in vivo* behaviors of the conjugates because the retention time of the prodrugs increased with the molecular weight of the carriers [30]. Prolonged retention of the prodrug is critical to the tumor accumulation of the therapeutic agents loaded. However, for linear PEG macromolecules, the number of available hydroxyl groups for drug coupling does not change with the length of the polymeric chain, which limits the application of PEG for drug conjugation purposes. Therefore,the development of new PEG derivatives to improve its drug loading efficiency has become a hot topic in material science and is of great significance to the tumor-targeted delivery of small molecular agents and 4-arm PEG derivatives were thus developed [39], and the 4-arm PEG based prodrugs have entered clinical trials with promising results [40–44]. For small molecular drugs such as 5-Fu, treatment requires a high therapeutic concentration, while the macromolecular based prodrugs have a relatively low drug loading efficiency. Thus, the modification of linear PEG creates derivatives with high drug loading efficiency which will have great significance for anticancer drug development [45].

In this study, a macromolecular prodrug, 5-fluorouracil-1 acid-PAE derivative (5-FA-PAE), was designed and synthesized to increase the drug loading efficiency, achieve delivery to the tumor and prolong the retention time. PEG with a molecular weight of 38 kDa was selected as the starting material to obtain the multi-hydroxyl PEG derivative, which was then coupled with 5-fluorouracil-1 acetic acid (5-FA), to afford the prodrug. The *in vitro* drug release, pharmacokinetics, *in vivo* distribution and antitumor effect of the prodrug were investigated, respectively.

Materials and Methods

Materials

Polyethylene glycol (PEG, average molecular weight ~38 kDa), allyl glycidyl ether (AGE), mercaptoethanol, 1-(3-dimethylamino-propyl)-3-ethylcarbodiimide hydrochloride (EDC·HCl) and N-hydroxysuccinimide (NHS) were purchased from Sigma-Aldrich (USA). Sodium hydride (NaH) was supplied by Damao Chemical Reagent Factory (Tianjin, China). 5-Fluorouracil (USP29) was purchased from Nantong Jinghua Pharmaceuticals Co., Ltd (Jiangsu, China). All other chemicals used were of reagent grade.

Synthesis of multi-hydroxyl polyethylene glycol derivative (polyethylene glycol-allyl glycidyl ether-mercaptoethanol, PAE)

Polyethylene glycol-allyl glycidyl ether (PA) was synthesized as described before [46,47] with some modifications. Briefly, 10.0 g of PEG was melted in an oil bath at 120°C with stirring under vacuum for about 3 h to remove the adsorbed moisture before adding 120 mg of NaH. The mixture was stirred for 4 h at 120°C, and 2.0 ml of AGE was added. The product was recrystallized with isopropanol to remove the micromolecular materials.

Synthesis of 5-FA-PAE prodrug

5-FA was synthesized as previously described [48,49] with some modification. Briefly, 6.5 g of 5-Fu was dissolved in 25 ml of aqueous solution of potassium hydroxide (4 M), then 15 ml of aqueous solution of chloroacetic acid (5 M) was added dropwise with stirring. The pH value of the reaction mixture was monitored and kept at 10 by adding an aqueous solution of potassium hydroxide (10 M) during the addition of chloroacetic acid and throughout the whole course of the reaction. The mixture was heated to 50°C in an oil bath with stirring for 8 h, and then acidified by HCl to obtain 5-FA.

A solution of 5-FA (0.496 g) in 1 ml of dimethylformamide was added dropwise to a solution of 0.5 g of PAE in 20 ml of dimethylformamide, then 0.196 g (1.7 mmol) of NHS and 0.4 g (2.09 mmol) of EDC·HCl were added sequentially. After a further 16 h of incubation at room temperature away from light, the mixture was precipitated with 150 ml of isopropanol. The obtained residue was recrystallized by isopropanol several times until the reagents and uncoupled 5-FA were totally removed (monitored by TLC and HPLC), then dried in vacuum at 40°C overnight.

HPLC analysis

HPLC assay was established for the determination of 5-FA in PBS, plasma or tissues homogenates, which was performed using Shimadzu instruments (Chiyoda-Ku, Japan) consisting of a CTO-10A column thermostat, two LC-10AT pumps and a SPD-10A UV detector. A Scienhome ODS column (5 μm, 150×4.6 mm, Tianjin, China) was used to separate samples. Phosphate buffer (0.05 M, pH 2.5) was used as the mobile phase at a flow rate of 1 ml/min. The temperature of the column was kept at 35°C and the effluent was detected at 270 nm. Studies showed that the precision, accuracy, and recovery of this HPLC method all met the measurement requirements.

Safety evaluation

All animal experiments were approved by the Institutional Animal Care and Ethic Committee of Sichuan University (Approved No. SYXK2013-185). All animals were fed on a light and dark cycle and allowed free access to standard chow and water. Temperature and relative humidity were kept at 25°C and 50%, respectively. After experiment, mice were sacrificed by neck dislocation, and all efforts were made to minimize suffering. Myelosuppression is one of the major side effects of 5-Fu [14]. To assess the suppression level, 60 male Kunming mice (20–25 g, purchased from Laboratory Animal Center of Sichuan University) were randomly divided into 5 groups (n = 12) and were intravenously administered with 5-Fu (27.66 mg/kg), 5-FA (40 mg/kg), PAE (338 mg/kg) or 5-FA-PAE (378 mg/kg) (equivalent to 0.213 mmol/kg 5-FA). The control group was given physiological saline (0.009 g/ml). Zero point one mL blood samples were collected at prearranged time intervals (one day before injection and 1, 4, 7, and 10 days post injection). The white blood cells (WBC) and the blood platelets number were counted by MEK-6318K Automated Hematology Analyzer (Nihonkohden, Shinjuku-ku, Japan) as an index of myelosuppression.

In vitro drug release

The *in vitro* drug release of 5-FA-PAE was investigated in physiological saline (0.009 g/ml), PBS with various pH values, 50% mouse plasma (diluted with PBS, pH 7.4, v/v) and 50% mouse tumor homogenate which was obtained from the H22 tumor loaded mice (homogenized and diluted with physiological saline). An aqueous solution of 5-FA-PAE (100 μl) was added to 4 ml of preheated release medium (physiological saline or PBS with pH = 3.04, 4.51, 6.02, 7.41, 8.99). The mixture was maintained in a water bath at 37°C under continuously stirring, and 100 μl of each sample was collected at fixed time intervals (i.e. 0.25, 1, 3, 6, 10, 24, 48, 72, 96 h). The samples from physiological saline and PBS was acidified by 100 μl hydrochloric acid (1 M), diluted with 300 μl mobile phase and analyzed by HPLC. The samples from mouse plasma and tumor homogenate were obtained in duplicate at each time point (100 μl each). For hydrolysis, samples were mixed with 50 μl of aqueous solution of 5-bromouracil (96 μg/ml, 50 μl) as the internal standard, and then supplemented with 100 μl sodium hydroxide (1 M) and acidified by 100 μl hydrochloric acid (1 M), and extracted by 3.3 ml of ethyl ester for 15 min. After centrifugation at 10,000 rpm for 5 min, 2.7 ml of the ethyl ester portion was collected, concentrated in a nitrogen gas flow, redissolved in 100 μl of the mobile phase and centrifuged at 10,000 rpm for 10 min before HPLC analysis. The other group was not subjected to hydrolysis by substituting sodium hydroxide solution with saline and acidifying with 50 μl hydrochloric acid. The differences of 5-FA in the two groups at the same time point was the unreleased 5-FA in each sample. The decrement method was used to calculate the release rate. All experiments were conducted in triplicate.

Pharmacokinetics study

Male Wistar rats were purchased from The laboratory Animal Center of Sichuan University. 12 Wistar rats (body weight: 200 g ± 20 g) were divided into two groups randomly (n = 6). The control group and the test group were administered intravenously with 20 mg/kg of 5-FA and 189 mg/kg 5-FA-PAE (equivalent to 20 mg/kg of 5-FA) dissolved in physiological saline, respectively. The blood samples were collected into heparinized centrifuge tubes at predetermined intervals (see Table S2 in file SI) by retroorbital puncture, and the plasma was separated by centrifugation. Each plasma sample of the test groups was divided into two portions. They were treated as hydrolyzed and unhydrolyzed as described in the "*In vitro* drug release" section. The two portions of the samples were analyzed by HPLC to determine the plasma concentrations of released 5-FA and total 5-FA of the conjugate whereas the plasma samples of the control group were treated as unhydrolyzed samples.

In vivo distribution

Murine H22 hepatocarcinoma cells (purchased from Type Culture Collection of Chinese Academy of Sciences) were maintained in RPMI 1640 medium supplemented with 2 mM L-glutamine and 10% fetal bovine serum (FBS) at 37°C with 5% CO_2, and were passaged every 2 or 3 days. The tumor-bearing animal model was established by subcutaneous injection of H22 cells (1×10^7 cells/ml, in 0.2 ml saline) into the right axillary region of Kunming mice. The sizes of tumors were monitored 7 days after inoculation and the tumor volumes were calculated as described in

the "*Antitumor activity in tumor-bearing mice*" section. The mice with tumor volumes between 0.35 cm^3 and 0.65 cm^3 were randomized into two groups (n = 30). The control group and the test groups were administered intravenously with 20 mg/kg of 5-FA or 189 mg/kg 5-FA-PAE (equivalent to 20 mg/kg of 5-FA) dissolved in physiological saline (0.009 g/ml), respectively. The mice were exsanguinated and sacrificed by neck dislocation at predetermined time points. Tissues including heart, liver, spleen, lung, kidney, brain and tumor were collected, washed with physiological saline, weighed and homogenized with two fold concentrated physiological saline. The samples of the test group were treated as hydrolyzed samples as described in the section "*In vitro* drug release*", whereas those of the control group were treated as unhydrolyzed samples. All data are presented as the concentration of 5-FA.

Antitumor activity in tumor-bearing mice

The tumor-bearing mice model was established as previously described in the "*In vivo distribution*" section. 72 h after inoculation, mice with no signs of tumor growth were exclude from this experiment. 48 tumor-bearing mice were randomly divided into 4 groups (n = 12). The control group was administered intravenously with 20 ml/kg of physiological saline. The other groups were administered intravenously with 30 mg/kg (0.160 mmol/kg) of 5-FA or 284 mg/kg 5-FA-PAE (equivalent to 0.160 mmol/kg 5-FA) dissolved in physiological saline. 5-Fu (20.47 mg/kg, 0.160 mmol/kg) was administered as a control. All animals were administered once on day 3, 5, 7, 9, 11, 13, 15 after the inoculation of H22 cells and sacrificed on day 20. Tumors and organs (heart, liver, spleen, lung, kidney, brain and thymus) were removed and weighed. The tumor volume and tumor control rate were evaluated. The tumor volume, organ/body weight index and tumor control rate were calculated as follows:

$$\text{Tumor volume (mm}^3) = 0.5 \times \text{Width}^2 \times \text{Length}$$

$$\text{Organ/body weight index} = \text{weight of each organ (tumor)} / \text{weight of mouse} \times 100$$

$$\text{Tumor control rate (\%)} = \left(\begin{array}{c} \text{average tumor weight of control group} - \\ \text{average tumor weight of test group} \end{array} \right) / \begin{array}{c} \text{average tumor weight} \\ \text{of control group} \end{array}$$

Data analysis

The data of pharmacokinetics and *in vivo* distribution study were processed using the Drug and Statistics Software 2.0 (DAS 2.0, Shanghai, China). The statistical analysis of the samples was performed by using one-way ANOVA and Student's *t*-test. *p*-values <0.05 were considered as statistically different.

Results and Discussion

Synthesis and characterization of 5-FA-PAE prodrug

As a polyether macromolecule, PEG is widely used for its suitable solubility and bioavailability in developing drug delivery systems [50–53]. However, as a drug carrier, the loading efficiency of prodrugs based on PEG is significantly constrained due to the limited positions for drug conjugation, *i.e.*, two hydroxy groups in the linear PEG molecule [45]. Thus, the modification of PEG to create derivatives with higher drug loading efficiency is greatly needed. PEG with a molecular weight of 38 kDa was selected as the starting material to synthesize the derivative (Fig. 1A). Allyl glycidyl ether was coupled to both ends of PEG under the catalysis of sodium hydride to form an intermediate, namely PA, with multi-double bonds on the side chains. PA was further reacted with small molecules through the addition reaction of the double bonds and the thiol group to afford various PEG derivatives with multi-hydroxyl groups. ^{1}H-NMR showed that the double bonds disappeared completely in PAE (Figure S1 in file SI). The GPC analysis demonstrated that PA and PAE had similar molecular weight distribution as the starting material PEG (Table 1). As a common drug carrier, the molecular weight of PEG greatly influenced the *in vivo* behaviors of prodrugs [54]. As the molecular weight increases, the *in vivo* clearance rate decreases. Thus, PEG with a higher Mw is likely to prolong the retention time of prodrugs and increase the drug accumulation in a tumor. It is suggested that the Mw of PEG should be no less than 30 kD to

prevent the prodrug from quick elimination from kidney [55]. Accordingly, PEG of 38 kD was used as the starting material.

However, 5-Fu could not be directly coupled with the carriers due to the lack of available hydroxyl groups in the structure. The derivative of 5-Fu, 5-fluorouracil-1-acetic acid (5-FA), was synthesized first. The macromolecular prodrug multi-hydroxyl polyethylene glycol-5-fluorouracil-1-acetic acid (5-FA-PAE) was obtained by covalently conjugating 5-FA with the PEG derivative under the catalysis of carbodiimide condensing agents (Figure 1B). The successful synthesis of the 5-fluorouracil derivative and the prodrug was confirmed by ^{1}H-NMR (Figure S1 in file SI). A higher molecular weight (Mw) and polydispersity (PDI) of 5-FA-PAE were observed compared with those of PAE (Table 1). HPLC analysis indicated that after the double bond-thiol addition reaction, multiple hydroxyl groups were introduced on the PEG backbone thus making it capable of loading more drugs. The drug loading efficiency of 5-FA-PAE was determined as 10.58%, much higher than the maximum drug loading efficiency of PEG with the same molecular weight, which was calculated as 0.98% theoretically. The drug loading efficiency of 5-FA-PAE was improved by

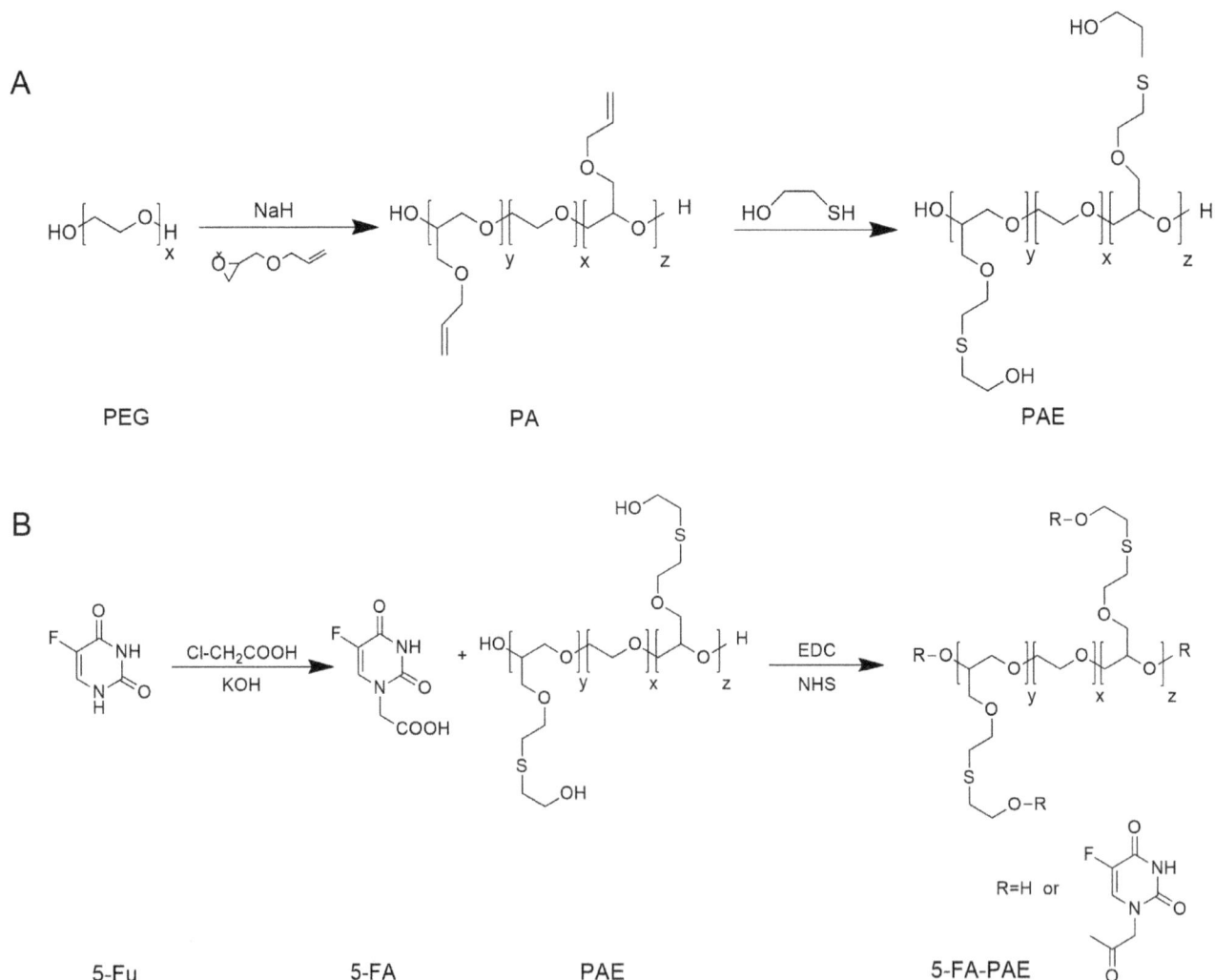

Figure 1. Synthesis routes of PAE (A) and 5-FA-PAE conjugates (B). (A) PA was synthesized by adding NaH to PEG and the mixture was stirred for 4 h at 120°C. Then PAE was obtained by adding AGE to the mixture. (B) 5-FA was added dropwise to PAE in dimethylformamide, then NHS and EDC·HCl were added. After incubation, the mixture was precipitated with isopropanol. The obtained residue was recrystallized by isopropanol several times and dried in vacuum at 40°C overnight to produce 5-FA-PAE.

Table 1. The molecular weight of the polymeric carrier (PEG, PA, PAE) and the prodrug (5-FA-PAE).

Compound	MP (Da)	Mw (Da)	Mn (Da)	PDI
PEG	38914	38045	27596	1.38
PA	33984	36039	21322	1.69
PAE	34282	36628	20842	1.76
5-FA-PAE	35413	44629	19998	2.23

PDI: polydispersity.

10.8-fold compared to that of 5-FA. The significant enhancement in drug loading efficiency would greatly increase the drug concentration within a tumor via the EPR effect.

Safety evaluation

To investigate the myelosuppression levels after 5-FA or 5-FA-PAE treatment, hematological parameters (i.e. the number of white blood cells and blood platelets) were measured at different time points after drug administration. Changes in these parameters presumably reflect the occurrence of myelosuppression and abnormality in the immune system. As shown in Table 2, the WBC count decreased after intravenous injection of 5-Fu, 5-FA and 5-FA-PAE. Only the group of 5-Fu exhibited significant reduction of WBC ($5.39 \pm 2.17 \times 10^9$/L one day after injection, $p < 0.05$). Then the WBC level increased gradually. Notably, the increase of WBC in the 5-Fu group was slower, leading to a lower WBC level at day 10 ($8.59 \pm 2.39 \times 10^9$/L) compared with the level before administration ($9.55 \pm 1.28 \times 10^9$/L), while the WBC level of other groups recovered within 4 days. Another major indicator of myelosuppression is the change in blood platelets number. Table S1 in file SI shows that though the platelets number of 5-Fu decreased 1 day after injection, the blood platelets of all groups didn't exhibit any significant changes, indicating that both 5-FA and 5-FA-PAE hardly affect the platelets level at such doses. Taken together, these results indicated that the prodrug of 5-Fu, 5-FA-PAE, showed a lower toxicity than 5-Fu.

In vitro drug release

The *in vitro* drug release behavior of 5-FA-PAE was investigated using phosphate buffered saline (PBS) of various pH values, physiological saline, mouse plasma and tumor homogenate as the release media. The release rate of 5-FA-PAE was pH-dependent. As the pH increased, the release rate increased significantly, reaching $94.1\% \pm 5.88\%$ at 96 h when the pH was 8.99 (Figure 2A). This is mostly likely due to the hydrolysis of ester bonds under basic conditions. However, if the conjugation with

the PEG derivative increased the retention time in plasma, this would possibly enhance the drug accumulation in a tumor (Figure 2B). The release rate of prodrug 5-FA-PAE in plasma was $89.46\% \pm 6.36\%$ at 10 h, and reached $98.15\% \pm 1.96\%$ at 24 h, while the rate was $55.9\% \pm 0.61\%$ in tumor homogenate at 24 h, suggesting that the ester bond can be easily degraded by easterases in plasma.

Pharmacokinetics study

A major drawback of 5-Fu is the relatively short half-life, which results in poor patient compliance and side effects. 5-FA, the derivative of 5-Fu, shows the same metabolism and clearance rate as 5-Fu. Moreover, after conjugation with PEG, the retention time in plasma was greatly prolonged, which might enhance tumor accumulation. After administration intravenously, 5-FA was rapidly eliminated from the blood circulation, which led to a complete removal at 6~8 h after administration, whereas the elimination rate of 5-FA-PAE was much lower than that of 5-FA, and the blood retention time of this macromolecular prodrug reached more than 96 h (Figure 3). The detailed plasma concentration of 5-FA and 5-FA-PAE at different time points are shown in Table S2 in file SI. Some pharmacokinetic parameters, such as the area under the curve (AUC), the mean retention time (MRT) and the elimination half-life ($t_{1/2}$) of 5-FA-PAE were much higher than those of 5-FA, *i.e.*, 25.6 times for AUC (546.6 ± 36.7 μg/ml ·h vs 21.37 ± 4.36 μg/ml ·h), 11.7 times for MRT (7.962 ± 0.400 h vs 0.679 ± 0.142 h) and 14.4 times for $t_{1/2}$ (22.10 ± 5.92 h vs 1.538 ± 0.419 h), indicating a much longer blood circulation times and a remarkably enhanced bioavailability of the macromolecular prodrug (Table 3). Meanwhile, the amount of 5-FA released from 5-FA-PAE in rat plasma was determined. Although the total amount of 5-FA-PAE in rat plasma was significantly higher than that of 5-FA, the concentration of released 5-FA from 5-FA-PAE was not as much as 5-FA. It was lower than the 5-FA group within 30 min after administration and then increased slightly afterwards (Table S2 in file SI). This may

Table 2. The number of white blood cells in mice administered with saline, 5-Fu, 5-FA, PAE or 5-FA-PAE ($\times 10^9$/L).

	1 day before injection	1 day after injection	4 days after injection	7 days after injection	10 days after injection
saline	9.77 ± 1.99	8.86 ± 2.79	11.19 ± 6.78	12.24 ± 4.37	12.06 ± 7.58
5-FA-PAE	9.35 ± 1.39	8.73 ± 1.90	11.73 ± 5.44	12.00 ± 2.02	12.52 ± 3.78
5-FA	9.13 ± 2.23	8.99 ± 1.86	10.32 ± 5.71	10.24 ± 4.50	11.55 ± 3.62
PAE	9.54 ± 1.64	8.46 ± 1.85	9.85 ± 3.09	10.74 ± 5.13	11.93 ± 3.40
5-Fu	9.55 ± 1.28	$5.39 \pm 2.17^*$	6.84 ± 5.76	7.34 ± 2.82	8.59 ± 2.39

Each value represents the mean $\pm$ SD (n = 12).
*$p < 0.05$ vs. 5-Fu,1 day before injection.

A

B

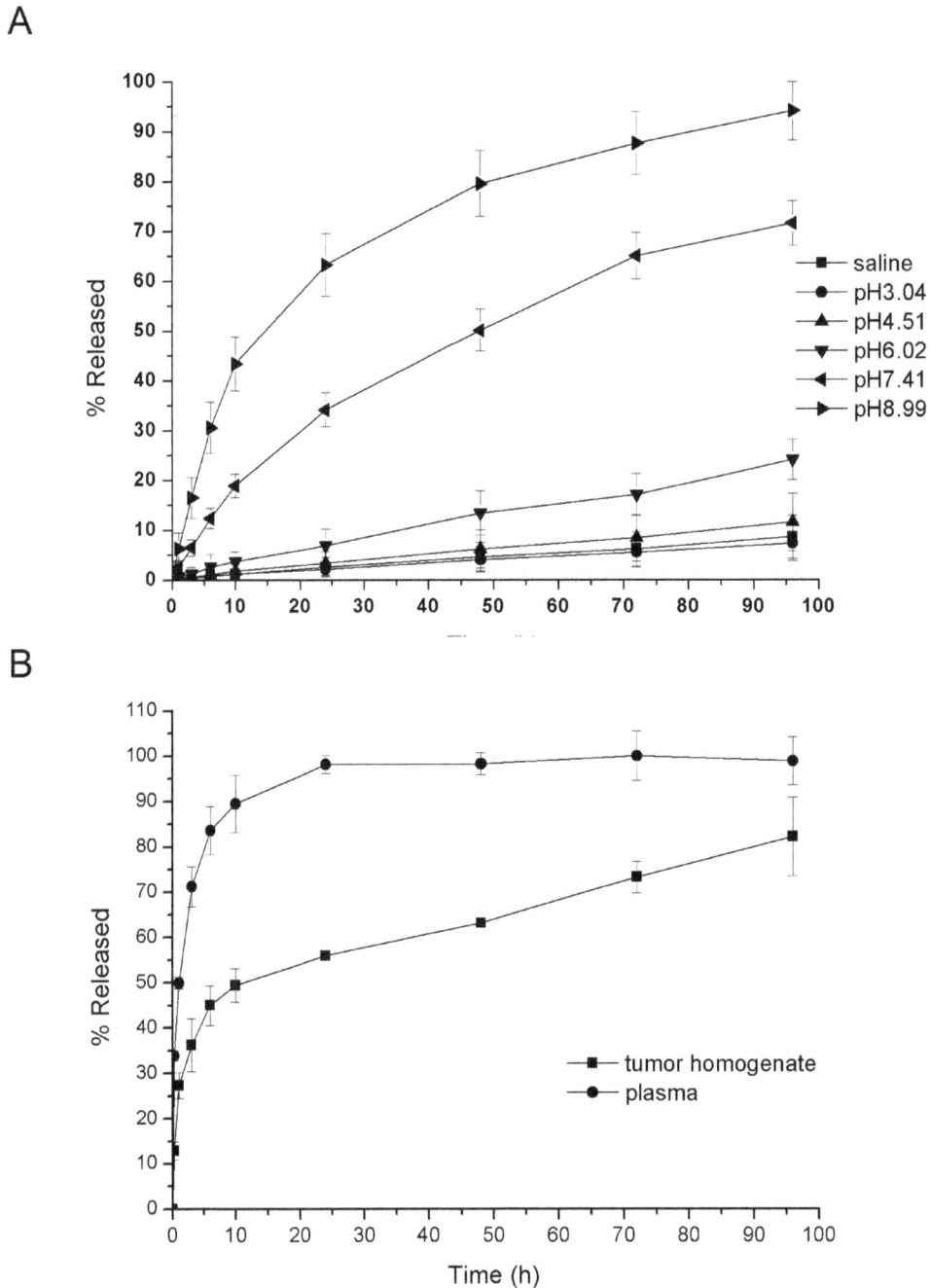

Figure 2. *In vitro* **drug release of 5-FA-PAE.** (A) Drug release profiles of 5-FA-PAE in PBS and saline. 100 μl 5-PA-PAE was added to preheated release media (PBS of different pH values or saline) and incubated at 37°C with stirring. Samples were collected at fixed time intervals, acidified by hydrochloric acid (1 M) and analyzed by HPLC. (B) Drug release profiles of 5-FA-PAE in murine tumor homogenate and plasma. The samples from mouse plasma and tumor homogenate were obtained in duplicate at each time point (100 μl each). For hydrolysis, 100 μl sodium hydroxide (1 M) were added to samples followed by 100 μl hydrochloric acid (1 M). The other group was not subjected to hydrolysis by substituting sodium hydroxide solution with saline and acidifying with 50 μl hydrochloric acid. The differences of 5-FA in the two groups at the same time point was the unreleased 5-FA in each sample. Each value represents the mean ± SD (n = 3).

have an impact on the antitumor efficacy of 5-FA-PAE, but could avoid certain possible side effects.

Due to the obvious discrepancy of retention time between 5-FA and 5-FA-PAE, two sets of different time points were adopted to fully describe the *in vivo* fate of 5-FA and 5-FA-PAE. The first time point for 5-FA and 5-FA-PAE was 1 min and 5 min after administration, respectively.

In the *in vitro* release study, about 98% of 5-FA was released from 5-FA-PAE in plasma at 24 h, in other words, 2% 5-FA-PAE remained intact, while in the pharmacokinetics study, the concentration of unreleased 5-FA-PAE was 228.276±5.441 μg/ml 5 min after administration (the difference between total concentration of 5-FA-PAE and free 5-FA released from 5-FA-PAE), and decreased to 2.439±0.258 at 24 h (about 1.1% of the

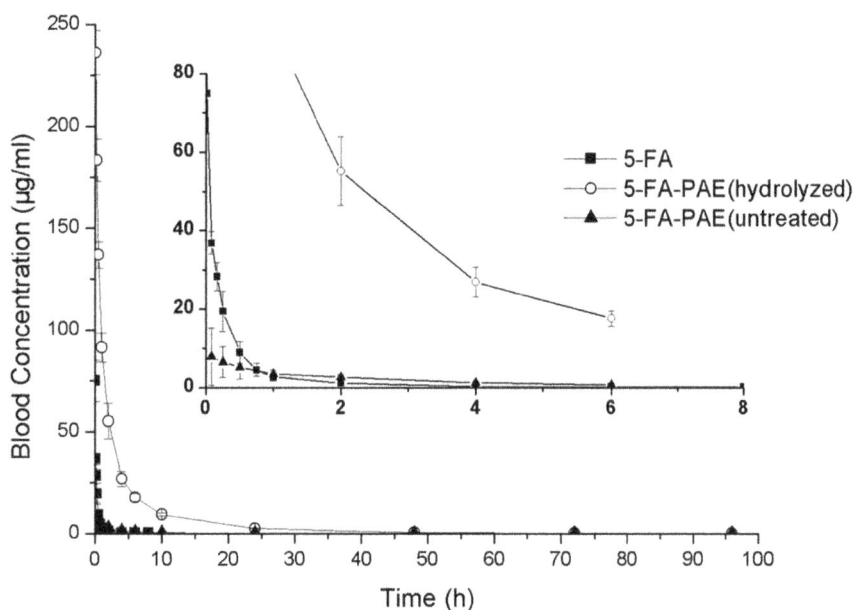

Figure 3. Pharmacokinetics of 5-FA and 5-FA-PAE after *i.v.* injection. The control group and the test groups were administered intravenously with 20 mg/kg of 5-FA or 189 mg/kg of 5-FA-PAE (equivalent to 20 mg/kg of 5-FA) dissolved in physiological saline, respectively. Each plasma sample of the 5-FA-PAE group was divided into two portions (treated as hydrolyzed and unhydrolyzed), which were analyzed by HPLC to determine the plasma concentrations of released 5-FA and total 5-FA of the conjugate whereas the plasma samples of the control group were treated as unhydrolyzed samples. Each value represents the mean ± standard deviation (n = 6).

concentration at 5 min), which is consistent with the previous *in vitro* release study. Comparing the concentration of the free 5-FA of unhydrolyzed and hydrolyzed 5-FA-PAE group, it can be concluded that the unreleased 5-FA-PAE was intact in the blood circulation, which could accumulate in tumor tissue in the form of prodrug and then slowly release 5-FA at the tumor site to achieve antitumor effect. 5-FA was shown to be rapidly eliminated from blood, while after conjugation with PAE, the retention time was significantly prolonged, which may be attributed to a protective role of PEG. Thus, the prolonged retention time of 5-FA not only extended the duration time and enhanced the bioavailability, but also improved the delivery of macromolecular drugs to a tumor.

In vivo distribution

Small molecular drugs eliminate quickly after intravenous administration, which could distribute them to normal tissues through capillaries nonspecifically. To analyze the *in vivo* biodistribution of 5-FA-PAE, the murine hepatic cancer cell line (H22) was used to establish the tumor-bearing animal model. The hepatoma H22 model has been widely use as a tumor model in the study of antitumor drugs and its mechanism. Generally, it is believed that the orthotopic tumor can better simulate the pathologic process of tumor development. However, due to the high mortality rate of animals and the complexity of operation, we

Table 3. Pharmacokinetic parameters of 5-FA and 5-FA-PAE after i.v. injection in rats.

Parameters	Unit	5-FA	5-FA-PAE
AUC $_{0-t}$	µg/ml·h	21.37±4.36	546.6±36.7
AUC $_{0-\infty}$	µg/ml·h	21.63±4.47	551.5±35.0
MRT $_{0-t}$	h	0.679±0.142	7.962±0.400
MRT $_{0-\infty}$	h	0.795±0.240	9.072±0.513
VRT $_{0-t}$	h^2	1.519±0.326	190.2±19.7
VRT $_{0-\infty}$	h^2	2.703±1.558	335.8±79.4
t$_{1/2}$	h	1.538±0.419	22.10±5.92
T$_{max}$	h	0.0167±0	0.097±0.034
V	ml/g	2.107±0.620	1.172±0.358
Cl	ml/g/h	0.967±0.259	0.036±0.002
C$_{max}$	µg/ml	74.92±10.16	232.4±13.5

AUC, area under the plasma concentration−time curve; MRT, mean residence time; VRT, variance of mean residence time; t$_{1/2}$: elimination half life; T$_{max}$, time of maximum concentration; V, apparent volume of distribution; CL, clearance; Cmax, the maximum of 5-FA concentration in plasma. Each value represents the mean ± SD (n = 5).

A

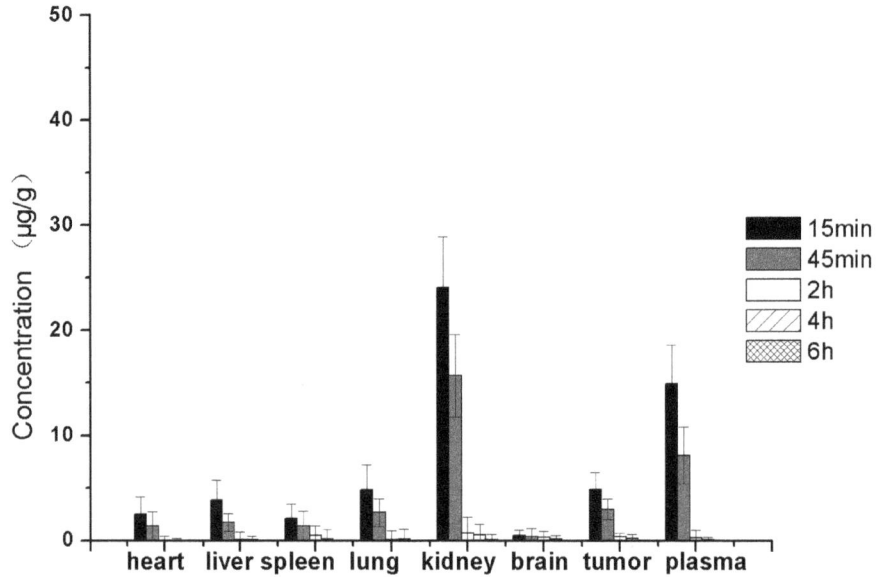

B

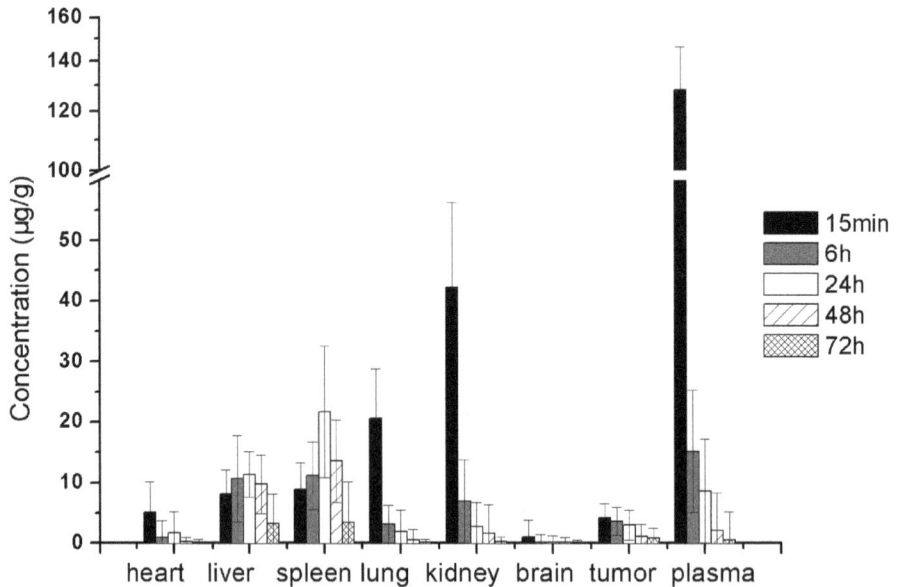

Figure 4. Biodistribution of 5-FA (A) and 5-FA-PAE (B) after *i.v.* injection. The tumor-bearing animal model was established by subcutaneous injection of H22 cells into Kunming mice. The control group and the test groups were administered intravenously with 20 mg/kg of 5-FA or 5-FA-PAE (equivalent to 20 mg/kg of 5-FA), respectively. The mice were exsanguinated and sacrificed at predetermined time points. Tissues (heart, liver, spleen, lung, kidney, brain and tumor) were collected, weighed and homogenized with two fold concentrated physiological saline. The samples of the test group were treated as hydrolyzed samples, whereas those of the control group were treated as unhydrolyzed samples. All data are presented as the concentration of 5-FA. Each value represents the mean ± standard deviation (n = 6).

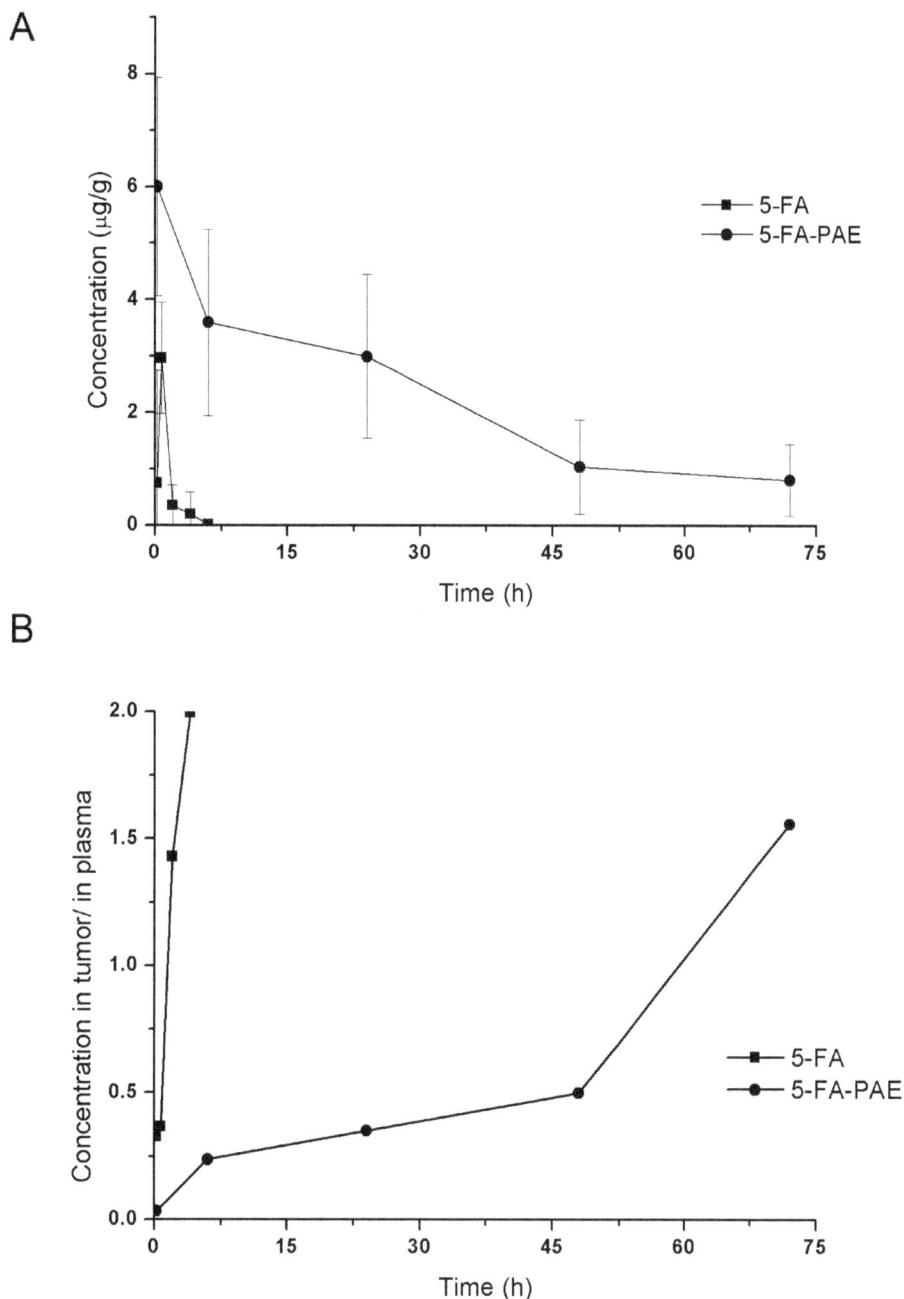

Figure 5. Drug concentration in tumor and plasma. The tumor-bearing mice model was described in the "In vivo biodistribution" section. The control group and the test groups were administered intravenously with 20 mg/kg of 5-FA and 5-FA-PAE (equivalent to 20 mg/kg of 5-FA), respectively. (A) Drug concentration of 5-FA and conjugated 5-FA-PAE in tumor at different time points. (B) Ratio of drug concentration in tumor vs. that in plasma of 5-FA and conjugated 5-FA-PAE.

adopted the ectopic model. After intravenous injection, at all time points, the concentration of 5-FA in kidney was significantly higher than other organs and in the tumor, suggesting that renal excretion was the major pathway of 5-FA elimination from the body. Other than kidney, 5-FA did not show any specificity in distribution with similar drug concentrations in heart, liver, spleen, lung and tumor. 15 min after the intravenous injection of 5-FA-PAE, the plasma concentration was the highest of all samples (128.1 ± 18.3 µg/g). However, as the time increased, the plasma concentration of 5-FA-PAE decreased rapidly, dropping to

$8,57 \pm 3.33$ µg/g at 24 h, while the concentration in liver and spleen increased gradually and peaked at 24 h (11.35 ± 3.78 µg/g in liver and 21.68 ± 10.83 µg/g in spleen). 5-FA-PAE was detectable in all organs and tumor at 72 h after injection (consistent with the pharmacokinetics study), indicating that the retention time of 5-FA-PAE was longer than 5-FA (Fig. 4A and 4B).

The concentration of 5-FA and 5-FA-PAE in tumor is shown in Fig 5A. The concentration of 5-FA decreased rapidly after administration and was undetectable after 6 h. Though the

A

B

saline   5-FA-PAE   5-FA   5-FU

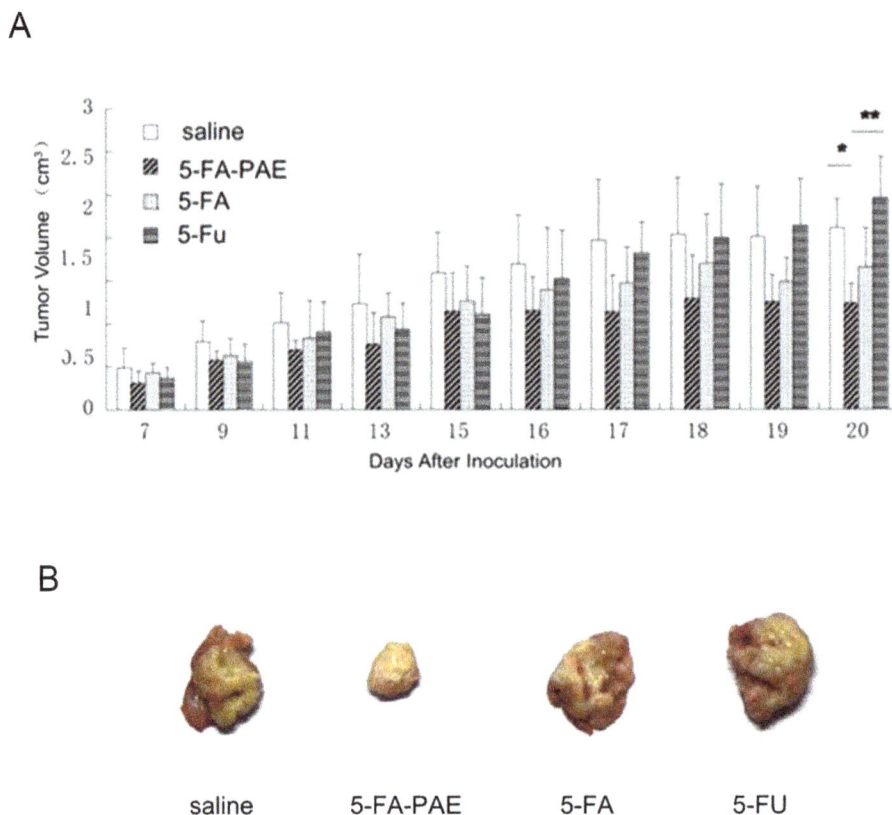

Figure 6. The antitumor effects on tumor-bearing mice. Mice were i.v injected with saline (20 mg/kg, 0.160 mmol/kg), 5-FA-PAE (284 mg/kg, 0.160 mmol/kg), 5-FA (30 mg/kg, 0.160 mmol/kg) or 5-Fu (20.47 mg/kg, 0.160 mmol/kg) on day 3, 5, 7, 9, 11, 13 and 15 after inoculation of H22 cells. On day 20, mice were sacrificed. Tumors and organs were removed and weighed. (A) The tumor volumes after inoculation (n = 6–12). * $p < 0.05$, ** $p < 0.01$. (B) Images of tumors in tumor-bearing mice on day 20 after inoculation of tumor cells (n = 6).

maximum concentration of 5-FA-PAE was slightly lower than 5-FA at 15 min after injection (4.22±2.3 µg/g for 5-FA-PAE and 4.86±1.62 µg/g for 5-FA), the concentration of 5-FA-PAE remained at a relatively high level and lasted for 72 h, indicating that 5-FA-PAE could slowly release 5-FA in the tumor and exert an antitumor effect. The concentration in the tumor vs. those in plasma of 5-FA-PAE and 5-FA is displayed in Fig. 5B. 45 min after administration, the concentration of 5-FA in tumor was lower than that in plasma, and then increased rapidly afterwards. 4 h after injection, the ratio of tumor/plasma concentration reached 1.99, suggesting that 5-FA could distribute from plasma to tumor within a short time, and that the clearance rate of 5-FA in plasma was higher than that in the tumor. 6 h after administration, the 5-FA concentration was almost undetectable in both plasma and tumor. The ratio of tumor/plasma concentration of 5-FA-PAE increased steadily within 48 h after injection and was lower than 0.5. Between 48 h to 72 h, the ratio increased quickly and reached 1.56 at 72 h, indicating that the clearance of 5-FA-PAE from tumor was much lower than that from the plasma. These results indicated that the amount of 5-FA-PAE in tumor lasted longer compared with that of 5-FA, exhibiting a sustained-release profile.

Table 4. Tumor weight and tumor control rate of mice administrated with saline, 5-Fu, 5-FA or 5-FA-PAE.

Treatment	Tumor weight (g)	Tumor control rate (%)
saline	2.229±0.521	-
5-FA-PAE	1.072±0.249 **	51.9±11.2$^\Delta$
5-FA	1.449±0.392 *	35.0±17.6$^\Delta$
5-Fu	2.383±0.841	−6.9±37.7

*$p < 0.05$ vs. saline group.
**$p < 0.01$ vs. saline group.
$^\Delta p < 0.05$ vs. 5-Fu group.
Each value represents the mean ± SD (n = 6).

Table 5. The organ/body weight index of mice administrated with saline, 5-Fu, 5-FA or 5-FA-PAE.

Tissue	saline	5-FA-PAE	5-FA	5-Fu
Heart	0.440±0.047	0.431±0.042	0.443±0.031	0.424±0.038
Liver	5.643±0.291	6.255±1.023	5.737±1.068	5.601±0.897
Spleen	1.226±0.390	1.360±0.543	1.398±0.478	1.264±0.694
Lung	0.978±0.236	0.955±0.141	1.068±0.407	0.900±0.109
Kidney	1.368±0.131	1.377±0.083	1.426±0.113	1.298±0.089
Brain	1.355±0.110	1.317±0.203	1.421±0.302	1.452±0.308
Thymus	0.192±0.097	0.261±0.070	0.221±0.155	0.167±0.086
Tumor	7.088±1.961	3.381±1.224*$^\Delta$	4.957±2.336	8.816±3.578

*$p < 0.05$ vs. saline group.
$^\Delta p < 0.05$ vs. 5-Fu group.
Each value represents the mean ± SD (n = 6).

Though the initial concentration and tumor/blood concentration ratio of 5-FA were higher than 5-FA-PAE, a high elimination rate of 5-FA severely limited its therapeutic effect in clinic. In comparison, the concentration of 5-FA-PAE in the tumor could be maintained at a relatively high level, which lasted for more than 70 h, despite the large variation (probably due to inter-individual difference). Similarly, the tumor/blood concentration ratio of 5-FA-PAE showed a gradually increasing trend.

Antitumor effect in tumor-bearing mice

5-Fu is the first-choice antimetabolite in the treatment of colon cancer and colorectal cancer. 5-FA, a derivative of 5-Fu, has been reported to be effective and safe [56–59]. To address the antitumor activity of the prodrug, 5-FA and 5-Fu were both used as controls. In the pharmacokinetics studies of anticancer drugs, two dosing regimens are commonly used. One is the preventive administration strategy in which drugs are administered at the beginning of the tumor growth. The other one is the therapeutic administration with drugs administered when the tumor growth reached a certain size. Since the relatively high mortality rate of the H22 tumor model in the later period of this experiment, we adopted a prophylactic administration scheme, i.e. 72 h after inoculation, mice with no signs of tumor growth were excluded from this experiment. Based on the pharmacokinetics and biodistribution results, we administered the drugs every other day (from day 3 to day 15 after inoculation). The antitumor effect of 5-FA-PAE was assessed by analyzing tumor volume, tumor control rate and the organ/body weight index of tumor-bearing mice. From the beginning of administration, the tumor volume of 5-FA-PAE group was smaller than that of the saline group, showing the highest antitumor activity (Figure 6A and 6B). The 5-FA and 5-Fu groups also displayed some antitumor effect. However, after the last administration on day 15, the tumor volume of these two groups increased obviously, while the tumor size of the 5-FA-PAE group did not, which suggested that the antitumor activity of 5-FA-PAE could last for a longer time. This is compatible with the pharmacokinetics results in which 5-FA-PAE showed a much longer retention time than that of 5-FA. 20 days after inoculation, the average tumor volume of 5-FA-PAE group was significantly smaller than that of the 5-Fu and saline groups ($p < 0.01$). However, no significant differences were observed between the 5-FA and 5-FA-PAE groups. This may be due to the large variation of the 5-FA group.

Though the tumor control rates of the 5-FA-PAE and 5-FA groups were not significantly different ($p > 0.05$), the tumor control rates of the 5-FA-PAE group (51.9±11.2%) and the 5-FA group (35.0±17.6%) were significantly higher than that of the 5-Fu and saline groups (Table 4). Since the tumor growth can affect the weight of normal organs, the organ/body weight index was used to assess the impact. The tumor/body index of the 5-FA-PAE (3.381±1.224) group was much lower than those of the 5-Fu (8.816±3.578) and saline groups (7.088±1.961, $p < 0.05$, Table 5). No significant differences were observed in other organ/body indices.

Owing to the conjugation with PEG, 5-FA-PAE exhibited a longer retention time, which led to a long-lasting antitumor effect. Notably, during the administration period, the death rate in the tumor-bearing mice of the 5-FA-PAE group is relatively high. This is probably due to the tumor growth and the toxicity of 5-FA-PAE, which is also a drawback of our present regimen and needs further refinement. However, after administration of all doses, no more deaths were observed in the 5-FA-PAE group, indicating that the toxicity caused by repeated administration of 5-FA-PAE was reversible. While in the 5-FA and 5-Fu groups, large number of animal deaths were observed after all administrations, suggesting a shorter duration of their antitumor effect.

Conclusion

To solve the paradox of drug loading and the molecular weight of PEG, we synthesized a PEG multi-hydroxyl derivative (PAE). PAE was coupled with 5-FA via ester bonds to afford 5-FA-PAE, and the drug loading efficiency was shown to be 10.8-fold higher than using unmodified PEG. Besides, the retention time and bioavailability of 5-FA-PAE were greatly improved compared to 5-FA, showing a prolonged half-life and improved antitumor efficacy *in vivo*. Owing to the improved drug loading efficiency and prolonged half-life, the multi-hydroxyl PEG derivative PAE proves to be an efficient carrier for 5-Fu. Future study should focus on further improving the tumor-targeting efficiency and the antitumor effect of 5-FA-PAE while reducing its toxicity. This paper provides some insights for the future development of antitumor drugs using PEG as a drug carrier.

Supporting Information

File S1 Supporting files. Figure S1, Identification of different polymers. The ^{1}H-NMR spectra of 5-Fu (A), 5-FA (B), PEG (C), the polymeric carrier PAE (D) and the prodrug 5-FA-PAE (E). **Table S1**, The number of blood platelets in mice administered with saline, 5-Fu, 5-FA, PAE or 5-FA-PAE. ($\times 10^9/$ L). **Table S2**, Plasma concentration of 5-FA and 5-FA-PAE at different time points.

Author Contributions

Conceived and designed the experiments: ZL XS TG ZZ. Performed the experiments: ZL. Analyzed the data: ML. Wrote the paper: ML.

References

1. Sarkar FH (2010) Recent trends in anti-cancer drug discovery. Mini Rev Med Chem 10: 357–358.
2. Na Y (2009) Recent cancer drug development with xanthone structures. J Pharm Pharmacol 61: 707–712.
3. Meada H (2001) SMANCS and polymer-conjugates macromolecular drug: advantages in cancer chemotherapy. Adv Drug Deliv Rev 46: 169–185.
4. Dang CT (2006) Drug treatments for adjuvant chemotherapy in breast cancer: recent trials and future directions. Expert Rev Anticancer Ther 6: 427–436.
5. Thompson N, Lyons J (2005) Recent progress in targeting the Raf/MEK/ERK pathway with inhibitors in cancer drug discovery. Curr Opin Pharmacol 5: 350–356.
6. Kelloff GJ, Boone CW, Malone W, Steele V (1993) Recent results in preclinical and clinical drug development of chemopreventive agents at the National Cancer Institute. Basic Life Sci 61: 373–386.
7. Sartor O, Halstead M, Katz L (2010) Improving outcomes with recent advances in chemotherapy for castrate-resistant prostate cancer. Clin Genitourin Cancer 8: 23–28.
8. Deeken JF, Figg WD, Bates SE, Sparreboom A (2007) Toward individualized treatment: prediction of anticancer drug disposition and toxicity with pharmacogenetics. Anti-cancer Drugs 18: 111–126.
9. Kintzel PE, Dorr RT (1995) Anticancer drug renal toxicity and elimination: dosing guidelines for altered renal function. Cancer Treat Rev 21: 33–64.
10. Duschinsky R, Pleven E, Heidelberger C (1957) The synthesis of 5-fluoropyrimidines. J Chem Soc 79: 4559–4560.
11. Ogiso T, Noda N, Asai N, Kato Y (1976) Antitumor agents. I. Effect of 5-fluorouracil and cyclophosphamide on liver microsomes and thymus of rat. Jpn J Pharmacol 26: 445–453.
12. Ogiso T, Noda N, Masuda H, Kato Y (1978) Antitumor agents. II. Effect of 5-fluorouracil and cyclophosphamide on immunological parameters and liver microsomes of tumor-bearing rats. Jpn J Pharmacol 28: 175–183.
13. Parker WB, Cheng YC (1990) Metabolism and mechanism of action of 5-fluorouracil. Pharmacol Ther 48: 381–395.
14. Macdonald JS (1999) Toxicity of 5-fluorouracil. Oncology 13: 33–34.
15. Shuey DL, Setzer RW, Lau C, Zucker RM, Elstein KH, et al. (1995) Biological modeling of 5-fluorouracil developmental toxicity. Toxicology 102: 207–213.
16. Van Kuilenburg AB, Meinsma R, Van Gennip AH (2004) Pyrimidine degradation defects and severe 5-fluorouracil toxicity. Nucleosides, Nucleotides and Nucleic Acids 23: 1371–1375.
17. Iyer L, Ratain MJ (1999) 5-fluorouracil pharmacokinetics: causes for variability and strategies for modulation in cancer chemotherapy. Cancer Invest 17: 494–506.
18. Milano G, Chamorey AL (2002) Clinical pharmacokinetics of 5-fluorouracil with consideration of chronopharmacokinetics. Chronobiol Int 19: 177–189.
19. Schalhorn A, Kühl M (1992) Clinical pharmacokinetics of fluorouracil and folinic acid. Semin Oncol 19: 82–92.
20. Pazdur R, Hoff PM, Medgyesy D, Royce M, Brito R (1998) The oral fluorouracil prodrugs. Oncology 12: 48–51.
21. Malet-Martino M, Martino R (2002) Clinical studies of three oral prodrugs of 5-fluorouracil (capecitabine, UFT, S-1): a review. Oncologist 7: 288–323.
22. Wang JX, Sun X, Zhang ZR (2002) Enhanced brain targeting by synthesis of 3′,5′-dioctanoyl-5-fluoro-2′-deoxyuridine and incorporation into solid lipid nanoparticles. Eur J Pharm Biopharm 54: 285–290.
23. Arias JL (2008) Novel strategies to improve the anticancer action of 5-fluorouracil by using drug delivery systems. Molecules 13: 2340–2369.
24. Menei P (1999) Local and sustained delivery of 5-Fluorouracil from biodegradable microspheres for the radiosensitization of glioblastoma. Cancer 86: 325–330.
25. Gupta Y, Jain A, Jain P, Jain SK (2007) Design and development of folate appended liposomes for enhanced delivery of 5-FU to tumor cells. J.Drug Targeting 15: 231–240.
26. Azori M (1987) Polymeric prodrugs. Crit Rev Ther Drug Carrier Syst 4: 39–65.
27. Hoste K, De Winne K, Schacht E (2004) Polymeric prodrugs. Int J Pharm 277: 119–131.
28. D'Souza AJM, Topp EM (2004) Release from polymeric prodrugs: linkages and their degradation. J Pharm Sci 93: 1962–1979.
29. Takakura Y, Hashida M (1995) Macromolecular drug carrier systems in cancer chemotherapy: macromolecular prodrugs. Crit Rev Oncol Hematol 18: 207–231.
30. Onishi H, Machida Y (2008) In vitro and in vivo evaluation of microparticulate drug delivery systems composed of macromolecular prodrugs. Molecules 13: 2136–2155.
31. Huang Y, Park YS, Wang J, Moon C, Kwon YM, et al (2010) ATTEMPTS system: a macromolecular prodrug strategy for cancer drug delivery. Curr Pharm Des 16: 2369–2376.
32. Goh PP, Sze DM, Roufogalis BD (2007) Molecular and cellular regulators of cancer angiogenesis. Curr Cancer Drug Targets 7: 743–758.
33. Maeda H, Fang J, Inutsuka T, Kitamono Y (2003) Vascular permeability enhancement in solid tumor: various factors, mechanisms involved and its implications. Int Immunopharmacol 3: 319–328.
34. Maeda H, Wu J, Sawa T, Matsumura Y, Hori K (2000) Tumor vascular permeability and the EPR effect in macromolecular therapeutics: a review. J Control Release 65: 271–284.
35. Maeda H, Bharate GY, Daruwalla J (2009) Polymeric drugs for efficient tumor-targeted drug delivery based on EPR-effect. Eur J Pharm Biopharm 71: 409–419.
36. Sawa T, Wu J, Akaike T, Maeda H (2000) Tumor-targeting chemotherapy by a xanthine oxidase-polymer conjugate that generates oxygen-free radicals in tumor tissue. Cancer Res 60: 666–671.
37. Pasut G, Veronese FM (2007) Polymer-drug conjugation, recent achievements and general strategies. Prog Polym Sci 32: 933–961.
38. Veronese FM, Harris JM (2002) Theme issue on "Peptide and Protein Pegylation I". Adv Drug Deliv Rev 54: 453–606.
39. Zhao H, Rubio B, Sapra P, Wu D, Reddy P, et al (2008) Novel prodrugs of SN38 using multiarm poly(ethylene glycol) linkers. Bioconjug Chem 19: 849–859.
40. Rowinsky EK, Rizzo J, Ochoa L, Takimoto CH, Forouzesh B, et al. (2003) A phase I and pharmacokinetic study of pegylated camptothecin as a 1-hour infusion every 3 weeks in pantients with advanced solid malignances. J Clin Oncol 21: 148–157.
41. Guo Z, Wheler JJ, Naing A, Mani S, Goel S, et al. (2008) Clinical pharmacokinetics (PK) of EZN-2208, a novel anticancer agent, in patients (pts) with advanced malignancies: a phase I, first-in-human, dose-escalation study. J Clin Oncol 26: 2556.
42. Ton NC, Parker GJ, Jackson A, Mullamitha S, Buonaccorsi GA, et al. (2007) Phase I evaluation of CDP791, a PEGylated di-Fab' conjugate that binds vascular endothelial growth factor receptor 2. Clin Cancer Res 13: 7113–7118.
43. Michallet M, Maloisel F, Delain M, Hellmann A, Rosas A, et al. (2004) Pegylated recombinant interferon-a lpha-2b vs recombinant interferon-alpha-2b for the initial treatment of chronic-phase chronic myelogenous leukemia: a phase III study. Leukemia 18: 309–315.
44. Hwu WJ, Panageas KS, Menell JH, Lamb LA, Aird S, et al. (2006) Phase II study of temozolomide plus pegylated interferon-alpha-2b for metastatic melanoma. Cancer 106: 2445–2451.
45. Pasut G, Veronese FM (2009) PEG conjugates in clinical development or use as anticancer agents: an overview. Adv Drug Deliv Rev 61: 1177–1188.
46. Koyama Y, Umehara M, Mizuno A, Itaba M, Yasukouchi T, et al. (1996) Synthesis of novel poly(ethylene glycol) derivatives having pendant amino groups and aggregating behavior of its mixture with fatty acid in water. Bioconjug Chem 7: 298–301.
47. Burton SC, Harding DRK (1998) Preparation of chromatographic matrices by free radical addition ligand attachment to allyl groups. J Chromatogr A 796: 273–282.
48. Hao AJ, Deng YJ, Li TF, Suo XB,Cao YH, et al. (2006) Degradation kinetics of fluorouracil-acetic-acid-dextran conjugate in aqueous solution. Drug Dev Ind Pharm 32: 757–763.
49. Udo K, Hokonohara K, Motoyama K, Arima H, Hirayama F, et al. (2010) 5-Fluorouracil acetic acid/beta-cyclodextrin conjugates: drug release behavior in enzymatic and rat cecal media. Int J Pharm 388: 95–100.
50. Smyth HF Jr Carpenter CP, Weil CS (1950) The toxicology of the polyethylene glycols. J Am Pharm Assoc 39: 349–354.
51. Richter AW, Akerblom E (1983) Antibodies against polyethylene glycol produced in animals by immunization with monomethoxy polyethylene glycol modified proteins. Int Arch Allergy Appl Immunol 70: 124–131.
52. Zalipsky S, Gilon C, Zilkha A (1983) Attachment of drugs to polyethylene glycols. Eur Polym J 19: 1177–1183.
53. Sheridan W, Menchaca D (1998) Overview of the safety and biologic effects of PEG-rHuMGDF in clinical trials. Stem Cells 16: 193–198.
54. Riebeseel K, Biedermann E, Löser R, Breiter N, Hanselmann R, et al. (2002) Polyethylene glycol conjugates of methotrexate varying in their molecular weight from MW 750 to MW 40000: synthesis, characterization, and structure-activity relationships in vitro and in vivo. Bioconjug Chem 13: 773–785.

55. Greenwald RB, Gilbert CW, Pendri A, Conover CD, Xia J, et al. (1996) Drug delivery systems: water soluble taxol 2'-poly(ethylene glycol) ester prodrugs-design and in vivo effectiveness. Med Chem 39: 424–431.

56. Chung SM, Yoon EJ, Kim SH, Lee MG, Heejoo L, et al. (1991) Pharmacokinetics of 5-fluorouracil after intravenous infusion of 5-fluorouracil-acetic acid-human serum albumin conjugates to rabbits. Int J Pharm 68: 61–68.

57. Zuo D, Jiang T, Guan H, Wang KQ, Qi X, et al. (2001) Synthesis, Structure and Antitumor Activity of Dibutyltin Oxide Complexes with 5-Fluorouracil Derivatives. Crystal Structure of [(5-Fluorouracil)-1-$CH_2CH_2COOSn(n$-Bu$)_2]_4O_2$. Molecules 6: 647–654.

58. Kang NI, Lee SM, Maeda M, Ha CS, Cho WJ (2002) Synthesis, antitumour and DNA replication activities of polymers containing vinyl-(5-fluorouracil)-ethanoate. Polym Int 51: 443–449.

59. Yang ZY, Wang LF, Yang XP, Wang DW, Li YM (2000) Pharmacological study on antitumor activity of 5-fluorouracil-1-acetic acid and its rare earth complexes. J Rare Earth 18: 140–143.

8

Intravenous Remifentanil versus Epidural Ropivacaine with Sufentanil for Labour Analgesia

Rong Lin[9], **Yiyi Tao**[9], **Yibing Yu**[9], **Zhendong Xu**, **Jing Su**, **Zhiqiang Liu***

Department of Anaesthesiology, Shanghai First Maternity and Infant Hospital, Tongji University School of Medicine, Shanghai, China

Abstract

Remifentanil with appropriate pharmacological properties seems to be an ideal alternative to epidural analgesia during labour. A retrospective cohort study was undertaken to assess the efficacy and safety of remifentanil intravenous patient-controlled analgesia (IVPCA) compared with epidural analgesia. Medical records of 370 primiparas who received remifentanil IVPCA or epidural analgesia were reviewed. Pain and sedation scores, overall satisfaction, the extent of pain control, maternal side effects and neonatal outcome as primary observational indicators were collected. There was a significant decline of pain scores in both groups. Pain reduction was greater in the epidural group throughout the whole study period (0~180 min) (P<0.0001), and pain scores in the remifentanil group showed an increasing trend one hour later. The remifentanil group had a lower SpO_2 (P<0.0001) and a higher sedation score (P<0.0001) within 30 min after treatment. The epidural group had a higher overall satisfaction score (3.8±0.4 vs. 3.7±0.6, P = 0.007) and pain relief score (2.9±0.3 vs. 2.8±0.4, P<0.0001) compared with the remifentanil group. There was no significant difference on side effects between the two groups, except that a higher rate of dizziness (1% vs. 21.8%, P<0.0001) was observed during remifentanil analgesia. And logistic regression analysis demonstrated that nausea, vomiting were associated with oxytocin usage and instrumental delivery, and dizziness was associated to the type and duration of analgesia. Neonatal outcomes such as Apgar scores and umbilical-cord blood gas analysis were within the normal range, but umbilical pH and base excess of neonatus in the remifentanil group were significantly lower. Remifentanil IVPCA provides poorer efficacy on labor analgesia than epidural analgesia, with more sedation on parturients and a trend of newborn acidosis. Despite these adverse effects, remifentanil IVPCA can still be an alternative option for labor analgesia under the condition of one-to-one bedside care, continuous monitoring, oxygen supply and preparation for neonatal resuscitation.

Editor: Sam Eldabe, The James Cook University Hospital, United Kingdom

Funding: These authors have no support or funding to report.

Competing Interests: The authors have declared that no competing interests exist.

* Email: drliuzhq@hotmail.com

[9] These authors contributed equally to this work.

Introduction

Epidural analgesia is efficient to relieve labour pain with fewer side effects on parturients and neonatus and regarded as the gold standard for obstetric analgesia [1]. However, some certain clinical conditions restrict its administration, such as maternal rejection or noncooperation, coagulation disorders, infection or tumor close to site of puncture, allergic reaction to local anesthetic, and spinal deformity [2]. It is clear that an effective and safe alternative should be established.

Remifentanil for intravenous patient-controlled analgesia (IVPCA) seems to be a promising option because of its particular pharmacokinetic and pharmacodynamic characteristics. Remifentanil as an ultra short-acting synthetic opioid has a very fast onset time (30~60 s), peak analgesic effect of 2.5 min, a high metabolic rate (context-sensitive half-life about 3~4 min), and no accumulated effect with repeated or long-term use [3–5]. Although it crosses the placental barrier with no difficulty, the drug can be degraded rapidly in the foetus [6].

A lot of studies with respect to the efficacy and complications of remifentanil for labour analgesia have been carried out. A prospective, randomised study from Douma et al. [7] on a group of only 20 patients discovered superior anesthetic effect was provided by epidural analgesia compared with remifentanil IVPCA. Volmanen et al. [8] designed a controlled, double-blinded study (42 parturients were randomly recruited) to observed analgesic efficacy of remifentanil and epidural analgesia just lasting for 60 min during the first stage of labour, and also reached similar conclusions. But they only evaluated fetal heart rate (FHR), umbilical artery pH and 1 min Apgar scores as fetal outcomes. Another randomised, controlled trial of Tveit et al. [9] (EA group 20, RA group 17) reported that remifentanil was more likely to cause sedation and oxygen desaturation, but was safe to neonates. In our recent meta-analysis involving 5 studies, remifentanil IVPCA was not found to afford better pain relief than epidural analgesia, but it did not bring serious adverse outcomes to mother and newborn [10]. Since most of these studies were somewhat limited by small sample sizes, a short observation period or inadequate assessment, it still remains controversial whether we can administrate remifentanil during labour without worry.

Thus we conducted this large sample study to retrospectively investigate maternal and neonatal outcomes of remifentanil IVPCA compared with epidural analgesia.

Materials and Methods

The study obtained approval from the Research Ethics Committee of Shanghai First Maternity and Infant Hospital. Written consent was obtained from each patient. All electronic medical records of parturients who had accepted intravenous remifentanil or epidural analgesia during labour in our institution from January 2013 to July 2013 were reviewed. Inclusion criteria were as follows: primipara (ASA status I or II), singleton pregnancy with cephalic presentation, gestational age of >36 weeks, spontaneous or induced labour. Records of women with request for caesarean section or stillbirth were excluded. In light of analgesia technique the eligible parturients elected, they were divided into two groups: the remifentanil group and the epidural group (Fig. 1).

Intravenous remifentanil analgesia regimen

Parturients were directed how to operate the PCA pump (Baxter 6060 Multi-Therapy infusion pump, Baxter Healthcare Corporation, Kista, Sweden) before the start of analgesia. The dosage regimen of remifentanil hydrochloride (Ultiva, GlaxoSmithKline, Oslo, Norway) diluted with saline to a concentration of $20~\mu g \cdot ml^{-1}$ was set to PCA bolus of $0.4~\mu g \cdot kg^{-1}$, a continuous background infusion at $0.04 \sim 0.05~\mu g \cdot kg^{-1} \cdot min^{-1}$ and a lockout time of 5 min. PCA doses were calculated according to estimated bodyweight (body height in centimeters -100) [9,11,12].

Epidural analgesia regimen

An epidural catheter was inserted in the epidural space at L2–3 or L3–4 with the patient in a lateral decubitus position by an anaesthesiologist. Then the same PCA pump was connected to the cannula. Parturients received a 10 ml initial loading dose of 0.068% ropivacaine and $0.3~\mu g \cdot ml^{-1}$ sufentanil, followed by a maintenance dose at $8~ml \cdot h^{-1}$ and a PCA bolus dose of 5 ml with a 15-min lockout interval. If necessary, the infusion dose could be adjusted (5–$10~ml \cdot h^{-1}$).

One-to-one nursing service was provided to every parturient entering into the delivery room. The analgesia was applied when the cervix dilated to 3 cm, and terminated before the beginning of the second stage of labor. Before administration of analgesia, intravenous infusion of lactated Ringers solution and oxygen inhalation through nasal tube were given by convention. Routine monitoring, including maternal noninvasive blood pressure (NIBP), heart rate (HR), pulse oxygen saturation (SpO_2), uterine activity and FHR by external tocodynamometry were accomplished and measured continuously. Numerical rating scale (NRS) pain score (an 11-point scale, $0 =$ no pain and $10 =$ worst pain imaginable) was used to assess the pain level. And the evaluation of sedation referred to the Ramsay sedation score ($1 =$ anxious, agitated, restless; $2 =$ cooperative, oriented, tranquil; $3 =$ responds to simple commands only; $4 =$ brisk response to light glabellar tap or loud auditory stimulation; $5 =$ sluggish response to light glabellar tap or loud auditory stimulation; $6 =$ no response to light glabellar tap or loud auditory stimulus). Non-invasive measurements mentioned above as well as pain and sedation scores were recorded before and immediately after treatment, afterwards every 30 min.

The day after delivery, parturients were asked about their overall satisfaction with analgesic therapy on a five-point verbal rating scale ($0 =$ very dissatisfied, $1 =$ dissatisfied, $2 =$ neutral [neither satisfied nor dissatisfied], $3 =$ satisfied, $4 =$ very satisfied), and to express the degree of pain relief likewise on a 5-point

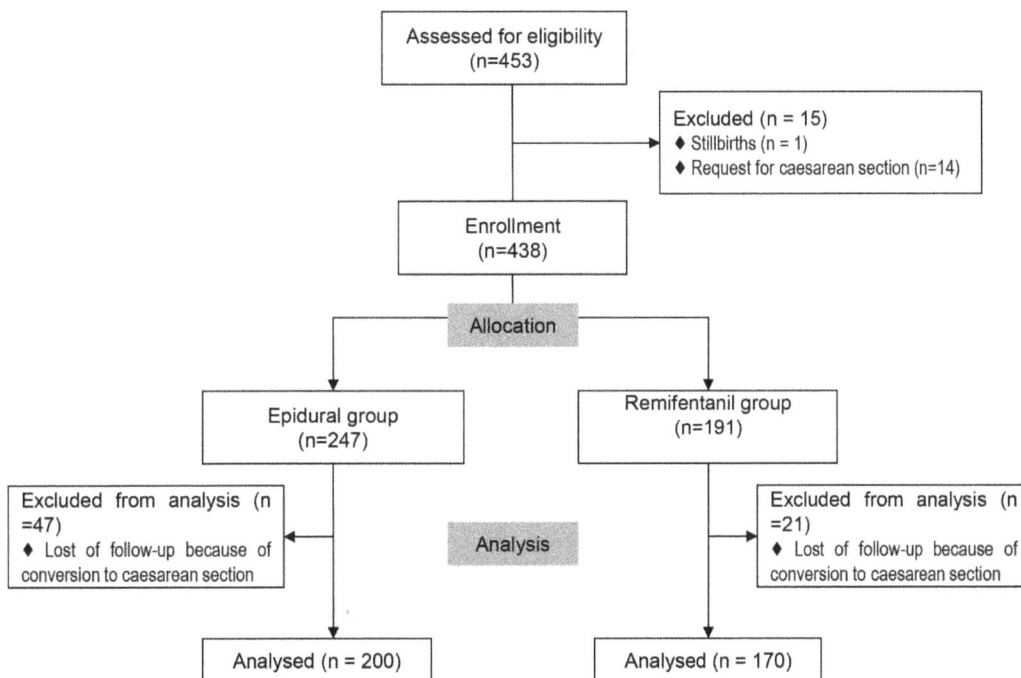

Figure 1. Flow-process diagram of the retrospective study.

categorical scale (0 = very poor, 1 = poor, 2 = moderate, 3 = good, 4 = very good) [9].

Excepting above, other data collected included: maternal demographic characteristics (age, gestational weeks, height, weight, BMI), delivery mode, oxytocin treatment, durations of analgesia, maternal adverse reactions (respiratory depression, excessive sedation, nausea and vomiting, skin pruritus), neonatal outcomes (Apgar scores at 1 and 5 min, umbilical-cord blood gas analysis, requirement for resuscitation).

Statistical analysis

SPSS version 18.0 (SPSS Inc., Chicago, IL, USA) was used for all data analysis. As a general rule, data were expressed as mean ± SD or frequency (percentage). P values less than 0.05 were considered statistically significant. Continuous variables were processed with Student's t-test. And Chi-square test was performed for categorical variables. To evaluate the relationship of side effects to other factors, logistic regression analysis was performed.

Results

Through reviewing the database, we identified 453 medical records that met inclusion criteria. Among them, fifteen subjects were ruled out on account of stillbirth (n = 1) or request for caesarean section (n = 14). Follow-ups of sixty-eight parturients were brought to a close due to their conversion to caesarean section. Finally, the following analysis was on the base of 370 observations (Epidural group 200, Remifentanil group 170) (Fig. 1). The conversive rate of caesarean section in the epidural group is significantly higher than in the remifentanil group (19.0% vs. 11.0%, P = 0.021). But there was no statistically significant difference between the two groups with regard to the indications for cesarean section (Table 1).

Table 1 demonstrated that parturients in the remifentanil group were taller in height and had a shorter duration of analgesia compared to those in the epidural group. Besides that, there was no statistically significant difference between the two groups as regards other demographic characteristics, mode of delivery and oxytocin utilization.

Comparing the two groups, pain scores were similar at baseline. After analgesic therapy, a significant decline in pain scores from baseline was discovered in both groups, and epidural pain scores decreased more at every given point in time (P<0.0001). One-hour treatment later, pain scores in the remifentanil group went steadily up but still inferior to the baseline. By comparison, the ascending tendency was minimal in the epidural group (Fig. 2).

Immediately after remifentanil analgesia, oxygen saturation reduced obviously compared to baseline (P<0.0001). And at that time point and 30 min after analgesia, mean SpO_2 of the remifentanil group was lower than that of the epidural group, with significant difference (P<0.0001). Nevertheless, those who suffered from desaturation could recover their original state rapidly by deep breaths and supplementary oxygen. By contrast, oxygen saturation of those receiving epidural analgesia remained stable throughout the whole childbirth (Fig. 3). No respiratory depression (RR<9 breaths/min or SpO_2<90%) was discovered in both groups.

The Ramsay sedation scores were significantly higher in the remifentanil group immediately and 30 min after treatment (P< 0.0001 and P<0.001, respectively) (Fig. 4). Six women following remifentanil regimen reached the maximum sedation score of 4.

The epidural group had a higher overall satisfaction score (3.8±0.4 vs. 3.7±0.6, P = 0.007) and pain relief score (2.9±0.3 vs. 2.8±0.4, P<0.0001) compared with the remifentanil group. Although more parturients receiving remifentanil reported nausea, vomiting and pruritus, the incidences of the above adverse reactions were similar between the two regimens. 21.8% of patients in the remifentanil group encountered dizziness, which was far higher than that in the epidural group (Table 2). Furthermore, logistic regression analysis demonstrated that nausea, vomiting were associated with oxytocin usage and

Table 1. Maternal demographic characteristics and labour data.

	Epidural Group (n = 200)	Remifentanil Group (n = 170)	P value
Age (years)	29.3±3.1	29.6±3.2	0.208
Gestational age (weeks)	39.6±1.1	39.6±1.0	0.817
Height (cm)	1.60±0.03	1.61±0.03	0.024
Weight (kg)	71.0±5.3	70.1±8.6	0.373
BMI (kg·m^{-2})	27.3±1.8	27.2±3.0	0.837
Duration of analgesia (min)	182.2±96.6	171.7±85.8	0.033
Oxytocin	88 (44%)	69 (40.6%)	0.508
Mode of delivery, n (%)			0.925
Spontaneous	191 (95.5%)	162 (95.3%)	
Instrumental	9 (4.5%)	8 (4.7%)	
Conversion to caesarean section, n (%)	47/247 (19.0%)	21/191 (11.0%)	0.021
Indications for cesarean delivery, n (%)			
Fetal distress	12/24 (25.5%)	8/21 (38.1%)	0.294
Prolonged labor	14/24 (29.8%)	7/21 (33.3%)	0.770
Cephalopelvic disproportion	13/24 (23.5%)	3/21 (14.3%)	0.230
Severe preeclampsia	3/24 (6.4%)	1/21 (4.8%)	0.793
Prenatal fever	5/24 (10.6%)	2/21 (9.5%)	0.889

Data are expressed as mean ± standard deviation or n (%). BMI = body mass index.

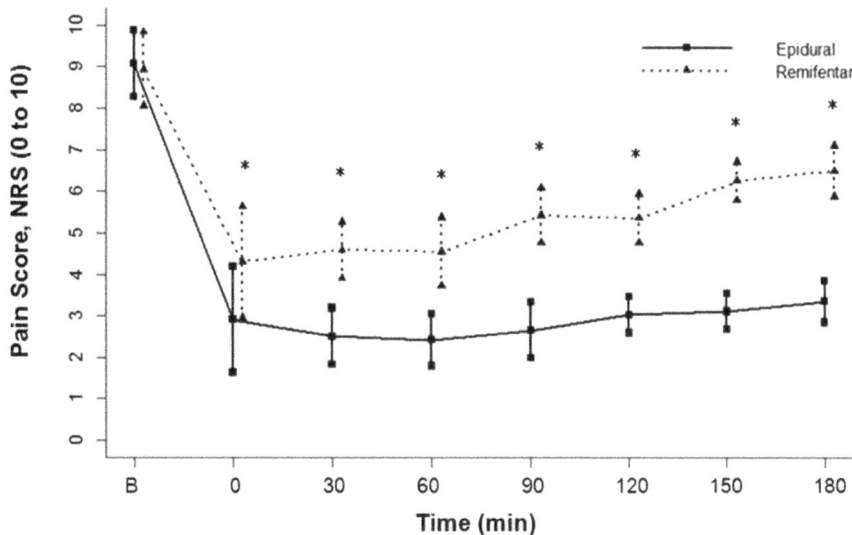

Figure 2. Comparisons in NRS pain scores between the two groups (Epidural group and Remifentanil group) at each time point. B represents baseline. NRS = numerical rating scale. *P<0.0001.

instrumental delivery, and dizziness was relative to the type and duration of analgesia (Table 3).

Neonatal data were summarized in Table 4. The analysis showed that there was no difference between the groups in relation to mean birth weight, Apgar scores and the incidence of abnormal FHR. FHR abnormalities included tachycardia, bradycardia, variable decelerations and late decelerations, and all were transient changes. The two groups were also similar with respect to the types of abnormal FHR. But umbilical pH and base excess of neonatus in the remifentanil group were significantly lower. Three newborns had 1 min Apgar scores <7, and all of them were from the epidural group. Two neonates were born after shoulder dystocia with Apgar score 4 and 5 for the 1st minute, and 8 and 7 for the 5th minute, respectively. The other had 1–5 min Apgar scores of 6–9 due to acute fetal distress. In addition, two neonates had an umbilical arterial pH<7.10, they were those who

experienced shoulder dystocia in the epidural group. But no umbilical venous pH<7.10 was registered.

Discussion

This research work shows that epidural analgesia appears to afford more preferable analgesia effect than remifentanil IVPCA. Pain scores reported from the epidural group were significantly lower at each set time-point (0, 30 min, 60 min, 90 min, 120 min, 150 min and 180 min after treatment), and epidural regimen produced more persistent contribution on labor analgesia. In relative terms, administration of remifentanil just had moderate pain reduction with gradual elevation of pain scores as the labor progressed. These findings were consistent with other recent studies [6,8,13–18]. Our previous meta-analysis has also demonstrated that there were higher pain scores at 1 h and 2 h for

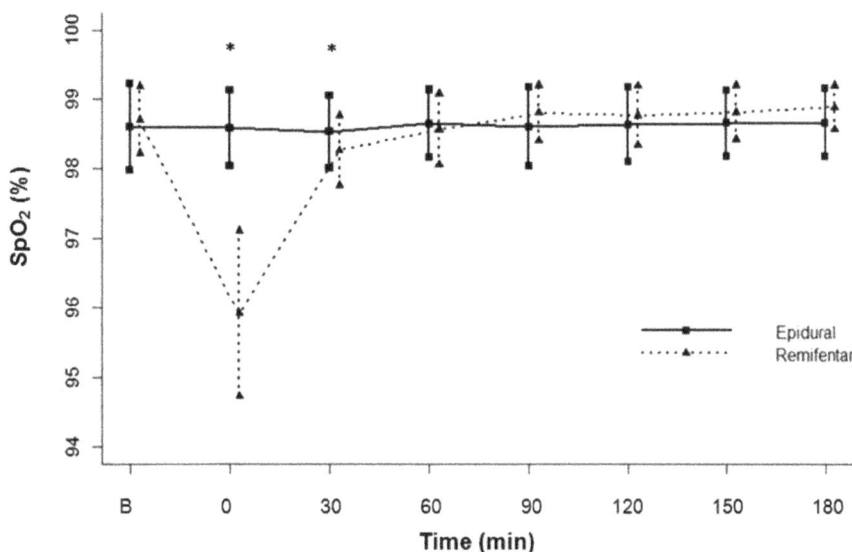

Figure 3. Comparisons in pulse oxygen saturation (SpO₂) between the two groups.

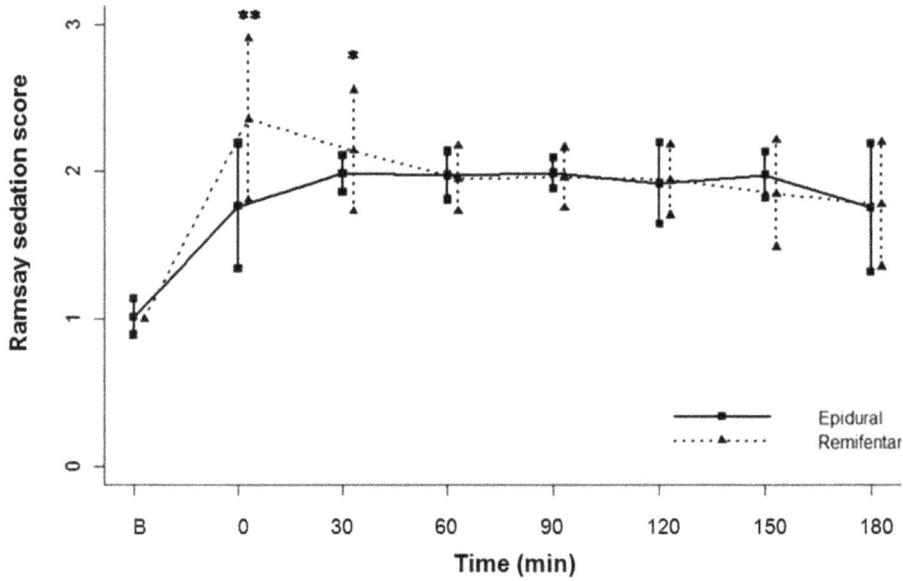

Figure 4. Comparisons in the Ramsay sedation score between the two groups (Epidural group and Remifentanil group) at each time point. B represents baseline. **P<0.0001, *P<0.001.

patients with remifentanil IVPCA compared with those receiving epidural analgesia [10]. At the beginning of remifentanil IVPCA, pain relief was still satisfactory because of its rapid onset. Progressive pain of uterus systole with the progress of labor and/or a tolerance to remifentanil after continuous use were probably responsible for the later rising pain scores in the remifentanil group [7,19]. Obviously, local anaesthetic by epidural had more control over the pain stress.

Although 92.4% of parturients with remifentanil IVPCA expressed satisfaction with analgesic effect (very satisfied: 77.1%, satisfied: 15.3%), the overall satisfaction scores and pain relief scores were lower in the remifentanil group, which seemed distinguished from those seen in other researches. Douma et al. [7] found there was no obvious distinction in satisfaction scores after delivery between the remifentanil group and the epidural group. Similarly, in the study of Stourac et al. [20], the level of the parturients' satisfaction with analgesia was similar both in the EA group and in the rPCA group (P = 0.24). One possible explanation for this was that these assessments carried subjective criteria to result in the difference. In addition, interindividual variation in the response to opioid [21,22] and the different administration schedules we adopted were likely to account for the disparity.

Table 2. Quality of analgesia and Side effects.

	Epidural Group (n = 200)	Remifentanil Group (n = 170)	P value
Overall satisfaction score	3.8±0.4	3.7±0.6	0.007
4- very satisfied	167 (83.5%)	131 (77.1%)	
3- satisfied	33 (16.5%)	26 (15.3%)	
2- neutral (neither satisfied nor dissatisfied)	0	13 (7.6%)	
1- dissatisfied	0	0	
0- very dissatisfied	0	0	
Pain relief score	2.9±0.3	2.8±0.4	<0.0001
4- very good	0	0	
3- good	185 (92.5%)	132 (77.6%)	
2- moderate	15 (7.5%)	38 (22.4%)	
1- poor	0	0	
0- very poor	0	0	
Dizziness	2 (1%)	37 (21.8%)	<0.0001
Nausea	11 (5.5%)	13 (7.6%)	0.403
Vomiting	9 (4.5%)	11 (6.5%)	0.404
Pruritus	3 (1.5%)	4 (2.4%)	0.548

Data are expressed as mean ± standard deviation or n (%).

Table 3. Multiple logistic regression analysis with side effects (nausea, vomiting and dizziness) as the dependent variable.

	OR	95% CI	P value
Nausea			
Oxytocin	0.23	0.09–0.59	0.0025
Instrumental	0.21	0.06–0.74	0.015
Vomiting			
Oxytocin	0.23	0.08–0.66	0.0064
Instrumental	0.17	0.05–0.59	0.0056
Dizziness			
Type of analgesia	32.35	7.52–139.18	<0.00015
Duration of analgesia	1.01	1.001–1.009	0.02

OR = odds ratio; CI = confidence interval.

Up to the present, the most suitable dosage regimen of remifentanil for labour still retains a controversial subject [23]. While the regimen without background infusion has been reported to produce superior effect on obstetric analgesia [14,24–28], recent researches indicated that fixed small PCA boluses with alterable infusion rate could provide effective analgesia with fewer adverse reactions [23]. Our dosage regimen of remifentanil ($0.04\sim0.05$ $\mu g \cdot kg^{-1} \cdot min^{-1}$ infusion and 0.4 $\mu g \cdot kg^{-1}$ PCA bolus) made reference to the previous studies and experiences from our institution. In clinical practice, we found remifentanil presented a delayed peak effect in spite of its quick onset. Thus PCA bolus alone could not act urgently to keep uterine contraction pain under control. Furthermore, a dose-related risk of respiratory depression and excessive sedation exist after remifentanil bolus injection, which has been discovered in healthy volunteers [29]. Some studies have recommended the bolus dose of 0.4 $\mu g \cdot kg^{-1}$ can be used effectively and securely [6,8,18,26,30], the infusion rate more than 0.05 $\mu g \cdot kg^{-1} \cdot min^{-1}$ may be connected with higher incidence of side effects [14].

In this study, a marked drop in maternal SpO_2 appeared within 30 min after using remifentanil. It may be related to a transient respiration inhibition at the onset of remifentanil. The oxygen desaturation (defined as $SpO_2 < 95\%$) episode persisted only for a brief duration, which could be reversed by deep breathing and oxygen inhalation through nasal tube. The incidence of oxygen desaturation we observed was 9.4%, far below other reported rates ($40\% \sim 74\%$) [14,16,18,31–33]. Perhaps that had something to do with preventive oxygen supply. And, continuous SpO_2 monitoring and bedside-monitor of the anaesthetist or midwife also contributed a great share in preventing desaturation, since hypoxia caused by remifentanil might still occur even in the situation of oxygen supply [8]. Besides, dehydration or exhaustion along with the application of remifentanil also could aggravate respiratory depression [34], so adequate transfusion treatment in advance is recommended.

Despite a higher level of sedation in the remifentanil group, all of patients could be awakened easily by a loud voice or the next uterine contraction pain. 21.8% of patients receiving remifentanil

Table 4. Neonatal outcomes.

	Epidural Group (n = 200)	Remifentanil Group (n = 170)	P value
Birth weight (g)	3399.8±382.9	3439.8±371.8	0.444
Apgar score			
1 min	9.7±0.8	9.7±0.6	0.984
5 min	9.9±0.3	9.9±0.3	0.712
Umbilical vein pH	7.31±0.07	7.29±0.07	0.015
Umbilical artery pH	7.28±0.07	7.26±0.06	0.001
Umbilical vein base excess (mol·l^{-1})	−4.50±2.13	−5.08±2.21	0.011
Umbilical artery base excess (mol·l^{-1})	−4.96±2.66	−6.13±2.33	<0.0001
Abnormal FHR changes, n (%)	27 (13.5%)	33 (19.4%)	0.124
During the analgesia period, n (%)	16/27 (59.3%)	24/33 (72.7%)	0.271
- Tachycardia, n (%)	3/16 (18.8%)	5/24 (20.8%)	0.601
- Bradycardia, n (%)	6/16 (37.5%)	11/24 (45.8%)	0.872
- Variable decelerations, n (%)	5/16 (31.3%)	7/24 (29.2%)	0.888
- Late decelerations, n (%)	2/16 (12.5%)	1/24 (4.2%)	0.327

Data are expressed as mean ± standard deviation or n (%). FHR = fetal heart rate.

reported dizziness, and we noted that a longer duration of remifentanil analgesia was more likely to cause dizziness. We speculated it might be related to a certain degree of cumulative effect. Yet, nobody complained uncomfortable for it. That being said, one-to-one nursing still needs to be ensured.

The frequencies of nausea, vomiting and pruritus were similar between the two groups, which were consistent with the results from previous studies [6,8,32,35]. Our analyses pointed out that some obstetric factors such as the usage of oxytocin and forceps may be associated with nausea and vomiting which are common during delivery. Studies showed that the occurance of nausea and vomiting is correlated to the degree of hypotension [36]. Higher doses of oxytocin or forceps delivery may lead to sudden haemodynamic change.

The impact of remifentanil on newborns has become a common concern. Neonatal outcomes observed in our study stayed at an acceptable level. Removed from two neonates with shoulder dystocia and one with acute fetal distress, other Apgar scores were normal. Besides, there were no significant differences in the incidence or types of abnormal FHR between the two groups. From the current data, systemic remifentanil seemed have no serious effect on FHR. However the fact that opioids have the capability of producing FHR abnormalities [6] cannot be taken lightly. We guessed close monitoring and routine oxygen supplementation should play a part in this. The mean umbilical cord gases in both groups were kept in normal range as well, whereas umbilical arterial/venous pH and base excess were lower in the remifentanil group. Our findings seemed to be different from previous studies [6,7,9,14,26,35], which found no effect from remifentanil on neonatal outcomes including umbilical pH and base excess. Despite the fact that remifentanil is easy to be metabolized in the neonates [30,37], it still has some influence on neonatal status. Therefore, we recommended neonatal resuscitation should be in train before birth for the neonates whose mothers have received remifentanil. 2010 American Heart Association Guidelines for Neonatal Resuscitation suggested that at least 1 person who must be capable of initiating resuscitation, including administration of positive pressure ventilation and chest compressions, should present at every delivery [38]. 2011 Chinese Neonatal Resuscitation Guidelines also have the same recommendations [39]. In our hospital, every delivery room keeps the necessary equipments and medications for resuscitation available. All practitioners in the delivery rooms including midwives are required to know the whole resuscitation process and have skills to perform the initial steps of resuscitation. The initial steps (about 60 s), which are called "the Golden Minute", will win precious rescue time for skilled personnel's arrival. Coordination between obstetrics and pediatrics, regular training, adequate preparation and prompt initiation of support are a forceful guarantee for successful neonatal resuscitation.

The demographics of two groups were matched except for height and duration of analgesia. The conversive rate and the indications of caesarean section are similar between the two groups. However, we have not been able to determine whether intravenous remifentanil for labour analgesia is helpful with lowering the conversive rate due to limited samples of our present study. As for the conversive rate of caesarean section in our study (15.5% [68/438]), it was really lower than figures reported in other studies. Ismail MT et al. [40] reported that the conversive rate in their study was 24.3%. We guessed it might be related to our inclusion criteria that only healthy primiparas without any obstetrics complications can be included. These patients were less likely to undergo caesarean section. Moreover, one-to-one bedside care, continuous monitoring, timely management and treatment may be also crucial to reduce the conversive rate of caesarean.

As a result of our retrospective study, the probability of missing data and selection bias is unavoidable. It is also the main limitation of our study. For instance, some data relating to blood pressure, heart rate, breathing rate and the quantities of drugs were not recorded completely and missing. A further prospective study will designed to refine the data. However, we believe the omissions and bias may be not big because we adopted a standardized analgesic procedure for labour and a detailed electronic recording system.

In this retrospective study, we confirmed that remifentanil IVPCA produced an observable improvement in pain scores, though not quite as efficacious as epidural analgesia. Furthermore, we also have reached some different conclusions from previous researches. For example, patients' satisfaction scores and neonatal umbilical cord gases in the remifentanil group were lower than those in the epidural group. As a systemic opioid, sedation, dizziness and desaturation were inevitable during using remifentanil. Fortunately, these adverse reactions were temporary and the effects on neonatal outcomes were small. We suggest that remifentanil analgesia can be implemented as an option for pain relief during childbirth under the precondition of ensuring one-to-one bedside care, continuous oxygen saturation monitoring, oxygen supply up front, and immediate availability of neonatal resuscitation.

Acknowledgments

The authors thank the three anonymous reviewers for their insightful comments and suggestions, which have led to a significantly improved paper.

Author Contributions

Conceived and designed the experiments: ZL. Performed the experiments: RL YT YY ZX JS. Analyzed the data: RL. Contributed reagents/materials/analysis tools: YT YY. Contributed to the writing of the manuscript: RL ZL.

References

1. Althaus J, Wax J (2005) Analgesia and anesthesia in labor. Obstet Gynecol Clin North Am 32: 231–244.
2. Miller RD (2010) Miller's anesthesia. Philadelphia, PA: Churchill Livingstone/ Elsevier.
3. Babenco HD, Conard PF, Gross JB (2000) The pharmacodynamic effect of a remifentanil bolus on ventilatory control. Anesthesiology 92: 393–398.
4. Egan TD (2000) Pharmacokinetics and pharmacodynamics of remifentanil: an update in the year 2000. Curr Opin Anaesthesiol 13: 449–455.
5. Kapila A, Glass PS, Jacobs JR, Muir KT, Hermann DJ, et al. (1995) Measured context-sensitive half-times of remifentanil and alfentanil. Anesthesiology 83: 968–975.
6. Volikas I, Butwick A, Wilkinson C, Pleming A, Nicholson G (2005) Maternal and neonatal side-effects of remifentanil patient-controlled analgesia in labour. Br J Anaesth 95: 504–509.
7. Douma MR, Middeldorp JM, Verwey RA, Dahan A, Stienstra R (2011) A randomised comparison of intravenous remifentanil patient-controlled analgesia with epidural ropivacaine/sufentanil during labour. Int J Obstet Anesth 20: 118–123.
8. Volmanen P, Sarvela J, Akural EI, Raudaskoski T, Korttila K, et al. (2008) Intravenous remifentanil vs. epidural levobupivacaine with fentanyl for pain relief in early labour: a randomised, controlled, double-blinded study. Acta Anaesthesiol Scand 52: 249–255.
9. Tveit TO, Seiler S, Halvorsen A, Rosland JH (2012) Labour analgesia: a randomised, controlled trial comparing intravenous remifentanil and epidural analgesia with ropivacaine and fentanyl. Eur J Anaesthesiol 29: 129–136.
10. Liu ZQ, Chen XB, Li HB, Qiu MT, Duan T (2014) A comparison of remifentanil parturient-controlled intravenous analgesia with epidural analgesia: a meta-analysis of randomized controlled trials. Anesth Analg 118: 598–603.

11. Egan TD, Huizinga B, Gupta SK, Jaarsma RL, Sperry RJ, et al. (1998) Remifentanil pharmacokinetics in obese versus lean patients. Anesthesiology 89: 562–573.

12. Tveit TO, Halvorsen A, Seiler S, Rosland JH (2013) Efficacy and side effects of intravenous remifentanil patient-controlled analgesia used in a stepwise approach for labour: an observational study. Int J Obstet Anesth 22: 19–25.

13. Balcioglu O, Akin S, Demir S, Aribogan A (2007) Patient-controlled intravenous analgesia with remifentanil in nulliparous subjects in labor. Expert Opin Pharmacother 8: 3089–3096.

14. Balki M, Kasodekar S, Dhumne S, Bernstein P, Carvalho JC (2007) Remifentanil patient-controlled analgesia for labour: optimizing drug delivery regimens. Can J Anaesth 54: 626–633.

15. D'Onofrio P, Novelli AM, Mecacci F, Scarselli G (2009) The efficacy and safety of continuous intravenous administration of remifentanil for birth pain relief: an open study of 205 parturients. Anesth Analg 109: 1922–1924.

16. Douma MR, Verwey RA, Kam-Endtz CE, van der Linden PD, Stienstra R (2010) Obstetric analgesia: a comparison of patient-controlled meperidine, remifentanil, and fentanyl in labour. Br J Anaesth 104: 209–215.

17. Evron S, Ezri T, Protianov M, Muzikant G, Sadan O, et al. (2008) The effects of remifentanil or acetaminophen with epidural ropivacaine on body temperature during labor. J Anesth 22: 105–111.

18. Volmanen P, Akural EI, Raudaskoski T, Alahuhta S (2002) Remifentanil in obstetric analgesia: a dose-finding study. Anesth Analg 94: 913–917, table of contents.

19. Olufolabi AJ, Booth JV, Wakeling HG, Glass PS, Penning DH, et al. (2000) A preliminary investigation of remifentanil as a labor analgesic. Anesth Analg 91: 606–608.

20. Stourac P, Suchomelova H, Stodulkova M, Huser M, Krikava I, et al. (2012) Comparison of parturient - controlled remifentanil with epidural bupivacain and sufentanil for labour analgesia: Randomised controlled trial. Biomed Pap Med Fac Univ Palacky Olomouc Czech Repub.

21. Landau R, Cahana A, Smiley RM, Antonarakis SE, Blouin JL (2004) Genetic variability of mu-opioid receptor in an obstetric population. Anesthesiology 100: 1030–1033.

22. Volmanen P, Alahuhta S (2004) Will remifentanil be a labour analgesic? Int J Obstet Anesth 13: 1–4.

23. Marwah R, Hassan S, Carvalho JC, Balki M (2012) Remifentanil versus fentanyl for intravenous patient-controlled labour analgesia: an observational study. Can J Anaesth 59: 246–254.

24. Blair JM, Dobson GT, Hill DA, McCracken GR, Fee JP (2005) Patient controlled analgesia for labour: a comparison of remifentanil with pethidine. Anaesthesia 60: 22–27.

25. Dhileepan S, Stacey RG (2001) A preliminary investigation of remifentanil as a labor analgesic. Anesth Analg 92: 1358–1359.

26. Evron S, Glezerman M, Sadan O, Boaz M, Ezri T (2005) Remifentanil: a novel systemic analgesic for labor pain. Anesth Analg 100: 233–238.

27. Hill D (2008) Remifentanil in obstetrics. Curr Opin Anaesthesiol 21: 270–274.

28. Volmanen PV, Akural EI, Raudaskoski T, Ranta P, Tekay A, et al. (2011) Timing of intravenous patient-controlled remifentanil bolus during early labour. Acta Anaesthesiol Scand 55: 486–494.

29. Egan TD, Kern SE, Muir KT, White J (2004) Remifentanil by bolus injection: a safety, pharmacokinetic, pharmacodynamic, and age effect investigation in human volunteers. Br J Anaesth 92: 335–343.

30. Kan RE, Hughes SC, Rosen MA, Kessin C, Preston PG, et al. (1998) Intravenous remifentanil: placental transfer, maternal and neonatal effects. Anesthesiology 88: 1467–1474.

31. Shahriari A, Khooshideh M (2007) A randomized controlled trial of intravenous remifentanil compared with intramuscular meperidine for pain relief in labor. J Med Sci 7: 635–639.

32. Thurlow JA, Laxton CH, Dick A, Waterhouse P, Sherman L, et al. (2002) Remifentanil by patient-controlled analgesia compared with intramuscular meperidine for pain relief in labour. Br J Anaesth 88: 374–378.

33. Volmanen P, Akural E, Raudaskoski T, Ohtonen P, Alahuhta S (2005) Comparison of remifentanil and nitrous oxide in labour analgesia. Acta Anaesthesiol Scand 49: 453–458.

34. Bonner JC, McClymont W (2012) Respiratory arrest in an obstetric patient using remifentanil patient-controlled analgesia. Anaesthesia 67: 538–540.

35. Blair JM, Hill DA, Fee JP (2001) Patient-controlled analgesia for labour using remifentanil: a feasibility study. Br J Anaesth 87: 415–420.

36. Ngan Kee WD, Khaw KS, Ng FF (2004) Comparison of phenylephrine infusion regimens for maintaining maternal blood pressure during spinal anaesthesia for Caesarean section. Br J Anaesth 92: 469–474.

37. Ngan Kee WD, Khaw KS, Ma KC, Wong AS, Lee BB, et al. (2006) Maternal and neonatal effects of remifentanil at induction of general anesthesia for cesarean delivery: a randomized, double-blind, controlled trial. Anesthesiology 104: 14–20.

38. Kattwinkel J, Perlman JM, Aziz K, Colby C, Fairchild K, et al. (2010) Neonatal resuscitation: 2010 American Heart Association Guidelines for Cardiopulmonary Resuscitation and Emergency Cardiovascular Care. Pediatrics 126: e1400–1413.

39. (2011) 2011 Neonatal Resuscitation Guidelines. Chin J Perinat Med 14: 415–419.

40. Ismail MT, Hassanin MZ (2012) Neuraxial analgesia versus intravenous remifentanil for pain relief in early labor in nulliparous women. Arch Gynecol Obstet 286: 1375–1381.

9

A Role of Supraspinal Galanin in Behavioural Hyperalgesia in the Rat

Diana Amorim[1,2], Ana David-Pereira[1,2], Patrícia Marques[1,2], Sónia Puga[1,2], Patrícia Rebelo[1,2], Patrício Costa[1,2], Antti Pertovaara[3], Armando Almeida[1,2], Filipa Pinto-Ribeiro[1,2]∗

1 Life and Health Sciences Research Institute (ICVS), School of Health Sciences (ECS), University of Minho, Braga, Portugal, 2 ICVS/3B's - PT Government Associate Laboratory, Braga/Guimarães, Portugal, 3 Institute of Biomedicine/Physiology, University of Helsinki, Helsinki, Finland

Abstract

Introduction: In chronic pain disorders, galanin (GAL) is able to either facilitate or inhibit nociception in the spinal cord but the contribution of supraspinal galanin to pain signalling is mostly unknown. The dorsomedial nucleus of the hypothalamus (DMH) is rich in galanin receptors (GALR) and is involved in behavioural hyperalgesia. In this study, we evaluated the contribution of supraspinal GAL to behavioural hyperalgesia in experimental monoarthritis.

Methods: In Wistar-Han males with a four week kaolin/carrageenan-induced monoarthritis (ARTH), paw-withdrawal latency (PWL) was assessed before and after DMH administration of exogenous GAL, a non-specific GALR antagonist (M40), a specific GALR1 agonist (M617) and a specific GALR2 antagonist (M871). Additionally, the analysis of c-Fos expression after GAL injection in the DMH was used to investigate the potential involvement of brainstem pain control centres. Finally, electrophysiological recordings were performed to evaluate whether pronociceptive On- or antinociceptive Off-like cells in the rostral ventromedial medulla (RVM) relay the effect of GAL.

Results: Exogenous GAL in the DMH decreased PWL in ARTH and SHAM animals, an effect that was mimicked by a GALR1 agonist (M617). In SHAM animals, an unselective GALR antagonist (M40) increased PWL, while a GALR2 antagonist (M871) decreased PWL. M40 or M871 failed to influence PWL in ARTH animals. Exogenous GAL increased c-Fos expression in the RVM and dorsal raphe nucleus (DRN), with effects being more prominent in SHAM than ARTH animals. Exogenous GAL failed to influence activity of RVM On- or Off-like cells of SHAM and ARTH animals.

Conclusions: Overall, exogenous GAL in the DMH had a pronociceptive effect that is mediated by GALR1 in healthy and arthritic animals and is associated with alterations of c-Fos expression in RVM and DRN that are serotonergic brainstem nuclei known to be involved in the regulation of pain.

Editor: Yvette Tache, University of California, Los Angeles, United States of America

Funding: This study was supported by grants from the Portuguese Science Foundation (FCT) Project n° PTDC/SAU-NEU/108557/2008, FEDER-COMPETE, by the Academy of Finland and the Sigrid Jusélius Foundation, Helsinki, Finland. DA was supported by FCT grant SFRH/BD/71219/2010 and ADP was supported by FCT grant SFRH/BD/90374/2012. The funders had no role in study design, data collection and analysis, decision to publish, or preparation of the manuscript.

Competing Interests: The authors have declared that no competing interests exist.

* Email: filiparibeiro@ecsaude.uminho.pt

Introduction

Galanin (GAL) is an injury-responsive peptide that is dramatically upregulated in the dorsal root ganglia and spinal dorsal horn interneurones during inflammation [1] or after nerve injury [2]. In healthy animals, GAL's action on nociceptive processing in the spinal cord is bidirectional, with low concentrations eliciting pronociceptive actions [3] and high concentrations promoting antinociception [4]. Differences in spinal actions of GAL also vary with the differential availability/activation of GAL receptor (GALR) subtypes. GALR1 has an inhibitory action and is more abundant than GALR2 (excitatory) and GALR3 (inhibitory) in the superficial dorsal horn [5]. Despite the considerable number of works evaluating its action in the peripheral nervous system and at

the spinal cord level, the role of GAL in pain modulation at the supraspinal level is mostly unknown.

In basal conditions several studies showed that, both in humans and rodents, GAL is expressed in the supraoptic nucleus, the paraventricular nucleus of the hypothalamus, the dorsomedial hypothalamic nucleus (DMH), the arcuate nuclei, the lateral hypothalamic area, the locus coeruleus (LC), the amygdala (AMY) and the median raphe nucleus [6], all areas involved in supraspinal pain modulation [7–11]. In relation to receptor expression, GALR1 is greatly expressed in the LC, dorsal raphe nucleus (DRN), the paraventricular nucleus of the hypothalamus, DMH, AMY, thalamus and medulla oblongata [12–15]. However, in the AMY, GALR2/R3 are also significantly expressed [12]. Similarly, all types of GAL receptors are expressed in the prefrontal cortex and the hippocampus but to a lesser extent [12,14,15]. GALR2 is highly expressed in the hypothalamus, dentate gyrus, piriform cortex and mammillary nuclei [14,15], while the expression of GALR3 has been reported mainly in the hypothalamus (preoptic, DMH, lateral and posterior hypothalamic, ventromedial and premammillary nuclei) [15], the bed nucleus of the stria terminalis, periaqueductal grey matter (PAG), lateral parabrachial nucleus and medial reticular formation [16]. Again, most brain areas mentioned above are involved in the codification and modulation of nociceptive inputs [7,10].

The administration of exogenous GAL to the arcuate [17], tuberomammillary [18], nucleus accumbens [19], central nucleus of the AMY [20,21] and PAG [22] decreases nociception in healthy rats, an effect that is mediated by GalR1 in rodents [23]. A similar effect is observed in some pathological conditions, such as acute inflammation or mononeuropathy [22], where the micro-injection of supraspinal exogenous GAL also decreases nociception. Albeit the apparent antinociceptive role of supraspinal GAL in pain modulation, the intracerebroventricular administration of a GALR1 agonist in rats increased c-Fos expression in the DMH [24], an area that facilitates nociception by promoting behavioural hyperalgesia [9,25]. As hyperalgesia is one of the hallmarks of chronic pain, activation of the DMH promotes behavioural hyperalgesia and GAL receptors are strongly expressed in the DMH, here we evaluated the contribution of GAL receptors in the DMH to the descending control of inflammatory hyperalgesia in monoarthritis as well as nociception in healthy controls.

Methods

1. Animals, ethical issues and anaesthesia

The experiments were performed in adult male Wistar Han rats with 175–250 g (Charles Rivers, Barcelona, Spain). A total of 96 animals (SHAM, n = 48 and ARTH, n = 48) were used in the experiments herein, 40 animals (SHAM, n = 20 and ARTH, n = 20) were used in the behavioural assessment, 32 animals (SHAM, n = 16 and ARTH, n = 16) in the c-Fos protocol and 24 animals (SHAM, n = 12 and ARTH, n = 12) in the electrophysiological evaluation. Animals were randomly assigned two by two to boxes upon arrival; a blue line was painted in the tail of one rat and a red line in the tail of the other. Each box was numbered from 1 to 48, no indication concerning if the animals were assigned to the SHAM or ARTH group was displayed. The list discriminating the boxes corresponding to the SHAM or ARTH groups was kept by an independent party. Each animal was considered a single unit within its experimental group. Animals were housed two per cage, except for animals with chronic intracerebral cannulae implanted that were housed individually. Food and water were available *ad libitum* and animals were maintained in a climate-controlled room, under $22\pm2°C$ of temperature, $55\pm5\%$ of humidity and under a 12 h light/dark cycle with lights on at 8:00am. The experimental protocol followed the European Community Council Directive 86/609/EEC and 2010/63/EU concerning the use of animals for scientific purposes and was approved by the Institutional Ethical Commission (Permit Number: 23248). All efforts were made to minimize animal suffering and to use only the number of animals necessary to produce reliable scientific data.

For cannula implantation the animals were anaesthetized i.p. with a mixture 1:1.5 of ketamine (Imalgene, Merial, Oeiras, Portugal) and medetomidine (Dorbene, Esteve, Carnaxide, Portugal). After the surgical procedure, the anaesthesia was reversed using atipamezole (Antisedan, Pfizer, Oeiras, Portugal, i.p.) and the animals were monitored until fully awake (grooming and eating).

Anaesthesia was induced by administering pentobarbitone (50 mg/kg, i.p., Eutasil, CEVA, Algés, Portugal) and maintained by infusing pentobarbitone (15–20 mg/kg/h, i.p.). The level of anaesthesia was frequently assessed by determining behavioural responses to noxious pinching. Body temperature was maintained within physiological range with the help of a warming blanket (DC Temperature Controller, FHC, Bowdoin, ME, USA). At the end of the experiment, animals received a lethal dose of pentobarbitone.

2. Induction of arthritis

The induction of monoarthritis (ARTH) was performed four weeks before the actual experiments, as described in detail elsewhere [9,26]. In order to maintain the researcher blind in relation to whether the animals from a specific box were assigned to the SHAM or ARTH groups, the animals were anaesthetized (section 2.1) by a third party in an adjacent room and then brought to the chirurgical table in groups of two for the injection of SAL or K/C in the right knee joint. Briefly, in anaesthetised animals a mixture of 3% kaolin and 3% carrageenan (K/C, Sigma-Aldrich, St. Louis, MO, USA) dissolved in saline was injected into the synovial cavity of the right knee joint at a volume of 0.1 mL. This model produces mechanical hyperalgesia, which begins a few hours after surgery and extends up to 8 weeks [27]. After the procedure, animals returned to the adjacent room, the anaesthesia was reversed and animals were monitored until fully recovered (eating and grooming). At the end of the induction session all boxes were returned to the animal house. In each animal, development of arthritis was verified again 1 h prior to each behavioural session. While confirming the arthritic status of the animals, through the flexion and extension of the right leg, the experimenter was handed the animals by a third party without any specific order and without prior knowledge of the box number. Only those rats that vocalized every time after five flexion–extension movements of the knee joint were considered to have arthritis, and they were included in the ARTH group. SHAM animals were injected with 0.1 mL saline in the synovial cavity of the right knee joint. SHAM animals did not vocalize to any of the five consecutive flexion–extension movements of the knee joint. After the test, the animals were returned to their home cages by a person other than the evaluator.

3. Behavioural assessment of nociception

All behavioural tests were performed during the day time, starting at 9:30am and ending at 1:30pm after which the animals were returned to the animal house.

3.1 Mechanical hyperalgesia. The application of noxious pressure to the primary site of injury is a classical approach to measure mechanical hyperalgesia [28], both in humans and animals [29]. Here, the pressure application measurement (PAM; Ugo Basile, Comerio, Italy) method was used. It allows an accurate behavioural measurement of mechanical hypersensitivity in rodents with chronic inflammatory joint pain [30] by the application of a force range of 0–1500 g. To perform the test and with the animal securely held, the force transducer unit (fitted to the experimenter's thumb) is placed on one side of the animal's knee joint and the forefinger on the other and an increasingly force is applied across the joint until a behavioural response is observed (limb-withdrawal, freezing of whisker movement, wriggling or vocalization) with a cut-off of 5 s. The peak force applied immediately prior to the behavioural response is recorded as the response threshold (RT). RT was measured twice in the ipsilateral and contralateral limbs at 1 min intervals. The mean RTs were calculated per animal. At the end of the session animals were returned to their home cage.

3.2 Thermal hyperalgesia (heat). Heat hyperalgesia was evaluated using the Hargreaves test [31]. The rats were habituated to the experimental conditions by allowing them to spend 1–2 h daily in the experimental room for the three days preceding any behavioural tests [9]. For assessing heat hyperalgesia, a radiant heat source was placed under the hindpaws in awake animals and the time spent between the heat application and the withdrawal response (Plantar Test Instrument, Model 37370, Ugo Basile, Varese, Italy) was registered as the paw-withdrawal latency (PWL). In each session, the PWL was assessed prior to drug administration in the DMH and 20 min after. In each time point, the PWL was repeated twice at an interval of 1 min and the mean of these values was used in further calculations. Cut-off time was 15 s.

4. Procedures for intra-DMH microinjections

Before the placement of the guide cannulas the animals were anaesthetized (section 2.1) by a third party in an adjacent room and then brought to the chirurgical table one at the time. For intra-DMH drug administration, four weeks before the actual experiments (at the same time that arthritis was induced), animals were anaesthetised and placed in a stereotaxic frame, and one stainless steel guide cannula (26 gauge; PlasticsOne, Roanoke, VA, USA) was then implanted in the DMH according to the coordinates of the atlas by Paxinos and Watson [32]. The tip of the guide cannula was positioned 1 mm above the desired injection site in the DMH [AP, −3.24 mm from bregma; LM, 0.4 mm lateral from the midline (right side); DV, 7.5 mm below the surface of the skull]. The guide cannula was kept in place through the use of two dental screws and dental cement. A dummy cannula was inserted into the guide cannula to close the top. After the procedure, the anaesthesia was reversed and animals were monitored until being fully recovered (eating and grooming) in the adjacent room and returned to the animal house.

In order for the experimenter to remain blinded in relation to which animals were SHAMs or ARTHs, prior to the beginning of the behavioural session, the cards displaying the number of the box were substituted by cards displaying letters. Test drugs were administered in the DMH through a 33-gauge injection cannula (PlasticsOne) inserted into and protruding 1 mm beyond the tip of the guide cannula. The microinjection was made using a 10.0-μL-Hamilton syringe connected to the injection cannula by a polyethylene catheter (PE-10; Plastics One). The injection volume was 0.5 μL and therefore, the spread of the injected drugs within the brain was expected to be 1 mm [33]. The efficacy of injection was monitored by observing the movement of a small air bubble through the tubing. The injection lasted 20 s and the injection cannula was left in place for additional 30 s to minimize the return of drug solution back to the injection cannula. Brain injection sites were histologically verified from post-mortem sections and plotted on standardized sections from the stereotaxic atlas [32] (**Fig. 1**). After the completion of the tests and animals were returned to the animal house, the cards were switch again. The attribution of the letter cards was recorded in a lab book separate from the one used to register the results. The order of attribution of the letter cards was random and changed in each experimental session. The order of the administration of the drugs to each animal was defined at the beginning of the experiment to avoid potential confounding effects related to this parameter. The results of the tests were only associated with the respective animal after the end of the experiment.

5. Drugs

Solutions for drug administration in the DMH were prepared in sterilized saline 0.9% (Unither, Amiens, France; pH 7.2). All the experimental drugs used in this work were acquired from Tocris (Bristol, UK). Each injection had a volume of 0.5 μL and contained either GAL (1.0 nmol), a non-specific GAL receptor antagonist (M40, 1.0 nmol), a specific GALR1 agonist (M617, 1.0 nmol) or a specific GALR2 antagonist (M871, 1.0 nmol) [17,20,23]. Control injections were performed with SAL in order to avoid any confounding effect that might result from injecting the liquid itself.

6. Course of the pharmacological study

Four weeks following induction of arthritis and insertion of the guide cannula for DMH injections, the efficacy of DMH-induced phasic and tonic modulation of nociception was determined by assessing the effect of DMH injection of exogenous GAL, M40, M671 and M871 upon the PWL in awake SHAM and ARTH animals. SAL was used in control injections. The latency of the withdrawal response was assessed 20 min [18,34] following the intra-DMH injections. The interval between behavioural assessments of different drug treatment conditions in the same animal was at least two days. The order of testing different drugs varied between the animals.

7. Recording of neuronal activity in nociceptive RVM cells

For the electrophysiological study, animals were removed from the animal house in a random order, one per day, already anaesthetized, by a person other than the experimenter. Anaesthesia (section 2.1) was administered at 9:30am, the electrophysiological recordings started between 10am and 10:30 am and lasted for 3 h. The order of the administration of the drugs varied between the animals. The electrophysiological recordings of the activity of RVM neurones followed a protocol described in Pinto-Ribeiro and colleagues [9]. In anaesthetised animals, a recording electrode was placed in the RVM (AP: 5.88 mm rostral to the interaural line, ML: −0.6 to 0.6 mm lateral from the midline, and DV: 10.0 mm below the surface of the skull) [32]. Single neurone activity was recorded extracellularly with tungsten electrodes (tip impedance 3–10 MΩ at 1 kHz), the signal was amplified and filtered and data sampling was performed through a CED Micro 1401 interface and Spike 2 software (Cambridge Electronic Design, Cambridge, UK).

Recording of RVM neurones was started after the animal was under light anaesthesia; i.e., the animals gave a brief withdrawal response to noxious pinch, but the pinch did not produce any longer lasting motor activity, nor did the animals have spontaneous limb movements. RVM neurones were classified based on their response to noxious heating of the tail with a tail-flick device (Ugo Basile). Heat stimulation of the tail was applied during 10 s. Functional classification of RVM neurones followed the scheme developed earlier by Fields and colleagues [35] and by Fields and Heinricher [36]. The neurones whose firing activity increased during heat stimulation of the tail were considered On-cells, those decreasing its activity were classified as Off-cells and finally, cells displaying only a negligible (<10%) or no alteration in discharge rates during noxious stimulation were considered Neutral-cells and were not analysed in this study. However, a significant difference with the classification scheme of Fields [35] is that in the present study the noxious stimulus-induced withdrawal reflex was not taken into account in the classification. Therefore, as in previous studies, RVM cells are here called On-like and Off-like cells [9,37,38] rather than On- or Off-cells.

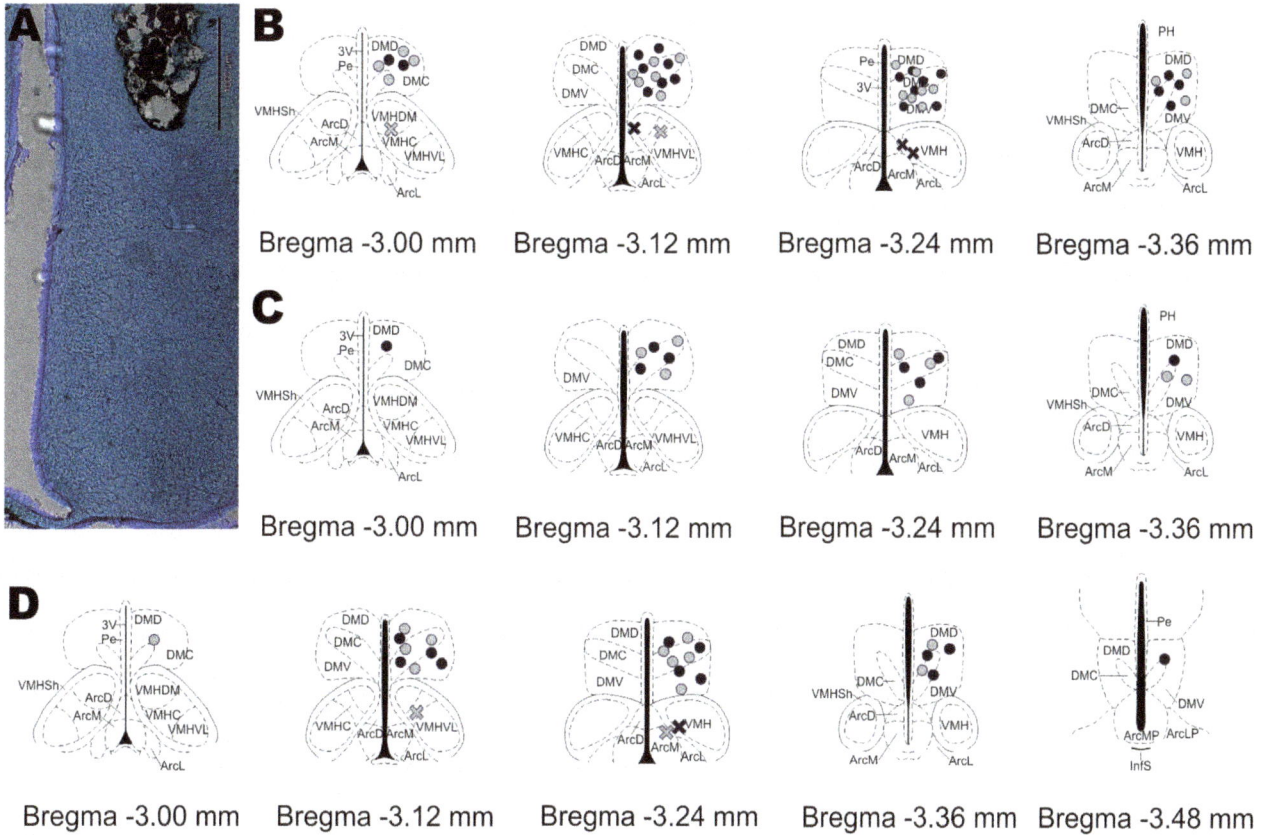

Figure 1. Anatomical confirmation of drug injection sites in the dorsomedial nucleus of the hypothalamus (DMH). (**A**) Photomicrograph of an example of the drug injection site in the right DMH of the rat brain (AP: −3.24 mm from bregma) superimposed with the appropriate plate of the Paxinos and Watson (2007) stereotaxic atlas. (**B**) Schematic representation of injection sites in the DMH during the behavioural study. The coordinates for the injection sites are as follow −3.00 mm, −3.12 mm, −3.24 mm and −3.36 mm from bregma. (**C**) Schematic representation of injection sites in the DMH during the protocol for the induction of c-Fos expression. The coordinates for the injection sites are as follow −3.00 mm, −3.12 mm, −3.24 mm and −3.36 mm from bregma. (**D**) Schematic representation of injection sites in the DMH during the electrophysiological study. The coordinates for the injection sites are as follow −3.00 mm, −3.12 mm, −3.24 mm, −3.36 mm and −3.48 mm from bregma. (Grey dots correspond to injection sites in the DMH of control (SHAM) animals and black dots show injection sites in the DMH of arthritic (ARTH) animals; grey and black crosses correspond to injection sites outside the DMH of SHAM and ARTH animals, respectively) ArcD- arcuate hypothalamic nucleus, dorsal; ArcL- arcuate hypothalamic nucleus, lateral; ArcM- arcuate hypothalamic nucleus, medial; DMC - dorsomedial hypothalamic nucleus, compact; DMD – dorsomedial hypothalamic nucleus, dorsal; DMV - dorsomedial hypothalamic nucleus, ventral; VMHDM - ventromedial hypothalamic nucleus, dorsomedial; VMHSh - ventromedial hypothalamic nucleus, shell; VMHVL - ventromedial hypothalamic nucleus, ventrolateral.

The characterization of the response properties of RVM cells consisted of the following assessments performed successively: (i) spontaneous activity; (ii) response to heating of the tail; (iii) recovery to the spontaneous activity level.

It should be noted that when analysing responses of RVM neurones to peripheral stimulation, the baseline discharge frequency (recorded just before the stimulation) was subtracted from the discharge frequency assessed during the stimulation using the following formula:

Evoked response

= (cell activity during acute noxious stimulation)

− (basal cell activity prior to stimulus application)

Thus, positive values represent an increase and negative ones represent a decrease in cell activity evoked by peripheral stimulation.

During the recordings, animals also had a guide cannula implanted for drug administration into the DMH. After determining the baseline spontaneous activity of RVM cells and their baseline noxious-evoked responses to peripheral stimulation, either exogenous GAL or a non-specific GALRs antagonist (M40) were microinjected in the DMH, in order to assess its phasic or tonic effect, respectively, upon the discharge rate of RVM neurones. All results from drug administrations were plotted for the variation in activity comparing baseline (before drug administration) and values obtained 20 min after the injection into the DMH. The results of the electrophysiological analysis were only associated with the respective animal after all recordings were performed.

8. Course of the electrophysiological study

Electrophysiological recordings of RVM neurones (SHAM: On-like cells, n = 58 and Off-like cells, n = 40; ARTH: On-like cells, n = 46 and Off-like cells, n = 47) were performed under pentobarbitone anaesthesia four weeks after the administration of K/C

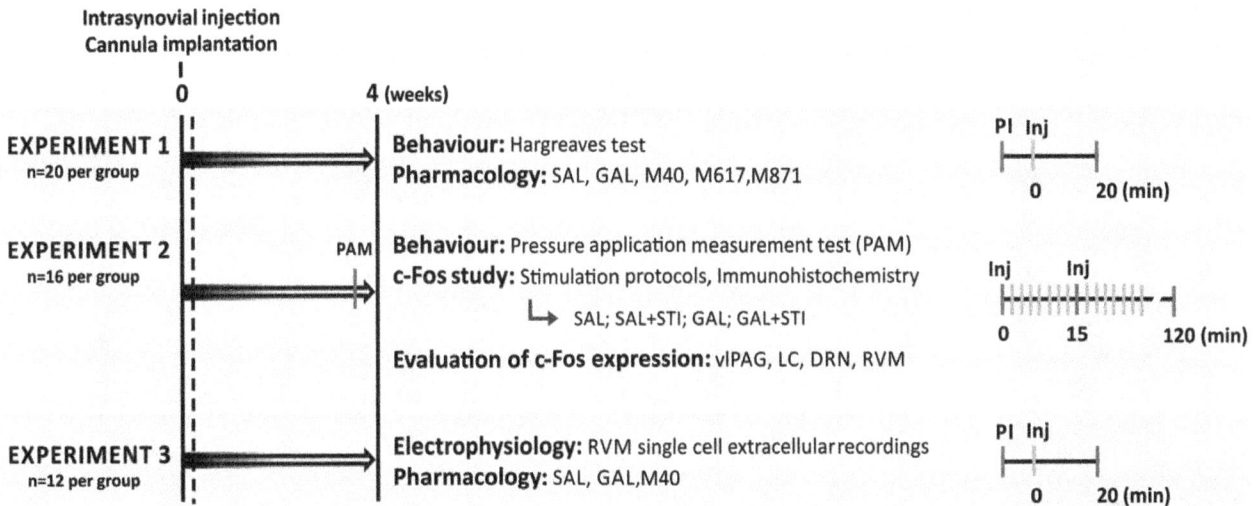

Figure 2. Schematic representation of the experimental design. In all experiments, animals were divided in two groups, control (SHAM) when injected with saline and arthritic (ARTH) when injected with a mixture of kaolin and carrageenan in the synovial capsule of the right knee joint. Three days after the intrasynovial injection, arthritis was confirmed by performing five consecutive movements of flexion/extension of the knee (dashed line). Animals in the ARTH group developed a clear swelling of the treated knee joint and all gave a vocalization response during a minor extension and flexion of the affected limb by the experimenter. SHAM animals displayed no obvious swelling of the knee joint and did not vocalize when the limb was flexed. Four weeks after the induction of monoarthritis animals were tested in three independent experiments. In experiment 1, the Hargreaves test was used to study the effect of exogenous galanin (GAL), a non-specific GAL receptor antagonist (M40), a specific GAL receptor-1 agonist (M617) and a specific GAL receptor-2 antagonist (M871) in the dorsomedial nucleus of the hypothalamus (DMH) upon paw-withdrawal latency (PWL) (n = 20 per experimental group). In each animal, the development of arthritis was confirmed again 1 h prior to each behavioural session by performing five consecutive movements of flexion/extension of the knee. During the experimental sessions, PWL was assessed before and 20 min after the administration of the drugs to the DMH. In experiment 2, two days prior the c-Fos study, the pressure application measurement (PAM) test was performed to confirm the arthritic state of the animals. c-Fos expression was evaluated in SHAM and ARTH animals after exogenous GAL or saline (SAL) administration in the DMH, peripheral noxious mechanical stimulation and the simultaneous application of noxious mechanical stimulation after the microinjection of exogenous GAL in the DMH (n = 16 per experimental group). Peripheral stimulation was applied each 2 minutes during 2 hours and two drug injections were made in the DMH, one at the beginning and another 15 minutes after the beginning of peripheral stimulation. Neurones expressing c-Fos were quantified bilaterally in the ventrolateral periaqueductal grey matter (vlPAG), locus coeruleus (LC), dorsal raphe nucleus (DRN) and rostral ventromedial medulla (RVM). In experiment 3, RVM neurones were recorded before and after the administration of exogenous GAL and M40 in the DMH. The assessment of neuronal activity includes a preliminary evaluation of spontaneous and noxious-evoked activity followed by the recording of these parameters 20 min after drug administration to the DMH (n = 12 animals per experimental group). PI – Pre-injection; Inj – Injection; SAL - saline microinjection in the dorsomedial nucleus of the hypothalamus; GAL - galanin microinjection in the dorsomedial nucleus of the hypothalamus; SAL+STI – saline microinjection in the dorsomedial nucleus of the hypothalamus and extension of right limb; GAL+STI – galanin microinjection in the dorsomedial nucleus of the hypothalamus and extension of right limb.

(ARTH) or SAL (SHAM) in the right knee of animals. In RVM recordings, the response properties of nociceptive neurones were assessed by determining their spontaneous activity and the response to noxious heating of the tail. Search for the next neurone to be studied started about 30 min after testing of the previous one was completed. At the end of the recording session, electrolytic lesions were made in the recording sites, the animals were given a lethal dose of pentobarbitone and the brains were removed for histological verification of the recording and injection sites.

9. c-Fos study

For the c-Fos induction protocol, animals were removed from the animal house in a random order, one per day, already anaesthetized, by a person other than the experimenter. Anaesthesia (section 2.1) was administered at 9:30 am; the protocol started between 10am and 10:30am and lasted for 2 h. To evaluate changes in brain activation after exogenous GAL administration in the DMH and/or peripheral noxious stimulation in SHAM and ARTH animals, c-Fos immunoreaction was performed following the protocol described elsewhere [39]. Animals were held in a stereotaxic frame. For drug administration, a guide cannula was placed in the DMH according to the

coordinates of the atlas by Paxinos and Watson [32] and one of the following protocols was performed: (i) SAL microinjection in the DMH of SHAM animals; (ii) exogenous GAL microinjection in the DMH of SHAM animals; (iii) SAL microinjection in the DMH and extension of right limb of SHAM animals; (iv) exogenous GAL microinjection in the DMH and extension of right limb of SHAM animals; (v) SAL microinjection in the DMH of ARTH animals; (vi) exogenous GAL microinjection in the DMH of SHAM animals; (vii) extension of right limb of ARTH animals; (viii) exogenous GAL microinjection in the DMH and extension of right limb of ARTH animals. Two exogenous GAL (or SAL) doses were injected in the DMH with a 15 min interval (**Fig. 2**). Extension of the paw was performed 5 times every 2 minutes for 2 h. Two hours after the first injection and first knee extension (beginning of the protocol), the animals were transcardially perfused with 4% paraformaldehyde in 0.1 M phosphate buffer saline (PBS, pH = 7.4), brains were removed and then post-fixed overnight in the same fixative and kept in a solution of 8% sucrose in PBS. One in three coronal vibratome (Leica, Carnaxide, Portugal) sections (50 μm thick) were treated with a solution of 3.3% H_2O_2 in PBS (30 min) to inhibit endogenous peroxidase activity, and then sequentially washed thrice (10 min) in PBS and PBS-Triton (PBS-T; 0.3% triton X-100; Sigma-Aldrich, Sintra,

Portugal). Sections were then incubated in a blocking solution of 2.5% fetal bovine serum (FBS; Biochrom, Cambridge, United Kingdom) in PBS for 2 h, followed by the incubation overnight at 4°C in rabbit anti-Fos antibody (1:2000 in PBST and 2% FBS; Calbiochem, Merck, Algés, Portugal). The following day, after three washes (10 min) in PBST, sections were incubated in biotinylated polyclonal swine anti-rabbit antibody (1:200 in PBST; Dako, Denmark) for 1 h and again washed thrice (10 min) in PBS-T. Sections were then incubated in avidin–biotin complex (ABC; 1:200 in PBST; Vectastain, Vector Laboratories, Peterborough, USA) for 1 h followed by a series of washing steps with PBST (twice, 10 min), PBS (twice, 10 min) and Tris-HCl (0.05 M, pH 7.6) (twice, 10 min). Finally, sections were stained with diaminobenzidine (0.0125% in a solution of Tris-HCl with 0.02% H2O2; Sigma Aldrich) and washed twice (10 min) with Tris-HCl and PBS. After staining, the sections were mounted on SuperFrost slides (Braunschweig, Germany). c-Fos levels were determined by counting the number of Fos-immunoreactive neurones occurring bilaterally in the brainstem with the aid of a Stereo Investigator 10 Software (Microbrigthfield Bioscience, Madgedurg, Germany) using a video camera (Microbrigthfield Bioscience) attached to a microscope (BX51, Olympus Iberia, Lisboa, Portugal).

10. Statistics

For the effect of drugs upon PWL, the minimum number of animals needed was determine à priori using the G power software (version 3.1.9.2, University of Kiel, Germany) considering a ANOVA-2-way test, α err probability of 0.05, power of 0.95 and an effect size of 0.80 was n = 23. For the effect of drugs upon RVM neuronal activity, the minimum number of animals needed was determine à priori using the G power software considering a ANOVA-2-way test, α err probability of 0.05, power of 0.95 and an effect size of 0.80 was n = 28. For the effect of drugs upon c-Fos expression, the minimum number of animals needed was determine à priori using the G power software considering a ANOVA-2-way test, α err probability of 0.05, power of 0.95 and an effect size of 0.80 was n = 32. The results of the RT analysis correspond to the mean ± SD of raw data; no method of data normalization was used. To assess the effect of the drugs upon PWL for each behavioural session, the value of the basal withdrawal latency (withdrawal latency prior to drug administration) was subtracted from the value of the withdrawal latency at the peak effect of the drug, a negative value indicated the withdrawal latency decreased while a positive value corresponded to an increase in withdrawal latency after drug administration to the DMH. To perform this evaluation, raw data was used. To assess the effect of the drugs upon spontaneous neuronal activity, the value of the activity of RVM On- and Off-like cells without noxious peripheral stimulation prior to the administration of drugs in the DMH was subtracted from the activity of these cells without noxious peripheral stimulation at the peak effect of the drug. Similarly, to assess the effect of the drugs upon the noxious-evoked neuronal activity the value of the activity of RVM On- and Off-like cells during noxious peripheral stimulation prior to the administration of drugs in the DMH was subtracted from the activity of these cells during noxious peripheral stimulation at the peak effect of the drug. Only raw data was used in this analysis. To compare the level of c-fos in each area, the total number of cells stained was registered per area studied and only raw data was used in this analysis. The GraphPad Prism 6 software (GraphPad Software Inc, La Jolla, CA, USA) was used to perform the statistical analysis. The comparison of differences between RT in the PAM test and between the baseline of RVM neuronal

spontaneous and heat-evoked activities of SHAM and ARTH animals were performed using a student's t-test for unpaired data. To compare differences in RT between the ipsilateral and the contralateral side in SHAM and ARTH animals a student's t-test for paired data was used. All other comparisons between groups were performed using a two-way ANOVA followed by a Bonferroni correction for multiple comparisons post-hoc test. Statistical significance was accepted for $P<0.05$.

Results

1. Monoarthritic animals developed ipsilateral mechanical allodynia

Three days after the intrasynovial injection, all animals in the ARTH group developed a clear swelling of the treated knee joint and all gave a vocalization response during a minor extension and flexion of the affected limb by the experimenter. SHAM animals displayed no obvious swelling of the knee joint and did not vocalize when the limb was flexed.

Mechanical hyperalgesia in the knee joint was assessed by determining RT to mechanical pressure over the knee joint. No differences were found between the RT of the ipsilateral and contralateral hindpaws in SHAM animals ($t_7 = 1.535$, $P = 0.169$) while in ARTH animals the ipsilateral RT was significantly lower than the contralateral ($t_7 = 3.377$, $P = 0.0118$). No differences were found between the contralateral RT of SHAM and ARTH animals ($t_{14} = 0.000$, $P>0.999$). Four weeks after induction of monoarthritis, RT was significantly different between SHAM and ARTH animals ($t_{14} = 2.883$, $P = 0.012$). This result indicates that K/C induced a significant RT decrease, i.e., mechanical hyperalgesia (**Fig. 3**).

2. Exogenous GAL in the DMH decreases paw-withdrawal latency, an effect reversed by the administration of a GAL receptors antagonist

To investigate a possible role of supraspinal GAL in phasic and tonic pain facilitation in SHAM and ARTH animals, paw withdrawal latencies (PWL) were assessed after exogenous GAL or M40 microinjection, respectively, in the DMH. The PWL of SHAM and ARTH animals 20 min after exogenous GAL microinjection in the DMH was significantly decreased when compared with SAL injection (main effect of the drug: $F_{1,76} = 61.880$, $P<0.001$). The exogenous GAL-induced decrease in PWL was of the same magnitude in the SHAM and ARTH groups (main effect of the group: $F_{1,76} = 2.704$, $P = 0.104$). *Post hoc* tests confirmed that the PWL of SHAM and ARTH animals treated with exogenous GAL was significantly lower than the PWL of SHAM and ARTH animals treated with SAL (**Fig. 4A**).

Non-specific inhibition of GAL receptors induced by administration of M40 in the DMH significantly altered the PWL when compared with SAL injection (main effect of the drug: $F_{1,76} = 13.830$, $P<0.001$). The effect of M40 was significantly different between SHAM and ARTH animals (main effect of the group: $F_{1,76} = 10.070$, $P = 0.002$). The M40-induced effect on PWL varied with the experimental group (interaction between group and drug: $F_{1,76} = 8.048$, $P = 0.006$). *Post hoc* tests indicated that M40 significantly increased PWL in SHAM animals, but did not alter PWL in ARTH animals (**Fig. 4B**).

3. Nociceptive facilitation after exogenous GAL in the DMH is mediated by GAL receptors type-1

To determine which GAL receptor is involved in pain facilitation induced by exogenous GAL in the DMH, PWL was

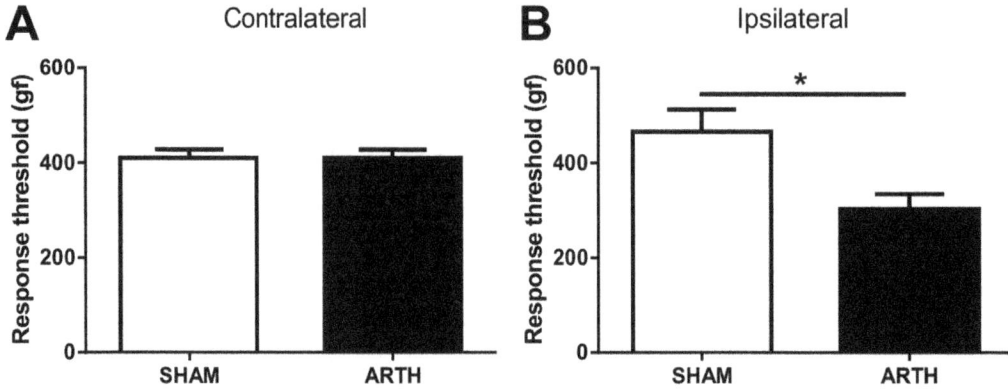

Figure 3. Response threshold. Four weeks after the induction of monoarthritis in the right hind limb, no differences were observed in the response threshold (RT) of the contralateral hindpaws between control (SHAM) and arthritic (ARTH) animals (**A**) in the pressure application measurement. In the ipsilateral side however ARTH animals displayed a decrease in RT during the pressure application measurement when compared to SHAM animals (**B**). Mean response threshold is presented as mean + SEM. (*$P<0.05$, t-test for unpaired data). gf – gram force.

assessed after the administration of M617 (a specific agonist of GAL receptor type-1 - GalR1) and M871 (a specific antagonist of GAL receptor type-2 - GalR2) into the DMH. Twenty minutes after microinjecting M617 in the DMH, PWL was significantly decreased when compared with SAL injection (main effect of the drug: $F_{1,76} = 39.530$, $P<0.001$). The effect of M617 was not

different between SHAM and ARTH groups (main effect of the group: $F_{1,76} = 0.357$, $P = 0.552$). *Post hoc* tests confirmed that PWL significantly decreased after M617 administration in the DMH both in SHAM and ARTH animals when compared to PWL after SAL administration (**Fig. 4C**).

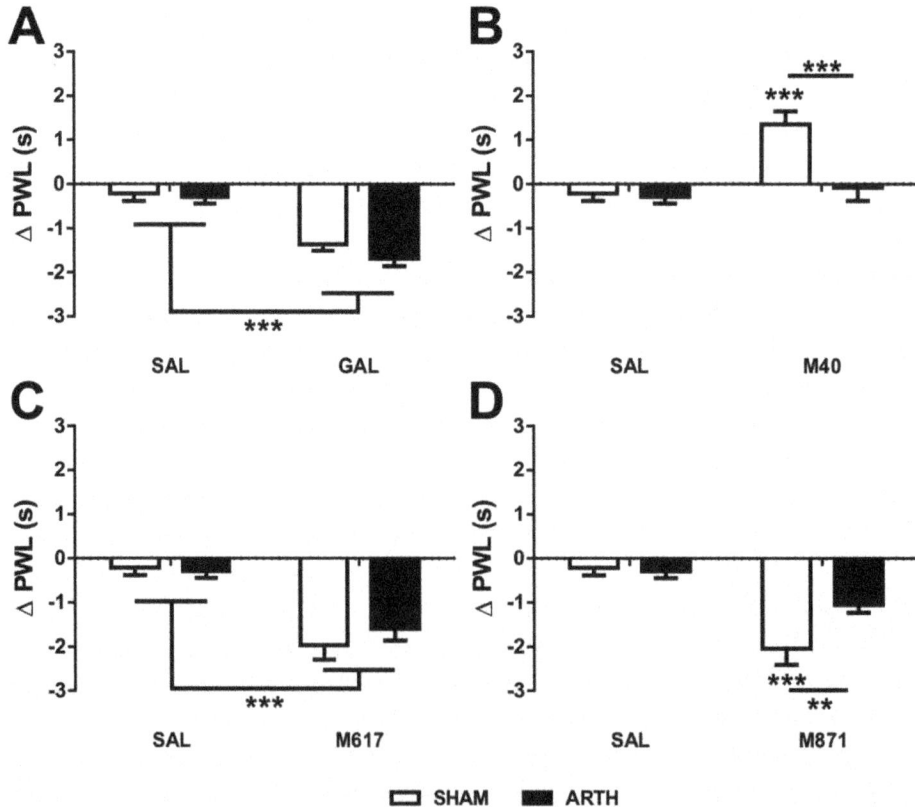

Figure 4. Paw-withdrawal latency after drug administration in the dorsomedial nucleus of the hypothalamus (DMH). In this experiment the analysis of the paw-withdrawal latencies in control (SHAM) and arthritic (ARTH) animals was performed 20 minutes after the intracerebral microinjection of either exogenous galanin (GAL) (**A**), a non-specific antagonist of GAL receptors (M40; **B**), a specific agonist of GAL receptor-1 (M617; **C**) or a specific antagonist of GAL receptor-2 (M871; **D**). Note that the pronociceptive action of exogenous GAL administration in the DMH in SHAM and ARTH animals (**A**) is only mimicked by the microinjection of M617 (**C**). Mean response latency is presented as mean + SEM. (*$P<0.05$, **$P<0.01$, ***$P<0.001$, t-test with a Bonferroni correction for multiple comparisons).

Administration of M871 in the DMH had a significant effect on PWL (main effect of the drug: $F_{1,76} = 29.820$, $P<0.001$), and the effect of M871 varied with the experimental group (interaction group x drug: $F_{1,76} = 5.089$, $P = 0.027$). Post hoc tests showed that M871 significantly decreased the PWL in SHAM animals but did not alter significantly the PWL of ARTH animals (**Fig. 4D**).

4. Expression of c-Fos in brainstem areas involved in pain control is altered by exogenous GAL in the DMH

Descending pain modulatory drive from the forebrain to the spinal cord may be relayed by multiple areas in the brainstem. To determine which brainstem areas mediate exogenous GAL-driven descending pain modulatory effects originating in the DMH, c-Fos expression was investigated in caudal brain areas that not only expressed GAL and/or its receptors but that are also involved in the descending modulation of nociception. Hence, we compared changes in c-Fos expression in the ventrolateral periaqueductal grey matter (VLPAG), the LC, the dorsal raphe nucleus (DRN) and the rostral ventromedial medulla (RVM) between SHAM and ARTH animals after (i) SAL microinjection in the DMH of SHAM animals; (ii) GAL microinjection in the DMH of SHAM animals; (iii) SAL microinjection in the DMH and extension of right limb of SHAM animals; (iv) GAL microinjection in the DMH and extension of right limb of SHAM animals; (v) SAL microinjection in the DMH of ARTH animals; (vi) GAL microinjection in the DMH of SHAM animals; (vii) extension of right limb of ARTH animals; (viii) GAL microinjection in the DMH and extension of right limb of ARTH animals.

Expression of c-Fos following injection of SAL in the DMH was considered to represent basal activation. The number of c-Fos positive neurones in the contralateral RVM varied with the stimulation protocol used (main effect of the protocol: $F_{3,24} = 22.570$, $P<0.001$) with different effects on SHAM and ARTH animals (interaction group x protocol: $F_{3,24} = 42.280$, $P<0.001$). Post-hoc testing showed that exogenous GAL in the DMH significantly increased c-Fos expression when compared to SAL-injected animals in both experimental groups, although a higher expression was observed in ARTH animals (**Fig. 5A**). The flexion-extension protocol (SAL+STI) increased c-Fos expression in SHAM animals when compared to SAL and GAL administration while it decreased its expression in ARTH animals when compared to GAL-Injected ARTH. The simultaneous infusion of GAL in the DMH and flexion-extension of the injected limb decreased c-Fos expression in SHAM when compared with its expression after the flexion-extension protocol and in ARTH when compared with GAL-injected ARTH (**Fig. 5A**). Similarly, in the ipsilateral RVM, the number of cells activated was significantly different depending on the protocols (main effect of the protocol: $F_{3,24} = 70.240$, $P<0.001$), an effect that varied with the experimental group (interaction group x protocol: $F_{3,24} = 20.240$, $P<0.001$). Post-hoc testing showed that GAL in the DMH increased the number of c-Fos expressing cells in both experimental groups when compared to SAL-injected animals, while its expression was different between SHAM and ARTH animals after repeated flexion-extension of the injected limb, with increased c-Fos expression in SHAM animals alone when compared with SAL and GAL-injected SHAM (**Fig. 5B**). The simultaneous injection of GAL in the DMH and flexion-extension of the injected limb significantly decreased the number of c-Fos positive cells in SHAM when compared to the flexion-extension protocol and in ARTH animals when compared with GAL administration and the flexion-extension protocols (**Fig. 5B**).

The number of c-Fos expressing neurones in the contralateral LC did not vary with the stimulation protocols (main effect of the

protocol: $F_{3,24} = 0.413$, $P = 0.745$) although it was significantly different between experimental groups (main effect of the group: $F_{3,24} = 16.410$, $P<0.001$). Post-hoc testing did not show a specific alteration between each stimulation protocol (**Fig. 5C**). In the ipsilateral LC, the number of c-Fos positive cells varied with the stimulation protocol (main effect of the protocol: $F_{3,24} = 7.462$, $P = 0.001$), an effect that depended on the experimental group (interaction group x protocol: $F_{3,24} = 14.310$, $P<0.001$). Post-hoc testing showed an increase in the number of c-Fos expressing neurones after the simultaneous infusion of GAL in the DMH and flexion-extension of the injected limb in ARTH animals when compared with the same protocol in SHAM and with the SAL/GAL/flexion-extension protocols in ARTH (**Fig. 5D**).

In the contralateral vlPAG, the number of c-Fos expressing cells varied with the stimulation protocol (main effect of the protocol: $F_{3,24} = 19.200$, $P<0.001$), an effect that depended on the experimental group (interaction group x protocol: $F_{3,24} = 40.030$, $P<0.001$). Post-hoc testing showed a significant increase in the number of c-Fos positive cells in ARTH animals when compared to SHAM and after exogenous GAL in the DMH of SHAM animals when compared to SAL injected SHAM (**Fig. 5E**). In addition, in ARTH animals the number of c-fos expressing neurones was significantly lower in all protocols when compared to SAL injected ARTH animals (**Fig. 5E**). Similarly, the number of cells activated in the ipsilateral vlPAG was different after the stimulation protocols (main effect of the protocol: $F_{3,24} = 22.920$, $P<0.001$) and depended on the experimental group (interaction group x protocol: $F_{3,24} = 47.100$, $P<0.001$). Post-hoc testing (**Fig. 5F**) showed increased c-Fos expression in SAL-injected ARTH animals when compared with SAL-injected SHAM. GAL in the DMH significantly increased c-Fos expression in SHAM animals while it significantly decreased its expression in ARTH animals. c-Fos expression after the flexion-extension of the injected limb was not significantly different when compared to SAL-injected SHAM although it was significantly decreased when compared to GAL-injected SHAM (**Fig. 5F**). This protocol also significantly decreased c-Fos expression in ARTH animals when compared to SAL-injected ARTH although its expression was significantly higher when compared to GAL-injected ARTH. The simultaneous infusion of GAL in the DMH and flexion-extension of the injected limb did not significantly alter c-Fos expression when compared to SAL-injected SHAM but was significantly decreased when compared to its expression after GAL injection in the DMH. In ARTH animals, c-Fos expression was significantly decreased after the simultaneous infusion of GAL in the DMH and flexion-extension of the injected limb when compared to SAL-injected ARTH and the flexion-extension protocol (**Fig. 5F**).

Finally, In the DRN, the number of c-Fos positive cells varied with the stimulation protocol (main effect of the protocol: $F_{3,24} = 24.690$, $P<0.001$) and this effect was dependent of the experimental group (interaction group x protocol: $F_{3,24} = 14.140$, $P<0.001$). Post-hoc testing showed an increased DRN activation after GAL in the DMH in both experimental groups when compared to SAL-injected animals (**Fig. 5G**). The flexion-extension of the injured limb significantly increased c-Fos expression in SHAM animals when compared to ARTH animals and when compared with SAL- and GAL-injected SHAM. The simultaneous infusion of GAL in the DMH and flexion-extension of the injected limb increased c-Fos expression in SHAM animals when compared to ARTH and to its expression after SAL, but decreased when compared to the flexion-extension protocol. Additionally, it decreased c-Fos expression in ARTH animals when compared to GAL-injected ARTH (**Fig. 5G**).

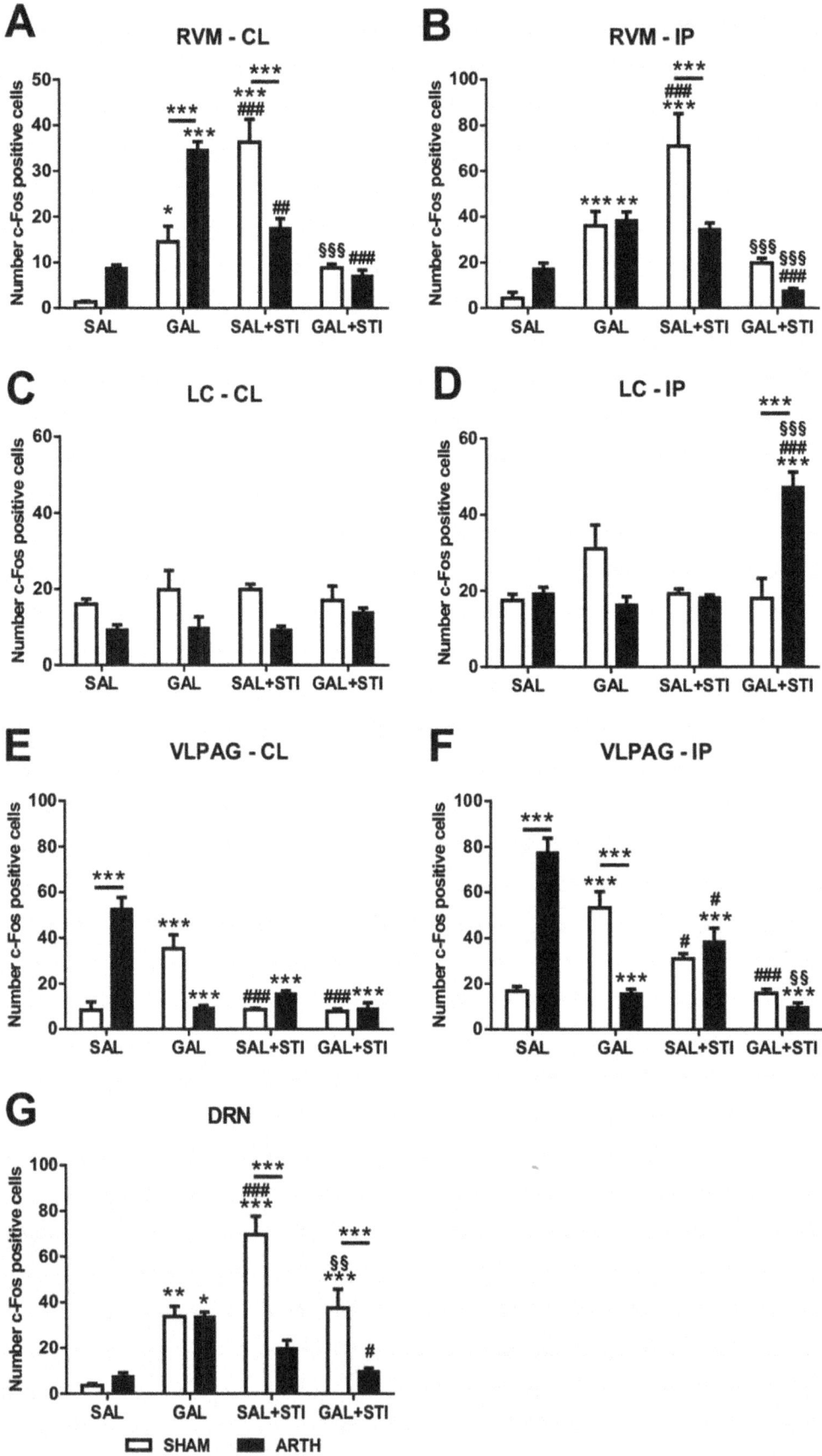

Figure 5. Brainstem c-Fos expression. Number of c-Fos positive cells in the contralateral (**A,C,E**) and ipsilateral (**B,D,F**) sides of the rostral ventromedial medulla (RVM; **A,B**), locus coeruleus (LC; **C,D**), ventrolateral periaqueductal matter (vlPAG; **E,F**) and dorsal raphe nucleus (DRN; **G**) after the administration of saline or exogenous galanin in the dorsomedial nucleus of the hypothalamus (DMH) with and without peripheral noxious stimulation. Data is presented as mean + SEM. SAL – Saline; GAL – Galanin; SAL+STI – SAL and peripheral noxious stimulation (limb flexion-extension); GAL+STI – GAL and peripheral noxious stimulation (limb flexion-extension). * indicates significant differences in c-Fos expression when compared to SAL injection in the DMH; * over line indicates differences in c-Fos expression between experimental groups; # indicates significant differences in c-Fos expression when compared to GAL injection in the DMH; § indicates significant differences in c-Fos expression when compared to the flexion-extension protocol (*, #$P<0.05$; **, ##, §§$P<0.01$; ***, ###, §§§$P<0.001$).

5. The activity of pain modulatory On- or Off-like cells in the RVM is not altered by exogenous GAL in the DMH

To evaluate the effect of exogenous GAL administration in the DMH upon the activity of RVM neurones, the spontaneous and heat-evoked activities of presumably pronociceptive RVM On-like cells and antinociceptive RVM Off-like cells were recorded in SHAM and ARTH animals before and after the administration of exogenous GAL, M40 or SAL.

Before drug administration, the spontaneous activity of RVM On-like cells was significantly decreased in ARTH animals when compared to SHAM animals (**Table 1**). The magnitude of the response evoked by noxious heating of the tail in RVM On-like cells was not different between SHAM and ARTH animals. In RVM Off-like cells, the spontaneous activity before drug treatments was significantly decreased in ARTH animals when compared to SHAM animals. Similarly, the magnitude of the heat-evoked response in RVM Off-like cells of ARTH animals was significantly lower when compared to that in SHAM animals (**Table 1**).

Microinjection of drugs into the DMH did not alter the spontaneous activity of RVM On-like cells (main effect of the drug: $F_{2,98} = 0.262$, $P = 0.770$). Overall, after drug injection, On-like cell spontaneous activity was different between ARTH and SHAM animals (main effect of the group: $F_{1,98} = 6.510$, $P = 0.012$) (**Fig. 6A**), although *post-hoc* tests failed to show a significant difference between experimental groups at a specific time point. The administration of drugs to the DMH did not alter the spontaneous activity of RVM Off-like cells (main effect of the drug: $F_{2,81} = 0.616$, $P = 0.543$) and the spontaneous activity was not different between experimental groups (main effect of the group: $F_{1,81} = 1.200$, $P = 0.277$) (**Fig. 6B**) 20 min after drug administration.

Microinjection of drugs into the DMH altered the heat-evoked activity of RVM On-like cells (main effect of the drug: $F_{2,98} = 5.010$, $P = 0.009$) but this effect did not vary with the experimental group (interaction group x drug: $F_{2,98} = 1.318$, $P = 0.272$). *Post hoc* testing failed to find significant drug treatment-induced effects on the heat-evoked response of On-like cells (**Fig. 6C**). Similarly, drug administration in the DMH changed the heat-evoked activity of RVM Off-like cells (main

effect of the drug: $F_{2,81} = 4.967$, $P = 0.009$) but these differences did not vary with the experimental group (interaction group x drug: $F_{2,81} = 2.230$, $P = 0.114$), 20 min after administration. Again, *post hoc* testing failed to find significant drug treatment-induced effects on the heat-evoked response of Off-like cells, except for the increase of response after exogenous GAL treatment in the SHAM group (**Fig. 6D**).

Discussion

This study demonstrates, for the first time, a pronociceptive role for supraspinal GAL, as the administration of this neuropeptide to the DMH significantly increased spinal nociception (as indicated by the decrease in PWL) in awake healthy and arthritic animals. Moreover, the microinjection of GAL receptor agonist/antagonist in the DMH showed that the exogenous GAL's pronociceptive effect was mediated by GALR1 but not GALR2. The analysis of c-Fos expression revealed the serotonergic RVM and DRN, particularly in SHAM animals, as caudal areas potentially involved in signalling this descending pronociceptive effect. The exogenous GAL-induced increase of c-Fos expression in the RVM may not be explained by action on RVM On-like or Off-like pain modulatory cells, as the discharge rates of these two non-serotonergic cell types remained unaltered during pharmacological manipulations in the present study.

1. Novel pronociceptive effect of supraspinal GAL

Administration of exogenous GAL into the DMH induced behavioural hyperalgesia (decreased PWL) in healthy and ARTH animals. This is a novel effect for GAL as previous studies had only reported an antinociceptive role of this neuropeptide after its administration in brain areas involved in pain modulation, such as the hypothalamic arcuate nucleus [40], central AMY [20] and the PAG [22]. Thus, and similarly to what is observed at the spinal cord level [41,42], GAL appears to have a bidirectional role in supraspinal descending pain modulation depending on the area where GALRs are activated. The demonstration of a tonic pronociceptive effect of GAL, by treatment of the DMH with a non-specific GALR antagonist, supports the proposal that the pronociceptive effect of GAL was mediated by GALRs.

Table 1. Spontaneous and heat-evoked baseline activities of rostral ventromedial medullary (RVM) On- and Off-like cells.

	Cell type	SHAM	ARTH	t	P
Spontaneous	On-like	1.86±0.39 Hz	0.77±0.19 Hz	$t_{102} = 2.689$	$P=0.008$**
	Off-like	4.77±0.46 Hz	3.37±0.26 Hz	$t_{85} = 2.833$	$P=0.006$**
Evoked	On-like	2.51±0.31 Hz	2.82±0.37 Hz	$t_{102} = 0.601$	$P=0.549$
	Off-like	-2.45±0.25 Hz	-1.72±0.26 Hz	$t_{85} = 2.782$	$P=0.007$**

Data presented as mean ± SEM.
**$P<0.01$.

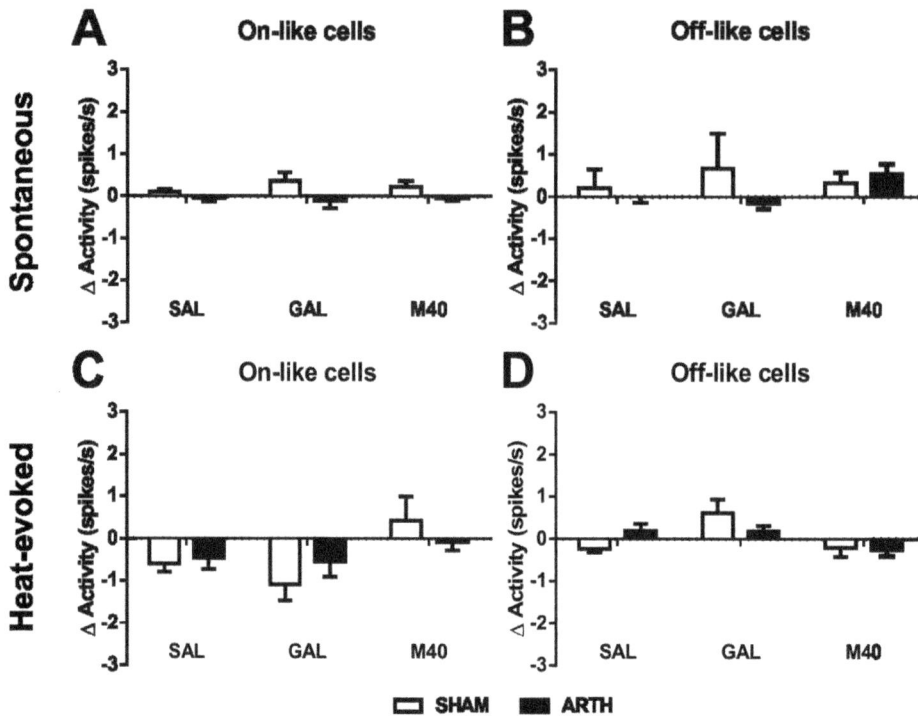

Figure 6. Spontaneous and noxious-evoked rostral ventromedial medulla (RVM) cell activity after the administration of exogenous galanin (GAL) or a non-selective GAL receptor antagonist (M40) in the dorsomedial nucleus of the hypothalamus (DMH). Overall, no changes were observed in the spontaneous (**A, B**) and noxious-evoked (**C, D**) activity of RVM pronociceptive On-like (**A, C**) and antinociceptive Off-like cells (B,D) before and 20 min after the intracerebral microinjection of exogenous GAL (**A–D**) and M40 (**A–D**). Data is presented as mean + SEM.

Administration of exogenous GAL in the DMH facilitated nociception in both ARTH and SHAM animals. This finding contrasts with the results of previous studies indicating that exogenous GAL is antinociceptive when administered in the hypothalamic arcuate nucleus of animals with inflammation [17], or in the PAG of animals with mononeuropathy [22]. Importantly, the present results show that the descending GAL-driven pathway originating in the DMH, unlike the glutamate-driven pathway [9], remains functional in animals with experimental monoarthritis. Administration of a non-specific GALR antagonist alone into the DMH of ARTH animals had no effect on nociception while it produced antinociception in SHAM controls. This finding suggests that the GAL-driven pathway descending from the DMH is not tonically active in ARTH as in SHAM animals, but its activation in ARTH animals depends on the activation of upstream pathways inducing the release of GAL in the DMH.

2. GAL-driven nociceptive facilitation is mediated by GALR1

Further analysis on the contributions of GALR1 and GALR2 to the pain modulatory role of GAL in the DMH demonstrated that the facilitatory effect of GAL is mediated by GALR1, a receptor that couples to the Gi/Go pathway to decrease adenylyl cyclase activity [43]. Once more, this result contrasts with the available literature, where the activation of this receptor at spinal and supraspinal levels is reported to elicit an antinociceptive effect [44–46]. In fact, in the spinal cord it was GALR2 that has been reported to have a pronociceptive effect [41]; however, the results on administration of a GALR2 antagonist in the present study indicated that endogenous GAL acting on GALR2 had a tonic antinociceptive action in SHAM animals, whereas blocking

GALR2 did not alter nociception in ARTH animals. Another possibility would be that the differential distribution of GALR1 and GALR2 receptors in the DMH could contribute to enhance GALR1-dependent effects, however as demonstrated by Mitchell and collaborators [47], not only does mRNAs analysis confirm an overlapping of GAL-R1 and GAL-R2 in the DMH but both receptors are also highly expressed in this nucleus. On the other hand, the expression of both receptors in the DMH does not account *per se* for the GAL/DMH pronociceptive effect since these receptors are also highly expressed and overlapping in the arcuate nuclei, an area where the intracerebral administration of exogenous GAL promotes antinociception [17]. Overall, it is probable that the facilitation of nociceptive behaviour by GAL in the DMH of ARTH animals results (i) from disinhibition of pronociceptive pathways driven by GALR1 and/or (ii) from a decrease in the activity of antinociceptive GALR2-driven circuits.

It is also possible that behavioural hyperalgesia in ARTH animals is reinforced by their emotional-like status. A recent study from our group [48] showed that animals with experimental monoarthritis displayed depressive-like behaviour. Interestingly, Blackshear *et al.* [24] showed that the intracerebroventricular injection of GAL and M617 increased c-fos expression in the DMH and the AMY, a nuclei involved the modulation of the emotional component of pain. Another work [49] showed that acute activation of GALR1 promoted the expression of 'prodepressive-like' behaviours, while GALR2 mediated the 'antidepressant-like' effects of GAL. Hence, taking into account that depressive states heighten pain perception in humans [50] and rodents [51], the pronociceptive GALR1 and the antinociceptive GALR2 effects observed in this study may be related to comorbid mood alterations known to be associated with chronic pain [52,53].

3. Activation of serotonergic nuclei is influenced both by exogenous GAL in the DMH and noxious peripheral stimulation

The analysis of c-Fos expression was restricted to the VLPAG, DR, LC and RVM since these areas have been previously demonstrated to be strongly modulated by the DMH [54–56], while simultaneously implicated in nociceptive processing [57–59]. The limb extension-induced increase in c-Fos expression in the VLPAG and RVM of SHAM animals suggests that repetitive extension of a non-arthritic knee joint for a period of two hours can be considered a noxious stimulus [60]. In addition, the increased c-for expression in the VLPAG and RVM also suggests that repetitive knee joint extension activated the feedback loop of nociception involving the PAG-RVM-spinal dorsal horn circuitry, which may either inhibit or facilitate nociception [11,61,62].

Administration of exogenous GAL into the DMH increased the expression of c-Fos ipsilaterally in the VLPAG and bilaterally in the RVM, which suggests that DMH neurones expressing GALR are able to activate descending nociceptive controls. However, our electrophysiological data shows that exogenous GAL in the DMH did not alter the activity of RVM On- and Off-cells that are non-serotonergic pain control neurones. Therefore, we propose that the RVM cells expressing c-Fos following exogenous GAL treatment may have been RVM Neutral-cells, a subpopulation of which are serotonergic [63] and which were not studied in the present electrophysiological experiment. The fact that the DMH GAL-driven descending pronociceptive drive is independent of RVM On- and Off-like cell activity is very interesting in terms of pain management, since many centrally acting analgesic compounds (opioids, cannabinoids and non-steroidal anti-inflammatory drugs) reduce pain by increasing the discharge rate of antinociceptive RVM Off-cells and/or by inhibiting the discharge rate of pronociceptive RVM On-cells [61].

In SHAM animals, repetitive limb extension alone or exogenous GAL administration alone in the DMH activated the descending PAG-RVM-spinal cord pathway as revealed by c-Fos expression. However, application of exogenous GAL simultaneously with repetitive extension of the limb failed to increase c-Fos expression in the PAG-RVM circuitry of SHAM animals, suggesting that together the two stimulation procedures counteracted each other's effect, leading to a general inhibition of this circuitry. The increased c-Fos expression in the RVM by the pronociceptive exogenous GAL treatment alone might reflect activation of RVM serotonergic cells. While the serotonergic system has a complex role in pain control, there is evidence suggesting that the net effect induced by RVM serotonergic neurones is facilitation of nociception [64]. It should be noted here that serotonergic RVM neurones are not On- or Off- cells [63] that were studied in the present electrophysiological experiment using noxious heat and shown not to be influenced by exogenous GAL. We propose that the GAL-induced descending action may have induced activation of medullo-spinal serotonergic neurones shown as increased c-Fos expression in the RVM and resulting in the relay of pronociceptive action to the spinal cord.

The increased expression of c-Fos in the serotonergic DRN after limb extensions is in line with a role of this nucleus in ascending [65] and descending [66] pain modulatory pathways. Similarly, increased expression of c-Fos of DRN after exogenous GAL in the DMH is not unexpected as the DMH projects directly to the DRN [67] and the activity of DRN serotonergic neurones is influenced by GALR1 present on their soma and proximal dendrites [68]. It still remains to be studied through which mechanisms the DRN might be involved in the relay of the descending pronociceptive effect driven by exogenous GAL in the DMH.

4. Activation of the noradrenergic LC by exogenous GAL in the DMH and noxious peripheral stimulation varies between SHAM and ARTH animals

Previous studies have demonstrated that the LC responds to noxious stimulation, as revealed e.g. by c-Fos expression [69], while it is a major source of spinal noradrenaline and descending noradrenergic control of nociception [70,71]. In the present study, exogenous GAL treatment of DMH alone failed to influence c-Fos expression of LC in SHAM or ARTH animals. However, following repetitive limb extensions, c-Fos expression of LC was increased in SHAM but not ARTH animals. Interestingly, the peripheral stimulation-induced increase of c-Fos expression in the LC was predominantly ipsilateral, while ascending nociceptive signals activate the LC contra- or bilaterally [71]. A potential explanation for the ipsilaterally increased c-Fos expression after peripheral stimulation in the present study is that it reflected activation of descending pain modulation pathways descending predominantly ipsilaterally rather than processing of the ascending afferent volley that is expected to be contra- or bilateral. The DMH has a strong galaninergic output to various brain areas [72], including the LC [65], and GAL has been shown to decrease neuronal firing in LC [73]. While these findings suggest that the DMH may directly modulate activity of the LC, they still leave open what is the underlying mechanism and functional significance of the finding that exogenous GAL treatment of the DMH together with repetitive limb extensions increased c-Fos activity in the LC of ARTH but not SHAM animals.

5. Influence of arthritis and repetitive limb movement

The increase of c-Fos expression in the VLPAG and to a lesser extent in the RVM of SAL-treated ARTH animals indicates an overall increase in the tonic activity of the PAG-RVM-spinal cord pathways after the induction of experimental monoarthritis, which is in accordance with the enhancement of descending inhibitory circuits during chronic inflammation [74–77]. Interestingly, limb extension in the ARTH group decreased c-Fos expression in the VLPAG suggesting that acute noxious mechanical stimulation of the injured knee dampens tonic descending inhibition mediated by the VLPAG. On the other hand, the increase in c-Fos expression in the RVM, taking into account that the RVM can either facilitate or inhibit nociception [78], could indicate that this nucleus is engaged in descending facilitation during acute noxious stimulation of ARTH animals, as shown for other chronic pain disorders [79–81].

Our electrophysiological results showed that before any drug treatments both the baseline and the peripheral stimulus-evoked response in antinociceptive RVM Off-like cells were lower in ARTH than SHAM animals, while there was no difference in the pre-treatment heat-evoked activity of pronociceptive RVM On-like neurones of ARTH and SHAM animals. This finding suggests that a decreased activity of RVM Off-like cells contributes to hyperalgesia in ARTH animals. However, it does not exclude the possibility that among descending facilitatory mechanisms contributing to hyperalgesia in ARTH animals were other cell types of the RVM, in particular medullospinal serotonergic neurones, or other brainstem nuclei.

Concerning the DRN, the expression of c-Fos after repetitive limb extensions was increased, when compared with SAL-treated ARTH animals, but similar to the expression in c-Fos in SHAM after limb extensions, suggesting that the nociceptive processing through this pathway is not enhanced after the induction of experimental monoarthritis. By contrast, it is possible that the noxious stimulation-evoked activation of the LC is impaired in

ARTH animals, since c-Fos expression was decreased when compared to SHAM animals after limb extensions and unaltered when compared to SAL-treated ARTH animals.

Without noxious stimulation, exogenous GAL in the DMH of ARTH animals appeared to dampen tonic descending inhibition (as indicated by decreased c-Fos expression in the VLPAG) while it enhanced the tonic activity of pronociceptive serotonergic (indicated by increased c-Fos expression in the DRN and RVM), but not noradrenergic (unaltered c-Fos expression in the LC) circuits. However, when combined with limb extensions, both tonic descending inhibition (decreased c-Fos expression in the VLPAG) and the activity of pronociceptive serotonergic areas (decreased c-Fos expression in the RVM and DRN) were diminished. This finding indicates that in ARTH animals, exogenous GAL in the DMH exerts differential effects under basal and noxious stimulation-evoked conditions. A differential effect has also been reported while studying the role of GAL in the presence/absence of stress [49].

By contrast, only the combination of exogenous GAL injection in the DMH and limb stimulation was able to enhance the activity of the noradrenergic pain system as evidenced by the strong increase of c-Fos expression in the LC. Although noradrenergic pathways were up to recently considered to exert mostly inhibitory influences on spinal nociception, Hickey and colleagues [59] recently demonstrated that a specific subpopulation of LC neurones enhances the processing of nociceptive information and could thus partly contribute to behavioural hyperalgesia in chronic inflammation. Further studies are needed to find out whether LC is involved in mediating the descending pronociceptive effect elicited by exogenous GAL in the DMH.

Conclusions

In the present study, we demonstrate a pronociceptive GALR1-mediated role for hypothalamic GAL in experimental monoarthritis. Exogenous GAL in the DMH appeared to exert differential effects upon the brainstem pain modulatory areas; the effect varied between the experimental group (healthy or arthritic animals), brainstem nucleus (PAG, RVM, DRN, or LC), and the presence or absence of concomitant noxious stimulation. Finally, the results suggest that further studies evaluating the potential applicability of GALR1 antagonists in the control of chronic inflammatory pain are needed.

Author Contributions

Conceived and designed the experiments: DA FPR. Performed the experiments: DA ADP PM SP PR. Analyzed the data: DA PC. Contributed reagents/materials/analysis tools: AA. Wrote the paper: DA FPR. Revised the manuscript: AP AA.

References

1. Jimenez-Andrade JM, Zhou S, Du J, Yamani A, Grady JJ, et al. (2004) Pronociceptive role of peripheral galanin in inflammatory pain. Pain 110: 10–21.
2. Liu HX, Hökfelt TG (2002) The participation of galanin in pain processing at the spinal level. Trends Pharmacol Sci 23: 468–474.
3. Reeve AJ, Walker K, Urban L, Fox A (2000) Excitatory effects of galanin in the spinal cord of intact, anaesthetized rats. Neurosci Lett 295: 25–28.
4. Yue H, Fujita T, Kumamoto E (2011) Biphasic modulation by galanin of excitatory synaptic transmission in substantia gelatinosa neurons of adult rat spinal cord slices. J Neurophysiol 105: 2337–2349.
5. Brumovsky P, Mennicken F, O'Donnell D, Hökfelt T (2006) Differential distribution and regulation of galanin receptors- 1 and -2 in the rat lumbar spinal cord. Brain Res 1085: 111–120.
6. Ch'ng JL, Christofides ND, Anand P, Gibson SJ, Allen YS, et al. (1985) Distribution of galanin immunoreactivity in the central nervous system and the responses of galanin-containing neuronal pathways to injury. Neuroscience 16: 343–354.
7. Millan MJ (2002) Descending control of pain. Prog Neurobiol 66: 355–474.
8. Pinto-Ribeiro F, Ansah OB, Almeida A, Pertovaara A (2008) Influence of arthritis on descending modulation of nociception from the paraventricular nucleus of the hypothalamus. Brain Res 1197: 63–75.
9. Pinto-Ribeiro F, Amorim D, David-Pereira A, Monteiro AM, Costa P, et al. (2013) Pronociception from the dorsomedial nucleus of the hypothalamus is mediated by the rostral ventromedial medulla in healthy controls but is absent in arthritic animals. Brain Res Bull 99: 100–108.
10. Pertovaara A, Almeida A (2006) Descending inhibitory systems. In: Cervero F, Jensen T, (eds) Handbook of Clinical Neurology, 3rd series, Elsevier, Amsterdam, pp 179–192.
11. Almeida A, Leite-Almeida H, Tavares I (2006) Medullary control of nociceptive transmission: reciprocal dual communication with the spinal cord. Drug Discov Today Dis Mech 3: 305–312.
12. Lu X, Lundström L, Langel Ü, Bartfai T (2005) Galanin receptor ligands. Neuropeptides 39: 143–146.
13. Mitchell V, Habert-Ortoli E, Epelbaum J, Aubert J, Beauvillain JC (1997) Semiquantitative distribution of galanin-receptor (GAL-R1) mRNA-containing cells in the male rat hypothalamus. Neuroendocrinology 66: 160–172.
14. Waters SM, Krause JE (2000) Distribution of galanin-1, -2 and -3 receptor messenger RNAs in central and peripheral rat tissues. Neuroscience 29: 265–271.
15. Webling KE, Runesson J, Bartfai T, Langel Ü (2012) Galanin receptors and ligands. Front Endocrinol 3: 146.
16. Mennicken F, Hoffert C, Pelletier M, Ahmad S, O'Donnell D (2002) Restricted distribution of galanin receptor 3 (GalR3) mRNA in the adult rat central nervous system. J Chem Neuroanat 24: 257–268.
17. Sun YG, Gu XL, Lundeberg T, Yu LC (2003) An antinociceptive role of galanin in the arcuate nucleus of hypothalamus in intact rats and rats with inflammation. Pain 106: 143–150.
18. Sun YG, Li J, Yang BN, Yu LC (2004) Antinociceptive effects of galanin in the rat tuberomammillary nucleus and the plasticity of galanin receptor 1 during hyperalgesia. J Neurosci Res 77: 718–722.
19. Xu SL, Li J, Zhang JJ, Yu LC (2012) Antinociceptive effects of galanin in the nucleus accumbens of rats. Neurosci Lett 520: 43–46.
20. Jin WY, Liu Z, Liu D, Yu LC (2010) Antinociceptive effects of galanin in the central nucleus of amygdala of rats, an involvement of opioid receptors. Brain Res 1320: 16–21.
21. Li J, Zhang JJ, Xu SL, Yu LC (2012) Antinociceptive effects induced by injection of the galanin receptor 1 agonist M617 into central nucleus of amygdala in rats. Neurosci Lett 526: 45–48.
22. Wang D, Lundeberg T, Yu LC (2000) Antinociceptive role of galanin in periaqueductal grey of rats with experimentally induced mononeuropathy. Neuroscience 96: 767–771.
23. Kong Q, Yu LC (2013) Antinociceptive effects induced by intra-periaqueductal grey injection of the galanin receptor 1 agonist M617 in rats with morphine tolerance. Neurosci Lett: 4–7.
24. Blackshear A, Yamamoto M, Anderson BJ, Holmes PV, Lundström L, et al. (2007) Intracerebroventricular administration of galanin or galanin receptor subtype 1 agonist M617 induces c-Fos activation in central amygdala and dorsomedial. hypothalamus. Peptides 28: 1120–1124.
25. Martenson ME, Cetas JS, Heinricher MM (2009) A possible neural basis for stress-induced hyperalgesia. Pain 142: 236–244.
26. Ansah OB, Pertovaara A (2007) Peripheral suppression of arthritic pain by intraarticular fadolmidine, an alpha 2-adrenoceptor agonist, in the rat. Anesth Analg 105: 245–250.
27. Radhakrishnan R, Moore SA, Sluka KA (2003) Unilateral carrageenan injection into muscle or joint induces chronic bilateral hyperalgesia in rats. Pain 104: 567–577.
28. Randall L, Selitto J (1957) A method for measurement of analgesic activity on inflamed tissue. Arch Int Pharmacodyn Thérapie 111: 409–419.
29. Rivat C, Richebé P, Laboureyras E, Laulin JP, Havouis R, et al. (2008) Polyamine deficient diet to relieve pain hypersensitivity. Pain 137: 125–137.
30. Barton NJ, Strickland IT, Bond SM, Brash HM, Bate ST, et al. (2007) Pressure application measurement (PAM): a novel behavioural technique for measuring hypersensitivity in a rat model of joint pain. J Neurosci Methods 163: 67–75.
31. Hargreaves K, Dubner R, Brown F, Flores C, Joris J (1988) A new and sensitive method for measuring thermal nociception in cutaneous hyperalgesia. Pain 32: 77–88.
32. Paxinos G, Watson C (2007) The rat brain in stereotaxic coordinates. 6th ed. Elsevier Inc.
33. Myers RD (1966) Injection of solutions into cerebral tissue: Relation between volume and diffusion. Physiol Behav 1: 171–174.
34. Sun YG, Gu XL, Yu LC (2007) The neural pathway of galanin in the hypothalamic arcuate nucleus of rats: Activation of beta-endorphinergic neurons projecting to periaqueductal gray matter. J Neurosci Res 85: 2400–2406.

35. Fields HL, Bry J, Hentall I, Zorman G (1983) The activity of neurons in the rostral medulla of the rat during withdrawal from noxious heat. J Neurosci 3: 2545–2552.
36. Fields H, Heinricher MM (1985) Anatomy and physiology of a nociceptive modulatory system. Philos Trans R Soc Lond B Biol Sci 308: 361–374.
37. Sanoja R, Tortorici V, Fernandez C, Price TJ, Cervero F (2010) Role of RVM neurons in capsaicin-evoked visceral nociception and referred hyperalgesia. Eur J Pain 14: 120.e1–9.
38. Song Z, Ansah OB, Meyerson BA, Pertovaara A, Linderoth B (2013) The rostroventromedial medulla is engaged in the effects of spinal cord stimulation in a rodent model of neuropathic pain. Neuroscience 247: 134–144.
39. Morgado C, Tavares I (2007) C-fos expression at the spinal dorsal horn of streptozotocin-induced diabetic rats. Diabetes Metab Res Rev 23: 644–652.
40. Gu XL, Sun YG, Yu LC (2007) Involvement of galanin in nociceptive regulation in the arcuate nucleus of hypothalamus in rats with mononeuropathy. Behav Brain Res 179: 331–335.
41. Liu H, Brumovsky P, Schmidt R, Brown W, Payza K, et al. (2001) Receptor subtype-specific pronociceptive and analgesic actions of galanin in the spinal cord: selective actions via GalR1 and GalR2 receptors. Proc Natl Acad Sci U S A 98: 9960–9964.
42. Hulse RP, Donaldson LF, Wynick D (2012) Differential roles of galanin on mechanical and cooling responses at the primary afferent nociceptor. Mol Pain 8: 41.
43. Wang S, Hashemi T, Fried S, Clemmons AL, Hawes BE (1998) Differential intracellular signaling of the GalR1 and GalR2 galanin receptor subtypes. Biochemistry 37: 6711–6717.
44. Blakeman KH, Hao JX, Xu XJ, Jacoby AS, Shine J, et al. (2003) Hyperalgesia and increased neuropathic pain-like response in mice lacking galanin receptor 1 receptors. Neuroscience 117: 221–227.
45. Hua XY, Hayes CS, Hofer A, Fitzsimmons B, Kilk K, et al. (2004) Galanin acts at GalR1 receptors in spinal antinociception: synergy with morphine and AP-5. J Pharmacol Exp Ther 308: 574–582.
46. Fu LB, Wanga XB, Jiao S, Wua X, Yua LC (2011) Antinociceptive effects of intracerebroventricular injection of the galanin receptor 1 agonist M 617 in rats. Neurosci Lett 491: 174–176.
47. Mitchell V, Bouret S, Howard AD, Beauvillain JC (1999) Expression of the galanin receptor subtype Gal-R2 mRNA in the rat hypothalamus. J Chem Neuroanat 16: 265–277.
48. Amorim D, David-Pereira A, Pertovaara A, Almeida A, Pinto-Ribeiro F (2014) Amitriptyline reverses hyperalgesia and improves associated mood-like disorders in a model of experimental monoarthritis. Behav Brain Res 265: 12–21.
49. Kuteeva E, Wardi T, Lundström I, Sollenberg U, Langel Ü, et al. (2008) Differential role of galanin receptors in the regulation of depression-like behavior and monoamine/stress-related genes at the cell body level. Neuropsychopharmacology 33: 2573–2585.
50. Murphy LB, Sacks JJ, Brady TJ, Hootman JM, Chapman DP (2012) Anxiety and depression among US adults with arthritis: prevalence and correlates. Arthritis Care Res (Hoboken) 64: 968–976.
51. Wang S, Tian Y, Song L, Lim G, Tan Y, et al. (2012) Exacerbated mechanical hyperalgesia in rats with genetically predisposed depressive behavior: role of melatonin and NMDA receptors. Pain 153: 2448–2457.
52. Verdu B, Decosterd I, Buclin T, Stiefel F, Berney A (2008) Antidepressants for the treatment of chronic pain. Drugs 68: 2611–2632.
53. Neugebauer V, Galhardo V, Maione S, Mackey SC (2009) Forebrain Pain Mechanisms. Brain Res Rev 60: 226–242.
54. Johnson P, Lowry C, Truitt W, Shekhar A (2008) Disruption of GABAergic tone in the dorsomedial hypothalamus attenuates responses in a subset of serotonergic neurons in the dorsal raphe nucleus following lactate-induced panic. J Psycopharmacology 22: 642–652.
55. Aston-Jones G, Chen S, Zhu Y, Oshinsky M (2001) A neural circuit for circadian regulation of arousal. Nat Neurosci 4: 732–738.
56. Wagner KM, Roeder Z, Desrochers K, Buhler AV, Heinricher MM, et al. (2013) The dorsomedial hypothalamus mediates stress-induced hyperalgesia and is the source of the pronociceptive peptide cholecystokinin in the rostral ventromedial medulla. Neuroscience 238: 29–38.
57. Wang QP, Nakai Y (1994) The dorsal raphe: an important nucleus in pain modulation. Brain Res Bull 34: 575–585.
58. De Luca MC, Brandão ML, Motta VA, Landeira-Fernandez J (2003) Antinociception induced by stimulation of ventrolateral periaqueductal gray at the freezing threshold is regulated by opioid and 5-HT2A receptors as assessed by the tail-flick and formalin tests. Pharmacol Biochem Behav 75: 459–466.
59. Hickey L, Li Y, Fyson SJ, Watson TC, Perrins R, et al. (2014) Optoactivation of locus ceruleus neurons evokes bidirectional changes in thermal nociception in rats. J Neurosci 34: 4148–4160.
60. Galbán CJ, Ling SM, Taub DD, Gurkan I, Fishbein KW, et al. (2007) Effects of knee injection on skeletal muscle metabolism and contractile force in rats. Osteoarthr Cartil 15: 550–558.
61. Ossipov MH, Dussor GO, Porreca F (2010) Central modulation of pain. J Clin Invest 120: 3779–3787.
62. Heinricher MM, Tavares I, Leith JL, Lumb BM (2009) Descending control of nociception: Specificity, recruitment and plasticity. Brain Res Rev 60: 214–225.
63. Potrebic SB, Fields HL, Mason P (1994) Serotonin immunoreactivity is contained in one physiological cell class in the rat rostral ventromedial medulla. J Neurosci 14: 1655–1665.
64. Wei F, Dubner R, Zou S, Ren K, Bai G, et al. (2010) Molecular depletion of descending serotonin unmasks its novel facilitatory role in the development of persistent pain. J Neurosci 30: 8624–8636.
65. Qiao JT, Dafny N (1988) Dorsal raphe stimulation modulates nociceptive responses in thalamic parafascicular neurons via an ascending pathway: further studies on ascending pain modulation pathways. Pain 34: 65–74.
66. Prado WA, Faganello FA (2000) The anterior pretectal nucleus participates as a relay station in the glutamate-, but not morphine-induced antinociception from the dorsal raphe nucleus in rats. Pain 88: 169–176.
67. ter Horst G, Luiten P (1986) The projections of the dorsomedial hypothalamic nucleus in the rat. Brain Res Bull 16: 231–248.
68. Larm JA, Shen PJ, Gundlach AL (2003) Differential galanin receptor-1 and galanin expression by 5-HT neurons in dorsal raphé nucleus of rat and mouse: evidence for species-dependent modulation of serotonin transmission. Eur J Neurosci 17: 481–493.
69. Voisin DL, Guy N, Chalus M, Dallel R (2005) Nociceptive stimulation activates locus coeruleus neurones projecting to the somatosensory thalamus in the rat. J Physiol 566: 929–937.
70. Jones SL (1991) Descending noradrenergic influences on pain. Prog Brain Res 88: 381–394.
71. Pertovaara A (2006) Noradrenergic pain modulation. Prog Neurobiol 80: 53–83.
72. Jacobowitz DM, Kresse A, Skofitsch G (2004) Galanin in the brain: chemoarchitectonics and brain cartography - a historical review. Peptides 25: 433–464.
73. Sevcik J, Finta EP, Illes P (1993) Galanin receptors inhibit the spontaneous firing of locus coeruleus neurones and interact with mu-opioid receptors. Eur J Pharmacol 230: 223–230.
74. Ren K, Dubner R (2002) Descending modulation in persistent pain: an update. Pain 100: 1–6.
75. Cervero F, Schaible HG, Schmidt RF (1991) Tonic descending inhibition of spinal cord neurones driven by joint afferents in normal cats and in cats with an inflamed knee joint. Exp Brain Res 83: 675–678.
76. Ren K, Dubner R (1996) Enhanced descending modulation of nociception in rats with persistent hindpaw inflammation. J Neurophysiol 76: 3025–3037.
77. Terayama R, Guan Y, Dubner R, Ren K (2000) Activity-induced plasticity in brain stem pain modulatory circuitry after inflammation. Neuro Rep 26: 1915–1919.
78. Heinricher MM, Barbaro NM, Fields HL (1989) Putative nociceptive modulating neurons in the rostral ventromedial medulla of the rat: firing of on- and off-cells is related to nociceptive responsiveness. Somatosens Mot Res 6: 427–439.
79. Porreca F, Ossipov MH, Gebhart GF (2002) Chronic pain and medullary descending facilitation. Trends Neurosci 25: 319–325.
80. Herrero JF, Cervero F (1996) Supraspinal influences on the facilitation of rat nociceptive reflexes induced by carrageenan monoarthritis. Neurosci Lett 209: 21–24.
81. Kovelowski CJ, Ossipov MH, Sun H, Lai J, Malan TP, et al. (2000) Supraspinal cholecystokinin may drive tonic descending facilitation mechanisms to maintain neuropathic pain in the rat. Pain 87: 265–273.

10

Comparison of Results from Different Imputation Techniques for Missing Data from an Anti-Obesity Drug Trial

Anders W. Jørgensen[1], Lars H. Lundstrøm[2], Jørn Wetterslev[2], Arne Astrup[3], Peter C. Gøtzsche[1,4]*

1 The Nordic Cochrane Centre, Dept 7811, Rigshospitalet, Copenhagen, Denmark, 2 Copenhagen Trial Unit, Copenhagen Centre of Clinical Intervention Research, Dept 7812, Rigshospitalet, Copenhagen, Denmark, 3 Department of Nutrition, Exercise and Sports, Faculty of Science, University of Copenhagen, Frederiksberg, Denmark, 4 Institute of Medicine and Surgery, Faculty of Health Sciences, University of Copenhagen, Copenhagen, Denmark

Abstract

Background: In randomised trials of medical interventions, the most reliable analysis follows the intention-to-treat (ITT) principle. However, the ITT analysis requires that missing outcome data have to be imputed. Different imputation techniques may give different results and some may lead to bias. In anti-obesity drug trials, many data are usually missing, and the most used imputation method is last observation carried forward (LOCF). LOCF is generally considered conservative, but there are more reliable methods such as multiple imputation (MI).

Objectives: To compare four different methods of handling missing data in a 60-week placebo controlled anti-obesity drug trial on topiramate.

Methods: We compared an analysis of complete cases with datasets where missing body weight measurements had been replaced using three different imputation methods: LOCF, baseline carried forward (BOCF) and MI.

Results: 561 participants were randomised. Compared to placebo, there was a significantly greater weight loss with topiramate in all analyses: 9.5 kg (SE 1.17) in the complete case analysis (N = 86), 6.8 kg (SE 0.66) using LOCF (N = 561), 6.4 kg (SE 0.90) using MI (N = 561) and 1.5 kg (SE 0.28) using BOCF (N = 561).

Conclusions: The different imputation methods gave very different results. Contrary to widely stated claims, LOCF did not produce a conservative (i.e., lower) efficacy estimate compared to MI. Also, LOCF had a lower SE than MI.

Editor: D. William Cameron, University of Ottawa, Canada

Funding: The authors have no support or funding to report.

Competing Interests: This trial was supported by Johnson & Johnson Pharmaceutical Research and Development, LLP, the producer of topiramate, to conduct the clinical trial from which the data for this paper originated (see reference 10). Arne Astrup is currently consultant or member of advisory boards for a number companies, including: Arena Pharmaceuticals Inc., USA; Basic Research, USA; BioCare Copenhagen, DenmarK; Boehringer Ingelheim Pharma, Germany; Gelesis, USA; Novo Nordisk, Denmark; Pathway Genomics Corporation, USA; S-Biotek, Denmark; Twinlab, USA; Vivus Inc., USA.

* Email: pcg@cochrane.dk

Introduction

Attrition has been described as the bane of clinical trials on anti-obesity drugs [1]. In most studies more than one third of the participants have dropped out after one year [2], and in most cases, missing data leads to bias [3]. Missingness can be classified as missing completely at random (MCAR), missing at random (MAR), or missing not at random (MNAR). In case of MCAR missingness is independent of any observed or unobserved data, e.g. a blood sample that is accidentally dropped on the floor. Only when missingness is MCAR, the use of a complete case analysis of the data, obtained exclusively from participants with all data observed, may give an unbiased result. However, in most studies MCAR is not the case [4]. When missingness is MAR, missingness depends on the observed data, e.g. people with the smallest treatment effect quit the trial. Finally, when missingness is MNAR,

it also depends on some unobserved data, e.g. people with an unregistered latent depression quit the trial due to mood changes.

One of the most commonly applied methods for handling attrition in obesity research is 'last observation carried forward' (LOCF) [2] where a missing weight measurement of a participant at the end of trial is replaced by the participant's last observed value. To assume that one's weight is unchanged after dropping out of a trial seems hard to justify, as participants tend to regain much of their lost weight within a short period of time after having stopped the intervention [5]. Therefore, 'baseline carried forward' (BOCF) has been proposed as a more reliable imputation strategy [6]. However, both BOCF and LOCF overestimate the precision of the effect estimate because the dataset is analysed, after single imputation of the missing data, as if it was a 'complete' dataset with no missing data [7]. Also intuitively, as one has doubts about the imputed data, the p-values and confidence interval should be larger than those computed. Therefore, BOCF and LOCF both provide undue certainty of the effect estimate even under MCAR assumptions.

There are more reliable techniques for handling missing data [8], and they can also be used when missingness is MAR. Attention has been drawn to the multiple imputation (MI) technique [9], which for some time has been recommended for handling missing data in obesity trials [2]. The multiple imputation technique is a stepwise procedure. First, based on the observed data, a plausible multivariable distribution for the missing values is estimated and they are being replaced by values randomly drawn from this distribution resulting in a complete dataset. Second, this procedure is repeated multiple times generating multiple datasets. Third, the datasets are then analysed separately producing multiple estimates, and fourth, the multiple estimates are pooled resulting in one single estimate. Compared to LOCF and BOCF, the precision will be more realistically estimated because the uncertainty of the imputed values is taken into account.

We had access to individual patient data from a large randomised three-armed weight loss maintenance trial that compared diet plus topiramate (96 mg or 192 mg) with diet plus placebo (clinicaltrials.gov PRI/TOP-INT-35) [10]. Our primary aim was to analyse the weight change and compare the results by using four different methods for handling missing data. We analysed the dataset of complete cases and datasets where missing weight measurements had been replaced using three different imputation methods LOCF, BOCF and MI. Our second aim was to report the results of the analysis of the primary outcome measure at the time-point specified in the trial protocol. These were not reported in the published paper [10], because of premature trial termination due to low tolerability of the drug.

Material and Methods

The trial was a randomised weight loss maintenance trial (n = 561) that compared placebo (n = 187) with topiramate 96 mg (n = 190) and 192 mg (n = 184) per day. It was designed to run for a total of 82 weeks; an 8-week non-pharmacological low-calorie diet run-in phase followed by randomisation, a 60-week intervention phase, a 2-week drug tapering period and 12-week follow-up period. The data included assessments of weight from 26 visits plus standard baseline values (age, height, sex, etc.), a variety of blood sample analyses and measures of hip and waist circumferences. Each visit corresponded to a specific number of weeks in the trial. More details about the methodology have been published previously [10]. The authors of the published trial report wanted to reduce the risk of bias due to premature trial termination and therefore chose to analyse only a subset of people who had received at least one dose of study drug, had provided at least one post-baseline efficacy evaluation, and had the opportunity to complete 44 weeks of treatment before the study closedown announcement. They only allowed data collected before the closedown announcement and up to week 44 to be included in the analysis of efficacy. The primary outcome was percent weight change from enrolment to the end of the intervention phase after 60 weeks of treatment, but this has not been published.

Data

Data was provided by the first author (AA) of a previous report of this trial [10] and imported to SPSS 18.0.

Missingness

We assessed the mechanism of missingness by using Little's test [11] and by plotting mean weights of people with missing data with those with data. Little's test is essentially a Chi-square test on whether the complete cases actually consist of a sample chosen completely at random (MCAR) from the intention-to-treat population considering the variables measured on the patients with missingness. $P<0.05$ excludes a scenario due to MCAR and makes the scenario missing at random (MAR, i.e. missingness is explained by measured variables) more likely, although a scenario of missing not at random (MNAR, i.e. missingness depending on some unobserved variable), can never be totally excluded.

Comparison of imputation methods

We used the data from baseline (randomisation, week 0) to end of treatment (week 60). For simplicity, we pooled the topiramate arms. We analysed the mean weight change in the placebo and the pooled topiramate group and the difference between the two from baseline to end of treatment. We also analysed percentage change in the same way. The results were plotted against time for comparisons between the four analysis methods. We used the t-test to calculate p-values.

Complete case analysis

This did not involve any imputation and was an analysis of data from participants on intervention, i.e. all available data from baseline to end of treatment.

Last observation carried forward

We substituted missing weight measurements with the last observed measurement. We allowed carrying forward the baseline value if this was the last observed measurement.

Baseline carried forward

We substituted missing weight measurements with the baseline weight.

Mutiple imputation

We imputed the missing weight measurements with values of weight obtained by the 'Fully conditional specification method' in SPSS ver. 18. This is an iterative Markov chain Monte Carlo method that can be used when the pattern of missing data is monotone (i.e. a subject attends all visits till a visit is missed and never returns) or none-monotone [12]. We used a linear regression model that contained the variables: intervention group, sex, race, age and baseline values (height, waist circumference, plasma glucose, triglycerides, HDL-cholesterol, HDL/LDL-ratio, insulin, haemoglobin and haemoglobin A1c). Additionally, we included body weight, but only at visits prior to the visit of interest. For example, we only included weight measurements from baseline to week 20 for the imputation at week 20. We log-transformed weight to satisfy the normality assumption which seemed to hold when we assessed Q-Q plots and used the Kolmogorov–Smirnov test (p> 0.2, df = 561), but not the Shapiro–Wilk test (p = 0.04, df = 561). We also assessed convergence by plotting the means and standard deviations by iteration and imputation. The default number of 10 iterations in SPSS 18 seemed to be too low (File S1) as the standard deviation gradually increased up till and stabilized at 400 iterations. Therefore we chose 500 iterations and 10 imputations assuring an efficiency of the imputation of 99%.

The primary outcome measure at 60 weeks in the trial protocol

We estimated the mean percent weight change from enrolment (week –8) to end of treatment using the same methods as described above. For completeness, we also re-analysed the data on the subset of people previously published [10]). Using the criteria above, it was not possible to get the exact same subset, but when we allowed data collected 3 days after the closedown announcement to be included in the analysis we came close.

Results

Details about the study population have previously been published [10]. Baseline characteristics are available in File S1 and include the variables used in our analyses after MI.

Missingness

Missing data on weight gradually increased from week 0 to 44 (from 0% to 27%), and then increased markedly (Figure 1); only 15% (n = 86) of the participants were still on treatment and had their weight recorded at the end of treatment. The reason for missingness varied, but although it was mostly caused by premature trial termination [10], the mechanism was unlikely to be MCAR (P<0.01; Little's test)(11). At most visits, participants who missed the following visit seemed to weigh more than those who attended (Figure 1).

Comparison of imputation methods over time and with increasing missingness

From baseline to week 44, the estimated difference in mean weight change between placebo and topiramate increased by all four methods. From week 44 to end of treatment, the difference increased in the complete case analysis and in LOCF, but decreased in MI and BOCF (Figure 2). From baseline to end of treatment the complete case analysis estimated the greatest difference in weight loss (9.5 kg) and BOCF the smallest (1.5 kg). MI and LOCF were similar with MI resulting in a slightly greater difference from the beginning and throughout most of the trial and

a slightly smaller difference at the end of treatment (6.4 kg) compared to LOCF (6.8 kg).

These differences were a result of an overall weight loss in the topiramate group (Figure 3) and weight gain in the placebo group (Figure 4). At the end of treatment the weight loss within the pooled topiramate group was again biggest in the complete case analysis (5.9 kg) and smallest in the BOCF (0.9 kg). Also, MI and LOCF estimated a similar weight loss in the beginning of the trial, but at the end of treatment MI (3.4 kg) showed a much smaller weight loss than LOCF (5.5 kg) (Figure 3). The change within the placebo group was similar in the complete case analysis and BOCF in the beginning, but at the end of treatment the complete case analysis estimated the biggest weight gain (3.7 kg) and BOCF the smallest (0.5 kg). In the placebo group, MI and LOCF were similar in the beginning, but at the end of treatment MI (3.0 kg) showed a greater weight gain than LOCF (1.3 kg at week 60) (Figure 4).

We got similar results when we analysed the percentage change from baseline (data not shown).

The trial's primary outcome measure at 60 weeks

The primary outcome measure at end of trial according to the trial protocol was the percentage change from enrolment (week –8) to end of treatment (week 60), and for placebo compared to topiramate 96 mg the mean difference in weight loss was 10.5% (SE = 2.2%) in the complete case analysis, 6.1% (SE = 0.7%) using LOCF, 5.5% (SE = 1.1%) using MI and 1.7% (SE = 0.4%) using BOCF. For placebo compared to topiramate 192 mg/day, the mean difference was 10.0% (SE = 1.9%), 7.5% (SE = 0.8%), 7.3% (SE = 1.0%) and 1.5% (SE = 0.4%) using complete case analysis, LOCF, MI and BOCF, respectively (Table 1). To check the robustness of the findings of this analysis, we also pooled the topiramate groups in a sensitivity analysis and the results were similar (File S1).

When we re-analysed the percentage change from enrolment to week 44 of the subset of participants, our results were similar to those published previously (File S1).

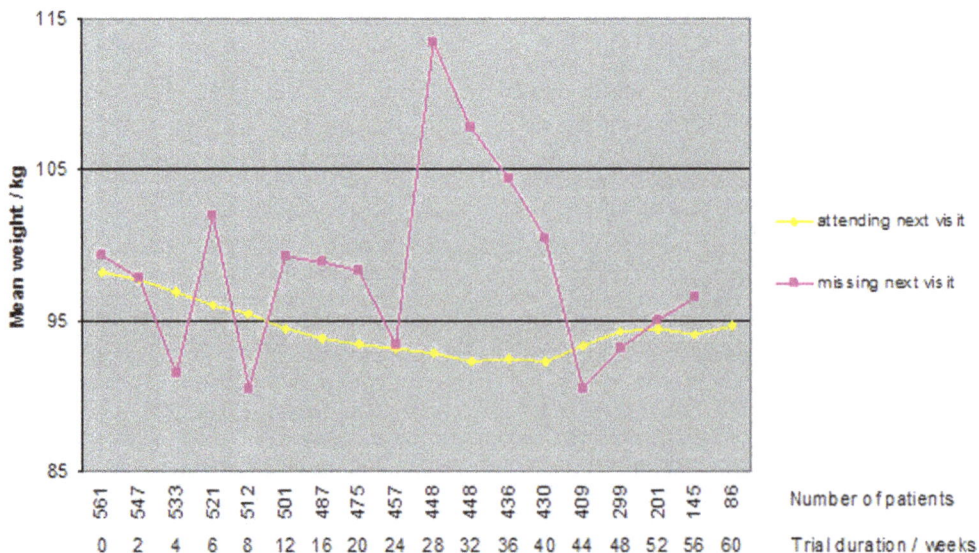

Figure 1. **Mean weight of participants attending or missing the next visit.** Some patients return after a missed visit. Therefore no change in number of patients at week 28 and 32.

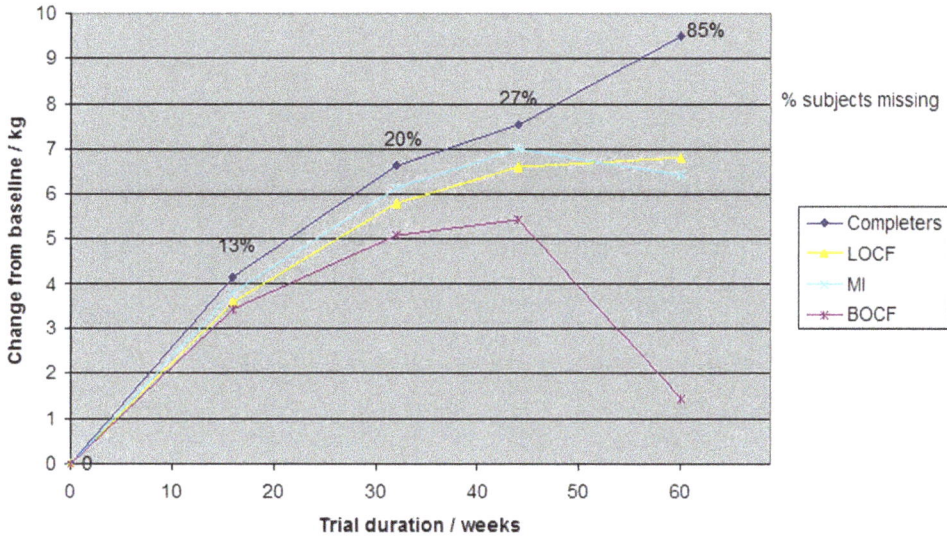

Figure 2. Analysis of difference in weight loss between placebo and topiramate pooled (96 and 192 mg/day) from baseline to week 60 using different methods.

Discussion

We compared 4 methods of analysing the effect of topiramate in a weight loss trial. We found that, in the beginning of the trial, LOCF and MI estimated similar body weight changes, but over time and with high attrition they estimated different changes. This, however, did not have a substantial impact on the difference in body weight change between topiramate and placebo, which was similar throughout the trial.

Complete case analysis estimated the greatest difference and BOCF the smallest. We also estimated the weight change as originally planned in the trial protocol as it was done in a previous publication of the trial [10], and our results confirmed, regardless of method, that in this trial topiramate produces a greater weight loss than placebo. Other placebo-controlled trials have also shown that topiramate reduces weight [13].

In several simulation studies, MI has been shown to provide a more accurate and broader confidence interval and a less biased estimate of the intervention effect than both complete case analysis and single imputations [14][15][16]. In these studies, the method has been to simulate missingness based on a complete dataset and to use different imputation techniques to calculate an estimate of the intervention effect from the imputed dataset. Thus, these studies have been able to evaluate how close the result of an imputation method comes to the correct estimate from the original complete dataset. The results of such simulation studies have been overwhelmingly in favour of MI.

In trials on anti-obesity drugs, it has previously been shown that the LOCF estimates similar effect sizes, but overestimates the

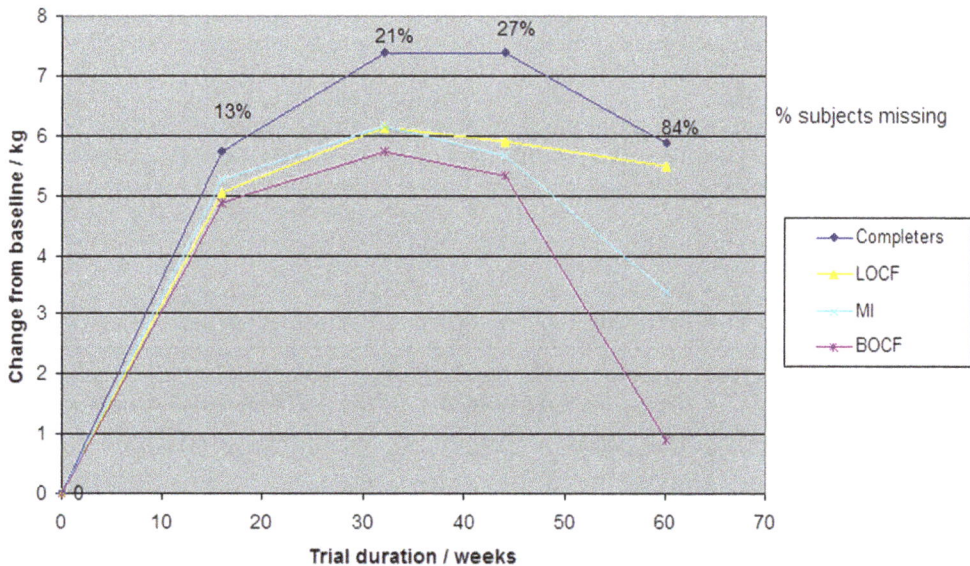

Figure 3. Analysis of weight loss over time in topiramate pooled (96 or 192 mg/day) group using different imputation methods.

Analysis of weight loss over time in placebo group using different imputation methods

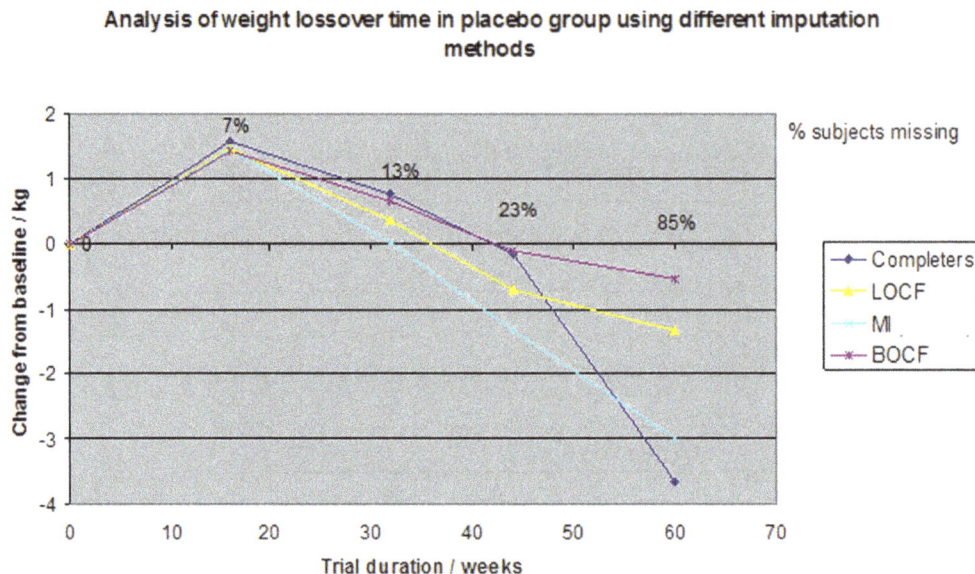

Figure 4. Analysis of weight loss over time in the placebo group using different imputation methods.

precision, compared to MI [2][8]. It is therefore wrong to describe LOCF as a conservative analysis, although this is often done.

Our results can be interpreted in relation to the *per-protocol (PP) assumption* that all participants adhere to treatment, which is an unrealistic scenario in trials on anti-obesity drugs, or the *intention-to-treat (ITT) method* that assumes that some participants do not adhere to treatment. Thus the PP analysis estimates the weight loss as if the participants adhere to the treatment and the ITT analysis estimates the weight loss of the intention to give the treatment regardless of adherence [17].

If a drug truly reduces the weight, the BOCF will yield a conservative estimate (smaller weight loss) than a PP analysis, but maybe a realistic estimate compared to an ITT analysis [6], as it is likely that participants regain some of their body weight when they stop treatment [5].

The interpretation of the LOCF analyses is difficult due to the course of weight change during a weight loss trial. Most of the weight loss occurs early on, then levels out and some is regained at the end of the trial [18]. Compared with a PP analysis, it may be reasonable to assume that LOCF underestimates the weight loss in the short term and overestimates it in the long term. On the other hand, compared with an ITT analysis, it is likely that LOCF overestimates the weight loss and therefore BOCF should be preferred for LOCF.

Our MI analysis is more compatible with the PP assumption than the ITT assumption [17], because the imputations were based on participants who were on treatment, topiramate or placebo. If we had had complete data on some of the participants that dropped out or did not adhere to the treatment, we could have used their data for MI, which would then have reflected an ITT analysis [17]. When no such data is available the MI analysis is clearly preferable to the biased PP analysis that only includes participants that have adhered to the protocol, but readers and researchers need to think carefully about the analytic assumption (e.g., PP versus ITT) used in an obesity trial.

Theoretically, the complete case analysis *can* occasionally be an unbiased PP analysis, but only when the participants in the analysis can be regarded as a random sample of the study population (when the missing mechanism is MCAR, which is rarely the case [4]). In our dataset, the missing mechanism was not MCAR. It seemed that those who had missing data weighed more than those without and thus the complete case analysis overestimated the weight loss.

Results from weight loss trials are often inadequately reported. The weight change within the treatment groups is stated and the p-value may be the only result reported from the comparison between the groups. Sometimes only the difference in weight change between the groups is stated. We have reported body weight change within the groups and between the groups, but also

Table 1. Percentage weight change from enrolment (- 8 week) to end of treatment (week 60).

	Placebo Mean (SE)	Topimarate 96 mg Mean (SE)	Topimarate 192 mg Mean (SE)
Completers	−7.1 (1.40) (n = 28)	−16.2 (1.58) (n = 31)	−16.1 (1.48) (n = 27)
LOCF	−9.2 (0.54) (n = 187)	−14.7 (0.52) (n = 190)	−16.2 (0.65) (n = 184)
MI	−7.7 (0.68) (n = 187)	−12.6 (0.75) (n = 190)	−14.6 (0.76) (n = 184)
BOCF	−9.8 (0.26) (n = 187)	−11.3 (0.33) (n = 190)	−11.5 (0.30) (n = 184)

SE: standard error.
For each difference (topiramate - placebo), P<0.001 (t-test).

p-values and CI-intervals. We found that MI and LOCF resulted in similar differences between topiramate and placebo, but that the weight change within the groups was smaller in the MI analysis than in LOCF and this difference increased over time and with increasing missing data. The most likely explanation for this is that LOCF, but not MI, ignores the course of weight change (described above) and that the bias LOCF introduces is more or less the same in both treatment groups. Further, MI introduced greater but more realistic uncertainty of the intervention effect estimate than LOCF and BOCF; analyses using LOCF and BOCF can therefore lead to spuriously significant results.

Limitations

As we do not know the true effect of topiramate or the body weight of the missing participants, it is impossible to validate our findings against a gold standard. Also, we do not know the exact mechanism of missingness. If the mechanism is MNAR, all imputation methods are likely to be biased. However, MI may provide less biased results in this situation as well [16].

Another limitation is that many data were missing simply because the trial was terminated prematurely, which is not a common reason for attrition in obesity trials. The reason for termination was harms. As we did not include harms in our imputation model, missingness could be related to data that are 'unobserved' by the MI procedure. On the other hand, the harms could be correlated to the variables we used; in fact, Figure 1 shows that missingness could be predicted by the weight of the participants. This suggests that people experiencing similar harms are more likely to stay in the trial if they have perceived an effect on their weight.

Suggestions for improved research

The major reason for missing data when participants quit the treatment is their lack of interest for having their weight measured and for obvious reasons trialists cannot force the patient to show up for a visit. Therefore we need weight loss trials that include incentives for participants to be followed up and other logistic methods for measuring the weight and side effects of those participants who decide to quit treatment.

Most trial protocols specify that investigators shall do their best to have a measurement at the end of the specified period, but usually do not provide incentives or methods. The protocol for the current trial stated that, "Participants withdrawn from the study prior to completion of treatment period will be encouraged [...] to attend study visits with assessments equivalent to those performed at Visit 23 [end of treatment]"

The protocol for the RIO-North America trial of rimonabant had a similar statement [19]: "For patients with premature treatment discontinuation or patients considered lost to follow-up, the [case report form] must be filled in up to the last visit performed. The Investigator should make every effort to re-contact and to identify the reason why the patient failed to attend the visit and to determine his/her health status and to retrieve study medication."

When the RIO-trial was published it was criticised in an editorial for only measuring those participants that completed the trial (53%) rather than all patients that were not lost to follow-up (93%) [18]. It is indeed possible to have a high follow-up as seen in a recently published weight loss trial of free meals and an intensive weight loss program. After 24 months the investigators had weight data on 92% of the study participants [20]. If participants don't attend the last visit, one might also contact them by phone and ask them to use their own scale at home. Despite a trend that self-reported weight is underestimated [22], this strategy may still be reliable when comparing intervention and control groups, because the bias introduced is likely to be similar in both groups.

Selective reporting of favourable analyses also occurs. In a placebo-controlled trial of long-term treatment with sibutramine, the authors only published an unadjusted ITT analysis (LOCF) (n = 464). Compared to placebo the body weight reduction with sibutramine 15 mg was 4.8 kg (p<0.001) and with 10 mg 2.8 kg (p<0.01) [21]. In a trial report of the same study submitted to the Danish Medicines Agency, an adjusted analysis of all available participants (including those who were withdrawn) that had their body weight measured at end of treatment (n = 305), showed smaller weight reductions, 3.0 kg (p<0.001) and 2.1 (p<0.01) kg, respectively.

When imputation is undertaken, more reliable techniques, such as MI, should be used and to make a proper ITT analysis, imputation should also be based on weight data collected after withdrawal In general, MI is considered one of the most reliable methods for imputing missing data. It has been available for more than 20 years and in standard statistical programs for about 10 years. But MI is rarely used in randomised trials and has only recently been proposed for trials on anti-obesity drugs [2]. There has been and still is a steadfast tradition of using LOCF in these trials, but policy is changing. The European Medicines Agency has from 2011 implemented a guideline for handling missing data in clinical trials [23] that the drug industry has to follow. The guideline does not find LOCF, (but BOCF) appropriate for chronic conditions such as obesity where the weight will be expected to return to baseline when the treatment is stopped and it describes MI as a more proper imputation technique. Therefore, we assume that we will see more trials using BOCF and MI in the future. With these changes, drug companies will be more motivated for minimising attrition and missing data because increasing attrition and missing data will result in a treatment effect that approaches zero when BOCF is used.

Conclusions

The different imputation methods gave different results, but all showed that topiramate reduced weight compared to placebo. In anti-obesity trials, imputation is obligatory due to the amount and type of missing data and because the complete case analysis is biased. However, the ITT analysis using LOCF, which in general is considered a conservative analysis, overestimated the precision. We suggest that post withdrawal weight data must be obtained to make a proper ITT analysis.

Author Contributions

Conceived and designed the experiments: AWJ JW PCG. Performed the experiments: AA. Analyzed the data: AWJ LHL JW. Contributed reagents/materials/analysis tools: AA. Wrote the paper: AWJ. Contributed to writing the paper: LHL JW AA PCG.

References

1. Fabricatore AN, Wadden TA, Moore RH, Butryn ML, Gravallese EA, et al. (2009) Attrition from randomized controlled trials of pharmacological weight loss agents: a systematic review and analysis. Obes Rev 10: 333–341.
2. Elobeid MA, Padilla MA, McVie T, Thomas O, Brock DW, et al. (2009) Missing data in randomized clinical trials for weight loss: scope of the problem, state of the field, and performance of statistical methods. PLoS ONE 4: e6624.
3. Sterne JAC, White IR, Carlin JB, Spratt M, Royston P, et al. (2009) Multiple imputation for missing data in epidemiological and clinical research: potential and pitfalls. BMJ 338: b2393.
4. Donders ART, van der Heijden GJMG, Stijnen T, Moons KGM (2006) Review: a gentle introduction to imputation of missing values. J Clin Epidemiol 5: 1087–1091.
5. Methods for voluntary weight loss and control (1992) NIH Technology Assessment Conference Panel. Consensus Development Conference, 30 March to 1 April 1992. Ann Intern Med 1993; 119: 764–770.
6. Ware JH (2003) Interpreting incomplete data in studies of diet and weight loss. NEJM 348: 2136–2137.
7. Beunckens C, Molenberghs G, Kenward MG (2005) Direct likelihood analysis versus simple forms of imputation for missing data in randomized clinical trials. Clin Trials 2: 379–386.
8. Molenberghs G, Kenward M (2007) Missing data in clinical studies. Wiley.
9. Gadbury GL, Coffey CS, Allison DB (2003) Modern statistical methods for handling missing repeated measurements in obesity trial data: beyond LOCF. Obes Rev 4: 175–184.
10. Astrup A, Caterson I, Zelissen P, Guy-Grand B, Carruba M, et al. (2004) Topiramate: long-term maintenance of weight loss induced by a low-calorie diet in obese subjects. Obes Res 12: 1658–1669.
11. Little RJA (1988) A Test of Missing Completely at Random for Multivariate Data with Missing Values. Journal of the American Statistical Association. 83: 1198–1202.
12. PASW Missing Values 18. http://support.spss.com/productsext/statistics/documentation/18/client/User%20Manuals/English/PASW%20Missing%20Values%2018.pdf. Accessed 14 Feb 2011.
13. Kramer CK, Leitão CB, Pinto LC, Canani LH, Azevedo MJ, et al. (2011) Efficacy and safety of topiramate on weight loss: a meta-analysis of randomized controlled trials. Obes Rev 12: e338–347.
14. Sinharay S, Stern HS, Russell D (2001) The use of multiple imputation for the analysis of missing data. Psychol Methods 6: 317–329.
15. Schafer JL, Graham JW (2002) Missing data: Our view of the state of the art. Psychological Methods 7: 147–177.
16. Schafer JL (1999) Multiple imputation: a primer. Stat Methods Med Res 8: 3–15.
17. Carpenter J, Kenward M Missing data in randomised controlled trials - a practical guide. http://www.haps.bham.ac.uk/publichealth/methodology/docs/invitations/Final_Report_RM04_JH17_mk.pdf. Accessed 14 Feb 2011.
18. Simons-Morton DG, Obarzanek E, Cutler JA (2006) Obesity research–limitations of methods, measurements, and medications. JAMA 295: 826–828.
19. Pi-Sunyer FX, Aronne LJ, Heshmati HM, Devin J, Rosenstock J (2006) Effect of rimonabant, a cannabinoid-1 receptor blocker, on weight and cardiometabolic risk factors in overweight or obese patients: RIO-North America: a randomized controlled trial. JAMA 295: 761–775.
20. Rock CL, Flatt SW, Sherwood NE, Karanja N, Pakiz B, et al. (2010) Effect of a free prepared meal and incentivized weight loss program on weight loss and weight loss maintenance in obese and overweight women: a randomized controlled trial. JAMA 304: 1803–1810.
21. Smith IG, Goulder MA (2001) Randomized placebo-controlled trial of long-term treatment with sibutramine in mild to moderate obesity. J Fam Pract 50: 505–512.
22. Gorber SC, Tremblay M, Moher D, Gorber B (2007) A comparison of direct vs. self-report measures for assessing height, weight and body mass index: a systematic review. Obes Rev 8: 307–26.
23. Guideline on Missing Data in Confirmatory Clinical Trials (2010) 10 July 2010. http://www.ema.europa.eu/ema/pages/includes/document/open_document.jsp?webContentId=WC500096793. Accessed 9 Nov 2012.

11

Measuring the Bright Side of Being Blue: A New Tool for Assessing Analytical Rumination in Depression

Skye P. Barbic[1], Zachary Durisko[1], Paul W. Andrews[2]*

1 Social Aetiology of Mental Illness (SAMI) Canadian Institute of Health Research (CIHR) Training Program, Centre for Addiction and Mental Health, Toronto, Ontario, Canada, **2** Department of Psychology, Neuroscience & Behaviour, McMaster University, Hamilton, Canada

Abstract

Background: Diagnosis and management of depression occurs frequently in the primary care setting. Current diagnostic and management of treatment practices across clinical populations focus on eliminating signs and symptoms of depression. However, there is debate that some interventions may pathologize normal, adaptive responses to stressors. Analytical rumination (AR) is an example of an adaptive response of depression that is characterized by enhanced cognitive function to help an individual focus on, analyze, and solve problems. To date, research on AR has been hampered by the lack of theoretically-derived and psychometrically sound instruments. This study developed and tested a clinically meaningful measure of AR.

Methods: Using expert panels and an extensive literature review, we developed a conceptual framework for AR and 22 candidate items. Items were field tested to 579 young adults; 140 of whom completed the items at a second time point. We used Rasch measurement methods to construct and test the item set; and traditional psychometric analyses to compare items to existing rating scales.

Results: Data were high quality (<1% missing; high reliability: Cronbach's alpha $= 0.92$, test-retest intraclass correlations >0.81; evidence for divergent validity). Evidence of misfit for 2 items suggested that a 20-item scale with 4-point response categories best captured the concept of AR, fitting the Rasch model ($\chi^2 = 95.26$; df $= 76$, $p = 0.07$), with high reliability ($r_p = 0.86$), ordered response scale structure, and no item bias (gender, age, time).

Conclusion: Our study provides evidence for a 20-item Analytical Rumination Questionnaire (ARQ) that can be used to quantify AR in adults who experience symptoms of depression. The ARQ is psychometrically robust and a clinically useful tool for the assessment and improvement of depression in the primary care setting. Future work is needed to establish the validity of this measure in people with major depression.

Editor: Ali Montazeri, Iranian Institute for Health Sciences Research, ACECR, Islamic Republic of Iran

Funding: Funding from the Social Aetiology of Mental Illness Funding Program, Centre for Addiction and Mental Health, TGF-96115. The role of the funder was to provide salary support for the two post-doctoral students who participated in the study (SB, ZD). The authors report that the funder had no role in study design, data collection and analysis, decision to publish, or preparation of the manuscript.

Competing Interests: The authors have declared that no competing interests exist.

* Email: pandrews@mcmaster.ca

Introduction

Depression affects approximately 350 million people worldwide and is a leading cause of global disability [1,2]. Alleviating depression assumes ever increasing importance as the individual and societal costs associated with depression rise every day [3]. Depression is associated with factors that increase mortality risk such as poor adherence to medical treatment and self-care for diabetes and cardiovascular disease [4] [5], health behaviors such as smoking and lack of physical activity [6], cognitive impairment [7] and disability [8]. It is also a common consequence of changes in health status (i.e., cancer [9] & stroke [10]), and/or new life roles (i.e., caregiving [11], immigration [12], and loss of employment [13]).

Primary care is a frequent entry point into the health care system for depressed patients. Since the 1980's gaps in quality of depression care in primary care systems have been noted and continue to be highlighted today [3,14–16]. Studies show that only 25% to 50% of patients with depression are accurately diagnosed by primary care physicians and, among those who are accurately diagnosed, few receive the recommended dosage and duration of either pharmacotherapy or evidence-based psychotherapy [16,17]. Confusing the picture, the medical community receives conflicting accounts of subclinical symptoms. Some argue that subclinical and clinical episodes are part of a single pathological continuum that should often be treated with medication [18], while others argue subclinical symptoms are often a normal response to stress [19].

In short, greater understanding of both clinical and subclinical depression will help primary care physicians, who are often the first line of treatment for depression, improve the overall health and quality of life of their patients.

Why does depression exist?

Despite decades of research, the molecular and physiological mechanisms underlying depression are not fully understood [20–22]. In addition, there is ongoing debate about the safety and efficacy of pharmacological and psychological treatments [23–28]. While efforts continue to understand *how* people become depressed, research from an evolutionary perspective (so-called "Darwinian Psychiatry" or "Evolutionary Medicine") asks *why* depression exists. Evolutionary medicine seeks to understand the difference between healthy and disordered states and why humans are susceptible to disease [29,30]. This perspective has informed our understanding of a broad range of psychiatric conditions and has been reviewed in detail previously [31,32]. Evolutionary hypotheses of the aetiology of depression are numerous [33,34], but typically suggest that depression has evolved as an adaptation to help regulate energy use and navigate adverse situations. If depression can indeed be adaptive, primary health care providers and researchers may need to consider different approaches to treatment.

The Concept of Interest: Analytical Rumination

One leading hypothesis of the origin of depression proposes that many depressions are the result of an ancient defence mechanism designed by natural selection to promote analytical thinking in response to complex life stressors [35]. The *analytical rumination hypothesis* [35] states that the symptoms of depression result in extended bouts of persistent, distraction-resistant cognitive analysis, which can function to help individuals resolve challenges in their lives. This hypothesis recognizes that the resolution of exceptionally complex problems, such as those associated with adverse life events and major stressors, can require prolonged and in-depth bouts of analysis that lead to impairment and disengagement from everyday life. Problems can occur in a variety of contexts, but analysis will involve thinking through the components of the problem such as (1) its cause; (2) the aspects that need solving; (3) potential solutions; and (4) the costs and benefits associated with implementing various solutions.

While the ruminative thoughts associated with depression are commonly considered maladaptive [36–38], several authors have argued that depressive ruminations may be useful, or at least may begin as a useful means to focus and analyze problems in order to gain insight [39–41]. A substantial body of evidence indicates that depressed mood is associated with increased cognitive processing, improved accuracy on complex tasks, and enhanced detail-oriented judgement on tasks that require deliberate information processing [42–46]. Individuals with depression have also been shown to consistently outperform non-depressed controls when the experimental tasks involve cost-benefit analysis [47–52].

Clinical implications for understanding analytical rumination

Understanding analytical rumination has important clinical implications for how to assess and treat depression. Rather than viewing depression as an impairment or malfunction of the brain, the evolutionary perspective hypothesizes that it may sometimes occur as an adaptive response to promote the cognitive analysis required to understand and resolve current problems. Depressive episodes associated with high levels of analytical rumination may be most usefully treated by facilitating rumination and analysis

rather than medications or psychotherapies that may treat rumination as unproductive.

The challenge to understanding analytical rumination

Research in this arena has been limited by the lack of a reliable and valid psychometric instrument for analytical rumination. Analytical rumination, similar to many other important health constructs (i.e, quality of life), is not directly measurable (i.e., it is *latent*). Primary health care providers must rely on patient-reported outcomes (PROs) to gain information about the patient that cannot be collected by means of traditional clinical metrics such as lab values. Recently, the use of PROs has been emphasized as a valuable means to enhance care management by helping providers to understand not just whether a clinical value is within range, but how patients' lives may be affected by the value [53]. In order to develop a PRO that can be integrated into routine care in a clinically meaningful way, development and testing needs to carefully consider the concept of interest, content of use, and measurement rigour (i.e., precision, standardization, and comparability of scores across studies and diseases) [53,54].

Based on a thorough review of the theoretical construct [35], we are unaware of any measure that captures the full range of analytical rumination in a clinically meaningful way. The objective of this study was to develop and test a conceptually and psychometrically sound measure of analytical rumination to inform fundamental decisions in primary care practice, health research, and treatment trials.

Methods

Measure design

We developed a conceptual model (Figure 1) based on an extensive review of published theory on analytical rumination and depression [35]. The analytical rumination hypothesis states that individuals with depression engage in analysis to understand at least four different parts (domains) of their problems: (1) understanding the cause (e.g., "I tried to understand why I had these problems"); (2) understanding the aspects of the problems that need to be solved (e.g., "I tried to understand what was wrong in my life"); (3) generating possible solutions (e.g., "I thought about all my options for dealing with my problems"); and (4) evaluating the advantages and disadvantages of possible solutions (e.g., "I thought about whether my options for dealing with one problem would make other problems worse"). From this model, we generated 22 candidate items to capture the full range of analytical rumination, which we refer to as the Analytical Rumination Questionnaire (ARQ).

As described below, each item of the ARQ candidate item pool was scored on a 5-point Likert scale. Scoring categories range from

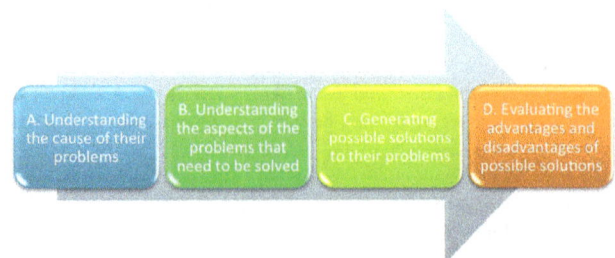

Figure 1. Working model describing the theoretical conceptualization of analytical rumination.

1 (none of the time) to 5 (all of the time). Possible scores ranged from 22–110, with a higher score indicating a higher level of analytical rumination (see Appendix S1 for candidate items in ARQ). We hypothesized that the four domains and the items themselves had a natural implicit ordering from low to high. Specifically, we hypothesized that people first attempt to understand why they have a problem (domain 1) and what needs to be solved (domain 2) before they attempt to generate (domain 3) and evaluate (domain 4) possible solutions.

Questionnaire administration

Participants, recruitment, and data collection. All participants were students at McMaster University taking undergraduate psychology courses. English-speaking adults aged 18 years and over were eligible to participate. We collected data in two studies. In the first, 439 participants filled out the ARQ at one time point, and in the second 140 participants filled it out at two time points. In order to encourage high response rates, we offered academic credit for participation. Both studies were approved by the McMaster Research Ethics Board and written informed consent was obtained prior to completing the ARQ.

Analysis Procedure

We used both traditional and Rasch psychometric analyses to evaluate the properties of the ARQ.

Traditional analyses

Traditional psychometric analyses have been described in detail elsewhere [55]. In brief, they use correlation and descriptive analyses to evaluate scaling assumptions (legitimacy of summing items), reliability, and validity [56]. Accordingly, we examined data from the ARQ for quality (percent missing for each item), scaling assumptions, scale to sample targeting (score means; standard deviation (SD); floor and ceiling effects), and internal consistency and reliability(Cronbach's alphas) [57]. We determined convergent and discriminant construct validity by examining correlations between the ARQ and other 3 other measures and variables (age and sex). For discriminant validity testing, we used the Beck Depression Inventory (BDI) [58] and the Positive and Negative Affect Scale (PANAS) [59]. For convergent validity testing we used the reflective pondering subscale of the Ruminative Response Scale (RRS) [37,38]. We hypothesized that correlations would be the highest with the ARQ and the reflective pondering subscale of the RRS, and the correlations of the ARQ with other variables would be lower.

Rasch Measurement Psychometric Testing

Rasch measurement is a paradigm commonly used to guide the development and testing of rating scales. Many statistical techniques for evaluating psychometric instruments attempt to develop a model from data that describes how people use an instrument. In contrast, a fundamental goal of Rasch measurement is to develop a psychometric instrument that reflects an *a priori* specified conceptual model [60]. One component of this conceptual model is *specific objectivity* (i.e., the instrument objectively measures the latent trait in the same way that a yardstick is an instrument for objectively measuring length). A specifically objective psychometric instrument must have several properties. First, all the items of the instrument must be related to a single latent trait (i.e., the instrument must be unidimensional) [61]. Second, for each item, there must be a monotonic relationship between the ordering of the responses of that item and the ordering of the latent trait [56]. For instance, for item 1 of

the ARQ, people who rank higher on the latent analytical rumination trait must be probabilistically more likely to endorse higher responses. Third, there must be local independence [62], which means that the answer to an item does not depend on the order in which items are presented. Finally, while a Rasch model allows items to differ in how diagnostic they are of the latent trait (i.e., some items indicate low levels of the latent trait while other items indicate high levels of the latent trait), the diagnostic ordering of items should not vary across the range of the latent trait [63]. For example, if a person who is low on the latent trait of analytical rumination is more likely to endorse item 1 of the ARQ than item 13, then this ordering must be preserved at higher levels of the latent trait. These assumptions are difficult to achieve in practice, so a psychometric instrument that fits the Rasch model has passed an important, rigorous test of measurement.

When a psychometric instrument satisfies the rigorous assumptions of the Rasch model, the sum of the scores of the individual items provides a complete description of the person's standing on the latent variable. An instrument that defines the full spectrum of the latent variable will range from -4 to +4 logits, corresponding to ±4 standard deviations of a standard normal distribution, and items will cover all levels of the latent distribution. Moreover, an instrument that fits the context of use is one that captures the full range of the latent distribution in a given population [64,65]. A range of parameters arising from the Rasch analysis can be used to judge the extent to which there is misfit between the items and people on this range, and as a result, the extent to which scoring and summing items is in fact, a valid and reliable approach [66].

For this analysis, we used all 22 candidate items. All assumptions were verified using the Masters' partial credit Rasch polytomous model [67], an appropriate mathematical derivation of the Rasch model suitable for investigating items with ordinal response options. All analyses were performed using RUMM 2030 [68].

Clinical Meaning. We examined the extent to which ARQ items were clinically cohesive and reflected our *a priori* hypothesis about how items covered the latent spectrum of low to high analytical rumination.

Thresholds for item response options. Each item of the ARQ was scored on a 5-point Likert scale, with five response categories (none of the time, some of the time, half of the time, most of the time, all of the time), and five integer scores assigned to each category (1, 2, 3, 4, and 5, respectively). The successive nature of the scores implies that there is a natural order to the assignment that reflects a continuum of increasing impact from less (i.e., 1 = not at all) to more (i.e., 5 = all of the time). We tested this assumption by statistical and graphical inspection of threshold locations and plots.

Item fit statistics. We tested the extent to which the participant's responses to an item fit the rigorous expectations of the Rasch model. Misfit of an item implies that the item is not working as intended and may not be measuring the intended construct. We used three indicators of fit: (1) log residuals (item-person interaction) (2) chi-square values (item-trait interaction), and (3) item characteristic curves. Rather than using absolute criteria for interpreting fit, these three indicators of fit were interpreted separately to understand the context of their use as a full item set capturing analytical rumination.

Item locations and targeting. We carefully looked at how items were distributed along the proposed latent analytical rumination continuum. We flagged items in similar locations as potentially redundant and warranting further investigation. We gauged the calibration of the instrument to the population by comparing graphically how closely the amount of analytical rumination displayed by the respondents was adequately measured by the items on the scale.

Person Separation Index (PSI) [69]. We used the PSI as a reliability statistic, analogous to Cronbach's alpha [57], to test the extent to which scale scores in the sample can be separated. Higher scores indicate higher reliability.

Differential Item Functioning (DIF). We determined whether each item's location on the latent analytical rumination construct was stable across groups using item characteristic curves and two-way analyses of variance with a Bonferroni correction of 0.05 for multiple comparisons. Groups included gender, age, ethnicity, and whether the individual reported a medical condition.

Unidimensionality. We tested the scale's ability to measure a single latent construct using a principal components analysis (PCA) of the residuals. We specifically tested the presence of a pattern of the residuals grouping into more than one subscale once the "Rasch factor" was extracted. We hypothesized that the response structure would be unidimensional and that, apart from a single variable and the item parameters mapped on this variable, the remaining variation was random. Depending on the factor loadings resulting from the PCA, we performed paired t-tests to assess whether person estimates derived from the subtests of items were significantly different from each other. If greater than 5% of t-tests were significant, explanation for the anomaly was put into question.

Dependency. We tested to see whether the responses to any of the items in the scale directly influenced the response to other items by examining item residual correlations.

Results

The sample consisted of 308 women (53%) and 271 men (47%) at enrollment with a mean age of 19 years (SD: 1.9). Thirty percent reported being of white-European descent, followed by 16% Asian, 9% East Asian, 5% African, 2% Aboriginal, and 14% reporting "Other". Thirty-three percent of the sample reported taking medication, with 28% of this sub-sample reporting contraceptive medication, and 7% reporting a form of anti-depressant medication.

Traditional Psychometric Results

Data satisfied criteria for all evaluated traditional psychometric properties. Missing data from all items ranged from <1%–2%. Scale scores were computable for 99% of respondents. Scale scores spanned the range of the scale and were not notably skewed. We did not observe any ceiling and floor effects.

Reliability and Validity. Internal consistency reliability was high (Cronbach alphas = 0.91), and the mean inter-item correlation was 0.83, supporting scale reliability. Scale validity was supported by the high Cronbach alpha coefficient and interscale correlations. Table 1 shows the results of the convergent and discriminant construct validity testing of the ARQ. Patterns of correlations were consistent with our predictions. Mean ARQ scores were correlated highest with the RRS subscale (r = 0.40), followed by the BDI and PANAS. As expected, the mean scores for men and women did not differ, nor did age impact ARQ scores.

Rasch Measurement Results

Clinical Meaning. The hierarchy of the items was clinically meaningful. Most (20/22) items mapped back to the a priori hypothesized analytical rumination continuum, with the expected order of item difficulty capturing a theoretical distribution of low

to high. Table 2 shows the ordering of the items from least to most difficult.

Threshold Response options. The item response options for 13/22 (59%) items were disordered. As shown in Figure 2b, we rescored disordered items by collapsing the middle category "half of the time" with the second category "some of the time". After rescoring, statistical and graphical evidence of misfit remained for only two items: "*I thought about all the bad things that could happen to me because of the situation I am in*" (item 13: fit residual = 5.95; $\chi^2 = 48.09$, df = 9, p<0.01); and "*I thought about how others were likely to respond to some of the actions I could take*" (item 9: fit residual = 4.33; $\chi^2 = 29.42$, df = 9, p<0.01). Both items had ICCs well below the theoretical curve, providing evidence of poor discrimination ability. After consultation with two content experts and two clinicians, and revision of conceptual model, the two items were removed.

Fit and targeting. Figure 2a shows the distribution of participants along the measurement continuum, ranging from −4.31 to +3.09, reflecting a broad, even spread. As shown in Table 3, overall person fit (i.e., mean person fit residual) was near the targeted level of 0 (mean location = 0.273, SD = 1.05) indicating the sample was representative of an expected population distribution. Person locations ranged from −4.50 to +3.20, with only 3 individuals lying outside of the individual fit residual range of −2.5 to +2.5. Item locations and their standard errors are reported in Table 2. Fit of the items was good. Figure 2c illustrates the item threshold range from −3.6 to +2.3 logits which covered 74% of the measurement continuum. Overall item fit was good with a mean (SD) of 0.28 (1.53) as shown in Table 2. Item residuals, χ^2 fit statistic, and the F-test after Bonferroni correction also were consistent with a reasonable fit.

Figures 2a and 2c show the targeting of the sample to the 20 remaining items, offering evidence of the strong targeting of our sample for evaluating ARQ performance. Scores spanned the range of the scale and were not notably skewed with little evidence of ceiling and floor effects. Of note was that a gap of items was observed >2.3, suggesting that individuals above this range are not as precisely measured as the remainder of the sample (n = 9, < 2% of the sample).

Person Separation Index. Scale reliability was high (PSI = 0.87), indicating the items adequately separated this sample along measurement continuum.

Unidimensionality. Examination of the eigenvalues from the principal component analysis suggested the presence of two or more subscales. This was also supported by the loadings in the first principle component that showed clear patterns of residuals on successive components, with 5 items with large positive correlations, and 5 others with negative loadings. The first set of items queried the first domain of our conceptual model (understanding the problem), whereas the second set queried the third domain (generating possible solutions to the problem). Evidence from grouping these items together in subtests provided some evidence of multi-dimensionality of borderline relevance, with 8% of the subtests (n = 55) showing significant differences in the estimated differences generated (t = 3.21, p = 0.04). This was a mild deviation from the 5% expected value, warranting further consideration and caution in future testing.

Differential Item Functioning. Both graphical and statistical evidence showed the difficulty level of the items was uniform across age, sex, ethnic background, self-report medication use, and time.

Table 1. Traditional psychometric methods: convergent and discriminant construct validity and group differences validity.

Instrument/variable	Scale/Variable	Correlation to the ARQ
RRS- Reflective Pondering	Sub Score	0.40*
RRS- Brooding	Sub Score	0.22
BDI	Total Score	0.25
PANAS	Total Score	0.20
Demographic variables		
	Age	0.13
	Sex	0.03
	Medication	0.15

*Significant <0.05; ARQ: Analytical Rumination Questionnaire, high scores indicate greater analytical rumination; RRS: Ruminative Response Scale, high scores indicate greater rumination; BDI: Beck Depression Scale, high scores indicate greater depression; PANAS: Positive and negative affect scale.

Discussion

The objective of this study was to provide evidence for the conceptual and measurement properties of a new concept of interest in health called *analytical rumination*. Our preliminary results support a set of 20 items, collectively called the Analytical Rumination Questionnaire (ARQ), that cover the full range of our conceptual model of analytical rumination[35]. By application of traditional psychometric and Rasch measurement testing, we have demonstrated that the ARQ is reliable, unidimensional, and meets

the criteria for objective rigorous measurement as outlined by the Rasch model. The Rasch model specifically confirmed the presence of a higher-order scale that consisted of 20 items reflecting each of the four theoretical domains previously mapped to the analytical rumination construct (see Figure 1) [35]. From a clinical perspective, our findings support a set of items that suggest a meaningful story of what it may mean to move from "low" analytical rumination to "high" analytical rumination (a fundamental prerequisite of measurement) [60,63]. For example, Table 1 shows that items on the lower end ask about problem

Table 2. Measures of fit and location (SE) of ARQ items.

Item	Item label	Location	SE	Fit Resid.	$\chi^{2\dagger}$	Prob*
22	I tried to think through my difficulties	−0.642	0.059	0.509	4.991	0.288
16	I tried to learn from my mistakes	−0.550	0.057	1.719	1.354	0.852
17	I tried to find a goal or purpose that was meaningful to me	−0.511	0.057	1.539	1.112	0.892
20	I tried to find a way to resolve an important issue	−0.405	0.059	−1.498	7.203	0.126
7	I tried to figure out the best option for dealing with my dilemma	−0.309	0.060	−0.929	7.268	0.122
19	I tried to figure out how to stick to my goals	−0.292	0.058	−1.577	9.721	0.050
18	I tried to find an answer to my problems	−0.273	0.055	1.077	1.362	0.850
6	I thought about all the options for dealing with my problems	−0.269	0.062	−1.169	10.407	0.034
12	I tried to figure out how to make the best out of a bad situation	−0.137	0.054	**−2.621**	12.412	0.023
8	I tried to figure out which of the problems I was facing were the most important and which I should do first	−0.006	0.056	−0.224	1.572	0.813
21	I tried to understand the past and the present	0.036	0.073	0.811	0.575	0.966
5	I thought about all the aspects of the problems I was facing that needed to be solved	0.053	0.057	−1.116	4.979	0.297
3	I thought about what I may have done to avoid these problems	0.081	0.054	0.116	1.583	0.812
1	I tried to understand why I had these problems	0.122	0.057	−0.468	4.708	0.319
2	I tried to figure out what I had done wrong	0.230	0.055	1.440	6.227	0.183
14	I tried to figure out how to best avoid future problems	0.278	0.057	1.027	0.388	0.983
10	I thought about whether some of the options I could take were likely to solve my problems or make things worse.	0.425	0.052	2.283	9.427	0.051
4	I thought about all the ways my life had become more difficult	0.496	0.052	2.048	12.494	0.015
15	I tried to figure out what was wrong in my life	0.509	0.052	1.474	2.426	0.658
11	I thought about whether my options for dealing with one problem would make other problems worse	1.028	0.055	1.277	8.768	0.067

Items are located in order of difficulty (from high AR to low AR). † degrees of freedom (620,4); *Bonferroni adjustment with a probability base of 0.01 (p = 0.005 for 20 items); note item 12 of borderline misfit. Included in the model because graphical fit was good and fit conceptual model.

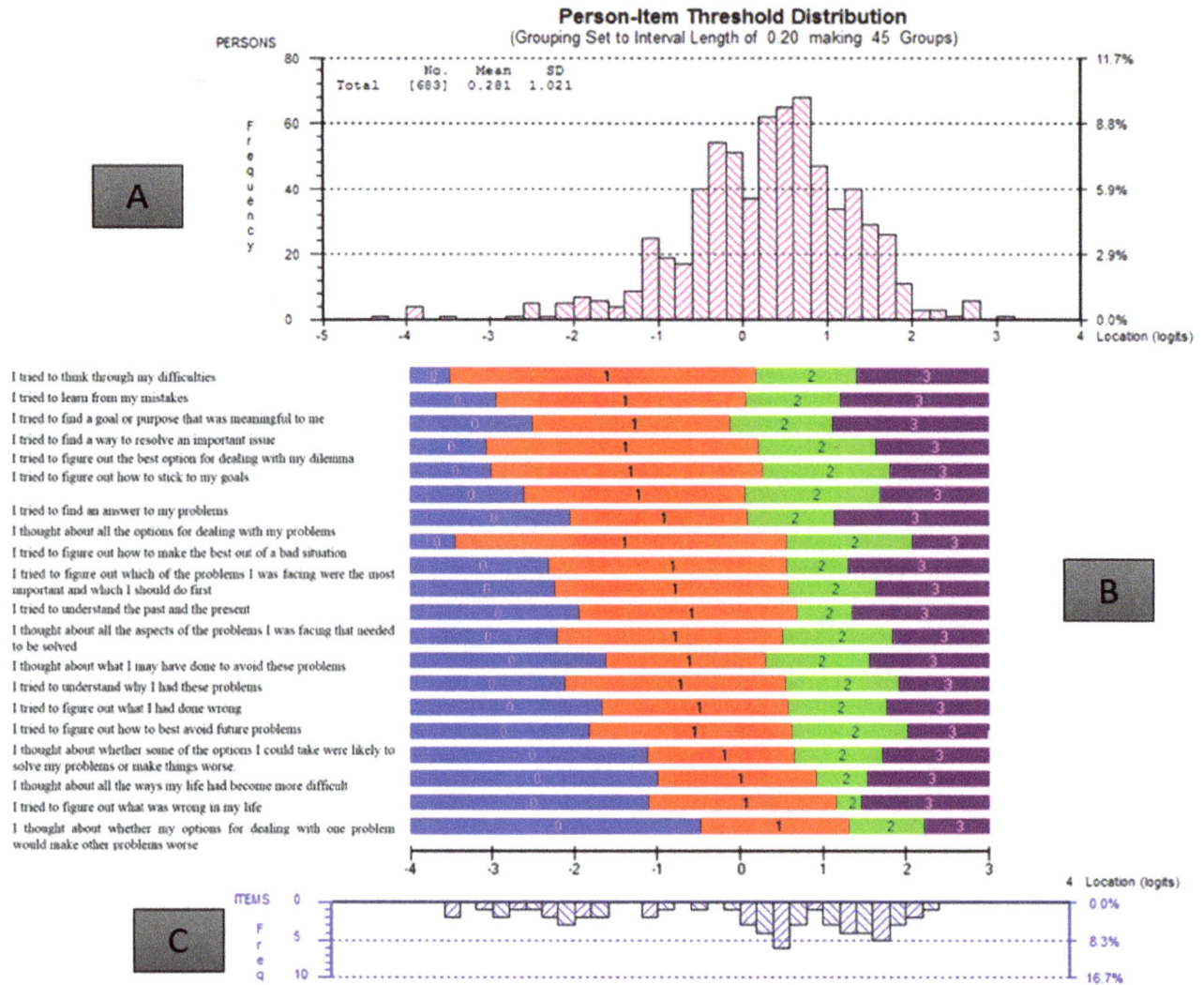

Person-Item Threshold Distribution
(Grouping Set to Interval Length of 0.20 making 45 Groups)

Figure 2. Summary of targeting to the sample of 20 items included in the Analytical Rumination Questionnaire. A. Distribution of items across the measurement continuum in the prototype analytical rumination questionnaire (ARQ). B. Item map showing expected score to each item, with items shown in order of difficulty. C. The location of the 20 items, relative to each other, on an interval scale.

Table 3. Indices of fit to a Rasch model.

ITEM-TRAIT INTERACTION	
Total Item χ	95.26
Total degrees of Freedom	76
Total χ² Probability	0.07
ITEM-PERSON INTERACTION	
ITEM	
Difficulty	0.00±0.43
Fit Residual	0.28±1.30
PERSON	
Measure	0.27 ±1.05
Fit Residual	−0.49 ± 1.91

identification ("I tried to think about my difficulties"). As difficulty increases, items capture domains hypothesized to reflect higher analytical rumination such as: identifying and understanding problems, generating possible solutions, evaluating the possible solutions, and learning how to prevent problem recurrence.

Given that recent meta-analyses indicate similar treatment efficacy for cognitive therapies (i.e., psychotherapy) and antidepressant medications [23,28], the development of the ARQ is timely. The ordering of the items supports the construct validity of analytical rumination, and could possibly be used as a guide to understand how individuals progress from problem identification to the problem resolution. At the level of primary care, family physicians or other health professionals may be able to use this information to engage in a dialogue with patients who experience depressive symptoms. We suggest that the effective assessment and treatment of depression could include helping patients (1) identify of a problems/stressor, (2) prioritize aspects that need solving, (3) identify potential solutions and plans for implementation, and (4) develop a plan to prevent further recurrence of the triggering problem. We hope that clinicians will use this perspective of the potentially adaptive aspects of depression in order to inform treatment. The evolutionary perspective suggests that there are many different aetiological pathways to the diagnostic symptoms of depression, each of which may be best suited to a different treatment strategy. One pathway is the functioning of adaptations designed to promote analytical rumination. The ARQ may be used to identify such cases, and to design personalized interventions that help patients make progress toward the resolution of their triggering problem.

The ARQ currently offers a quick and easy way to assess the stage and progress of a patient's problem-solving analysis. Interventions may therefore be tailored and personalized according to a patient's practical needs to resolve precipitating problems, rather than solely to treat symptoms. For example, psychiatrists and psychologists have developed several treatment strategies that may be effective at the low end of the ARQ spectrum, where patients have not yet identified aspects of their problems or the best solution. Current evidence-based interventions such as "exposure-based" therapies, mindfulness, and problem-solving therapy [70–75], that work to increase awareness of problems and reduce avoidance of stressors, may provide an alternative option for care for a population that is difficult to treat with medication alone. At the higher end of the spectrum, there may be more of a role for allied health professionals (e.g., occupational therapy) with expertise in goal-orientated cognitive therapies to help individuals who have identified the problem and goal, but are having difficulty implementing their plan of action. The ARQ developed in the present study will be an invaluable tool for future research to understand the effectiveness of these types of interventions.

From the original 22 candidate items, we found that 2 of the items functioned poorly. Further investigation of the anomalies revealed that each item consisted of more than one question per item (items 9 and 13). We removed these two items since the item

locations were close to other items on the scale, and were conceptually redundant. Rasch analysis also revealed inherent problems in the initial 5 option response scale. Upon reflection, we propose two possible explanations for the aberrant behaviour of this scoring structure. First, there may have been too many response options for the target population. A second possibility is that the scoring options were confusing because the categories included both qualitative (all the time, some of the time, etc.) and quantitative (half of the time) response options. Examination of the category frequencies and provided evidence that an optimal scoring structure for this scale would favour four response categories. The anomaly revealed in the scoring structure was resolved upon collapsing the middle category "half of the time", with the preceding category "some of the time."

Limitations of our study

The intended context of use for this scale is adults who experience depressive symptoms. For exploratory purposes, we began our conceptual and measurement testing with young adults in a university setting. Our preliminary results show that the ARQ targets this population very well and has excellent person separation. This sample may not generalise to patients who meet formal diagnostic criteria for clinical syndromes. However, as it currently stands, the ARQ may be useful in a primary care setting, where subclinical symptoms are often encountered. Future work in understanding this concept further in people with depression should include an iterative process of both qualitative and quantitative work to ensure the ARQ items are fit for purpose and measure what they purport to measure.

Conclusion

Our study provides preliminary results for a set of 20 items (Analytical Rumination Questionnaire) that collectively can be used as a reliable and valid instrument for the quantification of analytical rumination. The ARQ provides a starting point to provide insight into the conceptual underpinnings and measurement of analytical rumination for potential application in the self-management and clinical treatment of depression. Future analyses will further assess the construct validity of the scale by assessing the performance of the items in a clinical population of people with depression.

Author Contributions

Conceived and designed the experiments: SB ZD PA. Performed the experiments: PA ZD. Analyzed the data: SB. Contributed reagents/materials/analysis tools: SB. Wrote the paper: SB ZD PA.

References

1. Mathers C, Boerma T, Fat DM (2008) The global burden of disease: 2004 update. World Health Organization.

2. Ferrari AJ, Somerville AJ, Baxter AJ, Norman R, Patten SB, et al. (2013) Global variation in the prevalence and incidence of major depressive disorder: a systematic review of the epidemiological literature. 43Psychological Medicine.

3. Pickett YR, Ghosh SC, Rohs A, Kennedy GJ, Bruce ML, et al. (2014) Healthcare use among older primary care patients with minor depression. American Journal of Geriatric Psychiatry 22: 207–210.

4. Ciechanowski PS, WJ K, Russo JE (2000) Depression and diabetes: impact of depressive symptoms on adherence, function, and costs. Archives of Internal Medicine 160: 3278–3285.

5. Whooley MA, Wong JM Depression and Cardiovascular Disorders. Annual Review of Clinical Psychology 9: 327–354.

6. Freedland KE, Carney RM, Skala JA (2005) Depression and smoking in coronary heart disease. Psychosomatic Medicine 67: S42–46.

7. Alexopoulos GS, Meyers BS, Young RC, Kalayam B, Kakuma T (2000) Executive dysfunction and long-term outcomes of geriatric depression. Archives of General Psychiatry 57: 285–290.

8. Murray CLJ, Lopez AD (1996) The global burden of disease: a comprehensive assessment of mortality and disability from diseases, injuries, and risk factors in 1990 and projected to 2020. Boston, MA: Harvard University Press.

9. Krebber AMH, Buffart LM, Kleijn G, Riepman IC, de Bree R, et al. (2014) Prevalence of depression in cancer patients: a meta-analysis of diagnostic interviews and self-report instruments. Psycho-Oncology 23: 221–230.

10. Rochette A, Bravo G, Desrosier J, St.Cyr D, Bourget A (2007) Adaptation process, participation and depression over six months in first-stroke individuals and spouses. Clinical Rehabilitation 21: 554–562.

11. Cameron JI, Cheung AM, Streiner D, Coyte PC, Stewart DE (2011) Stroke Survivor Depressive Symptoms Are Associated With Family Caregiver Depression During the First 2 Years Poststroke. Stroke 42: 302–306.

12. Wong E, Miles JNV (2014) Prevalence and Correlates of Depression Among New U.S. Immigrants. Journal of Immigrant and Minority Health 16: 422–428

13. Olesen SC, Beutterworth P, Leach LS, LKelaher M, Pirkis J Mental health affects future employment as job loss affects mental health: findings from a longitudinal population study. BMC Psychiatry.

14. Whitebird RR, Solberg LI, Margolis KL, Asche SE, Trangle MA, et al. (2013) Barriers to Improving Primary Care of Depression: perspectives of Medical Group Leaders. Qualitative Health Research 23: 805–814

15. Katzelnick DJ, Kobak KA, Greist JH, Jefferson JW, Henk HJ (1997) Effect of primary care treatment of depression on service use by patients with high medical expenditures. Psychiatric Services 48: 59–64.

16. Katon W, Von Korff M, Lin E (1995) Collaborative management to achieve treatment guidelines. Impact on depression in primary care. JAMA 273: 1026–1031.

17. Mojtabai R, Olfson M (2011) Proportion Of Antidepressants Prescribed Without A Psychiatric Diagnosis Is Growing. Health Affairs 30: 1434–1442.

18. Pies R (2014) Grief and major depression. British Medical Journal 348: g179.

19. Dorwick C, Frances A (2013) Medicalising unhappiness: new classification of depression risks more patients being put on drug treatment from which they will not benefit. British Medical Journal 347: f7140.

20. Hamilton JP, Etkin A, Furman DJ, Lemus MG, Johnson RF, et al. (2012) Functional neuroimaging of major depressive disorder: A meta-analysis and new integration of baseline activation and neural response data. American Journal of Psychiatry 169: 693–703.

21. Krishnan V, Nestler EJ (2008) The molecular neurobiology of depression. Nature 455: 894–902.

22. Valenstein ES (1998) Blaming the brain: The truth about drugs and mental health. New York, NY: The Free Press.

23. Andrews PW, Thomson JA, Jr., Amstadter A, Neale MC (2012) Primum non nocere: An evolutionary analysis of whether antidepressants do more harm than good. Frontiers in Psychology 3: 117.

24. Barlow DH (2010) Negative effects from psychological treatments: A perspective. American Psychologist 65: 13–20.

25. Fournier JC, DeRubeis RJ, Hollon SD, Dimidjian S, Amsterdam JD, et al. (2010) Antidepressant drug effects and depression severity: A patient-level meta-analysis. Jama-Journal of the American Medical Association 303: 47–53.

26. Hollon SD, Thase ME, Markowitz JC (2002) Treatment and prevention of depression. Psychological Science in the Public Interest 3: 39–77.

27. Kirsch I, Deacon BJ, Huedo-Medina TB, Scoboria A, Moore TJ, et al. (2008) Initial severity and antidepressant benefits: A meta-analysis of data submitted to the Food and Drug Administration. Plos Medicine 5: 260–268.

28. Cuijpers P, Turner EH, Mohr DS, Hofmann SG, Andersoon G, et al. (2014) Comparison of psychotherapies for adult depression to pill placebo control groups: a meta-analysis. Psychological Medicine 44: 685–695.

29. Williams G, Nesse R (1991) The dawn of Darwinian medicine. Quarterly Review of Biology 66: 1–22.

30. Gluckman P, Beedle A, Hanson M (2009) Principles of evolutionary medicine. Oxford, UK: Oxford University Press.

31. Stevens A, Price J (2000) Evolutionary Psychiatry: A New Beginning: Routledge.

32. Brüne M (2008) Textbook of Evolutionary Psychiatry: The origins of psychopathology. New York: Oxford University Press.

33. Nesse RM (2000) Is depression an adaptation? Archives of General Psychiatry 57: 14–20.

34. Hagen EH (2011) Evolutionary theories of depression: a critical review. Canadian Journal of Psychiatry - Revue Canadienne de Psychiatrie 56: 716–726.

35. Andrews PW, Thomson JA (2009) The bright side of being blue: depression as an adaptation for analyzing complex problems. Psychological Review 116: 620–654.

36. Lyubomirsky S, Nolen-Hoeksema S (1993) Self-perpetuating properties of dysphoric rumination. Journal of Personality and Social Psychology 65: 339–349.

37. Nolen-Hoeksema S, Morrow J (1991) A prospective study of depression and posttraumatic stress symptoms after a natural disaster: the 1989 Loma Prieta Earthquake. Journal of Personality and Social Psychology 61: 115–121.

38. Nolen-Hoeksema S, Parker LE, Larson J (1994) Ruminative coping with depressed mood following loss. Journal of Personality and Social Psychology 67: 92–104.

39. Gut E (1985) Productive and Unproductive Depression: Interference in the Adaptive function of the Basic Depressed Response. British Journal of Psychotherapy 2: 95–113.

40. Martin L, Tesser A (1996) Some ruminative thoughts. In: Wyer J, Robert S, editors. Ruminative Thoughts Advances in Social Cognition. Hillsdale, New Jersey, England: Lawrence Erlbaum Associates. pp.1–47.

41. Papageorgiou C, Wells A (2001) Metacognitive beliefs about rumination in recurrent major depression. Cognitive and Behavioral Practice: 160–164.

42. Forgas J (1998) On being happy and mistaken: mood effects on the fundamental attribution error. Journal of Personality and Social Psychology 75.

43. Sinclair R (1998) Mood, categorization breadth, and performance appraisal: The effects of order of information acquisition and affective state on halo, accuracy, information retrieval. Organizational Behavior and Human Decision Processes 42: 22–46.

44. Sinclair RC, Mark MM (1995) The effects of mood state on judgemental accuracy: Processing strategy as a mechanism. Cognition and Emotion 9: 417–438.

45. Braverman J (2005) The effect of mood on detection of covariation. Personality & Social Psychology Bulletin 31: 1487–1497.

46. Storbeck J, Clore GL (2005) With sadness comes accuracy; with happiness, false memory: mood and the false memory effect. Psychological Science 16: 785–791.

47. Pietromonaco PR, Rook KS (1987) Decision style in depression: The contribution of perceived risks versus benefits. Journal of Personality and Social Psychology 52: 399–408.

48. Hertel G, Neuhof J, Theuer T, Kerr NL (2000) Mood effects on cooperation in small groups: Does positive mood simply lead to more cooperation? Cognition and Emotion 14: 441–472.

49. Au K, Chan G, Wang D, Vertinsky I (2003) Mood in foreign exchange trading: Cognitive processes and performance. Organizational Behavior and Human Decision Processes, 91: 322–338.

50. Smoski MJ, Lynch TR, Rosenthal MZ, Cheavens JS, Chapman AL, et al. (2008) Decision-making and risk aversion among depressive adults. Journal of Behavior Therapy and Experimental Psychiatry 39: 567–576.

51. Overall NC, Hammond MD (2013) Biased and accurate: depressive symptoms and daily perceptions within intimate relationships. Personality & Social Psychology Bulletin 39: 636–650.

52. von Helversen B, Wilke A, Johnson T, Schmid G, Klapp B (2011) Performance benefits of depression: sequential decision making in a healthy sample and a clinically depressed sample. Journal of Abnormal Psychology: 962–968.

53. Food and Drug Administration (2009) Patient reported outcome measure: use in medical product development to support labelling claims.

54. Mokkink LB, Terweea CB, Patrick D, Alonso J, Stratford JW, et al. (2010) The COSMIN study reached international consensus on taxonomy, terminology, and definitions of measurement properties for health-related patient-reported outcomes. Journal of Clinical Epidemiology 63: 737–745.

55. Streiner D, Norman G (2007) Health measurement scales: a practical guide to their development and use. Oxford: Oxford University Press.

56. Hobart JC, Cano SJ, Zajicek JP, Thompson AA (2007) Rating scales as outcome measures for clinical trials in neurology: problems, solutions, and recommendations. Lancet Neurology 6: 1094–1105.

57. Cronbach LJ (1951) Coefficient alpha and the internal structure of tests. Psychometrika 16: 297–334.

58. Beck AT, Ward CH, Mendelson M, Mock J, Erbaugh J (1961) An inventory for measuring depression. Archives of General Psychiatry 4: 561–571.

59. Watson D, Clark LA, Tellegen A (1988) Development and validation of brief measures of positive and negative affect: The PANAS scale. Journal of Personality and Social Psychology 54: 1063–1070.

60. Stone MH, Wright BD, Stenner AJ (1999) Mapping variables. Journal of Outcome Measurement 3: 308–322.

61. Marais I, Andrich D (2008) Effects of varying magnitude and patterns of response dependence in the unidimensional Rasch model. Journal of Applied Measurement 9: 105–124.

62. Sideridis GD (2011) The effects of local item dependence on estimates of ability in the Rasch Model. Rasch Measurement Transactions 25: 1334–1336.

63. Stenner AJ, Stone M, Burdick D (2011) How to model and test for the mechanisms that make measurement systems tick. Joint International IMEKO Jena, Germany.

64. Andrich D (2011) Rating Scales and Rasch Measurement. Expert Review of Pharmacoeconomics and Outcomes Research 11: 571–585.

65. Andrich D (1988) Rasch models for measurement. Beverly Hills: Sage Publications.

66. Andrich D, Sheridan B, Luo G RUMM 2030. 4.0 for windows (upgrade 4600.0109) edn Perth, WA. RUMM laboratory Pty Ltd 1997–2010.

67. Masters G (1982) A Rasch model for partial credit scoring. Psychometrika 47: 149–174.

68. Andrich D, Sheridan B, Luo G (2007) RUMM2020. Rasch unidimensional measurement models software. Perth, Western Australia: RUMM laboratory.

69. Andrich D (1982) An index of person separation in latent trait theory, the traditional KR20 index, and the Guttman scale response pattern. Educational Psychology Research 9: 95–104.

70. Nezu A (1986) Efficacy of a social problem-solving therapy approach for unipolar depression. Journal of Consulting and Clinical Psychology 54: 196–202.

71. Nezu A, Nezu C (2001) Problem solving therapy. Journal of Psychotherapy Integration 11.

72. Teasdale JD, Scott J, Moore R, Hayhurst H, Pope M, et al. (2001) How does cognitive therapy prevent relapse in residual depression? Evidence from a controlled trial. Journal of Consulting and Clinical Psychology 69: 347–357.

73. Hayes AM, Beevers CG, Feldman GC, Laurenceau J-P, Perlman C (2005) Avoidance and processing as predictors of symptom change and positive growth

in an integrative therapy for depression. International Journal of Behavioral Medicine 12.

74. Hayes AM, Feldman GC, Beevers CG, Laurenceau J-P, Cardaciotto L, et al. (2007) Discontinuities and cognitive changes in an exposure-based cognitive therapy for depression. Journal of Consulting and Clinical Psychology 75: 409–421.

75. Krpan KM, Kross E, Berman MG, Deldin PJ, Askren MK, et al. (2013) An everyday activity as a treatment for depression: the benefits of expressive writing for people diagnosed with major depressive disorder. Journal of Affective Disorders 150: 1148–1151.

12

Decitabine Rescues Cisplatin Resistance in Head and Neck Squamous Cell Carcinoma

Chi T. Viet[1,2], Dongmin Dang[2], Stacy Achdjian[2], Yi Ye[2], Samuel G. Katz[2], Brian L. Schmidt[1,2]*

1 Department of Oral Maxillofacial Surgery, New York University, New York, New York, United States of America, **2** Bluestone Center for Clinical Research, New York University, New York, New York, United States of America

Abstract

Cisplatin resistance in head and neck squamous cell carcinoma (HNSCC) reduces survival. In this study we hypothesized that methylation of key genes mediates cisplatin resistance. We determined whether a demethylating drug, decitabine, could augment the anti-proliferative and apoptotic effects of cisplatin on SCC-25/CP, a cisplatin-resistant tongue SCC cell line. We showed that decitabine treatment restored cisplatin sensitivity in SCC-25/CP and significantly reduced the cisplatin dose required to induce apoptosis. We then created a xenograft model with SCC-25/CP and determined that decitabine and cisplatin combination treatment resulted in significantly reduced tumor growth and mechanical allodynia compared to control. To establish a gene classifier we quantified methylation in cancer tissue of cisplatin-sensitive and cisplatin-resistant HNSCC patients. Cisplatin-sensitive and cisplatin-resistant patient tumors had distinct methylation profiles. When we quantified methylation and expression of genes in the classifier in HNSCC cells *in vitro*, we showed that decitabine treatment of cisplatin-resistant HNSCC cells reversed methylation and gene expression toward a cisplatin-sensitive profile. The study provides direct evidence that decitabine restores cisplatin sensitivity in *in vitro* and *in vivo* models of HNSCC. Combination treatment of cisplatin and decitabine significantly reduces HNSCC growth and HNSCC pain. Furthermore, gene methylation could be used as a biomarker of cisplatin-resistance.

Editor: Caterina Cinti, Institute of Clinical Physiology, c/o Toscana Life Sciences Foundation, Italy

Funding: This work was supported by NIH R01 DE19796 and Oral and Maxillofacial Surgery Foundation Research Support Grant. The funders had no role in study design, data collection and analysis, decision to publish, or preparation of the manuscript.

Competing Interests: The authors have declared that no competing interests exist.

* Email: vietc01@nyu.edu

Introduction

More than 60% of head and neck squamous cell carcinoma (HNSCC) patients present with advanced-staged disease, which is associated with a high mortality rate [1]. The current treatment for advanced-stage HNSCC is cisplatin and radiation for patients with good performance status; patients with limited performance status receive high-dose cisplatin alone [2–4]. Cisplatin resistance occurs in some patients and significantly reduces survival as there are no effective alternative therapies. The mechanism of cisplatin resistance is multifactorial and poorly understood [5]. In addition, none of the known mechanisms are reversible with drug therapy.

Aside from poor survival, HNSCC patients have significantly more pain than other cancer patients [6,7]. A meta-analysis of 52 studies evaluating prevalence of cancer pain shows that HNSCC has a higher prevalence of pain compared to all other sites [8]. HNSCC-induced pain limits orofacial functions such as swallowing, mastication and speech, which results in poor quality of life. In fact, outside of survival, pain-induced loss of function is the biggest concern for head and neck cancer patients [9,10]. Given the severe symptoms and reduced survival of HNSCC patients, a novel pharmacologic approach that both reduces cisplatin resistance and alleviates pain is needed.

DNA methylation is an epigenetic silencing mechanism that has recently been proposed as a mechanism for cisplatin resistance [11]. Unlike other chemotherapy resistance mechanisms, DNA methylation is reversible by demethylating drugs; decitabine is one of the most potent demethylating drugs. Decitabine has been used in clinical trials for hematological and solid malignancies, with the major side effect being transient and manageable myelosuppression [12–15]. We showed from previous studies in a preclinical HNSCC model that decitabine not only inhibits tumor growth, it also treats pain-induced loss of function [16].

Based on our preliminary studies we hypothesize that methylation is a reversible mechanism of cisplatin-resistance. Moreover, we propose that decitabine could be added to cisplatin chemotherapy to rescue cisplatin-resistance in HNSCC and alleviate cancer-induced pain. We use both *in vitro* and preclinical models to determine the anti-tumor and analgesic effects of decitabine on cisplatin-resistant HNSCC. To identify patients at risk for cisplatin resistance and those who would benefit from decitabine, we perform methylation profiling by analyzing biopsies from HNSCC patients treated with cisplatin.

Methods

Patient recruitment and tissue collection

All procedures were approved by the Institutional Review Board at New York University. A waiver of informed consent was granted in accordance with 45 CFR 46.116(d). We identified patients from 2005–2010 who had 1) biopsy-proven HNSCC, 2) no history of prior surgical or chemoradiation treatment for HNSCC, and 3) cisplatin-based chemotherapy with or without radiation. We obtained formalin-fixed, paraffin embedded (FFPE) initial incisional biopsies, performed prior to chemotherapy, for each patient. All patients received a CT scan pre-treatment and six months post-treatment; tumor progression was assessed by a radiologist by comparing pre- and post-treatment scans. Progression was classified with Response Evaluation Criteria in Solid Tumors (RECIST), with RECIST 1 signifying progressive disease (PD), RECIST 2 signifying stable disease (SD), RECIST 3 signifying partial response (PR), and RECIST 4 signifying complete response (CR).

Cell culture and drug treatments

SCC-25, a tongue SCC, and SCC-25/CP, which was made cisplatin-resistant by continuous cisplatin treatment [17], were obtained from Dr. John Lazo. The cells were cultured in Dulbecco's Modified Eagle Medium (DMEM), supplemented with 10% fetal bovine serum (FBS). For decitabine treatment, SCC-25 and SCC-25/CP were plated at 25% confluence on 10 cm plates and treated with 5 µM freshly-prepared decitabine (Sigma) in DMEM with supplements. Drug and media were changed every 24 hours until cells were confluent. Decitabine-treated cells were subsequently referred to as DAC-SCC-25 or DAC-SCC-25/CP.

Proliferation and apoptosis assays

SCC-25, SCC-25/CP, DAC-SCC-25, and DAC-SCC-25/CP were plated in 96-well plates at a density of 5,000 cells/well. Cells were treated with either cisplatin (1–300 µM) or drug vehicle (3% DMSO in DMEM supplemented with 2% FBS); drug and media were replenished after 24 hrs. Cell viability was quantified using the MTS assay (Promega) after 48 hours of drug treatment. Apoptosis was quantified with the Caspase-Glo-3/7 assay (Promega) after 24 hours of drug treatment.

Cancer mouse model

The cancer pain mouse model was produced as previously described [18]. Experiments were performed on female BALB/c, athymic mice weighing 16–20 g at the time of SCC inoculation. All the procedures were approved by the New York University Committee on Animal Research. Researchers were trained under the Animal Welfare Assurance Program. 5×10^6 SCC-25/CP cells were suspended in Matrigel (Becton Dickinson & Co.) to a volume of 50 µl and inoculated into the plantar surface of the right hind paw. 2–4% isoflurane inhalational anesthesia was used for inoculation. Twenty-four mice were divided into four groups, (1) combination treatment with decitabine (6 mg/kg) and cisplatin (6 mg/kg), (2) decitabine only (6 mg/kg), (3) cisplatin only (6 mg/kg), and (4) drug-vehicle control. Decitabine was dissolved in phosphate-buffered saline (PBS), filter-sterilized, and administered intraperitoneally (IP) at a volume of 200 µl on post-inoculation days (PID) 7 and 9. Cisplatin was dissolved in PBS with 1% dimethyl sulfoxide (DMSO), filter-sterilized, and injected IP at a volume of 200 µl on PID 12, 15, 18, and 21. Based on a previous study [19] the third-day, two week duration dosing of cisplatin is optimal in controlling tumor growth and minimizing normal tissue damage.

Paw volume measurements were performed to quantify cancer growth with a plethysmometer (IITC Life Sciences) as described [18]. Paw withdrawal testing was performed to evaluate mechanical allodynia as described [18]. Testing was performed by an observer blinded to the experimental groups between 0900 and 1200 h. Paw withdrawal thresholds were determined in response to pressure from an electronic von Frey anesthesiometer (IITC Life Sciences). The amount of pressure (g) needed to produce a paw withdrawal response was measured six times on each paw separated by 3 minute intervals. On PID 30 animals were euthanized with 4% isoflurane.

Sodium bisulfite modification and Methylight

5×10^6 cells were harvested from culture, homogenized with a Mini Beadbeater-1 (BioSpec Products) and subject to DNA/RNA extraction with AllPrep DNA/RNA Kit (Qiagen). Five 10 µm sections of formalin-fixed, paraffin embedded tissue from patients were subject to RNA/DNA extraction with the AllPrep DNA/RNA FFPE Kit (Qiagen). Methylight probes and primers for promoter regions of CRIP1, G0S2, MLH1, OPN3, S100 and TUBB2A were designed with Beacon Designer (Premier Biosoft). Sodium bisulfite conversion was performed according to manufacturer's recommendations using the EZ DNA Methylation Kit (Zymo Research). Methylight PCR was performed as previously described with COL2A1 as the internal control gene [20]. Percentage of methylated reference (PMR, i.e., degree of methylation) was calculated for each sample using M.SssI-treated, CpGenome universal methylated DNA (Millipore) as the positive control.

Quantitative reverse transcription PCR (RT-PCR) analysis

mRNA was reverse transcribed with Random Hexamers (Applied Biosystems). A 2 µl cDNA aliquot was amplified with the Taqman gene expression assay for the gene of interest, which did not detect residual genomic DNA. PCR was also performed to detect HPV16 E6 mRNA as described [21]. Human GAPDH was used as endogenous control. Delta-delta CT was used for relative quantification.

Statistical analysis

Statistical analysis was performed using Sigma Plot, version 11.0. Data was analyzed using Student's t-test, One-way ANOVA, Two-way ANOVA or Two-way RM ANOVA with Holm Sidak or Tukey post hoc testing as appropriate. Results were presented as mean ± standard error of the mean (SEM).

Results

Decitabine pre-treatment enhanced the cytotoxic and apoptotic effects of cisplatin on cisplatin-resistant cells

Based on the cell viability assay, we determined the effective dose-50 (ED-50) of cisplatin, which is the dose required to inhibit viability by 50%. The ED-50 of SCC-25 was 9.47 µM, whereas the ED-50 of SCC-25/CP was 21.1 µM. However, decitabine pre-treatment enhanced the cytotoxicity effect of cisplatin on the cisplatin-resistant SCC-25/CP line. The ED50 value of DAC-SCC-25 and DAC-SCC-25/CP were comparable at 6.55 µM and 6.96 µM, respectively (Figure 1A-D).

Additionally, we determined the effect of decitabine pre-treatment on cisplatin-mediated apoptosis. Figure 1E illustrates caspase 3/7 activity in SCC-25 and SCC-25/CP cells after cisplatin treatment, with higher activity denoting increased apoptosis. When compared to SCC-25 cells, SCC-25/CP had significantly lower apoptotic activity in response to cisplatin treatment at dose ranges of 3.6–100 µM, indicating resistance to cisplatin. Pre-treatment with decitabine restored the apoptotic activity of cisplatin on cisplatin-resistant cells, such that DAC-SCC-25/CP cells had significantly higher apoptotic activity than SCC-25/CP cells in response to cisplatin treatment. Decitabine pre-treatment also enhanced the apoptotic effects of cisplatin on

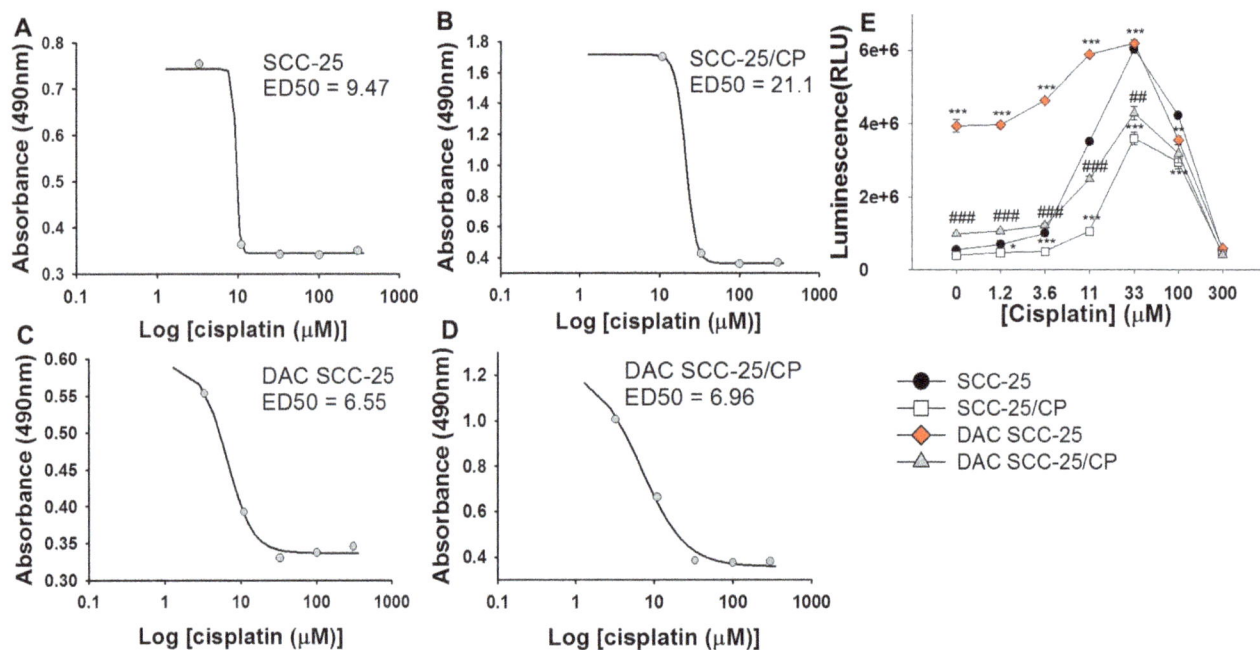

Figure 1. Decitabine pre-treatment enhances cytotoxic and apoptotic activity of cisplatin. (A-D) Cell viability is represented by absorbance (y-axis) and compared to common log of cisplatin concentration (μM). ED50, the concentration needed to inhibit viability by 50%, is listed for each cell line. **(E)** The graph depicts apoptosis activity (caspase 3/7 activity, measured as luminescence on y-axis) at different cisplatin concentrations (3-300 μM). A decrease in apoptotic activity at high dose ranges is an expected phenomenon in this assay due to early cell death from high drug doses prior to quantification. Decitabine pre-treatment in cisplatin-resistant SCC-25/CP cells increases apoptotic activity of cisplatin relative to non-treated SCC-25/CP cells. Decitabine pre-treatment in cisplatin-sensitive SCC-25 cells also increases apoptotic activity of cisplatin at lower doses. One Way ANOVA, Holm-Sidak test pairwise comparisons, *p<.05, **p<.01, ***p<.001, compared to SCC-25; #p<.05, ##p<.01, ###p< .001, compared to SCC-25/CP.

cisplatin-sensitive SCC-25 cells. DAC-SCC-25 cells had significantly higher apoptotic activity than SCC-25 cells, indicating an additional apoptotic benefit of decitabine treatment even when cancer cells are sensitive to cisplatin.

Decitabine and cisplatin combination treatment inhibited growth of cisplatin-resistant SCC in a mouse model

To determine whether including decitabine in the chemotherapy regimen augments the anti-tumor effect of cisplatin in cisplatin-resistant HNSCC *in vivo*, we created a mouse HNSCC model by inoculating SCC-25/CP cells into the right hind paw of BALB/c athymic mice. We chose the hind paw as the xenograft site because tumor volume and mechanical hypersensitivity could be reliably quantified at this site. SCC-25/CP inoculation resulted in tumor growth in the hind paw, represented by increased paw volume (Figure 2A) starting on PID 4. Decitabine treatment on PID 7 and 9 resulted in inhibition of tumor growth; however, this effect was not significant at the end of the experiment on PID 30, indicating that the effect of decitabine treatment alone could not be sustained. Cisplatin-only treatment also resulted in tumor growth inhibition, but the effect was not sustained after drug treatment was stopped on PID 21. Paw volume in the cisplatin-only group was not significantly different from the control group on PID 30. Combination treatment with decitabine and cisplatin was most effective in inhibiting tumor growth, and this inhibitory effect was sustained until PID 30. The mean paw volume change for the combination group was 10% on PID 30, compared to 65% in the control group. Body weight was not significantly different

among all four groups during weekly measurements, indicating that the drug doses used did not cause cachexia (data not shown).

Decitabine and cisplatin combination treatment resulted in the least mechanical allodynia in a cisplatin-resistant SCC mouse model

In addition to tumor growth inhibition we also determined the effects of drug treatment on cancer-induced pain. HNSCC patients most frequently complain of orofacial functional restriction due to pain [10]; we therefore quantified the effect of drug treatment on mechanical allodynia in our preclinical model. Figure 2B depicts the change in mechanical withdrawal threshold from baseline, with a decrease from baseline signifying increased mechanical allodynia. SCC-25/CP tumor growth resulted in increased mechanical allodynia, with a 58% decrease on PID 30 compared to baseline (4.22 g at baseline). When compared to the control group, combination treatment with decitabine and cisplatin resulted in the most significant reduction in mechanical allodynia. The mechanical threshold of the combination group only decreased by 36% on PID 30 (2.69 g from 4.23 g at baseline).

Methylation profiles were different between cisplatin-responsive and cisplatin-unresponsive HNSCC

We obtained FFPE tissue from 19 patients with biopsy-proven HNSCC who were treated with cisplatin. All 19 patients also received radiation in addition to cisplatin chemotherapy. Patient demographics are detailed in Table 1. None of the samples were positive for HPV16 E6 mRNA as detected by PCR (results not shown). We then categorized the tumors according to RECIST criteria, with RECIST 3 or 4 being "cisplatin responsive" (n = 7)

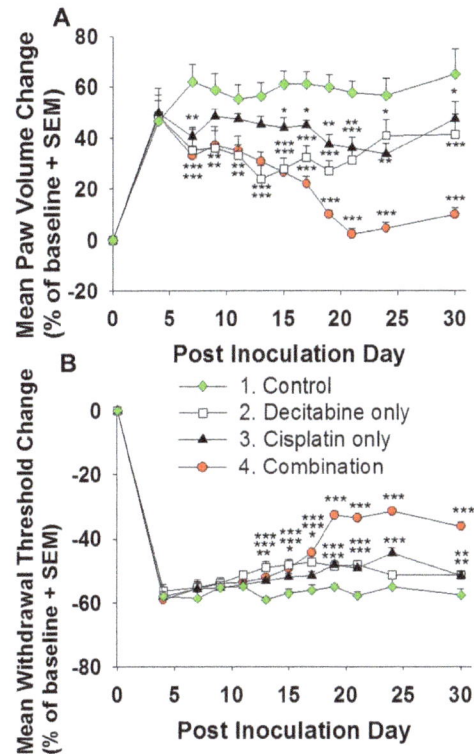

Figure 2. Combination treatment with decitabine and cisplatin results in significant anti-tumor and antinociceptive effects. (A) Combination treatment of decitabine and cisplatin produces a stronger anti-tumor effect in the preclinical model than either drug alone. Paw volume change from baseline (day 0 prior to cancer inoculation) are shown. Treatment with either decitabine or cisplatin alone produces a minor, non-sustained reduction in paw volume. Combination treatment with decitabine and cisplatin, however, produces sustained anti-tumor activity even after cessation of cisplatin treatment on PID 21. (B) The graph shows percent change in mechanical threshold from baseline. Mechanical threshold of mice treated with decitabine, cisplatin and combination treatment was significantly higher than the control groups on indicated days, signifying lower mechanical allodynia (*p<.05, **p< .01, ***p <.001, Two-way RM ANOVA, Holm-Sidak test, see Table 2).

and RECIST 1 or 2 being "cisplatin unresponsive" (n = 12). We quantified methylation within the promoter region of six genes: *CRIP1, G0S2, MLH1, OPN3, S100* and *TUBB2A*. These genes have been implicated in cisplatin resistance of carcinomas other than HNSCC [11,22,23]. We used the calculated PMR value to classify each sample as either "positive" or "negative" for methylation, using a cutoff of 10 based on our previous publication [24]. In the Figure 3A matrix, in which samples that were positively methylated for a gene were colored grey, the cisplatin unresponsive group had more methylated samples. 8 of 12 samples in the cisplatin unresponsive group, and no samples in the cisplatin responsive group, had positive methylation of at least 50% of the genes in the gene panel.

The same methylation trend was present *in vitro*. We compared methylation levels of the cell lines across the six genes with two separate statistical methods. Firstly we used the six genes as a single classifier (Two-way ANOVA, Tukey test, see Table 2 for statistical summary). Secondly we compared the methylation levels of the cell lines for each separate gene (Student's t test, Table 3). While methylation of the separate genes was not significantly different between SCC-25 and SCC-25/CP, the methylation

signature of the whole gene panel was significantly different between the two cell lines (Table 2). The methylation signature of the entire classifier was also significantly different between SCC-25/CP and DAC-SCC-25/CP cells.

To determine whether promoter methylation correlated with gene expression, we quantified mRNA of the six genes in SCC-25 and SCC-25/CP cells before and after decitabine treatment (*i.e.*, DAC-SCC-25 and DAC-SCC-25/CP cells). We compared relative expression of the cell lines using SCC-25 as the reference cell line (Figure 3B). We performed statistical analyses of the expression data for each separate gene (Table 3) and for the gene classifier of six genes (Table 2). SCC-25/CP cells had significantly lower expression than SCC-25 cells in four of the six genes. Decitabine treatment changed gene expression—such that expression of the gene classifier was significantly different between non-treated and decitabine-treated cells for both SCC-25 and SCC-25/CP cells (Table 2). When we analyzed each gene separately, decitabine resulted in either promoter demethylation or increase in gene expression of *CRIP1, G0S2, MLH1*, and *S100* in SCC-25 and *CRIP1, G0S2, MLH1*, and *TUBB2A* in SCC-25/CP.

Discussion

Decitabine restores cisplatin sensitivity and treats cancer-induced pain

The incidence of head and neck cancer is increasing, especially in younger people [25]. Chemoradiation with cisplatin remains the mainstay of primary or adjuvant treatment in these patients. Patients who are resistant to cisplatin suffer from cancer-induced pain and poor survival. While several mechanisms for cisplatin resistance have been established, none of the reported mechanisms are reversible. In this study we hypothesized that methylation of key genes is a molecular mechanism leading to cisplatin resistance. We decided to investigate DNA methylation as a resistance mechanism because it is reversible by available drugs. We used SCC-25 and its cisplatin-resistant counterpart, SCC-25/CP, and determined that pre-treatment with the demethylating drug decitabine enhanced the anti-proliferative and apoptotic effect of cisplatin on these cell lines. In our HNSCC mouse model, combination treatment with decitabine and cisplatin produced a more robust anti-tumor effect than either drug alone. Decitabine pre-treatment *in vitro* reversed cisplatin-resistance in SCC-25/CP cells, and lowered the dose of cisplatin required to produce anti-proliferative or apoptotic effects. Interestingly, decitabine pre-treatment also lowered the dose of cisplatin required for cisplatin-sensitive SCC-25 cells. The clinical significance of our results is that decitabine could salvage patients with cisplatin-resistant tumors; moreover, for those patients who have cisplatin-sensitive tumors, decitabine could lower the cisplatin dose required, allowing for reduced toxicity.

Previous studies have explored the effectiveness of epigenetic therapy in rescuing cisplatin resistance in other cancers. Adding hydralazine and valproate to cisplatin therapy significantly increased progression-free survival in advanced stage cervical cancer patients [26]. A phase I trial for patients with solid tumors showed that combination treatment of decitabine followed by carboplatin is safe [27]. A phase II study adding valproate and hydralazine to the same schedule of chemotherapy on which patients with solid cancers were progressing showed clinical benefit in 12 of 15 (80%) patients [28]. At the same time there have been studies adding demethylating agents to platinum-based chemotherapy with negative results. A phase II trial randomized ovarian cancer patients progressing 6–12 months after previous platinum therapy to one of two groups: one group would receive decitabine

A

RECIST 1/2   RECIST 3/4

1 2 3 4 5 6 7 8 9 10 11 12   13 14 15 16 17 18 19

CRIP1
GOS2
MLH
OP3
S100
TUBB2A

B

PMR

100

10

1

CRIP1   GOS2   MLH1   OP3   S100   TUBB2A

1. SCC-25
2. SCC-25/CP
3. DAC SCC-25
4. DAC SCC-25/CP

C

Relative expression

8
4
2
1
0.5
0.25
0.125
0.0625

CRIP1   GOS2   MLH1   OP3   S100   TUBB2A

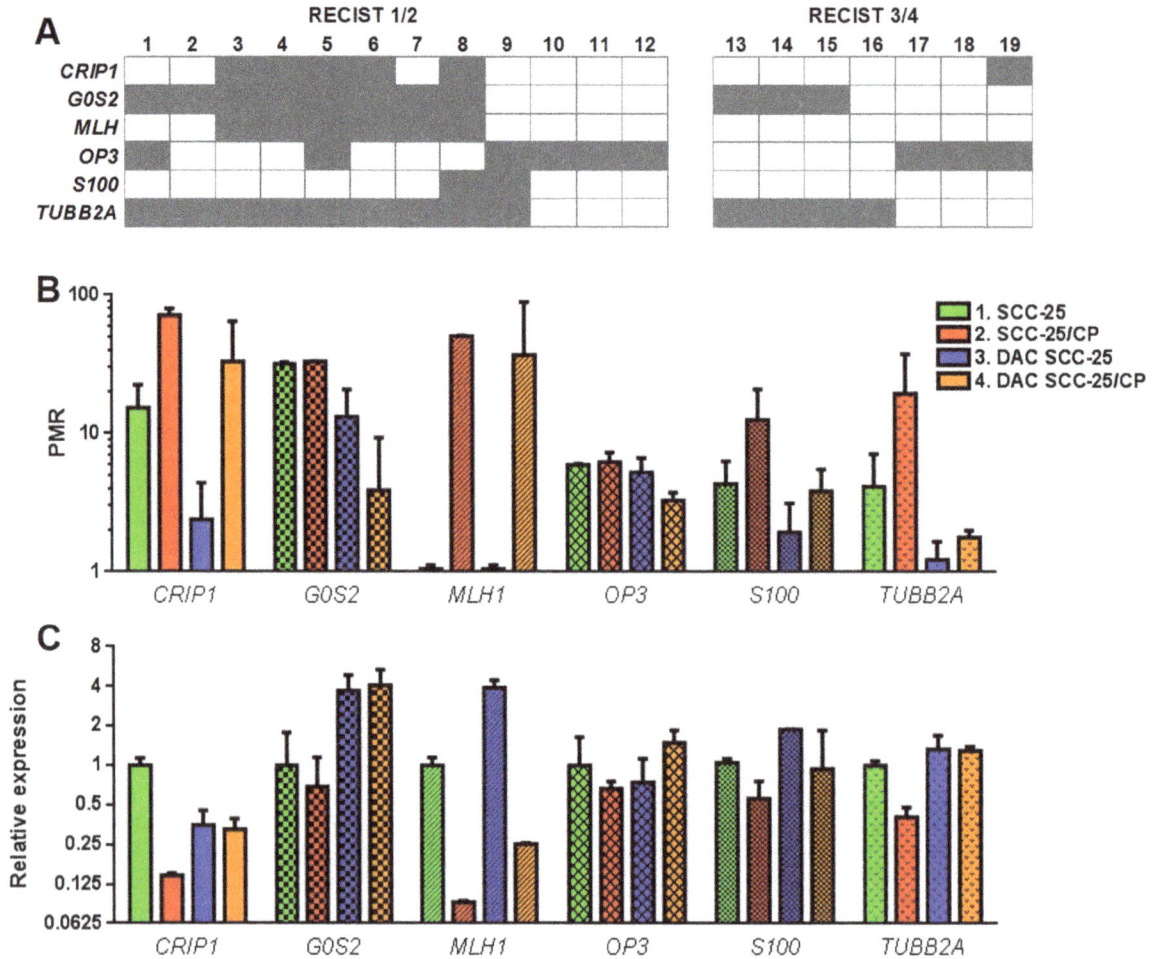

Figure 3. Methylation profiles were different between cisplatin-responsive and cisplatin-unresponsive HNSCC cancer tissues and cell lines. (A) A matrix of methylation profiles in cisplatin-unresponsive HNSCC tumors (RECIST 1 or 2) and cisplatin-responsive tumors (RECIST 3 or 4) was created using PMR = 10 as the cutoff for methylation positivity. Cisplatin-unresponsive tumors were more likely to be methylated at within the chosen gene panel (*CRIP1*, *GOS2*, *MLH1*, *OPN3*, *S100* and *TUBB2A*) than cisplatin-responsive tumors (66.7% cisplatin-unresponsive tumors vs 0% cisplatin-responsive tumors had 3 or more methylated genes). (B) The bar graph shows PMR values of SCC-25 and SCC-25/CP before and after decitabine treatment (*i.e.*, DAC-SCC-25 and DAC-SCC-25/CP) for each of the six genes. SCC-25/CP cisplatin-resistant cells had a significant hypermethylated methylation signature compared to SCC-25 cisplatin-sensitive cells. Decitabine treatment reversed methylation of SCC-25/CP cells toward a cisplatin-sensitive profile; the methylation signature of the six-gene classifier was significantly different between SCC-25/CP and DAC-SCC-25/CP cells. (C) The bar graph shows relative expression of the six genes for the two cell lines before and after decitabine treatment. SCC-25/CP cells had significantly lower expression levels for the six-gene classifier compared to SCC-25 cells. Decitabine treatment of SCC-25/CP cells (*i.e.*, DAC-SCC-25/CP) increased expression levels toward a cisplatin-sensitive expression profile. (See Tables 2 and 3 for statistical analysis.)

with carboplatin, and the second group would receive carboplatin alone. However the study closed after an interim analysis showed that the combination group had lack of efficacy and poor treatment deliverability [29]. Our dose scheduling of decitabine and cisplatin is based on previous work in ovarian and colon carcinoma [23] showing that multiple doses of decitabine are required prior to cisplatin administration to maximally sensitize xenografts to cisplatin.

In addition to reduced survival, head and neck cancer patients have significant function-limiting pain, which is either cancer-induced or treatment-induced. While survival and pain seem like unrelated issues, a recent randomized clinical trial shows that aggressive pain management in advanced-stage cancer patients significantly improves quality of life and increases survival [30]. Peripheral neuropathy is a major toxic side effect of cisplatin and contributes to pain [31]. The behavioral assay that we used on our preclinical model detects both cancer-induced pain and

neuropathic pain. We showed that combination therapy of decitabine and cisplatin resulted in significantly reduced mechanical pain. While nociception in our preclinical model was likely cancer-induced, decitabine treatment potentially reduces the required cisplatin dose, thus minimizing peripheral neuropathy.

Methylation classifier for cisplatin resistance

HNSCC survival has not dramatically improved, even in an era of burgeoning personalized medicine, for two reasons. The first reason is that no effective treatment has been developed to combat cisplatin resistance. The second is that there is no effective marker to predict cisplatin responsiveness. Therefore, in addition to re-purposing decitabine as a drug to rescue cisplatin-resistance, we developed a methylation and expression classifier that could differentiate between cisplatin-responsive and cisplatin-unresponsive HNSCC. The classifier must have the additional ability to

Table 1. Patient Demographics.

Case #	Sex	Age	Site	TNM	Disease burden at 6 months (RECIST)
1	F	58	retromolar trigone	T2N1M0	progressed (1)
2	M	56	tongue	T4aN2bM0	progressed (1)
3	M	48	retromolar trigone	T4aN0M0	progressed (1)
4	F	20	tongue	T4aN2bM0	progressed (1)
5	M	57	tongue	T4aN2bM0	progressed (1)
6	M	67	soft palate	T3N2bM0	progressed (1)
7	M	50	base of tongue	T2N2bM0	progressed (1)
8	M	59	base of tongue	T2N2cM1	progressed (1)
9	M	34	tongue	T1N1M0	progressed (1)
10	F	66	tongue	T1N1M1	progressed (1)
11	F	74	upper lip	T1N1M0	stable (2)
12	M	67	tongue	T2N0M0	stable (2)
13	M	61	tonsil	T1N2bM0	complete remission (4)
14	F	62	base of tongue	T4N2M0	complete remission (4)
15	F	71	base of tongue	T1N3M0	complete remission (4)
16	M	50	tonsil	T2N2aM0	complete remission (4)
17	F	51	tongue	T2N2M0	complete remission (4)
18	M	81	floor of mouth	T2N0M0	complete remission (4)
19	M	69	floor of mouth	T4aN1M0	complete remission (4)

predict decitabine efficacy in the setting of cisplatin-resistance. Previous studies have shown that although many genes are hypermethylated and downregulated in cisplatin resistant cancer, only a small proportion of these genes are re-expressed in response to decitabine treatment [32]. In developing a classifier that could potentially be used to monitor decitabine efficacy in patients with cisplatin-unresponsive HNSCC, we targeted genes that (1) are hypermethylated in cisplatin-unresponsive tumors and (2) can be re-expressed *in vitro* with decitabine treatment. We therefore combined methylation data from patient tumor tissues and cell lines following decitabine treatment to converge on six genes

(*CRIP1, G0S2, MLH1, OPN3, S100* and *TUBB2A*) as the classifier. These six genes have been shown in previous studies to be hypermethylated in cisplatin-resistant cell lines [11], but their methylation status in cancer tissue of HNSCC patients has not been quantified. One of the six genes, *MLH1*, has been shown to directly confer cisplatin sensitivity when re-expressed in ovarian cancer cells *in vitro* [23,32]. We showed that methylation of the six genes was higher in cisplatin-unresponsive tumors (RECIST 1/2) than cisplatin-responsive tumors (RECIST 3/4) of HNSCC patients. Moreover, when we assembled the six genes into a classifier and used the criterion of positive methylation in three or

Table 2. Statistical Summary of Two-way ANOVA and *Post Hoc* Analyses.

	Two-way ANOVA				*Post Hoc* Analysis	
	Effects	DF	F	P	Groups	P
Figure 2A	Tx	3	83.473	<0.001	4 vs. 1	<0.001
	Time	11	24.079	<0.001	2 vs. 1	<0.001
	Time × Tx	33	3.372	<0.001	3 vs. 1	<0.001
Figure 2B	Tx	3	17.841	<0.001	4 vs. 1	<0.001
	Time	11	875.806	<0.001	2 vs. 1	0.001
	Time × Tx	33	19.748	<0.001	3 vs. 1	0.007
Figure 3B	Cell line	3	12.37	<0.001	1 vs. 2	<0.001
	Gene	5	7.763	<0.001	1 vs. 3	ns
	Cell line × gene	15	2.652	0.0065	2 vs. 4	<0.05
Figure 3C	Cell line	3	9.96	<0.001	1 vs. 2	<0.01
	Gene	5	24.34	<0.001	1 vs. 3	<0.001
	Cell line × gene	15	3.999	0.001	2 vs. 4	<0.001

Table 3. Statistical Summary of Individual Gene Comparisons.

	CRIP1	G0S2	MLH1	OP3	S100	TUBB2A
Student's t tests comparing Percent of Methylated Reference						
SCC-25 vs. SCC-25/CP	0.0588	0.224	<0.0001	0.7096	0.1042	0.1456
SCC-25 vs. DAC SCC-25	0.016	0.0747	0.4228	0.5713	0.0884	0.1728
SCC-25/CP vs. DAC SCC-25/CP	0.2077	0.0172	0.004	0.068	0.0872	0.1595
Student's t tests comparing gene expression						
SCC-25 vs. SCC-25/CP	0.0126	0.6061	0.0127	0.0214	0.0813	0.0007
SCC-25 vs. DAC SCC-25	0.0027	0.0146	0.0189	0.3702	0.0037	0.2028
SCC-25/CP vs. DAC SCC-25/CP	0.0222	0.0566	0.0004	0.0835	0.6253	0.0002

more genes to categorize cisplatin sensitivity, we could differentiate cisplatin-responsive from cisplatin-unresponsive tumors with a sensitivity of 67% and a specificity of 100%. The modest sensitivity is in part due to our small sample size—it was difficult to obtain initial biopsy samples with adequate tissue for DNA extraction. Another limitation is that we could not correlate methylation with gene expression, since we had obtained limited quantities of formalin-fixed, paraffin-embedded tissue that could not be used to reliably quantify mRNA or perform immunohistochemical staining. We therefore used our cell lines to determine whether there was a functional correlation between gene methylation status and expression levels. We showed that the cisplatin-resistant (SCC-25/CP) cells had a significantly different methylation signature of the six gene classifier compared to cisplatin-sensitive (SCC-25) cells. We then treated the cell lines with decitabine. We showed that decitabine treatment produced either a significant decrease in methylation or increase in gene expression in four of the six genes for both SCC-25 and SCC-25/CP. When all six genes were used as a single classifier, we showed statistically significant differences between the decitabine-treated and non-treated cell lines. Therefore the six genes responded to decitabine treatment and could potentially be used to monitor decitabine efficacy in cisplatin-resistant HNSCC.

Chemotherapy with radiation is typically used for HNSCC, as adjuvant post-surgical treatment for tumors with worrisome features [33], or as primary treatment for advanced stage disease. Cisplatin remains the most frequently used and most effective chemotherapy, as it is thought to act synergistically with ionizing radiation by enhancing the formation of cluster damage to DNA [34]. One perceived limitation of the study is that the preclinical model did not accurately replicate HNSCC treatment, since radiation was not included in the treatment scheme. Our rationale for not including radiation was to isolate the effects of cisplatin on the cancer cells and to eliminate any synergy between cisplatin and radiation.

In summary, our study establishes methylation as a mechanism of cisplatin resistance, and pre-treatment with a demethylating drug as a possible strategy to reduce cisplatin resistance. While the role of gene methylation on cisplatin sensitivity has been explored *in vitro* [11], our study uses a preclinical cisplatin-resistant HNSCC model to determine the effect of decitabine on proliferation and pain. Furthermore, we utilize cancer tissues from HNSCC patients to create a classifier for cisplatin-resistance. Despite limited sensitivity of the classifier due to small sample size, we show in the cell lines that decitabine treatment reverses methylation and increases expression of genes within the classifier. Our current results lay the groundwork for future studies focused on demethylation therapy for cisplatin resistance and methylation markers as a method to identify patients with cisplatin resistance.

Author Contributions

Conceived and designed the experiments: CTV DD SA YY SGK BLS. Performed the experiments: CTV DD SA YY SGK. Analyzed the data: CTV BLS. Contributed reagents/materials/analysis tools: CTV BLS. Wrote the paper: CTV DD SA YY SGK BLS.

References

1. Vernham GA, Crowther JA (1994) Head and neck carcinoma–stage at presentation. Clinical otolaryngology and allied sciences 19: 120–124.
2. Pignon JP, le Maitre A, Maillard E, Bourhis J (2009) Meta-analysis of chemotherapy in head and neck cancer (MACH-NC): an update on 93 randomised trials and 17,346 patients. Radiotherapy and oncology: journal of the European Society for Therapeutic Radiology and Oncology 92: 4–14.
3. Pignon JP, le Maitre A, Bourhis J (2007) Meta-Analyses of Chemotherapy in Head and Neck Cancer (MACH-NC): an update. International journal of radiation oncology, biology, physics 69: S112–114.
4. Pignon JP, Bourhis J, Domenge C, Designe L (2000) Chemotherapy added to locoregional treatment for head and neck squamous-cell carcinoma: three meta-analyses of updated individual data. MACH-NC Collaborative Group. Meta-Analysis of Chemotherapy on Head and Neck Cancer. Lancet 355: 949–955.
5. Stewart DJ (2007) Mechanisms of resistance to cisplatin and carboplatin. Critical reviews in oncology/hematology 63: 12–31.
6. Fischer DJ, Villines D, Kim YO, Epstein JB, Wilkie DJ (2010) Anxiety, depression, and pain: differences by primary cancer. Supportive care in cancer: official journal of the Multinational Association of Supportive Care in Cancer 18: 801–810.
7. Viet CT, Schmidt BL (2012) Biologic mechanisms of oral cancer pain and implications for clinical therapy. Journal of dental research 91: 447–453.
8. van den Beuken-van Everdingen MH, de Rijke JM, Kessels AG, Schouten HC, van Kleef M, et al. (2007) Prevalence of pain in patients with cancer: a systematic review of the past 40 years. Annals of oncology: official journal of the European Society for Medical Oncology/ESMO 18: 1437–1449.
9. Kolokythas A, Connelly ST, Schmidt BL (2007) Validation of the university of california san francisco oral cancer pain questionnaire. J Pain 8: 950–953.
10. Connelly ST, Schmidt BL (2004) Evaluation of pain in patients with oral squamous cell carcinoma. J Pain 5: 505–510.
11. Chang X, Monitto CL, Demokan S, Kim MS, Chang SS, et al. (2010) Identification of hypermethylated genes associated with cisplatin resistance in human cancers. Cancer Research 70: 2870–2879.
12. Daskalakis M, Blagitko-Dorfs N, Hackanson B (2010) Decitabine. Recent Results Cancer Res 184: 131–157.
13. Blum W, Garzon R, Klisovic RB, Schwind S, Walker A, et al. Clinical response and miR-29b predictive significance in older AML patients treated with a 10-day schedule of decitabine. Proc Natl Acad Sci U S A 107: 7473–7478.
14. Cashen AF, Schiller GJ, O'Donnell MR, DiPersio JF (2010) Multicenter, phase II study of decitabine for the first-line treatment of older patients with acute myeloid leukemia. J Clin Oncol 28: 556–561.
15. Stewart DJ, Issa JP, Kurzrock R, Nunez MI, Jelinek J, et al. (2009) Decitabine effect on tumor global DNA methylation and other parameters in a phase I trial in refractory solid tumors and lymphomas. Clin Cancer Res 15: 3881–3888.

16. Viet CT, Dang D, Ye Y, Ono K, Campbell RR, et al. (2014) Demethylating Drugs as Novel Analgesics for Cancer Pain. Clin Cancer Res.

17. Teicher BA, Cucchi CA, Lee JB, Flatow JL, Rosowsky A, et al. (1986) Alkylating agents: in vitro studies of cross-resistance patterns in human cell lines. Cancer Res 46: 4379–4383.

18. Viet CT, Ye Y, Dang D, Lam DK, Achdjian S, et al. (2011) Re-expression of the methylated EDNRB gene in oral squamous cell carcinoma attenuates cancer-induced pain. Pain 152: 2323–2332.

19. Marcu LG, Bezak E (2012) Neoadjuvant cisplatin for head and neck cancer: Simulation of a novel schedule for improved therapeutic ratio. J Theor Biol 297: 41–47.

20. Ogino S, Kawasaki T, Brahmandam M, Cantor M, Kirkner GJ, et al. (2006) Precision and performance characteristics of bisulfite conversion and real-time PCR (MethyLight) for quantitative DNA methylation analysis. J Mol Diagn 8: 209–217.

21. Shi W, Kato H, Perez-Ordonez B, Pintilie M, Huang S, et al. (2009) Comparative prognostic value of HPV16 E6 mRNA compared with in situ hybridization for human oropharyngeal squamous carcinoma. J Clin Oncol 27: 6213–6221.

22. Ibanez de Caceres I, Cortes-Sempere M, Moratilla C, Machado-Pinilla R, Rodriguez-Fanjul V, et al. (2010) IGFBP-3 hypermethylation-derived deficiency mediates cisplatin resistance in non-small-cell lung cancer. Oncogene 29: 1681–1690.

23. Plumb JA, Strathdee G, Sludden J, Kaye SB, Brown R (2000) Reversal of drug resistance in human tumor xenografts by 2′-deoxy-5-azacytidine-induced demethylation of the hMLH1 gene promoter. Cancer Research 60: 6039–6044.

24. Viet CT, Schmidt BL (2008) Methylation array analysis of preoperative and postoperative saliva DNA in oral cancer patients. Cancer Epidemiol Biomarkers Prev 17: 3603–3611.

25. Shiboski CH, Schmidt BL, Jordan RC (2005) Tongue and tonsil carcinoma: increasing trends in the U.S. population ages 20–44 years. Cancer 103: 1843–1849.

26. Coronel J, Cetina L, Pacheco I, Trejo-Becerril C, Gonzalez-Fierro A, et al. (2010) A double-blind, placebo-controlled, randomized phase III trial of chemotherapy plus epigenetic therapy with hydralazine valproate for advanced cervical cancer. Preliminary results. Medical oncology.

27. Appleton K, Mackay HJ, Judson I, Plumb JA, McCormick C, et al. (2007) Phase I and pharmacodynamic trial of the DNA methyltransferase inhibitor decitabine and carboplatin in solid tumors. Journal of clinical oncology: official journal of the American Society of Clinical Oncology 25: 4603–4609.

28. Candelaria M, Gallardo-Rincon D, Arce C, Cetina L, Aguilar-Ponce JL, et al. (2007) A phase II study of epigenetic therapy with hydralazine and magnesium valproate to overcome chemotherapy resistance in refractory solid tumors. Ann Oncol 18: 1529–1538.

29. Glasspool RM, Brown R, Gore ME, Rustin GJ, McNeish IA, et al. (2014) A randomised, phase II trial of the DNA-hypomethylating agent 5-aza-2′-deoxycytidine (decitabine) in combination with carboplatin vs carboplatin alone in patients with recurrent, partially platinum-sensitive ovarian cancer. Br J Cancer 110: 1923–1929.

30. Temel JS, Greer JA, Muzikansky A, Gallagher ER, Admane S, et al. (2010) Early palliative care for patients with metastatic non-small-cell lung cancer. The New England journal of medicine 363: 733–742.

31. Amptoulach S, Tsavaris N (2011) Neurotoxicity caused by the treatment with platinum analogues. Chemother Res Pract 2011: 843019.

32. Zeller C, Dai W, Steele NL, Siddiq A, Walley AJ, et al. (2012) Candidate DNA methylation drivers of acquired cisplatin resistance in ovarian cancer identified by methylome and expression profiling. Oncogene 31: 4567–4576.

33. Cooper JS, Pajak TF, Forastiere AA, Jacobs J, Campbell BH, et al. (2004) Postoperative concurrent radiotherapy and chemotherapy for high-risk squamous-cell carcinoma of the head and neck. The New England journal of medicine 350: 1937–1944.

34. Rezaee M, Hunting DJ, Sanche L (2013) New insights into the mechanism underlying the synergistic action of ionizing radiation with platinum chemotherapeutic drugs: the role of low-energy electrons. Int J Radiat Oncol Biol Phys 87: 847–853.

13

Amyotrophic Lateral Sclerosis-Linked Mutant VAPB Inclusions Do Not Interfere with Protein Degradation Pathways or Intracellular Transport in a Cultured Cell Model

Paola Genevini[1], Giulia Papiani[1¤a], Annamaria Ruggiano[1¤b], Lavinia Cantoni[2], Francesca Navone[1]*, Nica Borgese[1,3]*

1 Institute of Neuroscience, Consiglio Nazionale delle Ricerche, and Department of Medical Biotechnology and Translational Medicine (BIOMETRA), Università degli Studi di Milano, Milano, Italy, 2 Department of Molecular Biochemistry and Pharmacology, Istituto di Ricerche Farmacologiche "Mario Negri", Milan, Italy, 3 Department of Health Science, Magna Graecia University of Catanzaro, Catanzaro, Italy

Abstract

VAPB is a ubiquitously expressed, ER-resident adaptor protein involved in interorganellar lipid exchange, membrane contact site formation, and membrane trafficking. Its mutant form, P56S-VAPB, which has been linked to a dominantly inherited form of Amyotrophic Lateral Sclerosis (ALS8), generates intracellular inclusions consisting in restructured ER domains whose role in ALS pathogenesis has not been elucidated. P56S-VAPB is less stable than the wild-type protein and, at variance with most pathological aggregates, its inclusions are cleared by the proteasome. Based on studies with cultured cells overexpressing the mutant protein, it has been suggested that VAPB inclusions may exert a pathogenic effect either by sequestering the wild-type protein and other interactors (loss-of-function by a dominant negative effect) or by a more general proteotoxic action (gain-of-function). To investigate P56S-VAPB degradation and the effect of the inclusions on proteostasis and on ER-to-plasma membrane protein transport in a more physiological setting, we used stable HeLa and NSC34 Tet-Off cell lines inducibly expressing moderate levels of P56S-VAPB. Under basal conditions, P56S-VAPB degradation was mediated exclusively by the proteasome in both cell lines, however, it could be targeted also by starvation-stimulated autophagy. To assess possible proteasome impairment, the HeLa cell line was transiently transfected with the ERAD (ER Associated Degradation) substrate CD3δ, while autophagic flow was investigated in cells either starved or treated with an autophagy-stimulating drug. Secretory pathway functionality was evaluated by analyzing the transport of transfected Vesicular Stomatitis Virus Glycoprotein (VSVG). P56S-VAPB expression had no effect either on the degradation of CD3δ or on the levels of autophagic markers, or on the rate of transport of VSVG to the cell surface. We conclude that P56S-VAPB inclusions expressed at moderate levels do not interfere with protein degradation pathways or protein transport, suggesting that the dominant inheritance of the mutant gene may be due mainly to haploinsufficiency.

Editor: Yanmin Yang, Stanford University School of Medicine, United States of America

Funding: This work was supported by the CARIPLO Foundation (http://www.fondazionecariplo.it/it/index.html) project 2007-5098 (NB), PNR-CNR Aging Program 2012–2014, and Università Statale di Milano. The funders had no role in study design, data collection and analysis, decision to publish, or preparation of the manuscript.

Competing Interests: The authors have declared that no competing interests exist.

* Email: f.navone@in.cnr.it (FN); n.borgese@in.cnr.it (NB)

¤a Current address: Oligomerix, Inc., New York, New York, United States of America
¤b Current address: Cell and Developmental Biology Programme, Centre for Genomic Regulation (CRG), Barcelona, Spain

Introduction

VAPB, and its homologue VAPA, are members of the highly conserved and ubiquitously expressed VAP (Vesicle-Associated Membrane Protein (VAMP)-Associated Protein) family of ER tail-anchored transmembrane proteins. The cytosolic N-terminal region, consists of a domain that is homologous to the nematode major sperm protein (MSP), followed by a central coiled-coil domain; the transmembrane segment is close to the C-terminus, and the last four C-terminal residues are probably exposed to the ER lumen [1].

By interacting with FFAT (two phenylalanines in an acidic tract) motif-containing polypeptides, VAPs are able to recruit a wide spectrum of proteins, and are thus implicated in a variety of physiological functions (reviewed in ref 1), including membrane trafficking [2,3], lipid transport and metabolism [4,5], membrane contact site formation [6,7,8,9,10], Ca^{2+} homeostasis [9], ER-cytoskeleton interactions [11], participation in the unfolded protein response [12], neurotransmitter release and neurite extension [13,14]. Specific roles that functionally distinguish the two mammalian VAP isoforms have not been identified so far.

The identification of a dominant missense mutation in the VAPB gene in patients affected by a slowly progressing form of familial motor neuron disease (ALS8) [15] greatly increased the interest in VAP proteins. The mutation, which causes substitution of proline 56 with serine in the MSP domain (P56S mutation), disrupts VAPB's three-dimensional structure and favors its aggregation [16,17,18]. Initially identified in eight Brazilian families with a shared Portuguese ancestor [19], the same mutation was subsequently detected in an unrelated German patient, carrying a haplotype distinct from the one linked to the mutation in the Brazilian families [20]. Three additional mutations of VAPB have since been identified in familial Amyotrophic Lateral Sclerosis (ALS) patients [21,22,23], however, in these cases, the segregation of the mutation with the disease was not demonstrated.

Like many proteins linked to neurodegenerative diseases, mutant VAPB forms intracellular inclusions. Work from our laboratory, however, revealed important differences between P56S-VAPB inclusions and other inclusion bodies. More specifically, we showed that, after insertion into the ER membrane, P56S-VAPB rapidly clusters to generate paired ER cisternae that give rise to a profoundly restructured ER domain and not to a cytosolic protein aggregate, as is generally the case [24]. Moreover, we demonstrated that, at variance with other inclusion bodies linked to neurodegenerative diseases, ER-derived ubiquitinated P56S-VAPB inclusions can be easily cleared by the proteasome, with no apparent involvement of basal macroautophagy (here referred to as autophagy) [25].

Although protein misfolding and aggregation are a common feature of several neurodegenerative diseases, including ALS, their precise pathogenic role is poorly understood, and both a toxic gain of function as well as loss of function by dominant negative effects are thought to be involved. In the case of ALS8, studies in transfected mammalian cells and in fly models have revealed that wild-type VAPB, as well as VAPA and other functionally important interactors, are sequestered within the VAPB inclusions, leading to the hypothesis that the dominant inheritance of ALS8 is due to a dominant negative effect of the mutant protein [12,16,26,27,28,29].

In addition to the loss of function mechanism, driven by sequestration of potentially functional proteins into inclusion bodies, evidence for a toxic gain-of-function of mutant VAPB has also been reported. P56S-VAPB inclusions are ubiquitin-positive both in transfected cells [25] and in motor neurons of transgenic animals [30], and both wild-type and P56S-VAPB, when overexpressed, have been observed to impair the activity of the proteasome [31]. These observations suggest that VAPB inclusions may disturb proteostasis, and are in line with the many studies pointing to alteration in protein degradation pathways as an important pathogenic mechanism underlying aggregated misfolded protein toxicity both in sporadic and familial ALS (reviewed in refs [32–35]).

One limitation of most of the studies on the mechanism of P56S-VAPB pathogenicity in mammalian systems has been the use of strongly overexpressing transfected cells, which may be inadequate to unravel the effects of the mutant protein expressed from a single allele, as in patients' cells. In our previous work, we developed a cell line inducibly expressing P56S-VAPB at levels comparable to those of the endogenous protein, and used this cell line to investigate the genesis, nature and clearance of the P56S-VAPB-containing aggregates [24,25]. In the present study, we have investigated whether the presence of P56S-VAPB-containing inclusions, generated by mutant VAPB expressed at levels comparable to those of the endogenous protein, interferes with physiological protein degradation pathways or impairs normal protein transport from the ER to the plasma membrane. We find that the inclusions neither interfere with general proteostasis nor with the intracellular transport of a model secretory membrane protein. We also confirm that P56S-VAPB inclusions are exclusively cleared by the proteasome under basal conditions both in neuronal and non-neuronal cells, but find that they can be degraded by stimulated autophagy. Our results are consistent with the idea that haploinsufficiency alone may underlie the dominant inheritance of P56S-VAPB.

Materials and Methods

Plasmids

The pTre Tight vectors (Clontech), coding for *myc*-wt VAPB or *myc*-P56S-VAPB have been described [24,25].

pGEX vectors coding for fragments 132–225 or 1–225 of VAPB fused to GST were provided by C.C. Hoogenraad (Utrecht University, NL). VAPA-pGEX2T coding for full-length VAPA fused to GST was generated from the rat VAPA sequence amplified from a pGEM4 recombinant plasmid. The VAPA clone was provided by Stephen Kaiser [36]. Specific restriction sites for subcloning in the pGEX2T vector were introduced into the PCR primers: upper 5′ ATCCCGGGAATGGCGAAACACGAGC 3′ (SmaI restriction site underlined) and lower 5′ TAGAATTCG-CAGGTCGACTCTAGAC 3′ (EcoRI restriction site underlined).

pTK-Hyg and pEGFP-N1 were from Clontech; pCINeoHA-CD3δ and pCDM8.1-ts045VSVG-EGFP were generously provided by A.M. Weissman (National Institutes of Health) and J. Lippincott-Schwartz (National Institutes of Health, Bethesda, MD) respectively.

All constructs generated in the laboratory were checked by sequencing.

Antibodies

The following primary antibodies were obtained from the indicated sources: anti-*myc* monoclonals (clone 9E10), Santa Cruz or Sigma; monoclonal anti-tubulin (clone B-5-1-2), monoclonal anti-actin, and polyclonal anti-LC3 (L8918), Sigma; polyclonal anti-p62 (ab91526), Abcam; monoclonal anti-VSVG (clone IE9F9), keraFAST; polyclonal anti-HA, Invitrogen (71-5500) or Santa Cruz (SC-805); polyclonal anti-GFP (ab290), Abcam. Polyclonal anti-giantin serum and anti-GM130 were kindly provided by Dr. M. Renz (Institute of Immunology and Molecular Genetics, Karlsruhe, Germany) [37] and A. de Matteis (Telethon Institute of Genetics and Medicine, Naples, Italy) [38], respectively.

Anti-VAPB polyclonal antibodies were produced in the laboratory as follows. The VAPB 132–225 fragment fused to GST was expressed in E. coli BL21 by induction with 0.5 mM Isopropyl β-D-1-thiogalactopyranoside (IPTG), following standard procedures. The expressed protein was purified with glutathione-Sepharose 4B resin (GE Healthcare) according to the manufacturer's protocol. A rabbit was immunized with the VAPB fragment excised from GST by thrombin digestion. The sera were first tested against lysates of E.coli BL21 induced to express either full-length VAPA-GST or VAPB 1-225-GST. Cross-reactive anti-VAPA antibodies were then eliminated by adsorption of 3 ml of sera with 1.60 mg of VAPA-GST immobilized on glutathione-sepharose beads. Finally, anti-VAPB antibodies were purified from the adsorbed sera using 1 mg of 132–225 VAPB fragment coupled to CNBr-activated Sepharose 4B as affinity ligand (see Fig. S1).

Peroxidase-conjugated anti-rabbit and anti-mouse IgG were from Sigma, anti-mouse IRDye 680 and anti-rabbit IRDye 800 from LI-COR Bioscience, Alexa Fluor 488 anti-rabbit and Alexa Fluor 568 anti-mouse IgG from Invitrogen, DyLight 549 or 633 anti-mouse and anti-rabbit IgG from Pierce.

Cell culture, transfection, and P56S-VAPB expression analysis

HeLa Tet-Off cell lines expressing *myc*-P56S-VAPB [24,25] were maintained in DMEM supplemented with 10% FBS Tet-free (Hyclone), 1% Pen/Strep, 1% L-Glut, G418 (100 µg/ml), Hygromycin (100 µg/ml), and doxycycline (Dox) (500 ng/ml). Expression of P56S-VAPB was induced by transferring the cells to Dox-free medium. Degradation of VAPB was followed after re-addition of Dox to the medium, as previously described [25]. Briefly, four days after removal of Dox, equal numbers of cells were seeded onto 35 mm Petri dishes containing a coverslip, and incubation in the absence of Dox was continued for another two days. At this time, the coverslips were fixed and stained with DAPI; nuclei from random fields were counted to assess that each dish contained an equal number of cells. Dox was then added back to the samples, and cells were collected after treatment with the indicated drugs and at the time intervals indicated in the figures. The collected cells were lysed with SDS-lysis buffer [2% SDS, 50 mM Tris-HCl, pH 8, plus Complete (Roche) protease inhibitors] and all samples were brought to the same volume. Equal aliquots were then analyzed by SDS-PAGE-Immunoblotting. The levels of VAPB were corrected for minor variations in the number of plated cells.

NSC34 Tet-Off cell lines were generated in the laboratory of L. Cantoni [39] and were maintained in DMEM supplemented with 10% FBS, 1% P/S, 1% L-Glut, 1% Na+Pyruvate and G418 (250 µg/ml). For most experiments, NSC34 Tet-Off cells were plated on Matrigel (BD Biosciences)-coated wells.

All transfections were carried out with JetPei (Polyplus transfection) according to the manufacturer's protocol. For the transient transfection of induced P56S-VAPB-HeLaTet-Off cells, incubation with JetPei DNA complexes was carried out in the presence of FBS from Gibco. After 24 h, the medium was replaced with complete medium supplemented with Tet-free serum, and the cells were treated as indicated in the figure legends.

To generate NSC34 Tet-Off VAPB clones, cells were co-transfected with pTK-hyg and pTre vector coding either for *myc*-wt VAPB or *myc*-P56S-VAPB. After transfection cells were selected with 150 µg/ml hygromycin. After approximately four weeks of growth in selection medium, individual clones were collected, amplified and induced to express the transgene by growth in the absence of Dox for 4–5 days. Increased expression was obtained by addition of 10 mM Na+butyrate for 12 h. For *myc*-P56S-VAPB, five positive clones were identified out of 41 tested, while for *myc*-wt-VAPB, two out of 23.

To investigate clearance of P56S-VAPB inclusions from the NSC34 lines, cells were induced to express P56S-VAPB by growth for 4 days in Dox-free medium followed by treatment with 10 mM Na+butyrate for 12 h. Cells were then transferred to Na+butyrate-free, Dox (0.5 µg/ml) -containing medium, and P56S-VAPB degradation was followed as described for the HeLa Tet-Off clones.

Drug treatments and starvation

Lactacystine and Torin 1 were from Cayman Chemical; MG132 was from Calbiochem. Other drugs were from Sigma. 3-Methyladenine (3-MA) and Cycloheximide (CHX) were dissolved in water and used at final concentration of 10 mM and 50 µg/ml, respectively. Na+butyrate was dissolved in complete medium and used at 10 mM final concentration. The following

drugs were dissolved in DMSO and used at the final concentrations indicated between brackets: Bafilomycin (200 nM), MG132 (10 µM), Lactacystin (10 µM) and Torin1 (250 nM). Control cells received equal volumes of the vector.

Cells were starved by replacing culture media with EBSS (Earle's Balanced Salt Solution).

SDS-PAGE and Immunoblotting

SDS-PAGE and blotting were performed by standard procedures. Protein content was assayed with the BCA Protein Assay Kit (Thermo Scientific). Before immunostaining, blots were stained for total protein with Ponceau S (Sigma); they were then incubated with antibodies diluted in TBS+5% milk+0.1% Tween. Peroxidase-conjugated secondary antibodies were revealed by ECL (Perkin Elmer). The films were digitized, and band intensities were determined with ImageJ software (National Institutes of Health) after calibration with the optical density calibration step table (Stouffer Graphics Arts). Alternatively, Infrared dye-conjugated secondary antibodies were used. In this case, blots were scanned with the Odyssey CLx Infrared Imaging System (LI-COR Biosciences), and band intensities were determined with Image Studio software (LI-COR Biosciences).

Fluorescence Microscopy

Cells grown on coverslips were fixed with 4% paraformaldehyde (PFA)+4% sucrose and processed for immunofluorescence as described previously [25]. Images were acquired with the Zeiss LSM 510 Meta confocal system equipped with a 405/488/543/ 633 dichroic (Carl Zeiss, Oberkochen, Germany) and using a 63xPlanApo lens. Alexa Fluor 488 and GFP were acquired using the 488 line of the Argon/2 laser, and a 505–550 band pass emission filter. For Alexa Fluor 568 and DyLight 549, the 544 line of the He/Ne laser was used in combination with a 560–615 band pass emission filter. For DyLight 633, the 633 line of the He/Ne laser was used in combination with a 650 long pass emission filter. DAPI was imaged using the 405 diode laser and a 420–480 band pass emission filter. Wide-field imaging was performed with an Axioplan microscope (Carl Zeiss, Oberkochen, Germany), using the 40× PlanNeofluar lens equipped with a phase contrast ring.

Image analysis was performed with ImageJ software.

VSVG transport

Cells induced or not induced to express P56S-VAPB were transfected with ts045VSVG-EGFP and immediately placed at 39.3°C. After 24 h, cells were brought to 32° in the presence of CHX and incubated for the times indicated in the figures.

To evaluate the amount of VSVG in the Golgi area at each time point, coverslips were fixed and processed for immunofluorescence with anti-giantin and anti-*myc* antibodies. 1.2 µm thick z-stacks (~20 cells for each condition and time point) were acquired centered around the plane with maximum giantin staining (x–y sections). For each section, a ROI corresponding to giantin staining was outlined; the integrated EGFP fluorescence intensity of this region was determined, and summed over the entire stack. This value was normalized to that of the entire cell, determined in each section in ROIs drawn around the periphery of the cell.

For determination of surface VSVG, cells were placed on ice, medium was replaced with pre-chilled PBS+0.5 mM CaCl2+ 1 mM MgCl2 and then samples were transferred to the cold room. After two washes, cells were blocked with 0.1% BSA in the same buffer, and then incubated with anti-VSVG primary antibody diluted in blocking buffer for 1 h. Cells were washed 3 times, fixed with chilled PFA (see above: *Fluorescence microscopy*) first at 4° for 10 min, then at RT for an additional 10 min. After blocking with

17% goat serum, the non-permeabilized cells were exposed to secondary anti-mouse antibody for 50 min at room temperature. After 5 washes, the cells were fixed again for 5 min with PFA, permeabilized with Triton-X100 and processed for immunofluorescence with polyclonal anti-VAPB and secondary anti-rabbit antibodies under standard conditions [25]. Z-stacks (15–30 cells for each condition and time point) comprising the total height of the cells were acquired (X–Y sections at 0.5 μm intervals) to measure EGFP and anti-VSVG fluorescence as described for the Golgi analysis.

For both the Golgi and the surface quantification of VSVG, images were acquired with identical parameters, taking care to remain below saturation in the EGFP and anti-VSVG channels.

Statistical Analyses

Significance of the difference in VAPB levels between treated and untreated cells and possible differences in the intracellular distribution of VSVG in cells induced or not induced to express P56S-VAPB were evaluated by Student's unpaired two-tailed t test. Two-way matched Anova, followed by Bonferroni's post-test, was used to simultaneously evaluate the effects of cycloheximide (CHX) treatment and P56S-VAPB induction on CD3δlevels, or of autophagocytosis stimulation and P56S-VAPB induction on the LC3-II/LC3-I ratio. To compensate for different absolute values of band intensities in different experiments, values were either normalized to the band intensities before drug treatment, or converted to logarithms. p values are given in the figure legends.

Results

P56S-VAPB is cleared exclusively by the proteasome under basal conditions, but can be degraded by stimulated autophagy

To investigate the mechanism of P56S-VAPB clearance, we used the previously characterized HeLa Tet-Off cell line [24,25], in which expression of mutant, *myc*-tagged, VAPB is repressed by tetracycline or Dox, and induced by removal of the antibiotic from the medium (compare lanes 1 and 6 of Fig. 1A with lanes 2 and 7). We previously showed that mutant VAPB in these cells is expressed at levels close to those of the endogenous protein, and that the expressed protein is detected exclusively within inclusions ([24,25], Fig. 2C). When induced cells were shifted to Dox containing medium, ~2/3 of P56S-VAPB was degraded within 9–10 h (Fig. 1A, B). Degradation was prevented by two different proteasomal inhibitors, MG132, used in our previous study [25], and lactacystin (Fig. 1A, B). In contrast, autophagy inhibitors (3-MA and the proton pump blocker Bafilomycin) were without effect on *myc*-P56S-VAPB (which we will refer to here as P56S-VAPB) clearance. We verified that Bafilomycin was active by evaluating its capability to inhibit the lysosomal degradation of the autophagosomal ubiquitin receptor p62/SQSTM1 (to which we refer here as p62). As shown in Fig. 1C, we found that indeed p62 levels were higher in Bafilomycin-treated cells compared to controls.

Our previous work demonstrated that P56S-VAPB is less stable than the wild-type protein [25]; furthermore, we found that the levels of endogenous VAPB are not affected by expression of the mutant protein, indicating that, although native VAPB may be sequestered within P56S-VAPB-generated inclusions [12,16], this sequestration does not result in an alteration of its rate of degradation. To extend these findings, we probed the levels of endogenous VAPB with anti-VAPB antibodies in experiments like the one illustrated in Fig. 1A. Using anti-VAPB antibodies, we could simultaneously visualize the transfected P56S-VAPB and the

endogenous wt protein. As shown in Fig. S2, endogenous VAPB levels were not affected either by P56S-VAPB expression or by proteasomal inhibitors, confirming its higher stability compared to the mutant protein as well as its insensitivity to the presence of the inclusions.

The results illustrated in Fig. 1A–C confirm and extend our previous results that indicated that under basal conditions P56S-VAPB is degraded exclusively by the proteasomal pathway, and that autophagy is not involved. We then asked whether the inclusions could become substrate for induced autophagy. To this end, we compared the rate of degradation of P56S-VAPB under normal or starvation conditions (Fig. 1D, E). Nine h after Dox addition, P56S-VAPB levels in starved cells were reduced to less than one half those of non-starved cells. Under starvation conditions, MG132 was less effective than under basal conditions in protecting mutant VAPB from degradation suggesting that the enhanced degradation was due to autophagy. This was confirmed by the observation that Bafilomycin rescued the excess degradation observed in starved cells, so that Bafilomycin-treated starved cells had P56S-VAPB levels similar to non-starved cells. Thus, whereas degradation of the P56S-VAPB is exclusively by the proteasomal pathway under basal conditions, the mutant protein may become an autophagosomal substrate under conditions that activate autophagy. The results of this biochemical analysis are in agreement with our previous morphological observations, showing close proximity of P56S-VAPB inclusions to p62 and LC3-positive autophagosomes in starved cells [25].

Neither proteasome-mediated degradation nor autophagic flux are altered by P56S-VAPB inclusions

Disturbance of proteostasis due to alterations in proteasomal function or autophagosomal flux represents an important mechanism of proteotoxicity of pathogenic aggregates [40]. Furthermore, interference with both these mechanisms by P56S-VAPB overexpressing cells has been reported [31,41]. We therefore investigated whether induction of the expression of P56S-VAPB inclusions in the HeLa Tet-Off cell line interferes with one or both of these pathways.

To investigate a possible interference with the proteasome, we analyzed the clearance of a substrate of ER associated degradation (ERAD), a pathway involving extraction of substrates from the ER, coupled to their ubiquitination and delivery to the proteasome [42]. Cells, induced or not to express P56S-VAPB, were transiently transfected with the CD3 complex δ chain (CD3δ), which, when expressed in the absence of the other subunits of the complex, is recognized by the quality control system of the ER and degraded by ERAD [43]. To follow CD3δ degradation, cells, grown in the presence or absence of Dox and co-transfected with EGFP and HA-tagged CD3δ, were treated with cycloheximide (CHX) for three h. This treatment did not affect EGFP nor tubulin (Fig. 2A), but strongly reduced CD3δ levels (Fig. 2A, B). Importantly, after CHX treatment, CD3δ levels were comparable in cells induced or not induced to express P56S-VAPB.

Since not all induced cells have detectable P56S-VAPB inclusions, we were concerned that the non-expressing cells might be preferentially transfected with CD3δ/EGFP, so that the results of Fig. 2A,B would be reporting on the situation in inclusion-negative cells. We therefore quantified the distribution of P56S-VAPB inclusions in transfected and non-transfected cells (Fig. 2C). In two separate experiments inclusions were detected in 52 and 44% of total cells and in 64 and 47% of EGFP-positive cells (~300 cells from random fields analyzed in each experiment). Thus, there is no bias towards P56S-VAPB low-expressing or negative cells in the efficiency of the transient transfection.

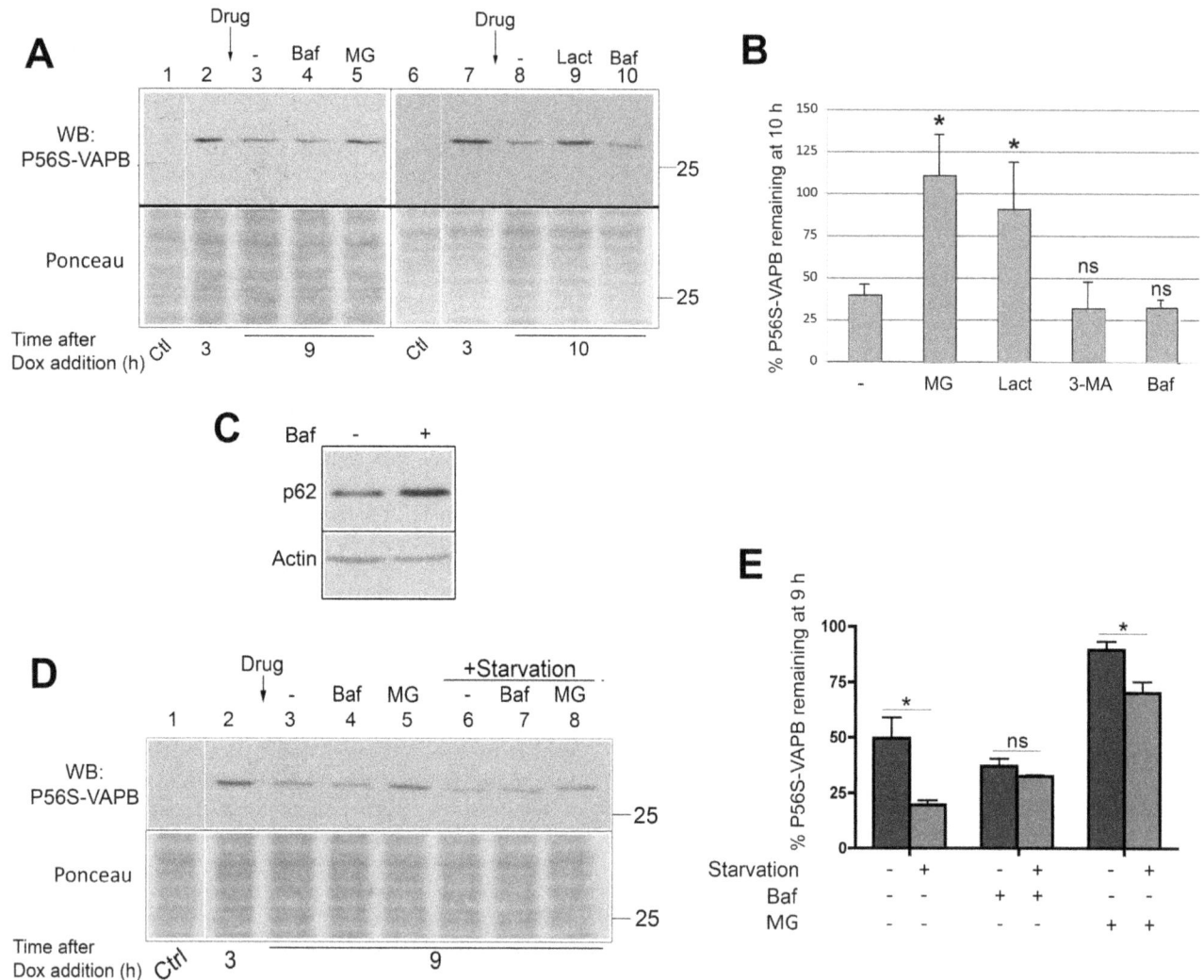

Figure 1. P56S-VAPB is degraded by the proteasome and by activated, but not basal, autophagy. A: Immunoblotting analysis of degradation of P56S-VAPB in the presence or absence of proteasome or autophagy inhibitors. 3 h after the inhibition of transcription of the P56S-VAPB transgene by addition of Dox to the media (lanes 2 and 7), cells were either left untreated (lanes 3 and 8), treated with the autophagy inhibitor Bafilomycin (Baf) or with the proteasome inhibitors MG132 (MG) or Lactacystin (Lact) for 6–7 h, as indicated. Control (Ctl) cells were grown in the presence of Dox. Equal aliquots of each sample were loaded (see Methods). The lower panel shows Ponceau staining of the blotted gel region, as loading control. The vertical white line (here and in panel D) juxtaposes lanes deriving from the same blot exposure. The position of the 25 kDa size marker is indicated. **B:** Quantification (means from 2–5 experiments +SEM) of P56S-VAPB remaining at 10 h after Dox addition in the presence or absence of drugs, as indicated, compared to levels measured at 3 h *: p = 0.013 and 0.025 for MG132 and lactacystin treated samples vs untreated by Student's t test. respectively. The difference between 3-MA or bafilomycin-treated samples and untreated was non-significant (ns). **C:** Equal amounts of protein of the samples of lanes 3 and 4 of panel A were analyzed for p62 by immunoblotting, to control for inhibition of autophagy by bafilomycin. Actin was probed as loading control. **D:** Effect of starvation on clearance of P56S-VAPB. 3 h after addition of Dox to the media (lane 2), cells were either left untreated (lane 3), or treated with bafilomycin (Baf) or MG132 (MG), as indicated, for 6 h; the samples of lanes 6–8 were also starved during the incubation with or without the drugs. Control (Ctl) cells were cultured in presence of Dox. Ponceau staining of the blotted region is shown in the lower panel. **E:** Quantification of three experiments (means +S.E.M.) of P56S-VAPB remaining 9 h after Dox addition under the indicated conditions compared to levels measured before drug treatment and/or starvation at 3 h after Dox addition. *: p = 0.036 by Student's t test; ns, non significant.

To investigate autophagosomal flux, we analyzed the behavior of two autophagosome markers after either pharmacological (torin 1) or starvation-induced autophagy [44]. The ubiquitin receptor p62 is degraded in autolysosomes; thus, its levels decrease under conditions of increased autophagy [44]. Analysis of autophagy-driven decrease of endogenous p62 levels in cells grown in the absence or presence of Dox showed that induction of P56S-VAPB expression did not interfere with p62 degradation (Fig. 2D, top). In similarly treated cells, we examined the generation of the lipidated form of LC3 (LC3-II), a reaction that occurs when LC3 is recruited to nascent autophagosomes [45]. In our HeLa cell line, the lipidated (LC3-II) form predominated already under basal conditions (Fig. 2D, lanes 1 and 4); the non-lipidated form (LC3-I) decreased both after torin 1 treatment and after starvation and differences between the ratio of the two forms were not detected between cells grown in the presence or absence of Dox (Fig. 2E).

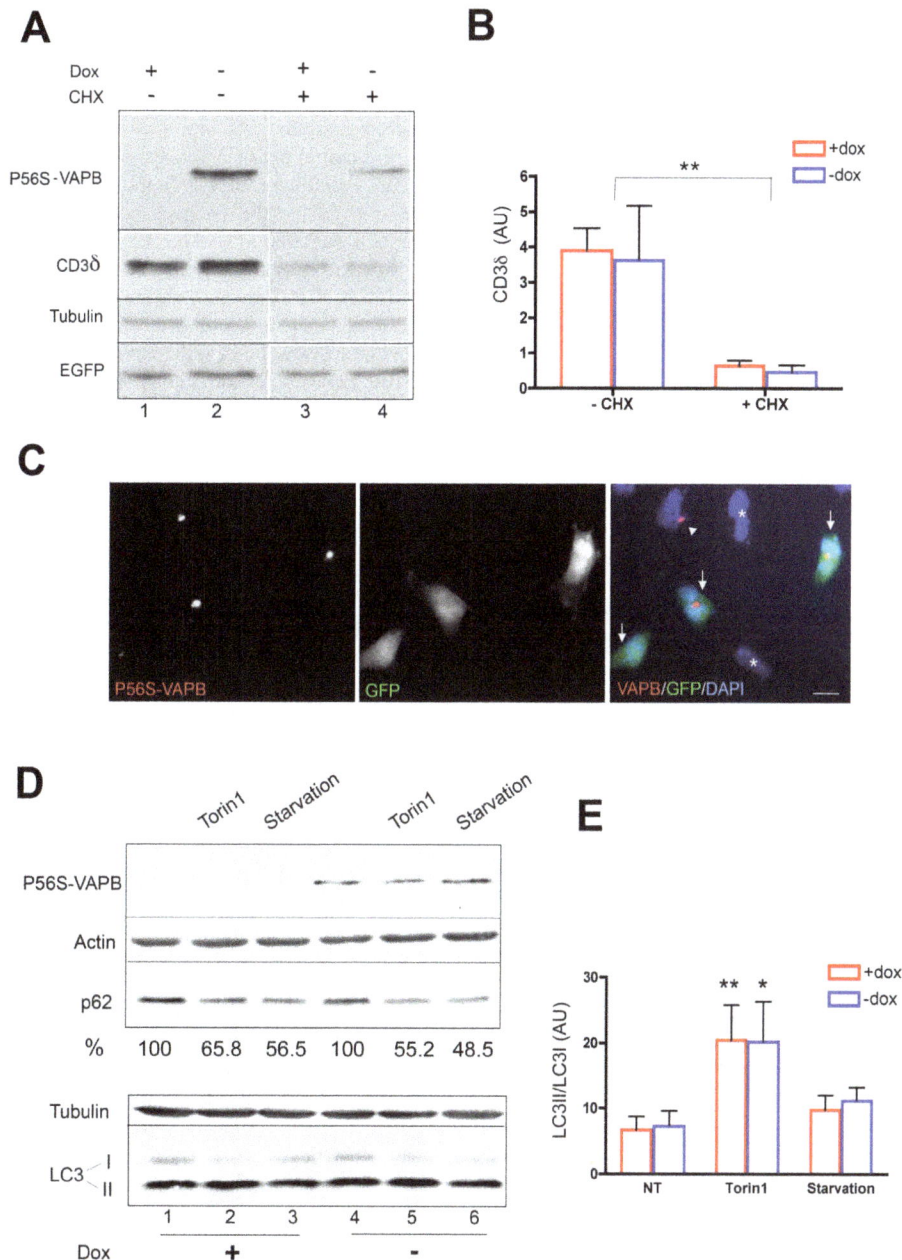

Figure 2. Lack of interference of P56S-VAPB inclusions with general proteostasis. A: Immunoblotting analysis of the degradation of the ERAD substrate CD3δ. Induced or not induced cells, co-transfected with plasmids specifying HA-CD3δ and EGFP, were treated with CHX for 3 h as indicated. Equal amounts of protein (30 μg) were loaded. B: Quantification of three experiments (means+SEM) of CD3δ remaining 3 h after CHX addition compared to untreated samples. Values were normalized to EGFP. By two-way Anova, the presence of Dox had no significant effect on CD3δ, while the effect of CHX was very significant (p = 0.0014). C: Immunofluorescence analysis of induced P56S-VAPB-Tet-Off cells co-transfected with HA-CD3δ and EGFP. The arrows in the merge panel indicate EGFP positive cells containing P56S-VAPB inclusions, revealed with anti-myc antibodies (left panel). Approximately equal proportions of cells with or without detectable inclusions were transfected (see text). The arrowhead indicates a non-transfected cell positive for P56S-VAPB. Asterisks indicate non-transfected cells negative also for VAPB. Nuclei were stained with DAPI (blue). Scale bar, 10 μm. D: Immunoblotting analysis of the effect of P56S-VAPB inclusions on autophagic flux. Cells expressing or not expressing P56S-VAPB where either left untreated or treated for 3 h with Torin1 or starvation medium (EBSS), as indicated. The levels of p62, as percentage of the values in untreated cells are indicated below the lanes. Values were normalized to actin content. E: Quantification of three experiments (means+SEM) of LC3II/LC3I ratio of cells treated either with Torin 1 or with starvation medium, in comparison to untreated cells. Two-way Anova analysis reported that the source of variation between samples was due to autophagocytosis induction (non-treated vs Torin 1: p<0.01 and <0.05 for non-induced and induced cells, respectively) and not to P56S-VAPB expression.

P56S-VAPB inclusions in a model motoneuronal cell line are degraded by the proteasome and not by basal autophagocytosis

To extend our findings to a cell line with characteristics closer to motor neurons, we created NSC34 cell lines stably expressing wild-type or P56S-VAPB under the tetracycline-repressible promoter. NSC34 is a mouse cell line created by fusion of a neuroblastoma line with spinal cord primary motor neurons, and currently represents the best characterized available cell line with motoneuronal characteristics [46]. As shown in Fig. 3A, wt *myc*-VAPB in these cells was distributed throughout the cytoplasm, in a dense reticular network, as expected for an ER protein, whereas the P56S mutant formed inclusions similar to those of HeLa cells and of transiently transfected NSC34 cells [24,28]. We then investigated the mechanism of degradation of mutant VAB by adding Dox to the medium in the presence of MG132 or Bafilomycin, as done for the HeLa cell line. As shown in Fig. 3B, the decrease of P56S-VAPB levels observed between three and ten h after exposure to Dox was nearly completely reversed by MG132, while Bafilomycin was without effect. The efficacy of Bafilomycin treatment was confirmed by the increase of p62 content. The degradation of P56S-VAPB determined by western blot correlated with the decrease in number and size of VAPB-positive inclusions visualized by immunofluorescence (Fig. 3C). Thus, under basal conditions, P56S-VAPB inclusions in NSC34 cells are cleared by the same proteasome-mediated mechanism as observed in HeLa cells.

Close relationship between P56S-VAPB inclusions and the Golgi Complex

Inspection of the localization of P56S-VAPB inclusions revealed that in most cases they were close to the nucleus, in a position similar to that of the Golgi apparatus. Since disruption of the Golgi in neurons is a hallmark of many neurodegenerative diseases, including ALS [47,48], we investigated the relationship of the inclusions to the Golgi, comparing their distribution with the one of two different Golgi markers, GM130, which is preferentially localized to the *cis* face of the Golgi ribbon, and giantin, which is present on Golgi vesicles. Remarkably, the inclusions appeared to be embedded within the Golgi complex (Fig. 4). The intricate relationship between the inclusions and the Golgi is better appreciated in the 3D reconstructions obtained from confocal stacks (Video S1).

P56S-VAPB inclusions do not interfere with the intracellular transport of Vesicular Stomatitis Virus Glycoprotein (VSVG)

The above observations suggested that the tight relationship between P56S-VAPB inclusions and the Golgi complex might underlie interference of the inclusions with transport through the secretory pathway, as reported in cells transiently transfected with mutant VAPB [49]. To investigate the functionality of the secretory pathway in cells expressing moderate levels of P56S-VAPB, we transfected the Tet-Off HeLa cell line with cDNA coding for the ts045 version of the secretory membrane protein VSVG. This protein presents the advantage of accumulating in the ER at 39°C, so that a synchronized wave of transport through the secretory pathway can be followed after release of the high temperature transport block [50]. We first compared the time course of accumulation in the Golgi of transfected VSVG in cells induced and not induced to express mutant VAPB. Random cells were imaged and Golgi localization was evaluated by superposition on the giantin-positive area of the cells. In the case of the

induced sample, cells lacking visible inclusions were not considered. As shown in Fig. 5, VSVG accumulated rapidly in the Golgi, with maximum accumulation at 30 min after release of the temperature block, with similar time course in induced and non-induced cells. At later times, Golgi fluorescence decreased, with concomitant appearance of surface staining.

The experiment of Fig. 5 indicates that transport of VSVG from the ER to the Golgi is not impaired by the presence of mutant VAP inclusions. To quantify transport to the cell surface, we incubated non-permeabilized cells with an antibody that recognizes the lumenal/extracellular domain of VSVG and determined cell surface fluorescence at various times after release of the temperature block. As shown in Fig. 6, arrival of VSVG at the cell surface was not delayed in the induced, compared to the non-induced cells, indicating that the intracellular transport of this model glycoprotein is not affected by the presence of P56S-VAPB inclusions in tight association with the Golgi complex.

Discussion

ALS is a rapidly progressive and devastating neurodegenerative disease characterized by loss of motor neurons from the brain and spinal cord and consequent fatal respiratory failure. Only 10% of ALS cases are inherited (Familial ALS, or FALS), but understanding the pathogenic mechanism of each of the over ten identified FALS-linked mutations [51,52] represents an important step towards unraveling the molecular basis of the much more common sporadic form of this fatal disease. Among the identified ALS-linked genes, the one coding for VAPB is rare and perhaps the least understood. Nevertheless, the observation that VAP levels are decreased in sporadic ALS patients [16,53] is consistent with a more general role of the VAPs in motor neuron pathophysiology, and suggests that clarification of the cellular effects of the mutant gene will bring important insights into the molecular pathogenesis of ALS.

Because of its interaction with many different protein partners, VAPB is involved in a variety of functions [1]; accordingly, a number of possible, not mutually exclusive, pathogenic mechanisms of mutant VAPB have been proposed. Many of these are based on the observation that P56S-VAPB forms intracellular inclusions that sequester both the wild-type protein and, to a lesser extent, VAPA [12,16,26,27,28], suggesting that loss of function by a dominant negative mechanism underlies mutant VAPB's mode of inheritance. In addition, it has been hypothesized that cellular dysfunction is caused by the sequestration within the inclusions of functionally important VAPB interactors, such as the ER-Golgi recycling protein Yif1A, involved in transport within the early secretory pathway [3], and the phosphoinositide phosphatase Sac1 [29]. The VAPs have also been implicated in modulation of the ER Unfolded Protein Response (UPR), and overexpression of P56S-VAPB is reported both to attenuate UPR signaling [12,54], and to increase ER stress in animal disease models [41,55,56].

In addition to these cellular dysfunctions attributable to specific interactions of the VAPs, mutant VAPB inclusions have been reported to inhibit the proteasome [31], possibly leading to a general dysregulation of proteostasis, as is the case for other ALS-linked mutant genes [33]. Thus, a combination of dominant negative effects and general proteotoxicity could act together to cause the reduction in cell viability that has been observed in a number of transfected cell models [16,17,21,28,57,58].

As pointed out in the Introduction, the different mechanisms proposed for P56S-VAPB pathogenicity have been based mainly on studies on cultured cells acutely overexpressing mutant VAPB, and are thus not clearly related to the situation in cells chronically

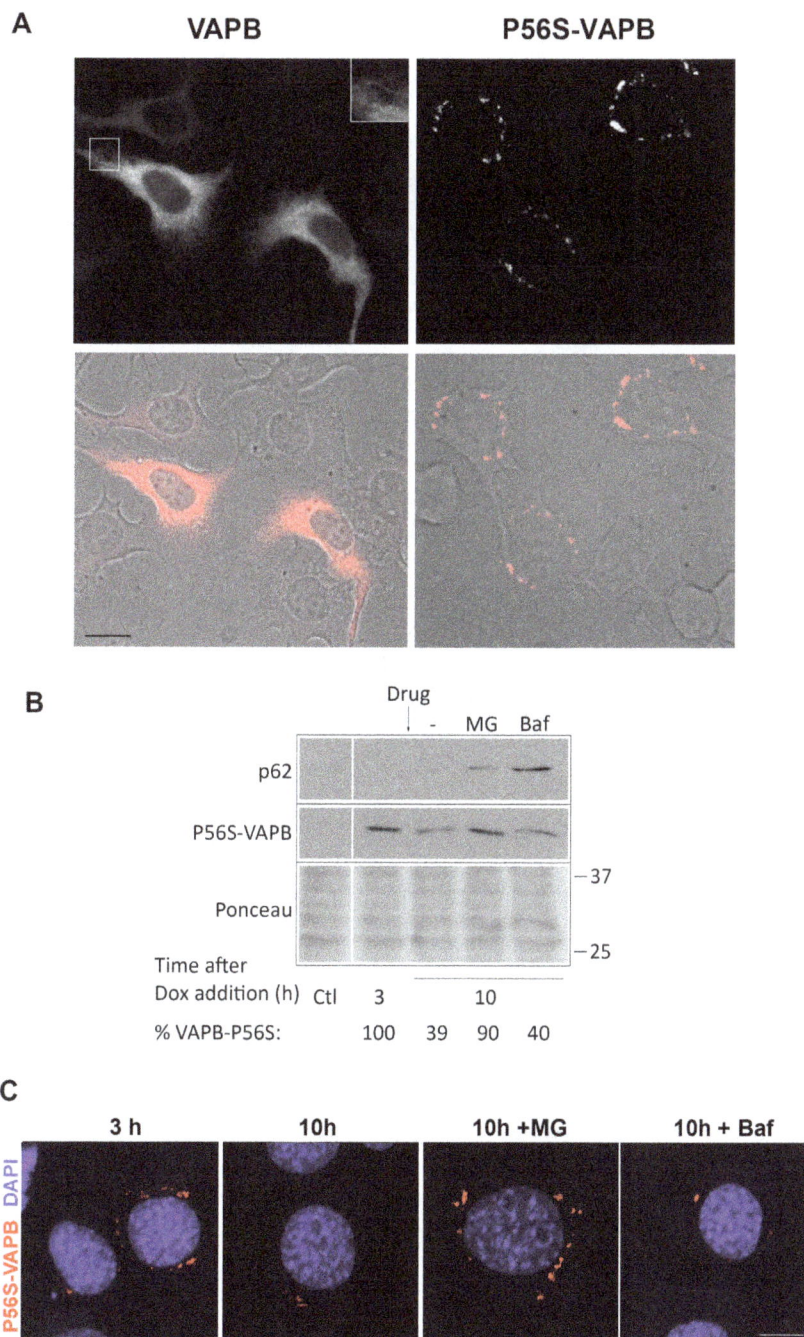

Figure 3. P56S-VAPB inclusions in a model motoneuronal cell line are degraded by the proteasome. A: Immunofluorescence analysis of NSC34 Tet-Off cells induced to express *myc*-wt-VAPB (left) or *myc*-P56S-VAPB (right). The upper panel shows anti-*myc* immunofluorescence, the lower one the superposition of *myc* staining with phase contrast. The inset of the upper left panel shows a 2 fold enlargement of the boxed area, and illustrates the web-like distribution of wt VAPB typical of an ER protein. Scale bar: 15 μm. **B:** Degradation of P56S-VAPB stably expressed in NSC34 cells. Induced cells were supplemented with Dox; 3 h thereafter the cells were either left untreated or treated with MG132 (MG) or Bafilomycin (Baf) for 7 h. Control (Ctl) cells were grown in the presence of Dox. Equal aliquots of each sample were loaded. The lower panel shows Ponceau staining of the blotted gel region; the positions of the 25 and 37 kDa size marker are indicated. The vertical white line indicates removal of irrelevant lanes form the image. The levels of P56S-VAPB, as percentage of values in untreated cells at 3 h after Dox addition, are indicated below the lanes. p62 immunoblotting was performed to check the efficacy of bafilomycin to inhibit autophagy (upper). **C:** Confocal analysis (single sections are shown) of P56S-VAPB inclusions stained with anti-*myc* antibody (red) at 3 h after Dox addition (left) and 7 h later in the presence or absence of the indicated drugs. Nuclei were stained with DAPI. The number and size of the inclusions decreased in the absence of drugs or in the presence of Bafilomycin, but remained similar to the 3 h cells when MG132 was present. Scale bar, 10 μm.

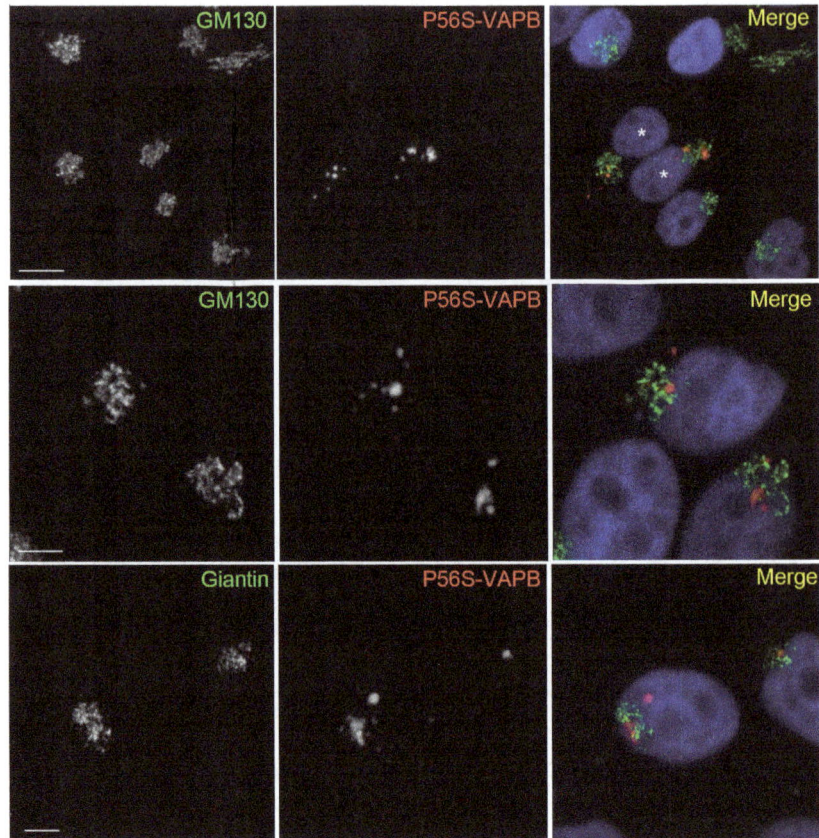

Figure 4. Close relationship between P56S-VAPB inclusions and the Golgi Complex. Induced HeLa Tet-Off cells were doubly immunostained with anti-*myc* antibodies, to reveal P56S-VAPB, and antibodies against the Golgi proteins GM130 or giantin, as indicated. Nuclei, stained with DAPI, are shown in the merge panel. Shown are maximum intensity projections of z-stacks. Scale bars: upper row, 10 μm; middle and lower row 5 μm.

expressing the mutant protein from a single allele. To investigate the effects of P56S-VAPB when expressed chronically at moderate levels, we turned to cell lines expressing mutant VAPB under the control of a Tet-repressible promoter. In Dox-free medium, these cells express P56S-VAPB at levels 2–3 fold higher than the endogenous protein ([24,25] and Figs. S1 and S2 of this study), and reach this steady state condition gradually over a period of several days after removal of Dox from the medium (unpublished results). Using these cells, we previously demonstrated that P56S-VAPB is unstable in comparison to the wt protein, and that its degradation is mediated by the proteasome and involves the participation of a key ERAD player, the AAA ATPase p97 [25]. Here, we have continued our investigation on the mechanism of degradation of P56S-VAPB inclusions as well as on their possible toxic effects on the cells.

First, we confirmed that under basal conditions mutant VAPB inclusions are cleared by the proteasome, both in HeLa and in a model motoneuronal cell line, but we also showed that autophagy, when stimulated, can further enhance degradation of the mutant protein. Thus, P56S-VAPB inclusions are available to degradation by both the major degradative pathways of the cell, and our results predict that, under conditions in which the cell potentiates autophagy, mutant VAPB inclusions will not become overrepresented in comparison to other compartments targeted by autophagy.

We then investigated whether P56S-VAPB inclusions interfere with two fundamental processes: (i) protein degradation mediated

by the proteasome and by autophagy; and (ii) protein transport through the secretory pathway.

Moumen et al. [31] reported that transient overexpression of wild-type and mutant VAPB results in an increase of polyubiquitinated proteins and stabilization of three different proteasomal substrates, among which the classical ERAD substrate CD3δ. However, in our cells, clearance of CD3δ, whose degradative pathway shares with the one of P56S-VAPB the involvement both of the proteasome and of p97, was unaffected by the expression of the mutant protein.

Autophagic dysfunction has been described in ALS, and both a significant autophagy upregulation and/or impairment with abnormal accumulation of autophagosomes have been observed (reviewed in ref 32). However, to our knowledge, the effect of P56S-VAPB inclusions on autophagic flow had yet not been investigated. We found that autophagy, stimulated either pharmacologically or by starvation, was unaffected by P56S-VAPB expression. Thus, it appears that cells can adjust the capacity of their degradative machinery to cope with moderate levels of mutant VAPB without consequent disturbances in proteostasis.

A second fundamental process in which the VAPs are implicated is intracellular transport through the secretory pathway, but contrasting results have been reported on the effect of P56S-VAPB expression on intracellular transport. In CHO cells, Prosser and collaborators [49] found a strong interference of overexpressed P56S-VAPB (and also of overexpressed wt VAPA) with VSVG transport, while no delay of the transport of the same

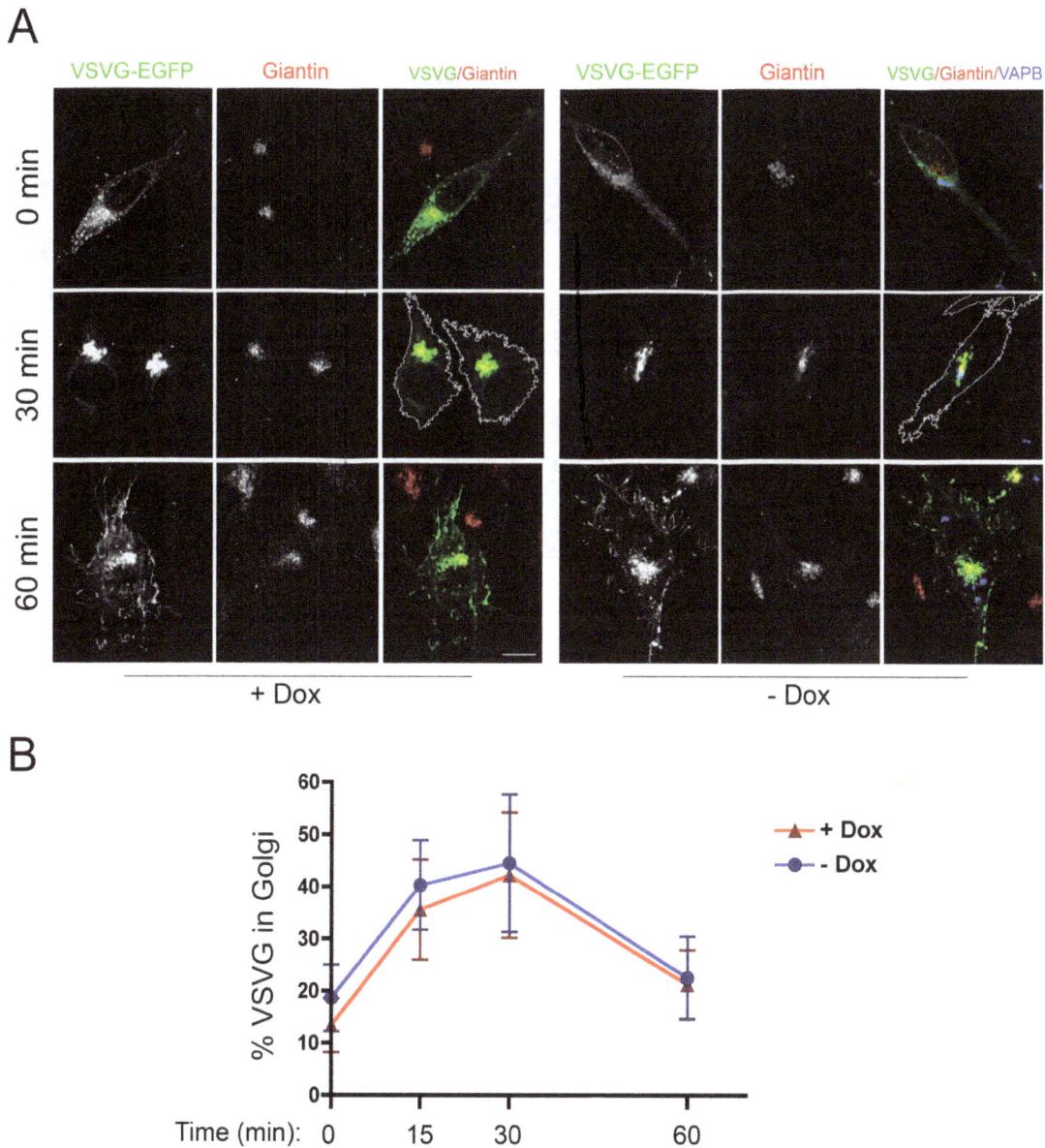

Figure 5. Transport of VSVG to the Golgi Complex occurs normally in cells expressing P56S-VAPB inclusions. A: HeLa-TetOff cells, induced (−Dox, right) or not induced (+Dox, left) to express *myc*-P56S-VAPB, were transfected with VSVG-EGFP at 39.3°C. After 24 h, one coverslip of each sample was fixed (0 min), while the others were shifted to 32°C and fixed after incubation for the indicated times. Cells were stained with anti-Giantin (red) and anti-*myc* (blue) antibodies. Maximum intensity projections of z-stacks are shown. The cell boundaries at the 30 min time point are indicated by the white line in the merge panel. Acquisition parameters were the same in all images. Scale bar, 10 μm. **B:** Time course (means ± SD) of VSVG transport through the Golgi. Significant differences between induced or non-induced samples were not detected by Student's t-test.

secretory membrane cargo was detected by Teuling et al. in primary hippocampal neuronal cultures [16]. In our system, we found that neither transport from the ER to the Golgi nor export to the cell surface were altered by the presence of P56S-VAPB inclusions. We conclude that cells can maintain secretory pathway function in the presence of P56S-VAPB inclusions, notwithstanding their close physical proximity to the Golgi apparatus demonstrated here.

The results reported in this study, showing a lack of interference of P56S-VAPB inclusions with basic cellular functions, are consistent with the outcome of analyses of transgenic animals. Restricting this discussion to mammals, four transgenic mouse lines have been reported so far [30,41,48,59]. Of these, only one,

in which the mutant protein was highly overexpressed (at seven fold higher levels than the endogenous protein), developed mild motor abnormalities and loss of cortical, but not spinal, motor neurons [41]. The other three strains, although presenting P56S-VAPB-containing inclusions in motor neurons, showed no motor abnormalities. These results suggest that the much lower levels of mutant protein expressed from a single allele in ALS8 patients may be devoid of pathogenic effect. Interestingly, in the study of Aliaga et al. [41], lower levels of mutant than of wild-type protein were detected in the brains of transgenic mouse strains that had comparable levels of mRNA expression. This observation demonstrates that the instability of the mutant protein first observed in cultured cells [25,31] is present also in animal tissues. P56S-VAPB

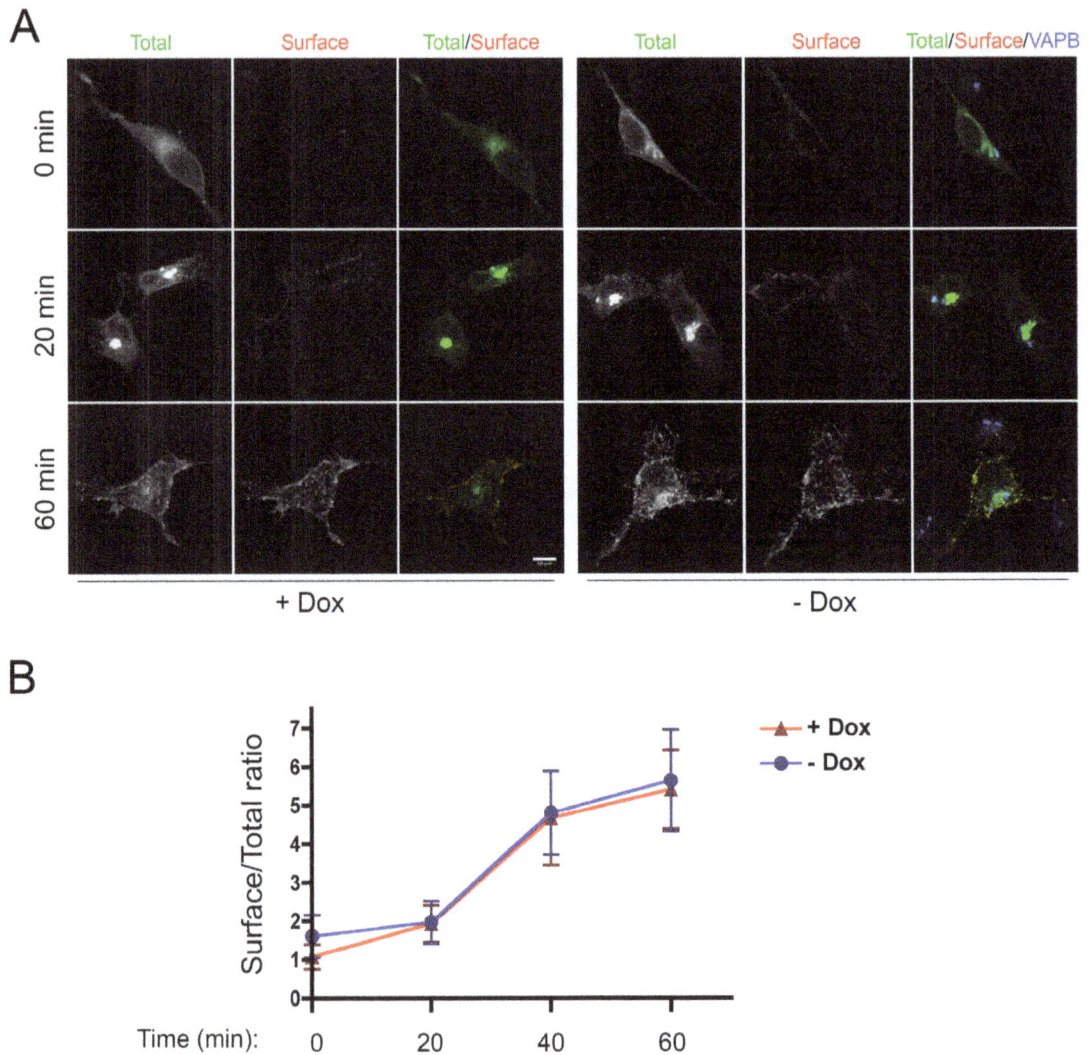

Figure 6. Transport of VSVG to the cell surface occurs normally in cells expressing P56S-VAPB inclusions. A: HeLa-TetOff cells, induced (−Dox) or not induced (+Dox) to express *myc*-P56S-VAPB, were transfected with VSVG-EGFP at 39.3°C. After 24 h, cells were shifted to 32°C. At the indicated times, the cells were chilled and incubated with anti-lumenal domain of VSVG under non-permeabilizing conditions (red). The cells were then permeabilized and stained with anti-VAPB antibodies (blue in merge panel - see Methods). Total VSVG (intracellular+surface) was revealed by GFP fluorescence (green). Maximum intensity projections of z-stacks are shown. The acquisition parameters were the same in all images. Scale bar, 10 μm. **B:** Time course (means ± SD) of VSVG surface labeling normalized to total EGFP fluorescence. Significant differences between induced or non-induced samples were not detected by Student's t-test.

instability most likely explains the lack of detectable VAPB inclusions in ALS8 (P56S-VAPB) patients' motor neurons generated from induced pluripotent stem cells (IPSC) [60].

In conclusion, our results provide an explanation for the discrepancy between the observations obtained in transiently transfected cells and transgenic mouse models, and support the hypothesis that haploinsufficiency alone underlies the dominant inheritance of VAPB mutations. In addition to the generally negative results obtained with the transgenic mice, this idea is supported also by the reduced levels of VAPB in iPSC-derived motor neurons of ALS8 patients [60] and in spinal motor neurons of sporadic ALS patients [16,53]. While strong effects of VAP deletion in cultured cells are obtained only when both homologues are silenced [3,5,16], the studies with mice specifically deleted for VAPB are in partial agreement with a pathogenic role of VAPB

haploinsufficiency in motor neuron disease. In one study, VAPB-deleted mice, although free from a full blown ALS phenotype, did develop mild, late onset defects in motor performance [22]; in another study, VAPB deletion was reported to cause alterations in muscle lipid metabolism [61]. To be noted, in the first of these studies [22], also the heterozygote mouse showed reduced motor performance in the Rotarod test, although the difference with respect to the controls was not statistically significant. This observation suggests that within the longer human lifespan, even a 50% reduction of the normal dosage of VAPB may affect motor neuron survival. Whether damage due to VAPB deficit is caused by the reduction of a unique VAPB function not carried out by VAPA, or whether long term motor neuron survival simply requires the full dosage of the sum of the two VAP homologues remains to be determined in appropriate cell and animal models.

Supporting Information

Figure S1 Purification of polyclonal anti-VAPB antibody. A: Western Blot analysis comparing the reactivity of anti-VAPB serum towards lysates from bacteria expressing GST-VAPA or GST-VAPB 1–225 (arrow) before and after adsorption to VAPA-coupled resin. Antibodies cross-reactive with VAPA are eliminated in this step of purification. The lower molecular weight bands recognized by the adsorbed antiserum in lysates from bacteria expressing the VAPB fusion protein are probably due to degradation products. **B:** Purification of adsorbed antiserum by affinity chromatography. Specificity of the antibodies was probed by western blotting against lysates from HeLa Tet-Off cells induced to express P56S-VAPB. Endogenous VAPB and P56S-VAPB induced by removal of Dox are indicated by the arrowhead and arrow, respectively. The asterisks indicate non-specific bands, of which the major ones are eliminated by the affinity purification.

Figure S2 Comparison of the effect of proteasome inhibitors on endogenous wild-type VAPB and on the transfected mutant protein. Cells were induced to express P56S-VAPB by Dox removal, and then returned to Dox-containing media, as described in the legend to Figure 1. At the indicated times, cells were collected, and the lysates were analyzed by SDS-PAGE - immunoblotting, with the use of an anti-VAPB antibody. The endogenous wild-type protein is distinguished from the transfected *myc*-tagged mutant by its faster migration. The

levels of endogenous wt VAPB are not affected by drug treatments. Control cells (ctr) were cultured in the presence of Dox.

Video S1 Maximum intensity projections of a field of P56S-VAPB- expressing HeLa Tet-Off cells doubly stained for VAPB with anti-*myc* antibodies (red) and for giantin (green). Shown are maximum intensity projections generated from rotation around the X-axis of a stack of 16 confocal sections acquired at 0.2 μm intervals. Each image is rotated by 5° with respect to the preceding one, for a total rotation of 180°.

Acknowledgments

In addition to the people who kindly supplied reagents (listed in Materials and Methods), we acknowledge the Monzino Foundation (Milan, Italy), for its generous gift of the Zeiss LSM 510 Meta confocal microscope. We are grateful to Sara Francesca Colombo and Angelo Poletti for helpful discussion and to Cecilia Gotti and Milena Moretti for help with rabbit immunization.

Author Contributions

Conceived and designed the experiments: PG FN NB. Performed the experiments: PG GP AR LC. Analyzed the data: PG GP FN NB. Contributed reagents/materials/analysis tools: LC. Wrote the paper: PG FN NB. Critical revision of the manuscript: LC.

References

1. Lev S, Ben Halevy D, Peretti D, Dahan N (2008) The VAP protein family: from cellular functions to motor neuron disease. Trends Cell Biol 18: 282–290.
2. Yang Z, Huh SU, Drennan JM, Kathuria H, Martinez JS, et al. (2012) Drosophila Vap-33 is required for axonal localization of Dscam isoforms. J Neurosci 32: 17241–17250.
3. Kuijpers M, Yu KL, Teuling E, Akhmanova A, Jaarsma D, et al. (2013) The ALS8 protein VAPB interacts with the ER-Golgi recycling protein YIF1A and regulates membrane delivery into dendrites. EMBO J 32: 2056–2072.
4. Kawano M, Kumagai K, Nishijima M, Hanada K (2006) Efficient trafficking of ceramide from the endoplasmic reticulum to the Golgi apparatus requires a VAMP-associated protein-interacting FFAT motif of CERT. J Biol Chem 281: 30279–30288.
5. Peretti D, Dahan N, Shimoni E, Hirschberg K, Lev S (2008) Coordinated lipid transfer between the endoplasmic reticulum and the Golgi complex requires the VAP proteins and is essential for Golgi-mediated transport. Mol Biol Cell 19: 3871–3884.
6. Levine T, Loewen C (2006) Inter-organelle membrane contact sites: through a glass, darkly. Curr Opin Cell Biol 18: 371–378.
7. Rocha N, Kuijl C, van der Kant R, Janssen L, Houben D, et al. (2009) Cholesterol sensor ORP1L contacts the ER protein VAP to control Rab7-RILP-p150 Glued and late endosome positioning. J Cell Biol 185: 1209–1225.
8. Stefan CJ, Manford AG, Baird D, Yamada-Hanff J, Mao Y, et al. (2011) Osh proteins regulate phosphoinositide metabolism at ER-plasma membrane contact sites. Cell 144: 389–401.
9. De Vos KJ, Morotz GM, Stoica R, Tudor EL, Lau KF, et al. (2012) VAPB interacts with the mitochondrial protein PTPIP51 to regulate calcium homeostasis. Hum Mol Genet 21: 1299–1311.
10. Alpy F, Rousseau A, Schwab Y, Legueux F, Stoll I, et al. (2013) STARD3 or STARD3NL and VAP form a novel molecular tether between late endosomes and the ER. J Cell Sci 126: 5500–5512.
11. Amarilio R, Ramachandran S, Sabanay H, Lev S (2005) Differential regulation of endoplasmic reticulum structure through VAP-Nir protein interaction. J Biol Chem 280: 5934–5944.
12. Kanekura K, Nishimoto I, Aiso S, Matsuoka M (2006) Characterization of amyotrophic lateral sclerosis-linked P56S mutation of vesicle-associated membrane protein-associated protein B (VAPB/ALS8). J Biol Chem 281: 30223–30233.
13. Saita S, Shirane M, Natume T, Iemura S, Nakayama KI (2009) Promotion of neurite extension by protrudin requires its interaction with vesicle-associated membrane protein-associated protein. J Biol Chem 284: 13766–13777.
14. Ohnishi T, Shirane M, Hashimoto Y, Saita S, Nakayama KI (2014) Identification and characterization of a neuron-specific isoform of protrudin. Genes Cells 19: 97–111.

15. Nishimura AL, Mitne-Neto M, Silva HC, Oliveira JR, Vainzof M, et al. (2004) A novel locus for late onset amyotrophic lateral sclerosis/motor neurone disease variant at 20q13. J Med Genet 41: 315–320.
16. Teuling E, Ahmed S, Haasdijk E, Demmers J, Steinmetz MO, et al. (2007) Motor neuron disease-associated mutant vesicle-associated membrane protein-associated protein (VAP) B recruits wild-type VAPs into endoplasmic reticulum-derived tubular aggregates. J Neurosci 27: 9801–9815.
17. Kim S, Leal SS, Ben Halevy D, Gomes CM, Lev S (2010) Structural requirements for VAP-B oligomerization and their implication in amyotrophic lateral sclerosis-associated VAP-B(P56S) neurotoxicity. J Biol Chem 285: 13839–13849.
18. Shi J, Lua S, Tong JS, Song J (2010) Elimination of the native structure and solubility of the hVAPB MSP domain by the Pro56Ser mutation that causes amyotrophic lateral sclerosis. Biochemistry 49: 3887–3897.
19. Nishimura AL, Al-Chalabi A, Zatz M (2005) A common founder for amyotrophic lateral sclerosis type 8 (ALS8) in the Brazilian population. Hum Genet 118: 499–500.
20. Funke AD, Esser M, Kruttgen A, Weis J, Mitne-Neto M, et al. (2010) The p.P56S mutation in the VAPB gene is not due to a single founder: the first European case. Clin Genet 77: 302–303.
21. Chen HJ, Anagnostou G, Chai A, Withers J, Morris A, et al. (2010) Characterization of the properties of a novel mutation in VAPB in familial amyotrophic lateral sclerosis. J Biol Chem 285: 40266–40281.
22. Kabashi E, El Oussini H, Bercier V, Gros-Louis F, Valdmanis PN, et al. (2013) Investigating the contribution of VAPB/ALS8 loss of function in amyotrophic lateral sclerosis. Hum Mol Genet 22: 2350–2360.
23. van Blitterswijk M, van Es MA, Koppers M, van Rheenen W, Medic J, et al. (2012) VAPB and C9orf72 mutations in 1 familial amyotrophic lateral sclerosis patient. Neurobiol Aging 33: 2950 e2951–2954.
24. Fasana E, Fossati M, Ruggiano A, Brambillasca S, Hoogenraad CC, et al. (2010) A VAPB mutant linked to amyotrophic lateral sclerosis generates a novel form of organized smooth endoplasmic reticulum. Faseb J 24: 1419–1430.
25. Papiani G, Ruggiano A, Fossati M, Raimondi A, Bertoni G, et al. (2012) Restructured endoplasmic reticulum generated by mutant amyotrophic lateral sclerosis-linked VAPB is cleared by the proteasome. J Cell Sci 125: 3601–3611.
26. Chai A, Withers J, Koh YH, Parry K, Bao H, et al. (2008) hVAPB, the causative gene of a heterogeneous group of motor neuron diseases in humans, is functionally interchangeable with its Drosophila homologue DVAP-33A at the neuromuscular junction. Hum Mol Genet 17: 266–280.
27. Ratnaparkhi A, Lawless GM, Schweizer FE, Golshani P, Jackson GR (2008) A Drosophila model of ALS: human ALS-associated mutation in VAP33A suggests a dominant negative mechanism. PLoS One 3: e2334.
28. Suzuki H, Kanekura K, Levine TP, Kohno K, Olkkonen VM, et al. (2009) ALS-linked P56S-VAPB, an aggregated loss-of-function mutant of VAPB, predisposes

motor neurons to ER stress-related death by inducing aggregation of co-expressed wild-type VAPB. J Neurochem 108: 973–985.

29. Forrest S, Chai A, Sanhueza M, Marescotti M, Parry K, et al. (2013) Increased levels of phosphoinositides cause neurodegeneration in a Drosophila model of amyotrophic lateral sclerosis. Hum Mol Genet 22: 2689–2704.

30. Tudor EL, Galtrey CM, Perkinton MS, Lau KF, De Vos KJ, et al. (2010) Amyotrophic lateral sclerosis mutant vesicle-associated membrane protein-associated protein-B transgenic mice develop TAR-DNA-binding protein-43 pathology. Neuroscience 167: 774–785.

31. Moumen A, Virard I, Raoul C (2011) Accumulation of wildtype and ALS-linked mutated VAPB impairs activity of the proteasome. PLoS One 6: e26066.

32. Chen S, Zhang X, Song L, Le W (2012) Autophagy dysregulation in amyotrophic lateral sclerosis. Brain Pathol 22: 110–116.

33. Robberecht W, Philips T (2013) The changing scene of amyotrophic lateral sclerosis. Nat Rev Neurosci 14: 248–264.

34. Blokhuis AM, Groen EJ, Koppers M, van den Berg LH, Pasterkamp RJ (2013) Protein aggregation in amyotrophic lateral sclerosis. Acta Neuropathol 125: 777–794.

35. Tan CC, Yu JT, Tan MS, Jiang T, Zhu XC, et al. (2014) Autophagy in aging and neurodegenerative diseases: implications for pathogenesis and therapy. Neurobiol Aging 35: 941–957.

36. Kaiser SE, Brickner JH, Reilein AR, Fenn TD, Walter P, et al. (2005) Structural basis of FFAT motif-mediated ER targeting. Structure 13: 1035–1045.

37. Seelig HP, Schranz P, Schröter H, Wiemann C, Renz M (1994) Macrogolgin - a new 376 kD Golgi Complex outer membrane protein as target of antibodies in patients with rheumatic disease and HIV infections. J Autoimmun 7: 67–91.

38. Marra P, Salvatore L, Mironov A Jr, Di Campli A, Di Tullio G, et al. (2007) The biogenesis of the Golgi ribbon: the roles of membrane input from the ER and of GM130. Mol Biol Cell 18: 1595–1608.

39. Babetto E, Mangolini A, Rizzardini M, Lupi M, Conforti L, et al. (2005) Tetracycline-regulated gene expression in the NSC-34-tTA cell line for investigation of motor neuron diseases. Brain Res Mol Brain Res 140: 63–72.

40. Powers ET, Morimoto RI, Dillin A, Kelly JW, Balch WE (2009) Biological and chemical approaches to diseases of proteostasis deficiency. Annu Rev Biochem 78: 959–991.

41. Aliaga L, Lai C, Yu J, Chub N, Shim H, et al. (2013) Amyotrophic lateral sclerosis-related VAPB P56S mutation differentially affects the function and survival of corticospinal and spinal motor neurons. Hum Mol Genet 22: 4293–4305.

42. Bernasconi R, Molinari M (2011) ERAD and ERAD tuning: disposal of cargo and of ERAD regulators from the mammalian ER. Curr Opin Cell Biol 23: 176–183.

43. Yang M, Omura S, Bonifacino JS, Weissman AM (1998) Novel aspects of degradation of T cell receptor subunits from the endoplasmic reticulum (ER) in T cells: importance of oligosaccharide processing, ubiquitination, and proteasome-dependent removal from ER membranes. J Exp Med 187: 835–846.

44. Klionsky DJ, Abdalla FC, Abeliovich H, Abraham RT, Acevedo-Arozena A, et al. (2012) Guidelines for the use and interpretation of assays for monitoring autophagy. Autophagy 8: 445–544.

45. Kabeya Y, Mizushima N, Ueno T, Yamamoto A, Kirisako T, et al. (2000) LC3, a mammalian homologue of yeast Apg8p, is localized in autophagosome membranes after processing. Embo J 19: 5720–5728.

46. Cashman NR, Durham HD, Blusztajn JK, Oda K, Tabira T, et al. (1992) Neuroblastoma x spinal cord (NSC) hybrid cell lines resemble developing motor neurons. Dev Dyn 194: 209–221.

47. Gonatas NK, Stieber A, Gonatas JO (2006) Fragmentation of the Golgi apparatus in neurodegenerative diseases and cell death. J Neurol Sci 246: 21–30.

48. van Dis V, Kuijpers M, Haasdijk ED, Teuling E, Oakes SA, et al. (2014) Golgi fragmentation precedes neuromuscular denervation and is associated with endosome abnormalities in SOD1-ALS mouse motor neurons. Acta Neuropathol Commun 2: 38.

49. Prosser DC, Tran D, Gougeon PY, Verly C, Ngsee JK (2008) FFAT rescues VAPA-mediated inhibition of ER-to-Golgi transport and VAPB-mediated ER aggregation. J Cell Sci 121: 3052–3061.

50. Bergmann JE (1989) Using temperature-sensitive mutants of VSV to study membrane protein biogenesis. Methods Cell Biol 32: 85–110.

51. Andersen PM, Al-Chalabi A (2011) Clinical genetics of amyotrophic lateral sclerosis: what do we really know? Nat Rev Neurol 7: 603–615.

52. Ferraiuolo L, Kirby J, Grierson AJ, Sendtner M, Shaw PJ (2011) Molecular pathways of motor neuron injury in amyotrophic lateral sclerosis. Nat Rev Neurol 7: 616–630.

53. Anagnostou G, Akbar MT, Paul P, Angelinetta C, Steiner TJ, et al. (2010) Vesicle associated membrane protein B (VAPB) is decreased in ALS spinal cord. Neurobiol Aging 31: 969–985.

54. Gkogkas C, Middleton S, Kremer AM, Wardrope C, Hannah M, et al. (2008) VAPB interacts with and modulates the activity of ATF6. Hum Mol Genet 17: 1517–1526.

55. Tsuda H, Han SM, Yang Y, Tong C, Lin YQ, et al. (2008) The amyotrophic lateral sclerosis 8 protein VAPB is cleaved, secreted, and acts as a ligand for Eph receptors. Cell 133: 963–977.

56. Moustaqim-Barrette A, Lin YQ, Pradhan S, Neely GG, Bellen HJ, et al. (2014) The amyotrophic lateral sclerosis 8 protein, VAP, is required for ER protein quality control. Hum Mol Genet 23: 1975–1989.

57. Langou K, Moumen A, Pellegrino C, Aebischer J, Medina I, et al. (2010) AAV-mediated expression of wild-type and ALS-linked mutant VAPB selectively triggers death of motoneurons through a Ca2+-dependent ER-associated pathway. J Neurochem 114: 795–809.

58. Chattopadhyay D, Sengupta S (2014) First evidence of pathogenicity of V234I mutation of hVAPB found in Amyotrophic Lateral Sclerosis. Biochem Biophys Res Commun 448: 108–113.

59. Qiu L, Qiao T, Beers M, Tan W, Wang H, et al. (2013) Widespread aggregation of mutant VAPB associated with ALS does not cause motor neuron degeneration or modulate mutant SOD1 aggregation and toxicity in mice. Mol Neurodegener 8: 1.

60. Mitne-Neto M, Machado-Costa M, Marchetto MC, Bengtson MH, Joazeiro CA, et al. (2011) Downregulation of VAPB expression in motor neurons derived from induced pluripotent stem cells of ALS8 patients. Hum Mol Genet 20: 3642–3652.

61. Han SM, El Oussini H, Scekic-Zahirovic J, Vibbert J, Cottee P, et al. (2013) VAPB/ALS8 MSP ligands regulate striated muscle energy metabolism critical for adult survival in caenorhabditis elegans. PLoS Genet 9: e1003738.

14

Enhanced Slow-Wave EEG Activity and Thermoregulatory Impairment following the Inhibition of the Lateral Hypothalamus in the Rat

Matteo Cerri*, Flavia Del Vecchio, Marco Mastrotto, Marco Luppi, Davide Martelli, Emanuele Perez, Domenico Tupone, Giovanni Zamboni, Roberto Amici

Department of Biomedical and NeuroMotor Sciences, Alma Mater Studiorum - University of Bologna, Bologna, Italy

Abstract

Neurons within the lateral hypothalamus (LH) are thought to be able to evoke behavioural responses that are coordinated with an adequate level of autonomic activity. Recently, the acute pharmacological inhibition of LH has been shown to depress wakefulness and promote NREM sleep, while suppressing REM sleep. These effects have been suggested to be the consequence of the inhibition of specific neuronal populations within the LH, i.e. the orexin and the MCH neurons, respectively. However, the interpretation of these results is limited by the lack of quantitative analysis of the electroencephalographic (EEG) activity that is critical for the assessment of NREM sleep quality and the presence of aborted NREM-to-REM sleep transitions. Furthermore, the lack of evaluation of the autonomic and thermoregulatory effects of the treatment does not exclude the possibility that the wake-sleep changes are merely the consequence of the autonomic, in particular thermoregulatory, changes that may follow the inhibition of LH neurons. In the present study, the EEG and autonomic/thermoregulatory effects of a prolonged LH inhibition provoked by the repeated local delivery of the $GABA_A$ agonist muscimol were studied in rats kept at thermoneutral (24°C) and at a low (10°C) ambient temperature (Ta), a condition which is known to depress sleep occurrence. Here we show that: 1) at both Tas, LH inhibition promoted a peculiar and sustained bout of NREM sleep characterized by an enhancement of slow-wave activity with no NREM-to-REM sleep transitions; 2) LH inhibition caused a marked transitory decrease in brain temperature at Ta 10°C, but not at Ta 24°C, suggesting that sleep changes induced by LH inhibition at thermoneutrality are not caused by a thermoregulatory impairment. These changes are far different from those observed after the short-term selective inhibition of either orexin or MCH neurons, suggesting that other LH neurons are involved in sleep-wake modulation.

Editor: Andrej A. Romanovsky, St. Joseph's Hospital and Medical Center, United States of America

Funding: This work has been supported by the grant PRIN 2008FY7K9S from the Ministero dell'Istruzione, dell'Università e della Ricerca (http://www.istruzione.it)- Italy (RA). The funders had no role in study design, data collection and analysis, decision to publish, or preparation of the manuscript.

Competing Interests: The authors have declared that no competing interests exist.

* Email: matteo.cerri@unibo.it

Introduction

The lateral hypothalamus (LH) is a complex network of several different kinds of neurons involved in many functions [1]. LH neurons are apparently able to evoke a behavioural response that is integrated and coordinated with an adequate level of autonomic activity. In fact, the pharmacological activation of LH neurons has been shown to promote active behaviour and locomotion [2], and to coherently induce an increase in sympathetic outflow [3]. Both effects can be the consequence of the activation of a subpopulation of LH neurons producing orexin [4].

Recently, it has been shown that the inhibition of LH neurons prevented rats from producing rapid eye movement (REM) sleep [5]. The cause of this complete absence of REM sleep was suggested to be the inhibition of the activity of a subpopulation of LH neurons which produces melanin-concentrating hormone (MCH) [5]. However, optogenetic inhibition of MCH neurons did not produce a significant reduction in REM sleep duration [6].

This supports the hypothesis that REM-on GABAergic (non-MCHergic/non-orexinergic) neurons, which have also been observed in the LH, play a role in the regulation of REM sleep appearance [7–9]. Additionally, the inhibition of neurons within the LH depressed waking and evoked an extended period of non-REM (NREM) sleep [5]. These observations partially fit with the reported effects of either optogenetic [8], or DREADD (designer receptors exclusively activated by designer drugs) silencing of orexin neurons [10], and the administration of a dual orexin receptor antagonist [11]. However, in these three cases of selective inhibition of orexinergic activity, wakefulness was not comparably suppressed to the level shown after muscimol injection within the LH [5], suggesting that the role played by LH neurons in arousal levels cannot be entirely ascribed to the orexin neurons. Furthermore, in the latter studies the increase in NREM sleep was not nearly as great as that shown after the inhibition of the entire LH neuronal population, and REM sleep was still present.

While the outcome of LH neurons inhibition (reducing wakefulness) fits well with the observed effect of LH neurons activation (promoting wakefulness), changes in autonomic functions induced by such inhibition have not yet been investigated.

Of particular interest is the role played by LH neurons in thermoregulation control. Since the activation of LH neurons produces an increase in thermogenesis [3], it can be hypothesized that LH neurons inhibition may result in a state of hypothermia. While a modest reduction in brain temperature (core temperature around 36°C), such as that described after peripheral injection of CCK [12], can favour both NREM sleep and REM sleep occurrence, during either spontaneous torpor [13–16] or centrally-induced deep hypothermia (Core temperature 22°C, 24°C) [17], [18], REM sleep appearance was inhibited. Therefore, the possibility that LH inhibition may induce a state of marked hypothermia could provide an alternative explanation for the inhibition of REM sleep appearance described by Clement et al., 2012.

In order to evaluate whether sleep changes induced by LH neurons inhibition are the mere consequence of a reduced thermogenesis and not of the inhibition of specific wake-sleep (WS) related neural substrates within the LH, the present study aims to investigate the effects induced on both the WS cycle and thermoregulation by the pharmacological inhibition of LH neurons. Moreover, since Clement and co-workers used a single administration of the GABA$_A$ agonist muscimol, leaving open the possibility that the relatively large vehicle volume and drug concentration might have caused an unwanted diffusion of the effects, we performed subsequent administrations of muscimol in small concentrations and volumes.

It is also critical to consider that neuronal inhibition can induce different effects according to the levels of neuronal activation preceding the inhibition. We therefore tested the effects of LH inhibition in different environmental conditions: at thermoneutrality, a condition that should not determine any specific activation of LH neurons, and during acute cold exposure, a condition that has been shown to increase the amount of wakefulness [19], and to induce a significant activation of LH neurons [20].

Here we show that the prolonged pharmacological inhibition of LH neurons almost abolished wakefulness and promoted a prolonged bout of NREM sleep characterized by an enhancement of slow-wave activity and by the absence of NREM-to-REM sleep transitions. A thermoregulatory impairment was observed when LH neurons were inhibited at an ambient temperature (Ta) of 10°C but not at Ta = 24°C.

Preliminary results of the experiments have been published in abstract form [21].

Materials and Methods

Ethical approval

The experiments were carried out with the approval of the Comitato Etico-Scientifico dell'Alma Mater Studiorum - University of Bologna (Ethical-Scientific Committee of the Alma Mater Studiorum - University of Bologna), in accordance with the European Union Directive (86/609/EEC) and under the supervision of the Central Veterinary Service of the Alma Mater Studiorum - University of Bologna and the National Health Authority. All efforts were made to minimize the number of animals used and their pain and distress.

Surgical Procedures

Male CD Sprague-Dawley rats (n = 12, Charles River Inc, Lecco, Italy) were deeply anaesthetized through the injection of diazepam (Valium; F. Hoffmann-La Roche ltd, Basel, Switzerland, 5 mg/kg, intramuscular) followed by ketamine-HCl (Ketavet; Parke-Davis, Detroit, MI, USA, 100 mg/kg, intraperitoneal), and placed in a stereotaxic apparatus (David Kopf Instruments, Tujunga, CA, USA) with the incisor bar set in order to keep the bregma and lambda on the same horizontal plane. Animals were surgically implanted with: i) electrodes for EEG and nuchal electromyographic (EMG) recording; ii) a catheter placed into the femoral artery for the telemetric recording of arterial pressure (AP) (PA-C40, DataSciences International, St.Paul, MN, USA); iii) a thermistor (B10KA303N, Thermometrics Corporation, Northridge, CA, USA) mounted inside a stainless-steel needle (21 gauge) stereotaxically implanted above the left anterior hypothalamus to record the deep brain temperature (T$_{brain}$); iv) two microinjection guide cannulas (C315G-SPC Plastics One Inc, Roanoke, VA, USA; internal cannula extension below guide: +3.5 mm), stereotaxically positioned in the left and the right LH. After surgery, animals received 20 ml/kg of saline subcutaneously and 0.25 ml of an antibiotic solution (penicillin G, 37500 IU; streptomycin-sulfate, 8750 IU) i.m. Animals recovered from surgery for at least one week, initially in their home cage and subsequently, for at least 3 days, in a Plexiglas cage with a stainless steel grid floor (wire diameter = 2 mm, inter-wire distance = 10 mm). The cage was positioned within a thermoregulated, sound-attenuated recording chamber where animals were kept throughout the experiment. The recording chamber was equipped with light and temperature controllers and acoustically insulated from the surroundings, so as to keep animals unaware of any activity outside the chamber. The recording chamber was located inside a Faraday-shielded room. Besides regular cage cleaning (at 9:00 am every day), operators entered the Faraday-shielded room only during the microinjection procedure. During recovery from surgery, animals were kept at an ambient temperature (Ta) of 24°C±0.5°C and under a 12:12 h light (L) - dark (D) cycle (light on at 09.00, 100 lux at cage level), and had free access to food and water. The recording chamber was also equipped with an infrared thermocamera (Thermovision A20, FLIR Systems, Boston, MA, USA) positioned under the stainless steel grid floor, to measure cutaneous temperature.

Experimental Protocols

After recovery from surgery (1 week to 10 days), animals were divided into two experimental groups. Animals in group A (n = 5) were recorded for 6 consecutive days in the following conditions: i) day 1, baseline, Ta = 24°C; ii) day 2, inhibitor injections (GABA$_A$ agonist muscimol, 1 mM, 100 nl, 1 bilateral injection/h starting at 11:00 h and ending at 16:00 h), Ta = 24°C; iii) day 3, recovery Ta = 24°C; iv) day 4, control, Ta = 24°C; v) day 5, saline vehicle injections (NaCl 0.9% w/v, 100 nl, 1 bilateral injection/h starting at 11:00 h and ending at 16:00 h), Ta = 24°C; vi) day 6, recovery, Ta = 24°C. Animals in group B (n = 7) were recorded for 6 consecutive days in the same conditions as those for group A with the exception that during both injection days (day 2 and day 5) animals were kept at Ta 10°C from 9:00 h to 17:00 h, the time period during which the injections were delivered.

Microinjection procedures

The microinjection system consisted of a Hamilton 5 μl gastight syringe (Hamilton Company, Bonaduz, Switzerland) positioned in an infusion pump (MA 01746, Harvard Apparatus, Holliston, MA, USA; infusion rate 0.3 μl/min) and connected to the internal cannula through one meter of microdialysis FEP tubing (ID

0.12 mm OD 0.65 mm, Microbiotech/se AB, Stockholm, Sweden).

The cannula and the tube were filled with either muscimol (Tocris Bioscience, Bristol, UK) dissolved in vehicle solution or vehicle solution only (commercially available sterile-pyrogen free saline for parenteral injection (0.9%), S.A.L.F. Bergamo, Italy), while the syringe and the initial part of the tube were filled with coloured mineral oil. The insertion of the internal cannula into the guide cannula was performed manually by an operator by opening the lid of the recording chamber, gently inserting the internal cannula in the guide cannula and locking the two together. Care was also taken to avoid removing the animal from the cage during the insertion of the cannula. Once the internal cannula was inserted, the lid of the recording chamber was closed. The pump and the syringe were located outside the recording chamber.

All microinjection procedures were performed as follows. At 10:55, the microinjecting cannula was inserted into the guide cannula. After closing the lid of the recording chamber, the first microinjection was performed. Ten minutes after the first injection, the lid of the recording chamber was opened again, the internal cannula extracted and inserted into the contralateral guide cannula. The lid was closed again, and the second microinjection was performed. After 10 more minutes, the recording chamber was opened and the cannula retrieved. This procedure was repeated for each of the 6 injections performed.

During each injection (average duration: 30 s±5 s), the volume injected (100 nl) was microscopically-assessed by the movement of the oil-liquid interface within the FEP tubing over a ruler. Compared to the single administration performed by Clement and co-workers [5] (muscimol, 1 µg/µl, 8.76 mM, in 300 nl), we thought that a sequence of injections (1 per hour) of a smaller volume (100 nl) and concentration (0.1 µg/µl, 1 mM) would reduce the possibilities of confounding effects induced by an unwanted diffusion to neuronal pools outside the LH.

Histology

At the end of the experiment, the injection site was marked with 80 nl of Fast Green 2% dye. Rats were anaesthetized with ketamine as described above and transcardially perfused (4% w/vol paraformaldehyde). The brain was extracted and postfixed overnight with 4% paraformaldehyde and then cryoprotected (30% w/vol sucrose). The brain was then sliced coronally on a cryostat (60 µm) and sections containing a dye spot were plotted on an atlas drawing [22] (Figure 1).

Signal Recording and Data Analysis

The EEG, EMG and T_{brain} signals were recorded by means of insulated copper wires connecting the headsocket to a swivel, amplified (Grass 7P511L, Astro-Med Inc, West Warwick (RI), USA), filtered (EEG: highpass 0.3 Hz, lowpass 30 Hz; EMG highpass 100 Hz, lowpass 1 KHz T_{brain} highpass 0.5 Hz), 12 bit digitalized (Micro MK 1401 II, CED, Cambridge, UK; acquisition rate: EEG: 1 KHz; EMG: 1 KHz; T_{brain}: 100 Hz) and acquired on a digital hard drive. AP signal was telemetrically recorded, amplified and digitally stored on a hard drive (acquisition rate: 500 Hz). Heart rate (HR) was derived from AP peak detection.

EEG power spectrum was calculated from a 4-sec-long 1-sec-sliding window. EEG total power and power bands (Delta (0.5–4.5 Hz), Theta (5.0–9.0 Hz), Sigma (11.0–15.0 Hz)) were normalized to the mean value (100%) of the day 1 (control) recording. A full EEG spectrum from 0.25 to 20 Hz for NREM sleep and wakefulness was also calculated and normalized according to the average state specific spectrum of day 1. Sleep stages were visually scored by an operator (one-second resolution), using a script

developed for Spike2 (sleepscore). Wakefulness, NREM sleep, and REM sleep were scored according to standard criteria based on EEG, EMG, and T_{brain} signals [19].

Digital images from the thermocamera were acquired at 1 frame/s and tail temperature (T_{tail}) was measured in the medial portion of the tail by analyzing the thermographic record (Thermocam Researcher, FLIR systems, Boston, MA, USA). Variations of T_{tail} were analyzed comparing the 10-min average value recorded one hour before the first injection with the 10-min average value recorded 1 hour after the first injection for all experimental groups. Paired t-test was used to compare the pre-injection levels of T_{tail} with the post-injection values. Unpaired t-test was used to compare T_{tail} variation induced by muscimol injection with the saline-induced variation.

Values are reported as mean ± SEM. A two-way ANOVA (SPSS 21.0) with repeated measures on both factors was used for the statistical analysis of the results of the injection day (i.e. day 2 or day 5) and, with a different time resolution, of the baseline day (i.e. day 1 or day 4) together with the recovery day (i.e. day 3 or day 6). The modified t-test (t*) was used for both the pre-planned orthogonal and the pre-planned non-orthogonal contrasts [23], [24]. The α level of the non-orthogonal contrasts was adjusted using the sequential Bonferroni method [25].

For the analysis of the injection day, the Main Factors were defined as follows: i) the Factor "time" (which was considered for repeated measures) had 48 levels, corresponding to each 30-min interval of the whole 24-h period; ii) the Factor "Experimental Condition" (which was considered for repeated measures) had two levels (saline and muscimol). For each 30-min interval of the Factor "time", data were compared by means of the following orthogonal contrast: saline vs. muscimol.

For the analysis of the baseline day and recovery day, the Main Factors were defined as follows: i) the Factor "time" (which was considered for repeated measures) had 4 levels, corresponding to the L and D periods of both days; ii) the Factor "Experimental Condition" (which was considered for repeated measures) had two levels (saline and muscimol). For each level of the "time" Factor, orthogonal contrasts were used to compare saline and muscimol results. For each level of the "Experimental Condition" Factor, the following pre-planned non-orthogonal contrasts were tested: recovery day_L vs. baseline day_L; recovery day_D vs. baseline day_D. The statistical analysis of the cumulative amount of wakefulness, NREM sleep, and REM sleep during the injection day was carried out with a t-test. The statistical analysis for T_{tail} was carried out comparing the 10 minutes T_{tail} average 1 hour before the beginning of the microinjection procedure with the 10 minutes T_{tail} average 1 hour later with a paired t-test. For all comparisons, statistical significance was set at p<0.05.

Results

Effects on sleep

The 6-h inhibition of the LH neurons was characterized by a significant increase in the amount of NREM sleep at both Ta 24°C and Ta 10°C (Figure 2). At Ta 24°C, the amount of NREM sleep increased significantly during the injection period with a peak after the second injection (93.6±3.1%, t*$_{(192)}$ = 4.43, p<0.05 compared to saline) and remained significantly higher compared to saline for the entire period of injections.

At Ta 10°C, the injections of muscimol induced a significant increase in the amount of NREM sleep that peaked after the third injection (90.5±4.9%, t*$_{(288)}$ = 5.52, p<0.05 compared to saline). A significant negative peak in the amount of NREM sleep was observed between 20:00 h and 21:00 h and was associated with a

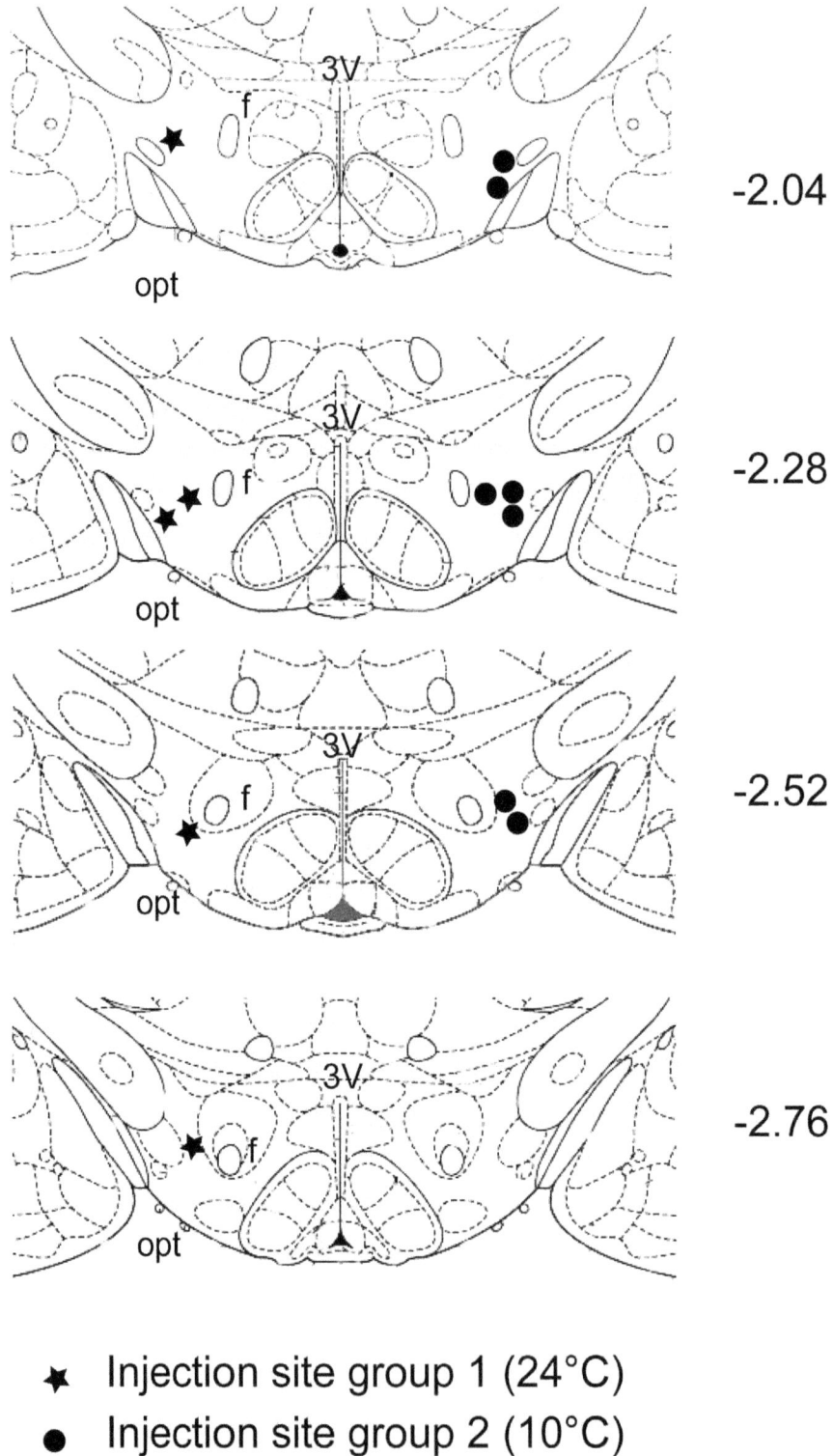

Figure 1. Injection Sites. The figure shows the location of the injection sites plotted on an atlas drawing [22]. Each injection was performed bilaterally but, for the sake of simplicity, is plotted monolaterally. Each slice refers to the antero-posterior distance in mm from Bregma, which is indicated on the right-hand side of each panel. The black stars, plotted on the left-hand side of each drawing, indicate the injection sites for group 1 animals (kept at an ambient temperature (Ta) of 24°C), while the black circles, plotted on the right-hand side of each drawing, indicate the injection sites for group 2 animals (exposed to Ta = 10°C during the injection period). 3V = third ventricle, f = fornex, opt = optic tract.

peak in the amount of wakefulness ($70.6 \pm 9.1\%$, $t^*_{(288)} = 4.15$, $p < 0.05$ compared to saline). On the recovery day after muscimol administration, no significant changes in the amount of NREM sleep were observed compared to the saline condition.

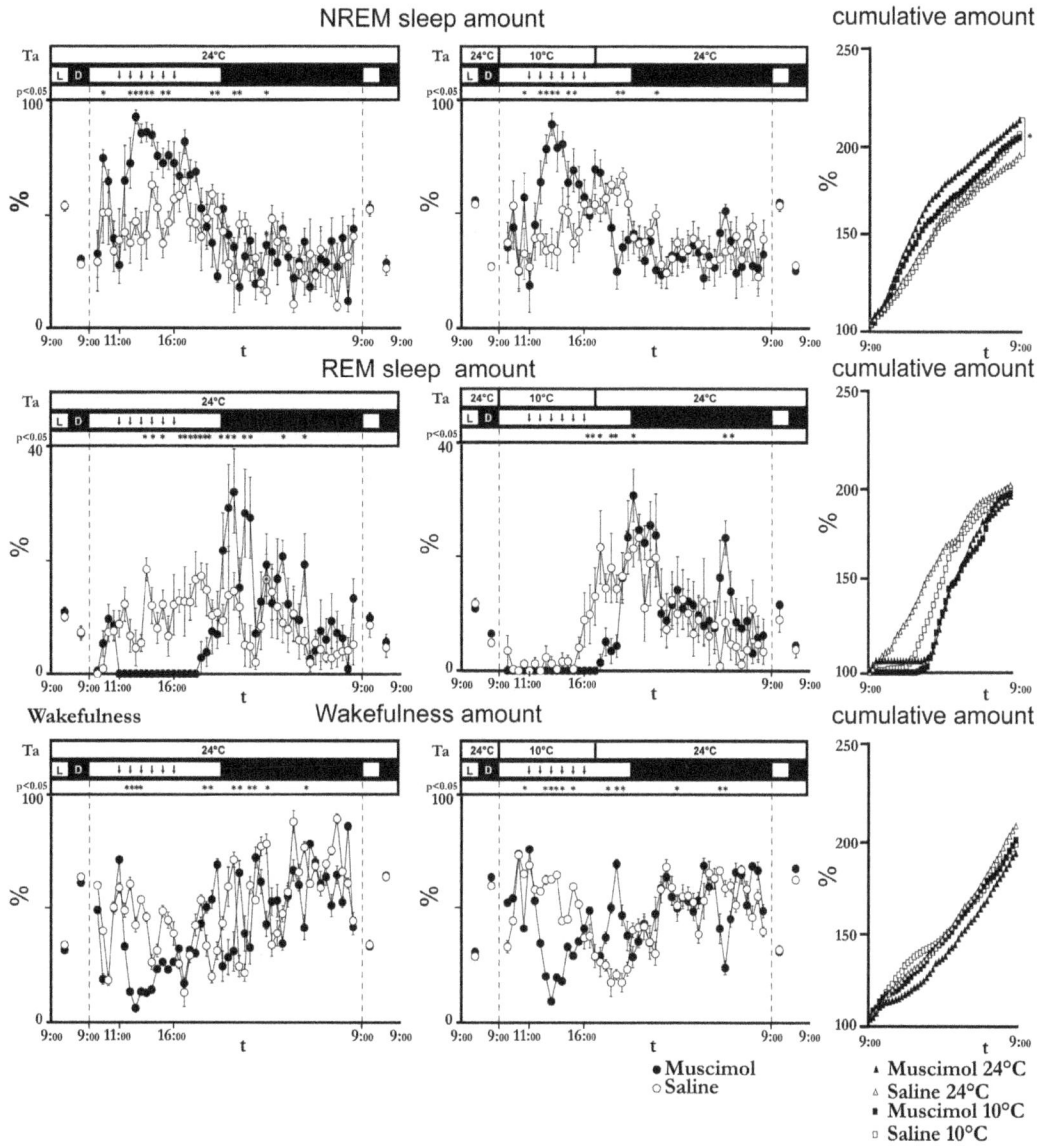

Figure 2. Sleep amount. The figure shows the time-course of the amount, expressed as the percentage of each epoch (12 h for Day 1, 3, 4, and 6; 30 min for day 2, and 5) of non-REM (NREM) sleep, REM sleep and wakefulness during the 6 experimental days (filled circles: days 1, 2 and 3; empty circles: days 4, 5 and 6) for group 1 animals (kept at an ambient temperature (Ta) of 24°C, left column) and group 2 animals (exposed to Ta = 10°C, from 9:00 to 17:00 of day 2, center column). The time resolution is 12 h for days 1, 3, 4, and 6 and 30 minutes for days 2 and 4. Vertical dashed lines divide consecutive experimental days. Each animal of each group was repeatedly injected with either the GABA$_A$ agonist muscimol (day 2, filled circles, 100 nl, 1 mM, 1 injection/h bilaterally) or saline (day 4, empty circles, 100 nl, 0, 9%, 1 injection/h bilaterally). Ta, light (L)/dark (D) cycle and statistical significance are plotted above each panel. Each down-pointing arrow marks an injection. Data are shown as mean ± SEM. * = p<0.05. In the right-hand column the cumulative amount (expressed as the percentage of the respective total amount during the day preceding the injection day) of NREM sleep, REM sleep and wakefulness during each injection day is shown. * = p<0.05.

During the 6-h period of LH neuron inhibition, the Delta power in NREM sleep was significantly higher both at 24°C and at 10°C, while Sigma power in NREM sleep was significantly lower compared to the saline condition (Figure 3). At Ta 24°C, Delta power increased rapidly after the first muscimol injection, reaching a peak after the third injection (138.3±12.0%, t*$_{(192)}$ = 2.59, p< 0.05 compared to saline), and returned to a normal level before the end of the injection period. On the other hand, Sigma power was drastically reduced after the first muscimol injection and remained very low for the entire period of injections (nadir: 40.3±5.8%, t*$_{(192)}$ = 5.48, p<0.05 compared to saline), slowly returning to normal at the end of the light period. At Ta 10°C, NREM sleep

Delta power rapidly increased after the first muscimol injection and remained significantly elevated for the entire injection period (peak 155.7±18.0%, t*$_{(240)}$ = 5.71, p<0.05 compared to saline). During the recovery day, Delta power showed a negative rebound; it was significantly lower compared to saline (Light period: 84.4±5.5%, t*$_{(20)}$ = 4.22, p<0.05 compared to saline; dark period: 83.9±7.3%, t*$_{(20)}$ = 3.32, p<0.05 compared to saline). Sigma power in NREM sleep was also drastically reduced, and remained significantly lower (nadir: 42.7±3.7%, t*$_{(288)}$ = 6.37, p<0.05 compared to saline) for a few hours after the last injection.

The EEG power spectrum in NREM sleep during the period of LH neuron inhibition showed a clear increase in the frequencies

Delta Power (NREM sleep)

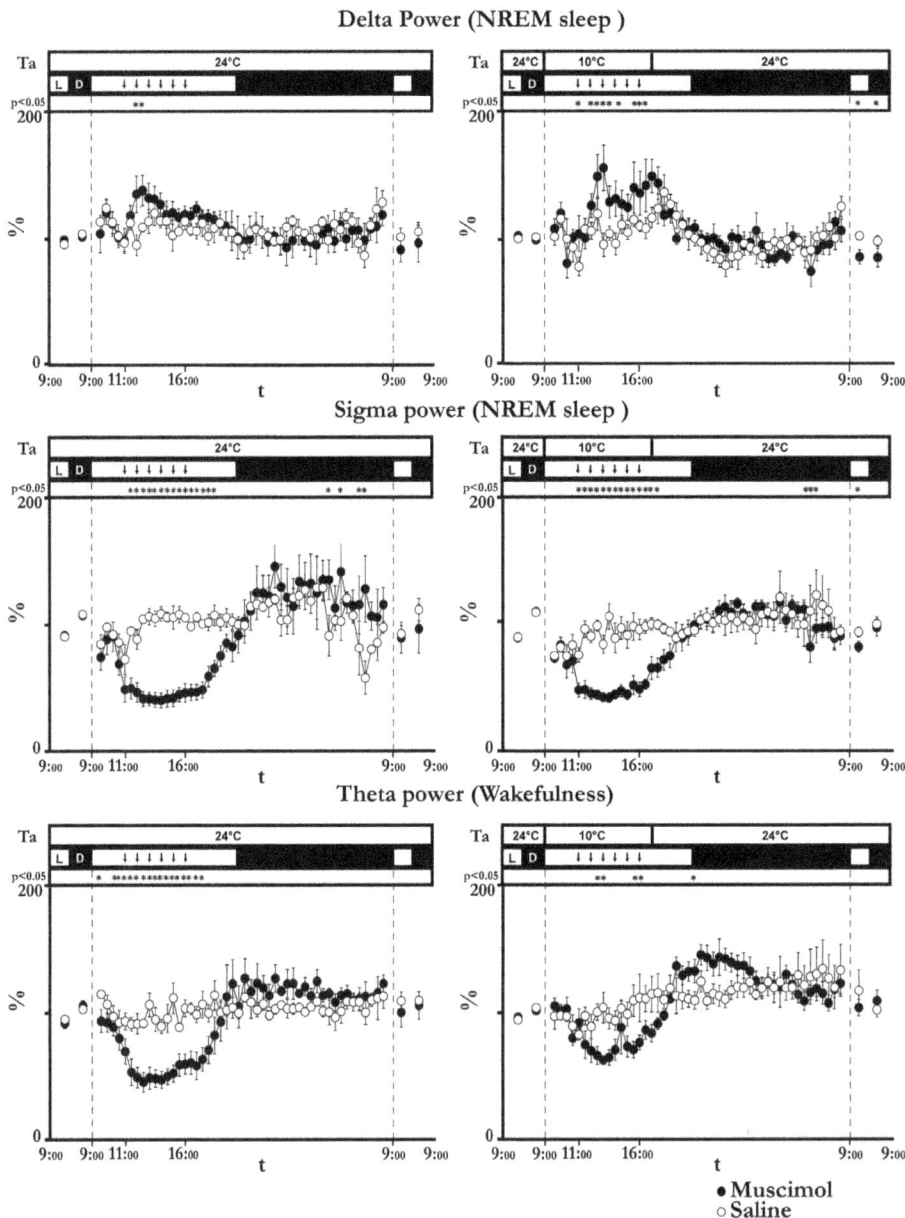

Sigma power (NREM sleep)

Theta power (Wakefulness)

● Muscimol
○ Saline

Figure 3. EEG power bands. The Figure shows the time-course of either Delta or Sigma power during non-REM (NREM) sleep and Theta power during wakefulness, during the 6 experimental days (filled circles: days 1, 2 and 3; empty circles: days 4, 5 and 6) for animals of group 1 (kept at an ambient temperature (Ta) of 24°C, left column) and for those of group 2 (exposed to Ta = 10°C from 9:00 to 17:00 of day 2, right column). Powers are normalized on the average EEG power of the day preceding the injection-day and expressed as percentages. The time resolution is 12 h for days 1, 3, 4, and 6 and 30 minutes for days 2 and 4. Vertical dashed lines divide consecutive experimental days. Each animal of each group was repeatedly injected with either the GABA$_A$ agonist muscimol (day 2, filled circles, 100 nl, 1 mM, 1 injection/h bilaterally) or saline (day 4, empty circles, 100 nl, 0, 9%, 1 injection/h bilaterally). Vertical dashed lines divide consecutive experimental days. Ta, light (L)/dark (D) cycle and statistical significance are plotted above each panel. Each downward arrow marks an injection. Data are shown as mean ± SEM. * = p<0.05.

below 2 Hz at Ta 24°C and below 3 Hz at Ta 10°C, and a drastic decrease in all the spectral components above 7 Hz was observed at both Tas (Figure 4).

REM sleep was totally suppressed during the prolonged inhibition of the LH neurons and for a few hours afterwards, at both Ta 24°C and Ta 10°C (Figure 2). Acute exposure to Ta 10°C with saline injections also resulted in an immediate drastic decrease in REM sleep amount, but at around 15:00 REM sleep appeared again. The amount of REM sleep lost during the injection period was fully recovered within the same day.

The changes in the amount of wakefulness induced by LH inhibition mirrored the effects on NREM sleep amount at both Ta 24°C and Ta 10°C (Figure 2). Theta power during wakefulness (Figure 3) was strongly decreased by the muscimol injections at both Ta 24°C (nadir: 47.4±6.8%, t*$_{(192)}$ = 4.21, p<0.05 compared to saline) and Ta 10°C (nadir: 63.2±3.1%, t*$_{(288)}$ = 2.13, p< 0.05 compared to saline), returning to normal levels a few hours after the last injections. Animals exposed to 10°C showed an increase in Theta power during the night following the LH

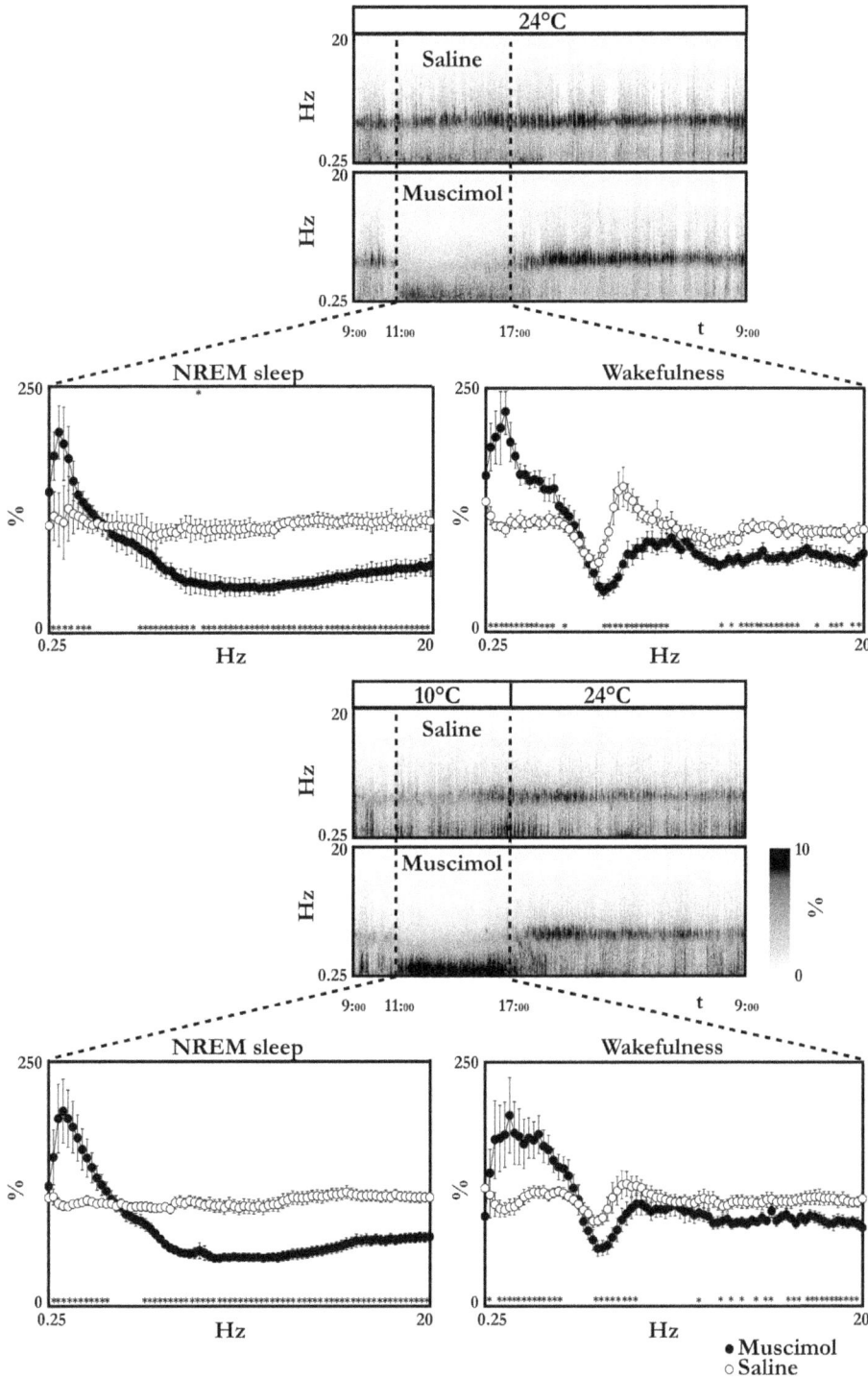

Figure 4. EEG spectra. The figure shows the time-course of the average EEG spectrum during the day of repeated injections of either the GABA$_A$ agonist muscimol (100 nl, 1 mM, 1 injection/h bilaterally) or saline (100 nl, 0, 9%, 1 injection/h bilaterally) for group 1 animals (A and B) and for group 2 animals (E and F). EEG power is normalized on the average EEG power recorded during the day before the injection day and expressed as percentages. Ambient temperature is indicated above each panel. Vertical dashed lines indicate the injection period, from the first injection to 1 hour after the last injection. Panels C, D, G and H show the average EEG spectrum in non-REM sleep and in wakefulness during the injection period. Data are shown as mean ± SEM. * = p<0.05.

inhibition. No significant differences were observed during the recovery day.

The EEG power spectrum in wakefulness during the period of LH neuron inhibition showed a clear increase in the frequencies

below 4 Hz at both Ta 24°C and Ta 10°C, and a drastic decrease in the frequency of the Theta band (Figure 4). Saline injections also produced a right-shift of the Theta region, which was around 1.5 Hz faster.

Effects on autonomic variables

At Ta 24°C, the repeated injection of saline produced a significant increase in T_{brain} compared to that observed during the injections of muscimol (peak: 37.8 ± 0.3°C, $t^*_{(192)} = 5.20$, $p<0.05$) (Figure 5). At Ta 10°C, saline injection still produced an increase in T_{brain}, while muscimol injections evoked a decrease in T_{brain}, that reached a nadir of 35.5 ± 0.2°C ($t^*_{(240)} = 8.42$, $p<0.05$ compared to saline) after 3 hours. T_{brain} returned rapidly towards physiological levels, but it remained significantly higher compared to the saline group for the rest of the day. No significant differences were observed in the recovery period. The decrease in T_{brain} was not caused by an increase in thermal dissipation, since the tail did not show any sign of vasodilation, but, rather, a modest but significant vasoconstriction (Figure 6), dropping from an average pre-injection value of 12.8 ± 1.1°C to 11.8 ± 1.1°C one hour after the first injection ($t_{(6)} = 2.59$, $p<0.05$). A significant reduction in T_{tail} was also observed at Ta 24°C, when T_{tail} dropped from an average pre-injection value of 31.1 ± 0.3°C to 29.6 ± 0.2°C one hour after the first injection ($t_{(4)} = 8.48$, $p<0.05$). The latter value was also significantly lower ($p<0.05$) compared to that observed one hour after the first saline injection (31.5 ± 0.4°C; $t_{(5)} = 3.55$).

At Ta 24°C, HR was significantly higher following saline injections than following muscimol administration (Figure 5). The increase in HR induced by saline may be the result of the repeated microinjection procedure that, despite the care taken in trying to minimize the handling of the animal, may have disturbed the animal, resulting in a modest stress-induced hyperthermia. This effect was completely blocked by muscimol injection. At Ta 10°C, the acute cold exposure caused a rapid increase in HR that was only partially reversed by muscimol injections in a limited time window. No major effects on AP levels were observed following either muscimol or saline injections at both Tas.

Discussion

The results of the present study show that, as previously described [5], in the rat kept at normal laboratory temperature (Ta, 24°C) the prolonged inhibition of LH neurons produced a pronounced increase in NREM sleep and a total suppression of REM sleep. These effects were not likely to be the mere consequence of changes in body temperature, since no decrease in T_{brain} was observed following muscimol injection in animals kept at Ta 24°C, suggesting that LH neurons do not play a role in the basic maintenance of body temperature in a thermoneutral environment.

A novel finding is that NREM sleep enhancement was characterized by an increase in Delta power, due to a large enhancement of slow wave activity (SWA), with almost no activity in the faster frequencies of the EEG spectrum. We categorized this state as NREM sleep, although its peculiar spectral EEG characteristics may call for an *ad hoc* denomination. Moreover, the results show that these effects were also produced when the inhibition of LH neurons occurred during acute cold exposure, a condition which is known to interfere with sleep processes [19].

The lack of relevant bodily thermal changes following muscimol injection at Ta 24°C suggests that the effects observed on either NREM sleep or REM sleep were the consequence of the inhibition of LH neurons specifically involved in the regulation of wake-sleep processes. Although the orexin and the MCH neurons within the LH may represent the best candidates [26], [27], a role for non-orexin/non-MCH neurons cannot be disregarded [9].

In fact, the features of the NREM sleep occurring after the inhibition of the entire population of neurons within the LH by muscimol substantially differ from those described after the selective inhibition of subpopulations of neurons in the same area, especially the orexin and the MCH neurons. As far as the orexin neurons are concerned, while their fast acute optogenetic inhibition was shown to be sufficient to rapidly induce SWA [28], and systemic pharmacological antagonism of orexin was shown to produce an increase in NREM sleep in several mammals [29], the 1-h optogenetically-mediated inhibition of these neurons in mice was effective in providing an increase in NREM sleep amount only when delivered during the dark period, but not during the light period of the LD cycle (i.e. the period in which the effect was observed in the present study) [8].

Also, while a pharmacological blockade of orexin receptors was not shown to induce significant changes in the NREM sleep EEG power spectrum in humans [30], [31], in the present study the spectral EEG characteristics of both NREM sleep and wakefulness during the period of muscimol injection appeared to be different from their physiological counterpart. Although the EEG trace during LH inhibition did not show evident abnormalities, the EEG power spectrum during NREM sleep, in particular, presented a large increase below 2 Hz and a drastic reduction in the faster frequency regions. In addition, the EEG spectrum of wakefulness was characterized by an increase in the power of the low-frequency region that was concomitant with a mild reduction in the power of the fast-frequency region. These findings, together with the observation that the activity of orexin neurons undergoes a circadian modulation that should be at its lowest level during our injection period [32], suggest that the increase in NREM sleep and in SWA induced by muscimol injections may be the results of the inhibition of a wider neuronal population within the LH rather than just the orexin neurons.

The inhibition of LH neurons at Ta 10°C induced a relevant hypothermia, confirming the role of LH neurons in thermoregulation and apparently providing an explanation for the suppression of REM sleep. However, the fact that after muscimol delivery at Ta 24°C brain temperature remained at baseline levels suggests that an impairment in thermogenesis was unlikely to be the cause of the absence of REM sleep. Interestingly, the almost complete suppression of Sigma power during NREM sleep indicates the absence of any attempt to enter REM sleep, since it is known that the NREM to REM sleep transition is marked by a strong increase in Sigma power [33].

The suppression of REM sleep may therefore be considered to be the consequence of the inhibition of the activity of MCH neurons [27]. However, the optogenetic inhibition of these neurons did not affect REM sleep duration [6], suggesting that other neurons in the area besides the MCH positive are involved in the regulation of REM sleep appearance. It can be suggested that this third population of neurons may be the population of GABA-positive/MCH-and-orexina-negative REM-on neurons [9]. These neurons may induce REM sleep by an inhibitory projection to the ventrolateral part of the periaqueductal gray and to the dorsal deep mesencephalic nucleus GABAergic REM-off neurons [27].

The REM sleep suppression caused by LH neurons inhibition may resemble the REM sleep suppression induced by an inflammatory state [34]. In both conditions the suppression of REM sleep is concomitant with an increase in NREM sleep and in Delta power, but LH inhibition does not induce any increase in brain temperature, as usually seen after cytokine injection [34]. In consideration of the fact that the increase in brain temperature during inflammatory response has been shown to be separable from the concomitant thermoregulatory effects [35], it is possible to hypothesize that the neuronal population within the LH may be one of the areas mediating the effects of cytokines on sleep.

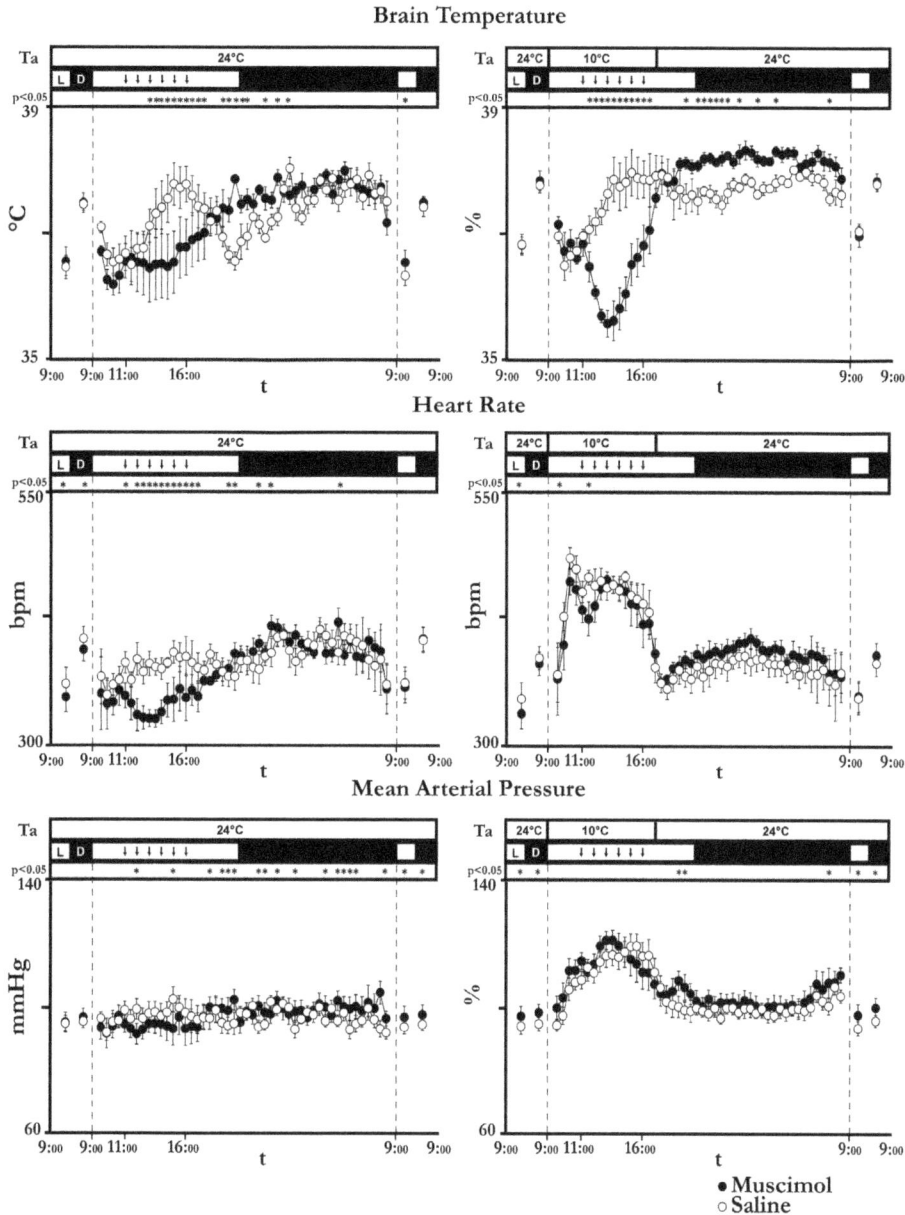

Figure 5. Autonomic parameters. The figure shows the time-course of brain temperature, heart rate and mean arterial pressure during the 6 experimental days (filled circles: days 1, 2 and 3; empty circles: days 4, 5 and 6) for animals of group 1 (kept at an ambient temperature (Ta) of 24°C, left column) and those of group 2 (exposed to Ta = 10°C from 9:00 to 17:00 of day 2, right column). The time resolution is 12 h for days 1, 3, 4, and 6 and 30 minutes for days 2 and 4. Vertical dashed lines divide consecutive experimental days. Each animal of each group was repeatedly injected with either the GABA$_A$ agonist muscimol (day 2, filled circles, 100 nl, 1 mM, 1 injection/h bilaterally) or saline (day 4, empty circles, 100 nl, 0, 9%, 1 injection/h bilaterally). Vertical dashed lines divide consecutive experimental days. Ta, light (L)/dark (D) cycle and statistical significance are plotted above each panel. Each downward arrow marks an injection. Data are visualized as mean ± SEM. * = p<0.05.

Our results also show that LH neurons have a limited role in regulating the activity of the autonomic nervous system.

LH inhibition failed to reverse the increase in HR and MAP caused by cold exposure and had limited effects on HR at Ta 24°C, suggesting that LH neurons are not involved in the thermoregulatory modulation of cardiovascular parameters.

Thermoregulation was more largely affected than cardiovascular regulation by LH neurons inhibition. At Ta 10°C, T$_{brain}$ decreased significantly during the delivery of the first three injections, but this decrease was quickly reversed, despite the fact that the LH neurons were still actively inhibited, suggesting the

activation of a compensatory system. Since the decrease in T$_{brain}$ was not caused by an increased thermal dissipation, it can only be explained by a reduced thermogenesis. It has been suggested that the orexin neurons within the LH are capable of amplifying an already active thermogenic drive, but have limited effects otherwise [4]. If this is the case, our data suggest that LH neurons, possibly the orexin neurons, are among the first responders that are activated to maintain a constant body temperature after cold exposure, potentiating the basic thermogenic drive, but they are not necessary for the maintenance of core temperature in a cold environment.

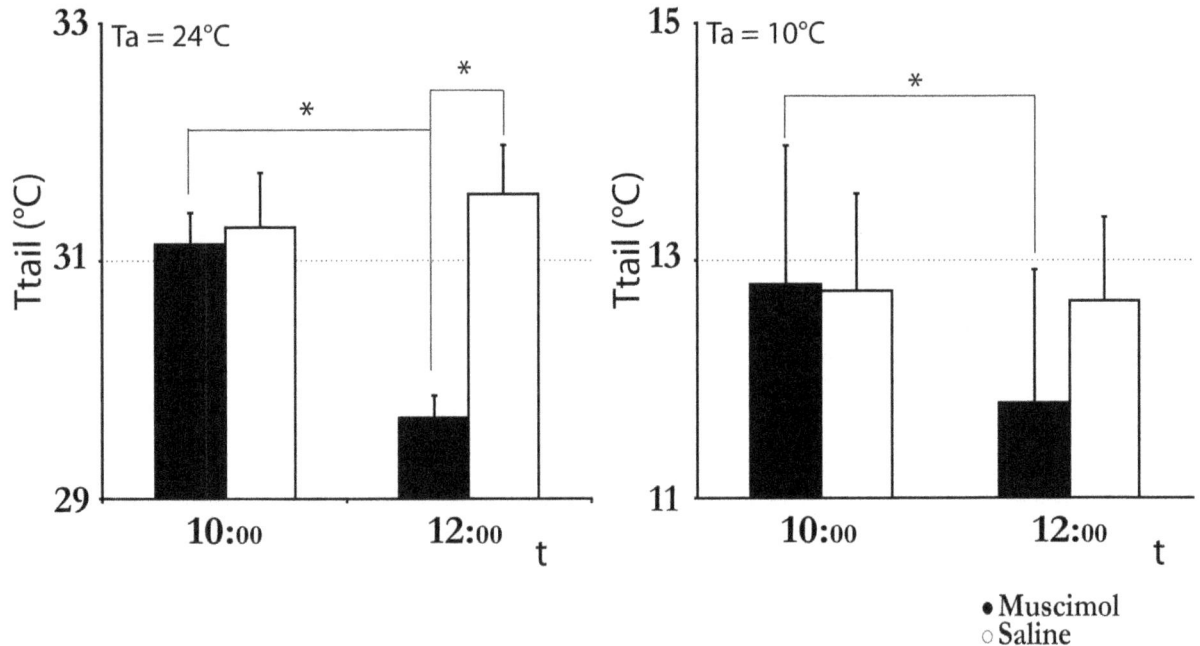

Figure 6. Tail temperature. The figure shows the average tail temperature measured from 9:50 to 10:00 (approximately 1 hour before the first injection) and from 11:50 and 12:00 (approximately 1 hour after the first injection of either muscimol (black bar) or saline (white bar)) at ambient temperature (Ta) = 24°C (on the left) or at Ta = 10°C (on the right). Data are shown as mean ± SEM. * = p<0.05.

At Ta 24°C, no decrease in T_{brain} was observed, suggesting that LH neurons may not play a role in the basic maintenance of body temperature in a thermoneutral environment. Unexpectedly, an increase in T_{brain} was observed during the injection of saline. This can be explained by the repeated injection procedure that, despite every effort on behalf of the experimenters, may have produced some distress in the animal. An alternative explanation may lie in the fact that orexin neurons have been shown to be activated by a decrease in pH [36]. Even if the volume of the saline injection was very small, the possibility that a transient reduction in extracellular pH may have resulted in an activation of orexin neurons cannot be ruled out, although it appears unlikely. It is worth noting that, whatever the cause of the saline-related increase in T_{brain}, the injection of muscimol suppressed it.

An increase in the vasoconstrictor tone in the tail blood vessels was induced by the muscimol injection both at Ta = 24°C and at Ta = 10 C°. The increased vasoconstriction may reveal the presence of a tonically-active inhibitory input originating in the LH and affecting other central areas involved in the regulation of cutaneous thermal conductance, such as the Preoptic Area [37] or the Raphe Pallidus [38]. Alternatively, it may be suggested that the reduction in the thermogenic drive induced by the inhibition of LH neurons immediately triggered a compensatory response that was sufficient to avoid hypothermia at Ta = 24°C but not at Ta = 10°C.

In conclusion, the results of our study show that: i) the acute inhibition of neurons within the LH induced a large increase in NREM sleep with enhanced SWA, and suppressed both REM sleep and the EEG activity characterizing the NREM to REM sleep transition; ii) these effects cannot be merely ascribed to the inhibition of either orexin or MCH neurons within the LH, suggesting a role for non-orexin/non-MCH neurons; iii) neurons located within the LH are involved in a first line of cold defense, but are not apparently essential for the maintenance of body temperature.

Acknowledgments

The authors wish to thank Ms. Melissa Stott for reviewing the English.

Author Contributions

Conceived and designed the experiments: MC GZ RA. Performed the experiments: MC FD MM DM. Analyzed the data: MC FD ML. Contributed to the writing of the manuscript: MC EP DT GZ RA.

References

1. Berthoud HR, Munzberg H (2013) The lateral hypothalamus as integrator of metabolic and environmental needs: from electrical self-stimulation to optogenetics. Physiol Behav 104: 29–39.
2. Li FW, Deurveilher S, Semba K (2011) Behavioural and neuronal activation after microinjections of AMPA and NMDA into the perifornical lateral hypothalamus in rats. Behav Brain Res 224: 376–386.
3. Cerri M, Morrison SF (2005) Activation of lateral hypothalamic neurons stimulates brown adipose tissue thermogenesis. Neuroscience 135: 627–638.
4. Tupone D, Madden CJ, Cano G, Morrison SF (2011) An orexinergic projection from perifornical hypothalamus to raphe pallidus increases rat brown adipose tissue thermogenesis. J Neurosci 31: 15944–15955.
5. Clement O, Sapin E, Libourel PA, Arthaud S, Brischoux F, et al. (2012) The lateral hypothalamic area controls paradoxical (REM) sleep by means of descending projections to brainstem GABAergic neurons. J Neurosci 32: 16763–16774.
6. Jego S, Glasgow SD, Herrera CG, Ekstrand M, Reed SJ, et al. (2013) Optogenetic identification of a rapid eye movement sleep modulatory circuit in the hypothalamus. Nat Neurosci 16: 1637–1643.

7. Hassani OK, Henny P, Lee MG, Jones BE (2010) GABAergic neurons intermingled with orexin and MCH neurons in the lateral hypothalamus discharge maximally during sleep. Eur J Neurosci 32: 448–457.

8. Tsunematsu T, Tabuchi S, Tanaka KF, Boyden ES, Tominaga M, et al. (2013) Long-lasting silencing of orexin/hypocretin neurons using archaerhodopsin induces slow-wave sleep in mice. Behav Brain Res 255: 64–74.

9. Sapin E, Berod A, Leger L, Herman PA, Luppi PH, et al. (2013) A very large number of GABAergic neurons are activated in the tuberal hypothalamus during paradoxical (REM) sleep hypersomnia. PLoS One 5: e11766.

10. Sasaki K, Suzuki M, Mieda M, Tsujino N, Roth B, et al. (2011) Pharmacogenetic modulation of orexin neurons alters sleep/wakefulness states in mice. PLoS One 6: e20360.

11. Betschart C, Hintermann S, Behnke D, Cotesta S, Fendt M, et al. (2013) Identification of a novel series of orexin receptor antagonists with a distinct effect on sleep architecture for the treatment of insomnia. J Med Chem 56: 7590–7607.

12. Kapas L, Obal F, Jr, Alfoldi P, Rubicsek G, Penke B, et al. (1988) Effects of nocturnal intraperitoneal administration of cholecystokinin in rats: simultaneous increase in sleep, increase in EEG slow-wave activity, reduction of motor activity, suppression of eating, and decrease in brain temperature. Brain Res 438: 155–164.

13. Walker JM, Garber A, Berger RJ, Heller HC (1979) Sleep and estivation (shallow torpor): continuous processes of energy conservation. Science 204: 1098–1100.

14. Harris DV, Walker JM, Berger RJ (1984) A Continuum of Slow-Wave Sleep and Shallow Torpor in the Pocket Mouse Perognathus longimembris. Physiological Zoology 57: 428–443.

15. Krilowicz BL, Glotzbach SF, Heller HC (1988) Neuronal activity during sleep and complete bouts of hibernation. Am J Physiol 255: R1008–1019.

16. Deboer T, Tobler I (1994) Sleep EEG after daily torpor in the Djungarian hamster: similarity to the effect of sleep deprivation. Neurosci Lett 166: 35–38.

17. Cerri M, Mastrotto M, Tupone D, Martelli D, Luppi M, et al. (2013) The inhibition of neurons in the central nervous pathways for thermoregulatory cold defense induces a suspended animation state in the rat. J Neurosci 33: 2984–2993.

18. Tupone D, Madden CJ, Morrison SF (2013) Central activation of the A1 adenosine receptor (A1AR) induces a hypothermic, torpor-like state in the rat. J Neurosci 33: 14512–14525.

19. Cerri M, Ocampo-Garces A, Amici R, Baracchi F, Capitani P, et al. (2005) Cold exposure and sleep in the rat: effects on sleep architecture and the electroencephalogram. Sleep 28: 694–705.

20. Takahashi Y, Zhang W, Sameshima K, Kuroki C, Matsumoto A, et al. (2013) Orexin neurons are indispensable for prostaglandin E2-induced fever and defence against environmental cooling in mice. J Physiol 591: 5623–5643.

21. Del Vecchio F, Al-Jahmany A, Amici R, Cerri M, Luppi M, et al. (2012) Effects on sleep of the inhibition of the lateral hypothalamus in the rat. J Sleep Res S358: 571.

22. Paxinos G, Watson C (2007) The rat brain in stereotaxic coordinates. San Diego: Elsevier.

23. Wallenstein S, Zucker CL, Fleiss JL (1980) Some statistical methods useful in circulation research. Circ Res 47: 1–9.

24. Winer BJ, Brown DR, Michels KM (1991) Statistical principles in experimental design. Boston: McGraw-Hill.

25. Holm S (1979) A simple sequentially rejective multiple test procedure. Scand J Stat 6: 65–70.

26. de Lecea L, Huerta R (2014) Hypocretin (orexin) regulation of sleep-to-wake transitions. Front Pharmacol 5: 16.

27. Luppi PH, Peyron C, Fort P (2013) Role of MCH neurons in paradoxical (REM) sleep control. Sleep 36: 1775–1776.

28. Tsunematsu T, Kilduff TS, Boyden ES, Takahashi S, Tominaga M, et al. (2011) Acute optogenetic silencing of orexin/hypocretin neurons induces slow-wave sleep in mice. J Neurosci 31: 10529–10539.

29. Brisbare-Roch C, Dingemanse J, Koberstein R, Hoever P, Aissaoui H, et al. (2007) Promotion of sleep by targeting the orexin system in rats, dogs and humans. Nat Med 13: 150–155.

30. Bettica P, Squassante L, Groeger JA, Gennery B, Winsky-Sommerer R, et al. (2012) Differential effects of a dual orexin receptor antagonist (SB-649868) and zolpidem on sleep initiation and consolidation, SWS, REM sleep, and EEG power spectra in a model of situational insomnia. Neuropsychopharmacology 37: 1224–1233.

31. Fox SV, Gotter AL, Tye SJ, Garson SL, Savitz AT, et al. (2013) Quantitative Electroencephalography Within Sleep/Wake States Differentiates GABAA Modulators Eszopiclone and Zolpidem From Dual Orexin Receptor Antagonists in Rats. Neuropsychopharmacology 38: 2401–2408.

32. Estabrooke IV, McCarthy MT, Ko E, Chou TC, Chemelli RM, et al. (2001) Fos expression in orexin neurons varies with behavioral state. J Neurosci 21: 1656–1662.

33. Capitani P, Cerri M, Amici R, Baracchi F, Jones CA, et al. (2005) Changes in EEG activity and hypothalamic temperature as indices for non-REM sleep to REM sleep transitions. Neurosci Lett 383: 182–187.

34. Krueger JM, Johannsen L (1989) Bacterial products, cytokines and sleep. J Rheumatol Suppl 19: 52–57.

35. Krueger JM, Takahashi S (1997) Thermoregulation and sleep. Closely linked but separable. Ann N Y Acad Sci 813: 281–286.

36. Williams RH, Jensen LT, Verkhratsky A, Fugger L, Burdakov D (2007) Control of hypothalamic orexin neurons by acid and CO2. Proc Natl Acad Sci U S A 104: 10685–10690.

37. Tanaka M, McKinley MJ, McAllen RM (2013) Role of an excitatory preoptic-raphe pathway in febrile vasoconstriction of the rat's tail. Am J Physiol Regul Integr Comp Physiol 305: R1479–1489.

38. Cerri M, Zamboni G, Tupone D, Dentico D, Luppi M, et al. (2010) Cutaneous vasodilation elicited by disinhibition of the caudal portion of the rostral ventromedial medulla of the free-behaving rat. Neuroscience 165: 984–995.

15

Prospective Randomized Trial of Enoxaparin, Pentoxifylline and Ursodeoxycholic Acid for Prevention of Radiation-Induced Liver Toxicity

Max Seidensticker[1,2]*, Ricarda Seidensticker[1,2], Robert Damm[1,2], Konrad Mohnike[1,2], Maciej Pech[1,2,7], Bruno Sangro[3], Peter Hass[4], Peter Wust[5], Siegfried Kropf[6], Günther Gademann[4], Jens Ricke[1,2]

1 Universitätsklinik Magdeburg, Klinik für Radiologie und Nuklearmedizin, Magdeburg, Germany, 2 International School of Image-Guided Interventions, Deutsche Akademie für Mikrotherapie, Magdeburg, Germany, 3 Clinica Universidad de Navarra, Liver Unit, Department of Internal Medicine, Pamplona, Spain, 4 Universitätsklinik Magdeburg, Klinik für Strahlentherapie, Magdeburg, Germany, 5 Charité Universitätsmedizin Berlin, Klinik für Radioonkologie und Strahlentherapie, Berlin, Germany, 6 Universitätsklinik Magdeburg, Institut für Biometrie und Medizinische Informatik, Magdeburg, Germany, 7 Medical University of Gdansk, 2nd Department of Radiology, Gdansk, Poland

Abstract

Background/Aim: Targeted radiotherapy of liver malignancies has found to be effective in selected patients. A key limiting factor of these therapies is the relatively low tolerance of the liver parenchyma to radiation. We sought to assess the preventive effects of a combined regimen of pentoxifylline (PTX), ursodeoxycholic acid (UDCA) and low-dose low molecular weight heparin (LMWH) on focal radiation-induced liver injury (fRILI).

Methods and Materials: Patients with liver metastases from colorectal carcinoma who were scheduled for local ablation by radiotherapy (image-guided high-dose-rate interstitial brachytherapy) were prospectively randomized to receive PTX, UDCA and LMWH for 8 weeks (treatment) or no medication (control). Focal RILI at follow-up was assessed using functional hepatobiliary magnetic resonance imaging (MRI). A minimal threshold dose, i.e. the dose to which the outer rim of the fRILI was formerly exposed to, was quantified by merging MRI and dosimetry data.

Results: Results from an intended interim-analysis made a premature termination necessary. Twenty-two patients were included in the per-protocol analysis. Minimal mean hepatic threshold dose 6 weeks after radiotherapy (primary endpoint) was significantly higher in the study treatment-group compared with the control (19.1 Gy versus 14.6 Gy, p = 0.011). Qualitative evidence of fRILI by MRI at 6 weeks was observed in 45.5% of patients in the treatment versus 90.9% of the control group. No significant differences between the groups were observed at the 12-week follow-up.

Conclusions: The post-therapeutic application of PTX, UDCA and low-dose LMWH significantly reduced the extent and incidence fRILI at 6 weeks after radiotherapy. The development of subsequent fRILI at 12 weeks (4 weeks after cessation of PTX, UDCA and LMWH during weeks 1–8) in the treatment group was comparable to the control group thus supporting the observation that the agents mitigated fRILI.

Trial Registration: EU clinical trials register 2008-002985-70 ClinicalTrials.gov NCT01149304

Editor: Vincent Wong, The Chinese University of Hong Kong, Hong Kong

Funding: This study was funded in full by Sirtex medical (http://www.sirtex.com.au/eu/), funding received by university hospital of Magdeburg. The writing of this paper was funded in part by Sirtex medical. Writing support was provided by Rae Hobbs and was funded by Sirtex medical. Apart from that, the funders had no role in study design, data collection and analysis, decision to publish, or preparation of the manuscript.

Competing Interests: M. Seidensticker has served as a speaker for Bayer Healthcare and Sirtex medical, and has received research funding from Sirtex medical. R. Seidensticker has served as a speaker for Bayer Healthcare and Sirtex medical, and has received research funding from Sirtex medical. J. Ricke has served as a speaker for Bayer Healthcare and Sirtex medical, and has received research funding from Sirtex medical, Bayer Healthcare and Siemens. M. Pech has served as a speaker for Sirtex medical. B. Sangro has served as a speaker and an advisory board member for Sirtex medical.

* Email: max.seidensticker@med.ovgu.de

Introduction

Highly targeted radiotherapy of liver malignancies has found to be effective in selected patients. Stereotactic radiotherapy, radio-embolization using yttrium-90 (^{90}Y) microspheres as well as image-guided brachytherapy (BT) have been described in the literature with promising results [1,2,3]. A key limiting factor of these therapies is the relatively low tolerance of the liver parenchyma to radiation leading to either subclinical focal or generalized injury of the liver parenchyma. When the intensity or the extent of radiation-induced liver injury (RILI) exceeds the functional reserve, clinical complications appear in the form of radiation (radioembolization) induced liver disease (RILD or REILD) [4,5,6,7]. Prior exposure or concomitant chemotherapy is thought to increase the risk of RILD (or REILD), and as a consequence is a relatively common complication, for example, after conditioning therapy prior to bone marrow transplantation (BMT) [5,8,9,10]. Liver damage whether associated with whole body irradiation or liver-directed radiotherapy have the same pathology, i.e. veno-occlusive disease (VOD) [5,11,12,13].

Medication designed to reduce RILI could improve the safety as well as enable more aggressive radiotherapy. Clinical studies have shown with varying strength of evidence that VOD/RILD after BMT can be ameliorated by pentoxifylline (PTX), ursodeoxy-cholic acid (UDCA) and low molecular weight heparin (LMWH) [14,15,16,17,18,19,20,21,22] (see Table 1). However, the equiv-ocal nature of the results from most studies probably reflect the heterogeneous study populations (including patients who have received prior chemotherapy or had underlying liver disease) [23]. Thus, a more standardized clinical model is needed to evaluate the protective effects of prophylactic regimens against VOD/RILD.

Image-guided, single-fractioned, high-dose-rate BT of liver malignancies is associated with a well-characterized focal RILI (fRILI), which can be visualized and quantified using functional hepatobiliary magnetic resonance imaging (MRI) (see Figure 1) [6,7]. Importantly, the histopathological evidence of fRILI (i.e. sinusoidal congestion with hepatocyte atrophy and increased reticulin deposits) correlates well with the absence of the hepatocyte uptake of hepatolbiliary MRI contrast media [24]. We have previously found that development of areas of fRILI were maximal at 6–8 weeks post-BT which correlates to the peak incidence of RILD/REILD after conditioning therapy/radio-embolization througout the first 2 months post-intervention [5,6,7,25]. We conducted a prospective study to quantify fRILI in patients who were randomized to BT with and without prophylactic PTX, UDCA and low-dose LMWH. To minimize the confounding effects of prior chemotherapy on radiation tolerability, only patients with liver metastases from colorectal cancer (mCRC) were included because these patients tend to have a more consistent pattern of prior exposition to chemotherapy. The cumulative effect of three drugs over a period of 8 weeks [26,27,28] was assessed and patients followed-up at 6 and 12 weeks.

Materials and Methods

The protocol for this trial and supporting CONSORT checklist are available as supporting information; see Checklist S1 and Protocol S1.

Study design

This was a prospective, randomised phase II, parallel-group, open-label study conducted at a single centre. The study was approved by the competent authorities (Federal Institute for Drugs and Medical Devices (in german: Bundesinstitut für Arzneimittel und Medizinprodukte - BfArM)) and the local ethics committee (Ethikkommission der Otto-von-Guericke-Universität der Medizi-nischen Fakultät). Trial registration: Eudra-CT: 2008-002985-70; ClinicalTrials.gov-identifier NCT01149304. Written informed consent was obtained from all patients prior to study entry. Group allocation approach was unrestricted randomization.

Patient characteristics

Consecutive patients (18–80 years) with liver metastases from mCRC, who were scheduled for local ablation with computed-tomography (CT)/MRI-guided BT between 2009 and 2012, were screened (Figure 2). (BT is the local standard ablative treatment in patients ineligible for surgical or all other appropriate interven-tion).

Women who were pregnant, lactating or of childbearing potential were excluded as were patients with liver cirrhosis, hepatitis B or C, severe coronary artery disease, autoimmune diseases, acute bacterial endocarditis, active major bleedings or high-risk of uncontrolled hemorrhage; severe or moderate renal impairment (GFR <60 mL/min), or known contraindication or hypersensitivity to any of the study treatments or procedures.

Treatment and follow-up

Patients received a single-fraction, CT- or MRI-guided BT of CRC liver metastases (see details below). In those randomized to prophylaxis, the following treatment was initiated during the evening of the day of BT: sc injection of 40 mg q.d. enoxaparin (Clexane, Sanofi Aventis, Paris, France) [20], oral 400 mg t.i.d. PTX (Trental, Sanofi Aventis) [16] and oral 250 mg t.i.d. UDCA (Ursofalk, Falk Pharma, Freiburg, Germany) [17,19]. Patients were discharged usually on the third day post-BT and continued to take study medication at home for 8 weeks. All patients were followed-up on day 3, week 6 and 12 with an optional follow-up at week 24. Within 24 hours of the procedure and at each subsequent visit, blood samples were taken for liver-specific and inflammato-ry/hemostatic laboratory parameters, and patients were assessed for ECOG-performance status and health-related quality-of-life (using the EQ5D-questionnaire). All adverse reactions related to the study medication or BT were recorded.

Compliance to the prophylactic regimen was evaluated during a dialogue at each visit and the evaluation of anti-Xa-activity at 6 weeks. Insufficient compliance was determined by: either anti-Xa-activity <0.1 IU/mL measured up to 4 hours after last enoxaparin injection, or two dose interruptions of the prophylactic regimen for more than 1 day/week. Non-compliant patients were withdrawn from the per-protocol analysis and study-specific medication stopped.

Image-guided interstitial brachytherapy

The technique of image-guided BT has been described previously [2]. Briefly, the placement of the introducer sheaths (6F Radiofocus, Terumo, Tokyo, Japan) with the BT applicators (Lumencath, Nucletron/Elekta, Veenendaal, The Netherlands) was performed using CT or MRI fluoroscopy. For treatment planning purposes, a spiral CT or T1-weighted MRI of the liver (reconstructed slice thickness: 3 mm) enhanced by intravenous application of iodine contrast media (CT) or Gd-EOB-DTPA (MRI) was acquired.

The high-dose-rate afterloading system (Microselectron, Nucle-tron/Elekta, Veenendaal, The Netherlands) employed an iridium-192 source with a nominal activity of 10Ci (i.e. 370GBq); decay correction was performed daily. Relative coordinates (x, y, z) of the catheters were determined in the CT/MRI-data set and trans-ferred to the treatment planning system (Oncentra, Nucletron/ Elekta). Using these coordinates, the clinical target volume and the predefined minimum dose (20 Gy, delivered as a single fraction [2]), the software calculated a dosimetry and the duration of the iridium-192 source inside the BT catheters. A planning CT with dosimetry is displayed in Figure 1B and F.

Table 1. Summary of published studies on drug treatments for the prevention of VOD/RILD.

Reference	Study design	N	Treatment regimen	Incidence of VOD	p-value*	Bilirubin (μmol/L)	p-value*
Attal et al. 1993 [14]	Prospective RCT	70	**Pentoxifylline** 1,600 mg/d day −8 to day+100 post-BMT	4%	NS	26.4 (mean max)	NS
		70	Control	3%		24.4 (mean max)	
Clift et al. 1993 [22]	Prospective RCT	44	**Pentoxifylline** 2,400 mg/d day −3 to day+70 post-allogeneic BMT	-		26.6 (mean max)	0.62
		44	Control	-		23.47 (mean max)	
Bianco et al. 1991 [16]	Phase 1–2	30	**Pentoxifylline** 1,200, 1,600, and 2,000 mg/d; day −10 to day+100 post-BMT	10%	0.001	-	-
		20	Control (retrospective)	65%		-	
Attal et al 1992 [15]	Prospective RCT	81	**Unfractionated heparin** 100 U/kg/d cont. infusion; day −8 to day+30 post-BMT	2.5%	0.01	7.4% exceeding 34	<0.05
		80	Control	14%		18.7% exceeding 34	
Forrest et al. 2003 [18]	Prospective single-arm	40	**LMWH:** dalteparin 2500 anti-Xa i.u; day −1 to day +30 post-BMT or hospital discharge	22.5%, 2.5% severe			
Or et al. 1996 [20]	Prospective RCT, pilot	61	**LMWH:** enoxaparin 40 mg/day; day+1 to day+40 post-BMT or hospital discharge		0.01	(duration of elevated levels)	0.01
		33	Control				
Essel et al. 1998 [17]	Prospective RCT	34	**UDCA** 600–1200 mg/d; day at least −1 to day +80 post-BMT	15%	0.03	102.6 (mean max)	0.13
		32	Control	40%		188.1 (mean max)	
Ohashi et al. 2000 [19]	Prospective RCT	67	**UDCA** 600 mg/d; day −21 to day+80 post-BMT	3%	0.004	Not reported in detail	NS
		65	Control	18.5%		Not reported in detail	

Table 1. Cont.

Reference	Study design	N	Treatment regimen	Incidence of VOD	p-value*	Bilirubin (µmol/L)	p-value*
Park et al. 2002 [28]	Prospective RCT	82	**UDCA** 600 mg/d + **unfractionated heparin** 5–50 U/kg/d adjusted aPTT of 50 s; day +1 to day +30 post-BMT or hospital discharge (but a minimum of 15d)	16%	0.348	148.8 (mean max)	0.725
		83	**Unfractionated heparin** 5–50 U/kg/d adjusted aPTT of 50 s; day +1 to day +30 post-BMT or hospital discharge (but a minimum of 15d)	19%		173.6 (mean max)	

*Group comparison; LMWH: Low molecular weight heparin; BMT: Bone marrow transplantation; Max: Maximum; NS: Not significant; VOD: Veno-occlusive disease; RCT: Randomized controlled trial; UDCA: ursodeoxycholic acid (ursodiol); aPTT: activated Partial Thromboplastin Time.

Magnetic resonance imaging

MRI (Achieva 1.5T, Philips, Best, The Netherlands) using the hepatobiliary contrast medium Gd-EOB-DTPA (Primovist, Bayer Healthcare, Leverkusen, Germany) was performed 1 day before and 6 and 12 weeks post-BT. MR-sequence of events was as follows: axial 3D T1-weighted (T1-w) gradient echo THRIVE (T1-High-Resolution-Isotropic-Volume-Excitation) (Time-to-Echo/Time-to-Repetition 4/10 ms, flip-angle 10°) with fat-suppression pre-contrast, at 20 s, 60 s and 120 s and 20 minutes after iv 0.1 mL/kg bodyweight Gd-EOB-DTPA. The slice thickness was 3 mm. For the study-specific MRI volumetry, dynamic THRIVE at 60 s (for the exclusion of tumor progression/local recurrence) and hepatobiliary phase THRIVE 20 min after application of Gd-EOB-DTPA (for the determination of area of fRILI) were mandatory.

Identification of the radiation isodose (minimal hepatic threshold dose) that demarcated the border between the fRILI and functioning liver tissue (as defined by non-uptake and uptake of Gd-EOB-DTPA enhanced MRI, respectively) was performed as follows in a blinded matter.

The hepatobiliary phase THRIVE was transferred to the BT-planning software. Image registration of the hepatobiliary phase THRIVE to the contrast-enhanced planning CT/MRI (including the dosimetry) was performed by an isoscalar local semi-automated point-based 3D-3D image registration using predefined match points (3 or 4 corresponding landmarks restricted to liver structures). Registration was only accepted if the target area merged perfectly by visual assessment. As a result of this procedure, the software simultaneously displayed the treatment dosimetry and anatomical structures/fRILI of the hepatobiliary phase THRIVE. The volume of the liver parenchyma with radiation-induced impaired uptake of Gd-EOB-DTPA (i.e. fRILI) was determined. The isodose of the dosimetry encircling this volume was determined at five different axial levels and the mean of these values recorded. This dose resembles the dose which was formerly applied at the now demarcated rim of the fRILI, corresponding to the assumed minimal hepatic tolerance dose. To ensure a negligible registration error, the volume of fRILI was inserted into the dose-volume-histogram of the dosimetry. The corresponding isodose was stored. Results of the two methods showed a high correlation of 0.899 and 0.562 (p<0.001 and p = 0.006) for 6 and 12 weeks, respectively. To minimize methodological errors, the mean isodose value of the two methods was taken. In case of more than one treated lesion, the mean of the determined isodoses was used. If no detectable fRILI was seen in follow-up, the minimal mean hepatic threshold dose was defined as the dose which was previously administered at the tumor margin (since an effect on the liver parenchyma above this dose level cannot be excluded). Figure 1 illustrates the development and appearance of the fRILI in hepatobiliary phase THRIVE.

Endpoints and statistical analyses

The aim of the study was to assess if a combination regimen of PTX, UDCA and low-dose LMWH for 8 weeks provided a preventive effect regarding irradiation damage to liver parenchyma (as resembled by the minimal mean threshold dose of the fRILI volume) at 6 weeks (primary endpoint) and at 12 weeks (secondary endpoint) after BT.

As additional descriptor, detectable fRILI in Gd-EOB-DTPA MRI (yes/no) was recorded at each follow-up. Further secondary objectives included the safety of the study treatment after BT including changes in bilirubin and albumin which were graded according to Common Terminology Criteria for Adverse Events version 3 (CTCAE3.0).

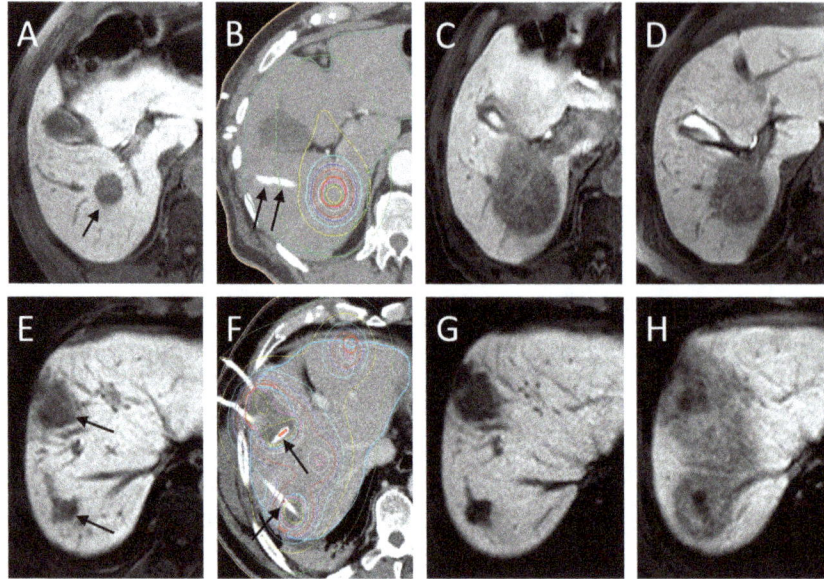

Figure 1. T1w-axial THRIVE 20 min after application of Gd-EOB-DTPA (A, C–E and G, H) and BT planning CT with dosimetry (B and F). A–D, control group. A: pre-treatment MRI displaying a metastasis scheduled for BT treatment (black arrow). B: Planning-CT after introduction of the brachytherapy catheters (black arrows). Clinical target volume (CTV) represented by bold red circle and dosimetry by coloured lines (red: 20 Gy-, blue: 12 Gy-isodose). C: MRI at 6 weeks showing substantial reduction in Gd-EOB-DTPA uptake by liver parenchyma adjacent to treated metastases (i.e. focal radiation-induced liver injury, fRILI). Note: The area of fRILI matches the geometry of the dosimetry (B). Determined threshold dose: 9.75 Gy. D: MRI at 3 months showing shrinkage of the fRILI. Determined threshold dose: 11.9 Gy. E–H, treatment group. E: pre-treatment MRI displaying two metastases (black arrow); two more treated lesions are not displayed in the plane. F: Planning-CT (annotations: see B). G: MRI at 6 weeks showing no fRILI. H: MRI at 3 months after radiotherapy (and 1 month after finishing study treatment) showing a substantial region of fRILI. Determined threshold dose: 15.8 Gy.

The relation between hepatocyte dysfunction and changes in the following liver-specific and inflammatory/hemostatic laboratory values were analysed: fibrinogen, factor-VIII-activity, interleukin-6, protein-C-activity, protein-S-activity, von-Willebrand-factor-activity and antithrombin-III-activity [29].

Determination of sample size was based on the expected minimum between-group difference of 2.1 Gy (SD 2.3 Gy) for minimal mean hepatic threshold dose at 6 weeks after BT (from 9.9 Gy to 12 Gy) [7]. A sequential test with 2 stages according to the Pocock-design was used which yielded a total of 22 observations per group with a scheduled interim analysis after 11 observations per group when a = 0.025 and power 1-b = 0.8. Interim-analysis showed a significant difference between the groups regarding the primary variable with a one-sided p-value of 0.011. A one-sided p of <0.0148 was necessary to terminate the study prematurely.

Statistical analysis was performed using SPSS (SPSS21, IBM, Chicago, Il, USA). Descriptive analysis of patient characteristics and laboratory findings was performed. The primary analysis was evaluated in the per protocol cohort and repeated in the intention-to-treat population as sensitivity analysis. Between-group differences in minimal mean hepatic threshold after BT at 6 and 12 weeks were compared using a two-sample t-tests, and evidence of detectable fRILI were compared using the Fisher's-exact-test. Possible confounding factors were evaluated using the Mann-Whitney-U-test for metric variables and the Fisher's-exact-test for categorical variables, and then between-group differences for the primary endpoint were evaluated with inclusion of the covariables (ANOVA and ANCOVA). The relationship between the minimal mean hepatic threshold dose and laboratory values was tested by Pearson's correlation and ANCOVA. Group comparison regarding ECOG and EQ5D was made by Mann-Whitney-U-test.

Median overall survival was estimated by Kaplan-Meier (group comparison by log-rank test). A p-value of <0.05 was statistically significant.

Results

Of 129 patients screened with liver metastases from colorectal cancer scheduled for BT, 30 patients were included in the study and 22 patients (11 per group) in the primary analyses of the per-protocol group (see CONSORT diagram, Figure 2). Demographic characteristics of randomized patients at screening are summarized in Table 2 and the baseline liver function and other laboratory parameters are presented in Table 3. Group comparison revealed a similar distribution of possible confounders. A tendency towards a larger volume of significantly radiation exposed liver parenchyma (>10 Gy) in the study treatment group (Table 2) may have potentially lowered the hepatic tolerance dose in this group instead of increase it [25].

The minimal mean hepatic threshold dose at 6 weeks after BT (primary endpoint) was significantly higher in the study treatment group than the control (19.1 Gy versus 14.6 Gy, p = 0.011, Table 4) with comparable results with the intention-to-treat analysis (Table 4). Correspondingly, fewer patients in the study treatment group than the control had evidence of fRILI at 6 weeks (45.5% versus 90.9%); this difference was also significant in the intention-to-treat analysis (Table 4). However at 12 weeks after BT (and 4 weeks after cessation of study treatment), these between-group differences were not observed (in neither the per-protocol nor intention-to-treat analyses) for the minimal mean hepatic threshold dose and the proportion of patients with fRILI (Table 4). Results from the optional follow-up at 24 weeks after BT continually showed no between-group differences for the minimal

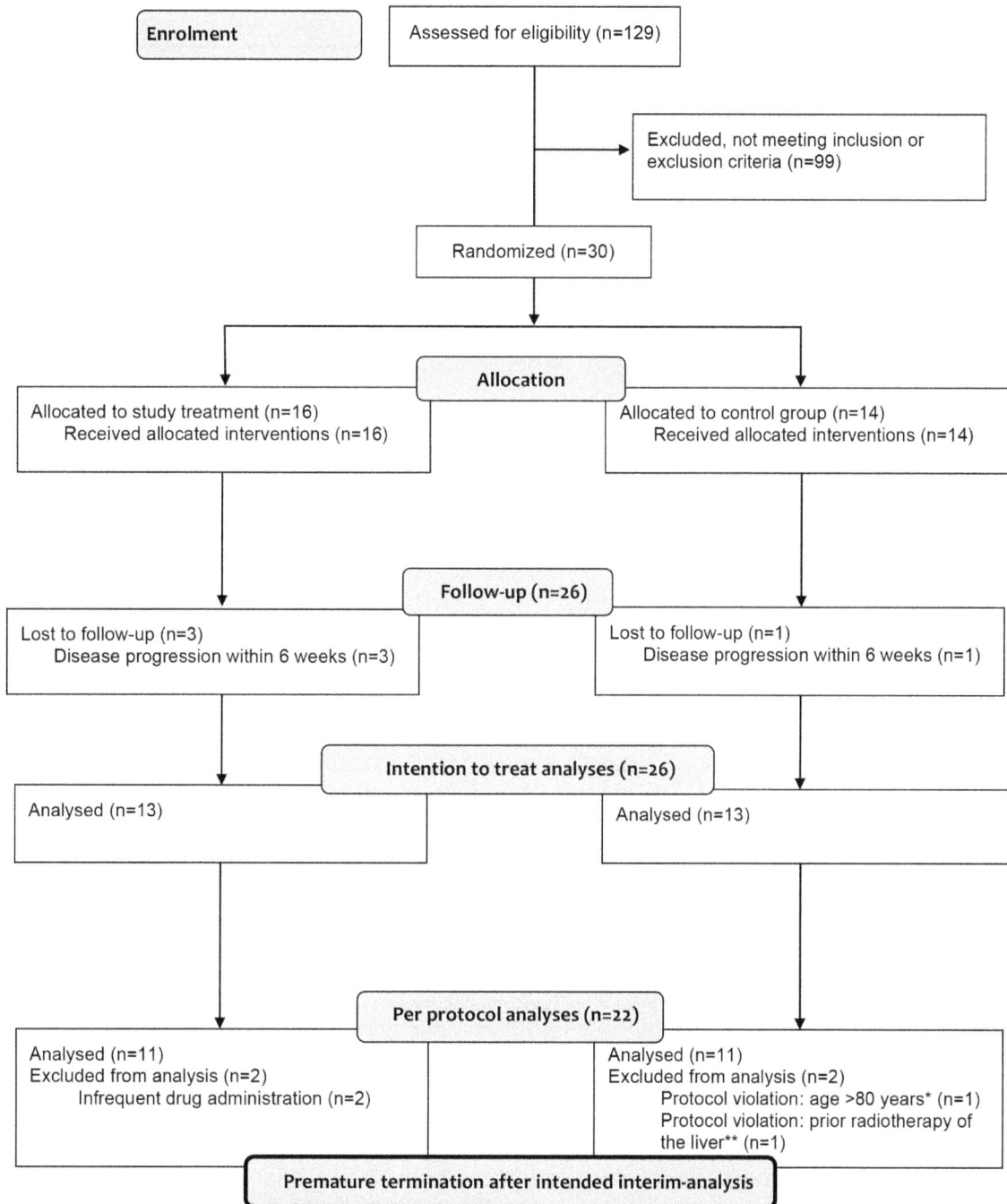

Figure 2. CONSORT-diagram. *Exclusion criterion age was initially disregarded by error in this patient (aged 82). **Exclusion criterion prior radiotherapy was initially disregarded by error in this patient (prior radiotherapy was performed 2 years earlier with location in the contralateral liver lobe).

mean hepatic threshold dose and the proportion of patients with fRILI (no change of the proportion of patients with fRILI as compared to 12 weeks follow-up; the minimal mean hepatic threshold dose for treatment group was 20.1 Gy (1 patient missing) and for the control group 21.0 Gy; p>0.05, per-protocol analysis (with comparable results with the intention-to-treat analysis)).

Covariate analyses also showed no influence of recorded covariables on the primary endpoint; only group allocation was significant (Table 5).

EQ5D (as a descriptor of quality of life) and distribution of ECOG performance status were not significantly different at baseline (Table 2) or at any follow-up visit (Table S1). Median overall survival from time of BT on was not different between the groups with 30.0 months (95%CI: 8.7–51.3) in the treatment group and 39.5 months (27.5–51.5) in the control group (p = 0.430).

Safety analyses were conducted in all 30 patients who received BT. The following mild-to-moderate adverse events CTCAEv3 grade 1–2 were reported (in the treatment/control groups) on day

Table 2. Patient characteristics (per protocol analysis).

Variable	Treatment group (n = 11)	Control (n = 11)	p-value (between group)*
Sex (m/f)	9/2	8/3	1.000
Age (years)	71.09±5.47	65.09±12.55	0.408
Weight (kg)	84.64±11.68	83.91±12.89	0.592
Height (cm)	174.09±6.79	172.64±6.90	0.834
ECOG at baseline (0/1/2)	6/4/1	4/5/2	0.370
EQ5D visual analogue score	72.36±14.56	76.36±13.02	0.446
History of liver surgery	45.5%	45.5%	1.000
Steatosis hepatis	36.4%	18.2%	0.635
Diabetes mellitus	18.2%	27.3%	1,000
Chemotherapy pretreatment			
Applied lines	1.00±0.63	1.00±0.45	1.000
no chemotherapy	18.2%	9.1%	NA
1 line	63.6%	81.8%	0.672
2 lines	18.2%	9.1%	NA
Prior chemotherapy			
Oxaliplatin	63.6%	63.6%	1.000
Irinotecan	36.4%	36.4%	1.000
Biologicals	54.5%	54.5%	1.000
Number of treated metastases	1.91±1.04	1.45±0.52	0.382
Maximum diameter of metastases (mm)	37.18±12.91	29.45±11.79	0.146
Clinical target volume (cm³)	42.82±29.26	31.36±37.14	0.156
Number of used brachytherapy catheters	3.18±1.78	2.27±1.74	0.079
Liver volume (cm³)	1296.1±226.6	1451.3±278.6	0.401
Interval between BT and 6 weeks FU (days)	43.91±4.76	45.09±4.68	0.757
Interval between BT and 3 months FU (days)	87.34±4.52	89.55±6.15	0.505
Liver volume with a dose exposure >10 Gy (%)	22.55±14.45	11.95±10.43	0.056
Chemotherapy during follow-up	18.2%	9.1%	1.000

Continuous data: mean ± standard deviation, frequencies: counts or percent.
*Group comparison, continuous data compared by Mann-Whitney U test, frequency data compared by Pearson's chi square test.

3 after BT: pain (1 patient/1 patient) and fatigue (0/1); at week 6: pain (2/0), fatigue (0/1), nausea (1/0) and diarrhea (2/0); nausea and diarrhea was probably related to PTX or UDCA. One grade 3 subacute bleeding episode from the bile duct, related to BT, occurred in the study treatment group which was successfully managed by endoscopic coagulation.

Analysis of the laboratory data revealed no grade 3/4 changes in bilirubin or albumin. One grade 1 reduction of albumin in the treatment group at 6 weeks was unchanged at week 12. One patient in control group with elevated (grade 1) bilirubin at baseline remained stable throughout follow-up. RILD was not observed on either group.

Laboratory analysis regarding liver-specific and inflammatory/hemostatic parameters found no relevant findings at baseline (Table 3). At week 6, slightly higher gamma-glutamyl-transferase levels and protein-S-activity were recorded in the control group compared with the treatment group. At 6 and 12 weeks, there was slight but significant mean decrease from baseline in cholinesterase in the treatment group. Additionally, mean fibrinogen and von-Willebrand-factor-activity increased significantly from baseline in the treatment group at 6 and 12 weeks; while significant increases

from baseline were recorded with mean fibrinogen, factor-VIII-activity and aspartate-transaminase in the control group at 6 weeks.

No correlation between the minimal mean hepatic threshold and liver-specific and inflammatory/hemostatic laboratory values was found at either week 6 or 12 (data not shown).

Discussion

In this prospective study, we were able to show a significant reduction in fRILI (as measured by hepatobiliary MRI) at 6 weeks after BT of colorectal liver metastases in patients who received low-dose LMWH, PTX and UDCA. Re-assessment of patients at 12 weeks (4 weeks after cessation of study treatment) found that the extent and incidence of fRILI was comparable to the control group, thereby supporting the reliability of our findings. This is further authenticated by the results of the (optional) 24 weeks follow-up. According to our results we believe that we were able to mitigate rather than delay the fRILI by the prophylactic regimen. The finding that the positive effect of the medication to the liver parenchyma as seen at the 6 weeks follow-up vanished after discontinuation of the medication (after 8 weeks) in the 3 months

Table 3. Laboratory parameters at baseline and follow-up (per protocol analysis).

Variable (normal range)		Treatment group (n = 11)	Control (n = 11)	p-value (between group)*	p-value (baseline vs. follow-up)**
Bilirubin	baseline	8.27±2.92	8.39±5.61	0.594	
(<21.0 µmol/L)	6 weeks	9.58±9.94	9.56±7.18	0.641	0.182 (0.350)
	12 weeks	8.71±4.27	8.75±5.95	0.735	0.594 (0.505)
Albumin	baseline	44.21±3.46	44.05±2.45	0.833	
(35.0–52.0 g/L)	6 weeks	42.49±5.16	42.67±3.17	0.743	0.197 (0.060)
	12 weeks	42.84±4.94	43.66±2.31	0.743	0.212 (0.332)
Cholinesterase	baseline	149.26±47.97	144.73±21.73	0.718	
(88–215 µmol/s.L)	6 weeks	136.27±51.65	143.82±29.10	0.433	**0.023** (0.929)
	12 weeks	132.94±49.22	153.36±30.96	0.088	**0.010** (0.423)
Aspartate transaminase	baseline	0.56±0.18	0.46±0.17	0.211	
(0.17–0.83 µmol/s.L)	6 weeks	0.59±0.17	0.55±0.23	0.533	0.373 (**0.016**)
	12 weeks	0.63±0.47	0.54±0.17	0.974	0.563 (0.056)
Alanine transaminase	baseline	0.44±0.20	0.51±0.36	1,000	
(0.17–0.83 µmol/s.L)	6 weeks	0.50±0.18	0.62±0.45	0.742	0.443 (0.109)
	12 weeks	0.53±0.43	0.52±0.27	0.718	0.508 (0.722)
Gamma glutamyltransferase	baseline	1.61±2.62	1.49±1.21	0.189	
(0.17–1.19 µmol/s.L)	6 weeks	0.82±0.83	2.21±1.71	**0.011**	0.100 (0.050)
	12 weeks	1.25±1.17	1.97±1.49	0.139	0.722 (0.306)
Glutamate dehydrogenase	baseline	104.36±91.47	108.82±94.84	0.844	
(<120 nmol/s.L)	6 weeks	67.55±31.43	123.27±105.88	0.490	0.328 (0.308)
	12 weeks	128.11±108.79	126.09±95.19	0.849	0.674 (0.374)
International normalized	baseline	93.9±3.03	95.55±2.98	0.053	
ratio (0.85–1.27)	6 weeks	94.11±2.71	94.8±2.44	0.399	0.438 (0.502)
	12 weeks	94.63±2.50	95.33±3.61	0.732	0.334 (0.498
Interleukin 6	baseline	4.54±3.31	3.71±3.09	0.245	
(<7.0 pg/mL)	6 weeks	8.44±8.53	7.62±4.41	0.809	0.266 (0.038)
	12 weeks	10.50±9.24	4.06±2.42	0.229	0.139 (0.515)
Fibrinogen	baseline	3.72±0.53	3.99±0.46	0.377	
(1.50–4.00 g/L)	6 weeks	4.50±1.17	4.77±0.84	0.365	**0.014 (0.017)**
	12 weeks	4.65±1.04	4.23±0.49	0.416	**0.037** (0.214)
Factor VIII activity	baseline	169.09±41.51	160.60±42.12	0.756	
(70–150%)	6 weeks	195.45±61.02	218.91±60.77	0.490	0.130 (0.093)
	12 weeks	199.7±67.26	257.09±150.23	0.360	0.169 (**0.017**)
Protein C activity	baseline	107.36±33.99	109.70±12.46	0.145	
(>70%)	6 weeks	108±32.68	106.55±18.67	0.767	0.799 (0.475)
	12 weeks	101.5±27.26	114±19.76	0.084	0.113 (0.540)
Protein S activity	baseline	85.36±12.26	86.80±12.55	0.848	
(>60%)	6 weeks	82.18±15.16	104.36±27.09	**0.036**	0.266 (0.086)
	12 weeks	87.3±14.54	91±10.6	0.549	0.799 (0.507)
von Willebrand factor	baseline	164.09±42.81	174.90±71.14	0.973	
activity (70–130%)	6 weeks	222.27±59.75	201.73±71.76	0.554	**0.013** (0.075)
	12 weeks	209.5±77.35	215.27±75.31	0.883	**0.013** (0.333)
Antithrombin III activity	baseline	92.73±13.72	98.90±11.50	0.191	
(>80%)	6 weeks	96.73±15.31	98.2±9.78	0.944	0.082 (0.779)
	12 weeks	96.4±12.08	96.73±9.51	0.751	0.407 (0.681)

*Between group comparison, Mann-Whitney U test;
**Comparison versus baseline (in brackets p-value of control group), Wilcoxon test.

Table 4. Minimal mean hepatic tolerance dose (Gy) and evidence of detectable focal radiation-induced liver injury (fRILI) after BT, group comparison.

Variable	Group			p-value (between groups)
Minimal mean hepatic tolerance dose (primary endpoint)		**Dose (Gy)**	**SD**	
At 6 weeks	Control	14.64 [14.15]	4.01 [3.93]	
	Treatment	19.06 [18.46]	3.35 [3.59]	**0.011 [0.007]**
At 12 weeks	Control	16.38 [16.10]	3.57 [3.60]	
	Treatment	19.04 [18.50]	2.88 [3.11]	0.069 [0.082]
Detectable fRILI		**Counts**	**Frequency**	
At 6 weeks	Control	10 [12]	90.9% [92.3%]	
	Treatment	5 [7]	45.5% [53.8%]	**0.022 [0.027]**
At 12 weeks	Control	10 [12]	90.9% [92.3%]	
	Treatment	10 [12]	90.9% [92.3%]	1.000 [1.000]

Per protocol analysis (n = 22); Intention-to-treat analysis (n = 26) in square brackets.

follow-up, make us believe that the fRILI was in fact mitigated in that period. Further on, the extent of the fRILI at 6 weeks in the treatment group and at 3 months (and 6 months) in both groups was less in size compared to the fRILI in the control group at 6 weeks (the peak of the fRILI in our study). Thus, the maximum extent of the fRILI at 6 weeks was skipped in the treatment group as compared to the control group. However, the radiation damage could not be suppressed completely by the prophylactic regimen with a rebound after cessation of the treatment to the level of the control group in later follow-ups. Thus, it is possibly right to assume additionally a delay on the development of the fRILI by the prophylactic regimen. This delay is considered to be advantageous as well since a rapid formation of the fRILI can be delayed (and mitigated) allowing the liver remnant to compensate for the fRILI. However, although appropriately powered, the study should be understood as a pilot due to the small sample size. To compensate for the rebound of the fRILI after cessation of the prophylactic regimen and for a better understanding of the dynamics of the fRILI, a study concept with a prolonged course for the prophylactic regimen is planned.

RILI remains a challenge in the treatment of liver malignancies by radiotherapy (whether percutaneous, interstitial or by radio-embolization) because it may eventually translate into RILD or REILD. Further on, life-threatening VOD associated with combined-modality induced liver disease occurs in 5–60% of patients undergoing BMT [18,23,26]. For this reason, the potentially protective effects of a number of treatments including low-dose LMWH, PTX and UDCA have been evaluated. Although the efficacy appears equivocal in some studies [14,15,16,17,18,19,20,21,28] (Table 1), we determined that the combination of low-dose LMWH, PTX and UDCA appeared to be the most promising option for further evaluation with BT. We believe that our success in showing a benefit in ameliorating fRILI with this combination is based on the following factors: a highly homogeneous patient cohort; attention to patient compliance to the prophylactic regimen; and direct measurement of damage to the liver parenchyma rather than clinical endpoints.

The treatment course of 8 weeks for the medication was determined on the assumption that occurrence of RILD and fRILI

peaks around 2 months after radiation-exposure [5,6,7,25]. However, our findings suggest that the radiation-induced injury to the liver structures and cell endothelial continues beyond 8 weeks and that discontinuation of the medication at this time allows the development of a veno-occlusive state/liver cell dysfunction. Endothelial cell damage, which triggers local thrombotic mechanisms, leading to microvascular flow insufficiency, production of cytotoxic substances, and ultimately hepatocellular necrosis, has been thought to be an early event in the development of RILD/VOD [5,10,11,30,31]. The current evidence indicates that PTX, low-dose LMWH and UDCA may act through a variety of mechanisms to alleviate these effects. PTX, for example, down regulates tumor-necrosis factor-α (TNF-α), a prime suspect in either the initiation or amplification of tissue injury following radiation. PTX also stimulates vascular endothelial production of non-inflammatory prostaglandins of the E- and I-series, enhancing loco-regional blood flow and promoting thrombolysis [16].

LMWHs are assumed to prevent subsequent thrombosis of hepatic venules after endothelial damage and therefore decrease the risk of VOD/RILD [18].

By oral administration of UDCA the concentration of potentially liver toxic hydrophobic bile acids can be reduced [32]. Several *in vitro* studies suggest that potential attenuating effects of UDCA on the pathogenesis of VOD is achieved through the down-regulation of inflammatory cytokine such as TNF-α and interleukin-1 [33]. These cytokines not only induce and amplify liver damage but are also associated with apoptosis in endothelial cells [34] and the development of VOD. UDCA also appears to have a direct effect on programmed-cell death, inhibiting apoptosis and protecting against the membrane damaging effects associated with hydrophobic bile acids in both hepatocytes and non-liver cells [35].

The rationale for this combined treatment approach is based on the assumption that LMWH, PTX and UDCA, which act through a variety of different mechanisms, may act synergistically or in a complimentary fashion to protect the liver [26,27,28]; although further study is needed to fully evaluate this hypothesis. However, based on the low toxicity profile of these medications, we believe

Table 5. Covariate analysis of minimal mean hepatic tolerance dose 6 weeks after BT (per protocol, n = 22).

Covariate*	p-value (group influence)	p-value (co-variate influence)
Sex (m/f)	0.015	0.458
Age (y)	0.016	0.864
Weight (kg)	0.010	0.117
Height (cm)	0.011	0.485
ECOG at baseline (0 and 1 vs 2)	0.008	0.310
EQ5D visual analogue score	0.015	0.868
History of liver surgery	0.007	0.064
Steatosis hepatis	0.014	0.845
Diabetes mellitus	0.015	0.627
Chemotherapy pre treatment	0.012	0.373
Used chemotherapeutic agents		
Oxaliplatin	0.013	0.991
Irinotecan	0.011	0.327
Biologicals	0.012	0.459
Number of treated metastases	0.013	0.681
Maximum diamter of metastases (mm)	0.023	0.669
Clinical target volume (cm³)	0.013	0.815
Liver volume (cm³)	0.018	0.937
Interval from BT to 6 weeks FU (days)	0.008	0.258
Liver volume with a dose exposure >10 Gy (%)	0.013	0.598
Chemotherapy during follow-up	0.015	0.191
Bilirubin baseline	0.030	0.401
Albumin baseline	0.020	0.784
Aspartate transaminase baseline	0.025	0.263
Alanine transaminase baseline	0.006	0.092
Cholinesterase baseline	0.013	0.425
Gamma glutamyltransferase baseline	0.012	0.317
Glutamate dehydrogenase baseline	0.011	0.352
International normalized ratio baseline	0.008	0.783
Interleukin 6 baseline	0.030	0.401
Fibrinogen baseline	0.002	0.232
Factor VIII activity baseline	0.005	0.615
Protein C activity baseline	0.004	0.868
Protein S activity baseline	0.004	0.831
von Willebrand factor activity baseline	0.004	0.763
Antithrombin III activity baseline	0.008	0.261

*Two-way ANOVA for categorical factors, ANCOVA for metric covariables.

that this initial approach can be justified. Although the patient numbers are small, the absence of severe toxicities acccords with experience of other published data [15,16,17,19,20,21,28].

Regarding changes of laboratory values, no clinically relevant (grade 3/4) toxicities were observed. The observed slight increases (varying over time and group) of fibrinogen, factor-VIII-activity, protein-S-activity and von-Willebrand-factor-activity correspond most likely to an unspecific increase in acute-phase proteins after radiotherapy or/and to a consequence of radiation-induced endothelial damage of the hepatic veins and sinuses with subsequent platelet aggregation. Regarding the course of liver specific laboratory paramters after BT, it might be argued that the

induced fRILI was possibly too small to induce a significant overall increase of these parameters. However, the slight but significant increase of aspartate transaminase in the control group indicates a parenchymal damage. Interestingly, this increase was not seen in the treatment group, indicating a decreased parenchymal damage under preventive medication.

The primary endpoint in our analysis is based on a surrogate i.e. fRILI visualized and quantified using hepatobiliary contrast agent (Gd-EOB-DTPA)-enhanced MRI. Hepatobiliary contrast agents differ from other gadolinium chelates in that they are selectively taken up by functioning hepatocytes through an organic-anion-transporter-polypeptide (mainly OATP1B1 and 3) and excreted into the bile by the multidrug-resistance-protein-2. For Gd-EOB-DTPA, the biliary excretion rate is approximately 50% in humans [36,37]. Regardless of the mechanism of damage to liver, the hepatobiliary contrast media in functionally altered liver parenchyma is significantly reduced [38]. This is also true for fRILI since a loss of uptake of hepatobiliary contrast media is clearly evident in the liver parenchyma adjacent to the clinical target volume after local radiotherapy (Figure 2) [6,7]. Importantly, an agreement has been found between the histopathological evidence of fRILI/VOD and loss of hepatocellular uptake of hepatobiliary contrast agent [24].

Unlike the reduced uptake of hepatobiliary contrast agents in sinusoidal-obstruction-syndrome observed after platinum-containing chemotherapy (which is reticular in geometry and generalized all over the liver) [39], the reduced uptake of hepatobiliary contrast media after BT is focal, homogenous and circumferential around the clinical target volume (Figure 1) [6,7]. Thus, we believe that we can exclude underlying sinusoidal-obstruction-syndrome as a confounder of our results. Additionally, the history of platinum-containing chemotherapy was equal between the groups and without influence on the endpoint.

We suggest that our study results can be transferred to other established radiation treatment methods of liver malignancies such as ^{90}Y-radioembolization. According to conversion calculations, the dose ranges in the liver parenchyma associated with ^{90}Y-radioembolization and BT are comparable, if re-calculated with respect to the standard fractionation. We therefore hypothesize that preventive treatment approaches against RILD/REILD should be equally effective for both ^{90}Y-radioembolization and BT.

Conclusions

In summary, our results show a highly significant reduction in fRILI after BT of colorectal liver metastases in patients who received low-dose LMWH, PTX and UDCA. Further on, we believe that these findings can be adopted for the prevention of radiation-induced liver damage after other radiotherapeutic approaches as ^{90}Y-radioembolization and that further clinical studies in this area are warranted.

Supporting Information

Table S1   ECOG, EQ5D dimensions and EQ5D VAS, baseline and follow-up; group comparison (per-protocol only).

Checklist S1   Consort Checklist regarding the present study.

Protocol S1   Study protocol as submitted to the competent authorities.

Author Contributions

Contributed to the writing of the manuscript: MS PW JR. Statistical planning and analysis: SK RD MS. Conceived and designed the experiments: MS RS RD BS JR. Performed the experiments: MS RS RD PH GG JR. Analyzed the data: MS RD KM MP RS SK. Contributed reagents/materials/analysis tools: PH GG SK.

References

1. Boda-Heggemann J, Dinter D, Weiss C, Frauenfeld A, Siebenlist K, et al. (2012) Hypofractionated image-guided breath-hold SABR (stereotactic ablative body radiotherapy) of liver metastases–clinical results. Radiation oncology 7: 92.
2. Ricke J, Mohnike K, Pech M, Seidensticker M, Ruhl R, et al. (2010) Local response and impact on survival after local ablation of liver metastases from colorectal carcinoma by computed tomography-guided high-dose-rate brachytherapy. International journal of radiation oncology, biology, physics 78: 479–485.
3. Seidensticker R, Denecke T, Kraus P, Seidensticker M, Mohnike K, et al. (2012) Matched-pair comparison of radioembolization plus best supportive care versus best supportive care alone for chemotherapy refractory liver-dominant colorectal metastases. Cardiovascular and interventional radiology 35: 1066–1073.
4. Emami B, Lyman J, Brown A, Coia L, Goitein M, et al. (1991) Tolerance of normal tissue to therapeutic irradiation. International journal of radiation oncology, biology, physics 21: 109–122.
5. Lawrence TS, Robertson JM, Anscher MS, Jirtle RL, Ensminger WD, et al. (1995) Hepatic toxicity resulting from cancer treatment. International journal of radiation oncology, biology, physics 31: 1237–1248.
6. Ricke J, Seidensticker M, Ludemann L, Pech M, Wieners G, et al. (2005) In vivo assessment of the tolerance dose of small liver volumes after single-fraction HDR irradiation. International journal of radiation oncology, biology, physics 62: 776–784.
7. Seidensticker M, Seidensticker R, Mohnike K, Wybranski C, Kalinski T, et al. (2011) Quantitative in vivo assessment of radiation injury of the liver using Gd-EOB-DTPA enhanced MRI: tolerance dose of small liver volumes. Radiation oncology 6: 40.
8. McDonald GB, Sharma P, Matthews DE, Shulman HM, Thomas ED (1985) The clinical course of 53 patients with venocclusive disease of the liver after marrow transplantation. Transplantation 39: 603–608.
9. Sangro B, Gil-Alzugaray B, Rodriguez J, Sola I, Martinez-Cuesta A, et al. (2008) Liver disease induced by radioembolization of liver tumors: description and possible risk factors. Cancer 112: 1538–1546.
10. Farthing MJ, Clark ML, Sloane JP, Powles RL, McElwain TJ (1982) Liver disease after bone marrow transplantation. Gut 23: 465–474.
11. Fajardo LF, Colby TV (1980) Pathogenesis of veno-occlusive liver disease after radiation. Archives of pathology & laboratory medicine 104: 584–588.
12. Reed GB, Jr., Cox AJ, Jr (1966) The human liver after radiation injury. A form of veno-occlusive disease. The American journal of pathology 48: 597–611.
13. Shulman HM, Gown AM, Nugent DJ (1987) Hepatic veno-occlusive disease after bone marrow transplantation. Immunohistochemical identification of the

material within occluded central venules. The American journal of pathology 127: 549–558.
14. Attal M, Huguet F, Rubie H, Charlet JP, Schlaifer D, et al. (1993) Prevention of regimen-related toxicities after bone marrow transplantation by pentoxifylline: a prospective, randomized trial. Blood 82: 732–736.
15. Attal M, Huguet F, Rubie H, Huynh A, Charlet JP, et al. (1992) Prevention of hepatic veno-occlusive disease after bone marrow transplantation by continuous infusion of low-dose heparin: a prospective, randomized trial. Blood 79: 2834–2840.
16. Bianco JA, Appelbaum FR, Nemunaitis J, Almgren J, Andrews F, et al. (1991) Phase I-II trial of pentoxifylline for the prevention of transplant-related toxicities following bone marrow transplantation. Blood 78: 1205–1211.
17. Essell JH, Schroeder MT, Harman GS, Halvorson R, Lew V, et al. (1998) Ursodiol prophylaxis against hepatic complications of allogeneic bone marrow transplantation. A randomized, double-blind, placebo-controlled trial. Annals of internal medicine 128: 975–981.
18. Forrest DL, Thompson K, Dorcas VG, Couban SH, Pierce R (2003) Low molecular weight heparin for the prevention of hepatic veno-occlusive disease (VOD) after hematopoietic stem cell transplantation: a prospective phase II study. Bone marrow transplantation 31: 1143–1149.
19. Ohashi K, Tanabe J, Watanabe R, Tanaka T, Sakamaki H, et al. (2000) The Japanese multicenter open randomized trial of ursodeoxycholic acid prophylaxis for hepatic veno-occlusive disease after stem cell transplantation. American journal of hematology 64: 32–38.
20. Or R, Nagler A, Shpilberg O, Elad S, Naparstek E, et al. (1996) Low molecular weight heparin for the prevention of veno-occlusive disease of the liver in bone marrow transplantation patients. Transplantation 61: 1067–1071.
21. Ruutu T, Eriksson B, Remes K, Juvonen E, Volin L, et al. (2002) Ursodeoxycholic acid for the prevention of hepatic complications in allogeneic stem cell transplantation. Blood 100: 1977–1983.
22. Clift RA, Bianco JA, Appelbaum FR, Buckner CD, Singer JW, et al. (1993) A randomized controlled trial of pentoxifylline for the prevention of regimen-related toxicities in patients undergoing allogeneic marrow transplantation. Blood 82: 2025–2030.
23. McDonald GB, Sharma P, Matthews DE, Shulman HM, Thomas ED (1984) Venocclusive disease of the liver after bone marrow transplantation: diagnosis, incidence, and predisposing factors. Hepatology 4: 116–122.
24. Seidensticker M, Burak M, Kalinski T, Garlipp B, Koelble K, et al. (2014) Radiation-Induced Liver Damage: Correlation of Histopathology with Hepatobiliary Magnetic Resonance Imaging, a Feasibility Study. Cardiovascular and interventional radiology.

25. Wybranski C, Seidensticker M, Mohnike K, Kropf S, Wust P, et al. (2009) In vivo assessment of dose volume and dose gradient effects on the tolerance dose of small liver volumes after single-fraction high-dose-rate 192Ir irradiation. Radiation research 172: 598–606.

26. Shulman HM, Hinterberger W (1992) Hepatic veno-occlusive disease–liver toxicity syndrome after bone marrow transplantation. Bone marrow transplantation 10: 197–214.

27. Lakshminarayanan S, Sahdev I, Goyal M, Vlachos A, Atlas M, et al. (2010) Low incidence of hepatic veno-occlusive disease in pediatric patients undergoing hematopoietic stem cell transplantation attributed to a combination of intravenous heparin, oral glutamine, and ursodiol at a single transplant institution. Pediatric transplantation 14: 618–621.

28. Park SH, Lee MH, Lee H, Kim HS, Kim K, et al. (2002) A randomized trial of heparin plus ursodiol vs. heparin alone to prevent hepatic veno-occlusive disease after hematopoietic stem cell transplantation. Bone marrow transplantation 29: 137–143.

29. Lee JH, Lee KH, Kim S, Lee JS, Kim WK, et al. (1998) Relevance of proteins C and S, antithrombin III, von Willebrand factor, and factor VIII for the development of hepatic veno-occlusive disease in patients undergoing allogeneic bone marrow transplantation: a prospective study. Bone marrow transplantation 22: 883–888.

30. Catani L, Gugliotta L, Vianelli N, Nocentini F, Baravelli S, et al. (1996) Endothelium and bone marrow transplantation. Bone marrow transplantation 17: 277–280.

31. Geraci JP, Mariano MS (1993) Radiation hepatology of the rat: parenchymal and nonparenchymal cell injury. Radiation research 136: 205–213.

32. Kowdley KV (2000) Ursodeoxycholic acid therapy in hepatobiliary disease. The American journal of medicine 108: 481–486.

33. Neuman MG, Shear NH, Bellentani S, Tiribelli C (1998) Role of cytokines in ethanol-induced cytotoxicity in vitro in Hep G2 cells. Gastroenterology 115: 157–166.

34. Lindner H, Holler E, Ertl B, Multhoff G, Schreglmann M, et al. (1997) Peripheral blood mononuclear cells induce programmed cell death in human endothelial cells and may prevent repair: role of cytokines. Blood 89: 1931–1938.

35. Rodrigues CM, Fan G, Ma X, Kren BT, Steer CJ (1998) A novel role for ursodeoxycholic acid in inhibiting apoptosis by modulating mitochondrial membrane perturbation. The Journal of clinical investigation 101: 2790–2799.

36. Pascolo L, Cupelli F, Anelli PL, Lorusso V, Visigalli M, et al. (1999) Molecular mechanisms for the hepatic uptake of magnetic resonance imaging contrast agents. Biochemical and biophysical research communications 257: 746–752.

37. Schuhmann-Giampieri G, Schmitt-Willich H, Press WR, Negishi C, Weinmann HJ, et al. (1992) Preclinical evaluation of Gd-EOB-DTPA as a contrast agent in MR imaging of the hepatobiliary system. Radiology 183: 59–64.

38. Watanabe H, Kanematsu M, Goshima S, Kondo H, Onozuka M, et al. (2011) Staging hepatic fibrosis: comparison of gadoxetate disodium-enhanced and diffusion-weighted MR imaging–preliminary observations. Radiology 259: 142–150.

39. Shin NY, Kim MJ, Lim JS, Park MS, Chung YE, et al. (2012) Accuracy of gadoxetic acid-enhanced magnetic resonance imaging for the diagnosis of sinusoidal obstruction syndrome in patients with chemotherapy-treated colorectal liver metastases. European radiology 22: 864–871.

16

Attitudes about Tuberculosis Prevention in the Elimination Phase: A Survey among Physicians in Germany

Christian Gutsfeld[1,2◕], Ioana D. Olaru[1◕], Oliver Vollrath[3], Christoph Lange[1,4,5,6]*

1 Division of Clinical Infectious Diseases, German Center for Infection Research Tuberculosis Unit, Research Center Borstel, Borstel, Germany, **2** Department of Psychosomatic Medicine, Sachsenklinik, Bad Lausick, Germany, **3** Institute of Medical Informatics and Statistics, University Hospitals Schleswig-Holstein, Campus Kiel, Kiel, Germany, **4** International Health/Infectious Diseases, University of Lübeck, Lübeck, Germany, **5** Department of Internal Medicine, University of Namibia School of Medicine, Windhoek, Namibia, **6** Department of Medicine, Karolinska Institute, Stockholm, Sweden

Abstract

Background: Targeted and stringent measures of tuberculosis prevention are necessary to achieve the goal of tuberculosis elimination in countries of low tuberculosis incidence.

Methods: We ascertained the knowledge about tuberculosis risk factors and stringency of tuberculosis prevention measures by a standardized questionnaire among physicians in Germany involved in the care of individuals from classical risk groups for tuberculosis.

Results: 510 physicians responded to the online survey. Among 16 risk factors immunosuppressive therapy, HIV-infection and treatment with TNF-antagonist were thought to be the most important risk factors for the development of tuberculosis in Germany. Exposure to a patient with tuberculosis ranked on the 10th position. In the event of a positive tuberculin-skin-test or interferon-γ release assay only 50%, 40%, 36% and 25% of physicians found that preventive chemotherapy was indicated for individuals undergoing tumor necrosis factor-antagonist therapy, close contacts of tuberculosis patients, HIV-infected individuals and migrants, respectively.

Conclusions: A remarkably low proportion of individuals with latent infection with *Mycobacterium tuberculosis* belonging to classical risk groups for tuberculosis are considered candidates for preventive chemotherapy in Germany. Better knowledge about the risk for tuberculosis in different groups and more stringent and targeted preventive interventions will probably be necessary to achieve tuberculosis elimination in Germany.

Editor: Antonio G. Pacheco, FIOCRUZ, Brazil

Funding: The study was funded by the German Center for Infection Research (DZIF). The funders had no role in study design, data collection and analysis, decision to publish or preparation of the manuscript.

Competing Interests: The authors have declared that no competing interests exist.

* Email: clange@fz-borstel.de

◕ These authors contributed equally to this work.

Introduction

Tuberculosis (TB) remains a major global health problem. In 2012, an estimated 8.6 million people developed TB and 1.3 million died from the disease (including 320,000 deaths among HIV-positive people) [1]. However in most of the low-prevalence countries in Western Europe and North America overall notification rates for TB have been declining for the last decades. With a total incidence of 5.3 cases per 100,000 population in 2011, TB has become a rare disease in Germany [2].

Due to the current absence of vaccines for the prevention of TB with a higher efficiency than the *Mycobacterium bovis* Bacille Calmette Guérin (BCG) vaccine, TB control primarily relies on the prevention of transmission of active TB by identification and treatment of patients with active disease. In order to further reduce

transmissions rates and ultimately eradicate TB, low incidence countries such as Germany eventually rely on contact investigations by public health services and physicians for active case finding and identification of contacts with latent infection with *Mycobacterium tuberculosis* (LTBI) [3,4].

In clinical practice, LTBI is defined by the presence of an adaptive immune response to antigens specific for *M. tuberculosis*, ascertained by a positive tuberculin-skin-test (TST) or interferon-γ release assay (IGRA) result, in the absence of active TB [4]. According to the Infection Protection Act (IFSG) in Germany close contacts of TB patients are required to be subject to a TST or IGRA testing by the public health authorities [5]. In case of positive test results national recommendations suggest preventive chemotherapy with isoniazid for a duration of nine months [6]. A contact person with LTBI will usually be referred to a private physician with the recommendation to initiate preventive chemotherapy [7]. In contrast to neighboring Switzerland [8], most of the contacts with LTBI referred to private pulmonologists or general practitioners in Germany by the public health authorities are left untreated. A recent survey in the state of Lower Saxony demonstrated that only 29% of healthy contacts with a positive TST or IGRA test result at the time of contact investigation received preventive chemotherapy [9]. In a large observational cohort study performed by the public health authorities in the city of Hamburg, even under study conditions only 21% of contacts with LTBI received preventive chemotherapy [10]. The low acceptance of preventive chemotherapy contradicts the expenses and efforts by the public health authorities in Germany to identify individuals at risk for the future development of TB.

To develop a basis for improvement of TB prevention we aimed to gain a better insight about the knowledge of physicians working within the German health care system about risk factors for TB and their attitude towards preventive chemotherapy.

Materials and Methods

To evaluate the knowledge and attitude of physician decision makers in Germany about current methods for the diagnosis of LTBI and preventive chemotherapy, we developed a standardized questionnaire that was initially revised by two independent international reviewers. Feasibility of this survey tool was evaluated in an anonymized pilot study involving distribution of paper questionnaires to 500 physicians. The return rate by mail was 130 questionnaires (26%). Results from the feasibility study were not included in the final analysis. Upon the experience with the pilot survey, it was decided to distribute the questionnaire by email via an internet-link leading to a web-based survey platform (www.surveymonkey.com). Instructions about the study background, design and participation were found in the study invitation and on the web-based survey platform. In February 2012 email invitations were send to physicians from the registries of the German Society for Pulmonology (DGP e.V.), the German working group of private physicians caring for HIV-infected patients (DAGNÄ e.V.), the network for rheumatic diseases (DGRh), the German network of occupational medicine physicians (ArbMedNet), and to TB officers at municipal or regional health care departments in Germany. Physicians were asked to participate in the survey within 30 days of notice. In order to ensure the participants anonymity the gathered results were encrypted by an independent code system.

The web-based questionnaire was composed of 8 main parts with 26 questions and a free commenting section for further remarks:

Part 1: Six single item questions about specific data of participating physicians (age, working area, expertise and patients collective).

Part 2: Three single item questions about past, current and future use and evaluation of diagnostic tools for LTBI such as TST and/or IGRAs.

Part 3: One multiple answer question with the opportunity to select three risk groups among sixteen options to estimate the risk of patients at risk for developing TB if diagnostic tools are positive.

Part 4: Five single item questions concerning risk groups and the implementation of national guidelines towards LTBI (offering testing and treatment to patients at risk).

Part 5: One single item question about favored therapy regimes for patients with LTBI.

Part 6: Nine questions about the attitudes of physicians towards TB prevention in Germany using six-point adjectival scales that included the response categories full and minimal agreement.

Part 7: One single item question about the necessity of improvement towards management of LTBI using a ranking scale in order to prioritize between diagnostics, period of therapy and effectiveness.

Eligible respondents included physicians who were involved in the diagnosis and/or therapy of LTBI. We excluded physicians who had no contact to a suspected case LTBI within the last 12 months.

Statistical analysis

The collected data consisted only of categorical variables. They were summarized using frequencies and percentages.

The paired sample McNemar Test was used to test the difference of proportions between past and future application of several diagnostic devices by German physicians (sample size N = 510). All tests were two-sided. A difference was considered statistically significant when the p-value was smaller than 0.05. All p-values were adjusted according to Bonferroni.

In addition to the p-values 95% confidence intervals (95% CI) for differences between past and future applications were calculated.

All data were analyzed using SPSS 19.0 for Windows (SPSS Inc., Chicago, Illinois, USA) and BIAS 9.16 for Windows (epsilon-Verlag; Dr. rer. med H. Ackermann, Goethe-University Frankfurt/Main, Germany).

The study was reviewed and approved by the Ethical Board of the University of Lübeck (#14-167). The study was a voluntary survey of German physicians and all data entered and analyzed were anonymous. There were no patients involved and consent from physicians providing data anonymously was not required. We have been in touch with the Ethical Board at the University of Lübeck and have received the written information that the Ethical Board of the University of Lübeck has no reservations against publication of the study results.

Results

Characteristics of German physicians participating in the survey

We contacted 1840 pulmonologists and 354 public health officers directly via email requesting participation in the survey. In addition, approximately 1000 rheumatologists, physicians caring for HIV-infected patients and physicians working in occupational medicine were addressed via the DGRh, DAGNÄ and ArbMed-Net email registers. 510 physicians responded to the survey (table 1). Only 15.2% (n = 76) of participating physicians were under the age of 40 and 6.0% (n = 30) were older than 60 years of age. More than one third (38.5%/n = 190) of the participating physicians were working in a hospital setting and almost one quarter (23.9%/n = 118) were working in a private practice. One-hundred and thirty-four physicians (26.3%) were employed as TB officers at municipal or regional health care departments and 11.5% (n = 55) of the physicians were working in the field of occupational medicine. Overall, 250 participants (49.0%) were specialized as pulmonologists.

Experience and future intention to use different tests for diagnosing LTBI

The changes of the attitude towards the methods for the diagnosis LTBI are shown in table 2. Physicians intend to use the

Table 1. Characteristics of German physicians participating in the survey.

Physicians data		Frequency	Percent (%)	n
Age	21–30 years	8	1.6	501
	31–40 years	68	13.6	
	41–50 years	205	40.9	
	51–60 years	190	37.9	
	>60 years	30	6.0	
Work Place	Established practitioner	118	23.9	493
	Teaching hospital	99	20.1	
	Non-teaching Hospital	49	10.0	
	University Hospital	42	8.5	
	Other	185	37.5	
Specialty	Internal Medicine	236	49.2	480
	General Practitioners	26	5.4	
	Occupational Medicine	55	11.5	
	Other	163	33.9	
Subspecialisation	Respiratory Medicine	250	49.0	510
	Public Health Medicine	134	26.3	
	Other	81	15.9	
	none	45	8.8	

ELISPOT IGRA (T-Spot.TB test) significantly more often and the TST significantly less often in the future when compared to the past. There is no significant change in the anticipated behavior for the use of the ELISA IGRA (QFT-GIT test) which is already in frequent use in the county.

Estimated risk by physicians for persons at risk to develop TB

When physicians were asked to prioritize groups with the highest risk for the future development of TB, patients with an immunosuppressive therapy, HIV-seropositive patients and pa-tients with a TNF-antagonist-therapy, were ranked on positions 1–3 among 16 risks groups (figure 1-right). Interestingly, contact persons of patients diagnosed with TB were ranked on position 10/16. Physicians' attitude of groups at risk for the future development of TB and data from the published literature (figure 1-left) did not match.

Intensity of testing vs. intensity of treatment

The majority of physicians recommend immunodiagnostic testing for LTBI (figure 2). For close contacts of patients with TB 94% of pulmonologist and 91% of non-pulmonologists suggest

Table 2. Experience and future intention to use different tests for diagnosing latent infection with Mycobacterium tuberculosis.

Diagnostic device	Past	Future	Difference	95% CI for difference	p-value	p-value adjusted
	p1	p2	p1–p2			
Tuberculin-Skin-Test	57.1%	34.1%	23%	[18.6; 27.3]	<0.001*	<0.001*
IGRA QuantiFeron Gold in tube	69.4%	67.7%	1.7%	[-1.2; 4.7]	0.298	1.000
IGRA T-Spot.TB	27.5%	32.2%	-4.7%	[-7.9; -1.5]	0.005*	0.0196*
Other technologies (e.g. flow cytometry)	5.9%	4.5%	1.4%	[-0.2; 2.9]	0.143	0.572

The sample size was N = 510.
p1: percentage of physicians using the corresponding test in the past.
p2: percentage of physicians using the corresponding test in future.
p1–p2: difference of percentages p1 and p2.
95% CI: 95% confidence interval for difference.
p-value: paired sample McNemar Test to test the difference of proportion between past and future application of several diagnostic devices by german physicians.
p-value adjusted: adjusted p-value according to Bonferroni.
The asterisk (*) indicates significant differences.

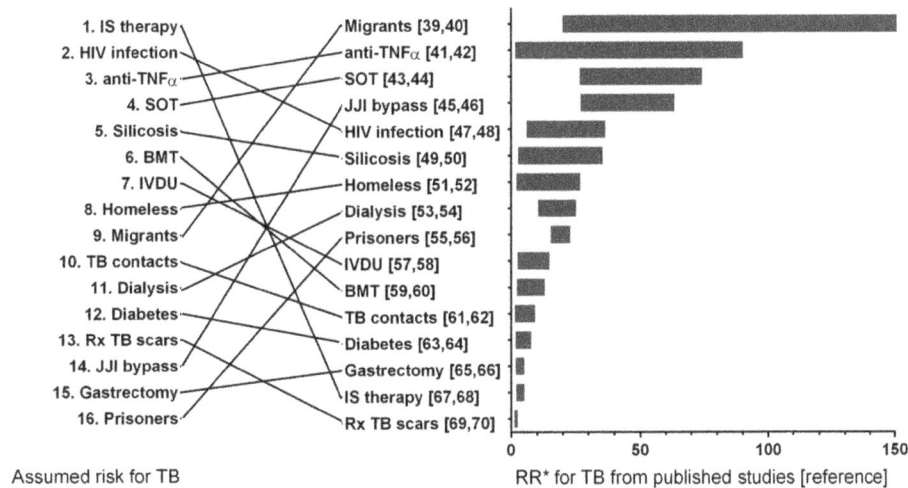

Figure 1. Subjective ranking (1 = highest risk; 16 = lowest risk) of risk groups for the future development of tuberculosis according to German physicians involved in LTBI testing (left) in comparison with the range of reported relative risks (RR) for the development of tuberculosis in the same risk groups according to published studies ranked according to the highest risk reported (right). References are shown in square brackets (max. to min.) [39–70]. *Risk is expressed as relative risk for cohort studies or controlled trials, odds ratio for case-control studies and incidence rate ratio when incidence in cases was compared to that in the general population. In the case of migrants the highest value for risk is not plotted on the graph (relative risk of 315.5). TNFα – tumor necrosis factor α, SOT – solid organ transplant, JJI bypass – jejunoileal bypass, IVDU – intravenous drug users, BMT – bone marrow transplant, IS therapy – immunosuppressive therapy, Rx – radiological.

testing. Similar results can also be observed for other risk groups such as patients undergoing TNF-antagonist therapy or migrants. However, there is a substantial discrepancy between the intention to test and the intention to treat. Physicians in Germany intend to treat only 50% of individuals undergoing TNF-antagonists therapy, 40% of close contacts of patients with TB, 36% of individuals with HIV-infection and 25% of migrants with a positive result in the TST and/or IGRA. Remarkably, for most risk groups no difference can be identified in the attitudes of pulmonologists vs. non-pulmonologists towards the intention to treat. The only significant difference was found towards individuals with HIV-infection and those undergoing immunosuppressive therapy.

Choice of preventive treatment of latent infection with *M. tuberculosis*

Physicians were able to choose between five different TB preventive treatment regimens or enter manually a treatment regime of their choice. Three hundred and sixty-two of 510 (71%) physicians answered the questions. The preferred preventive treatment is isoniazid for 9 months (n = 194; 54.4%), followed by isoniazid for 6 months (n = 85; 23.5%) and treatment with the combination of daily treatment with isoniazid and rifampicin for 3 months (n = 46; 12.7%). Fifteen physicians (4.1%) favored daily treatment with isoniazid monotherapy for 12 months and 5 physicians (1.4%) daily treatment with rifampicin monotherapy for 4 months. Fourteen physicians (3.9%) entered alternative treatment options.

Attitudes of decision makers towards TB prevention

Participants had the opportunity to express their attitudes by answering nine questions (q1–q9) concerning TB prevention and treatment (table 3). While 81.1% of the physicians agree that immunodiagnostic testing for LTBI in risk groups and treatment of individuals with a positive test result is an efficient method of TB prevention, more than 30% disagree to the principle "intention to

test is intention to treat!". The physicians who responded in the survey agreed that more than 40% of physicians and more than 55% of patients have no insight into the efficacy of preventive treatment. A large proportion of physicians (58.4%) and patients (69.0%) are thought to be hesitant to enter treatment for fear of adverse drug events.

Measures to improve TB prevention

Finally, physicians were asked to prioritize three statements concerning optimizing TB prevention. Most physicians (n = 173; 57.5%) favored improvements in the diagnostics of LTBI, while there was an equal proportion of physicians that favored a stronger efficacy of preventive treatment regimens (n = 129; 41%) or improvements to shorten the duration of preventive chemotherapy (n = 117; 39%).

Discussion

TB has become a rare disease in Germany and most other Western European Countries. As the World Health Organization (WHO) and the European Center for Disease Prevention and Control (ECDC) now aim for TB elimination [11,12], prevention of TB will focus especially on risk groups. However, currently available tests are poor prognostic markers for the identification of individuals who will develop TB in the future and the definitions of "risk groups for TB" are not universally applicable [13,14].

We evaluated the knowledge about TB risk factors and attitudes towards TB prevention among physicians involved in TB prevention and care in Germany. The key findings of this study are a surprisingly low proportion of individuals with LTBI belonging to classical risk groups for TB receiving preventive therapy and substantial gaps in the knowledge on the risk for TB in a country of low TB incidence resulting in uncertainties and non-stringent management of TB prevention.

Pulmonologists are more likely to note that physicians have no insight into the efficacy of preventive therapy than non-pulmo-

Table 3. Attitudes of German physicians involved in LTBI testing and/or the decision for the initiation of tuberculosis preventive chemotherapy.

Questions towards decision makers concerning tuberculosis prevention	Agreement			Chi-Square Test p-value
	Pulmonologists	Non Pulmonologists	All	
q1 Testing persons at risk with TST/IGRA and treating individuals with a positive test result is an efficient method of prevention.	78.3% (n = 148)	84.1% (n = 143)	81.1% (n = 291)	0.179
q2 "Intention to test is intention to treat!"	67.4% (n = 128)	71.6% (n = 121)	69.4% (n = 249)	0.423
q3 A risk analysis through TST and/or IGRA should be performed with all individuals belonging to a risk group	66.8% (n = 125)	68.3% (n = 114)	67.5% (n = 239)	0.821
q4 "Tuberculosis is on the decline in Germany and prevention is not necessary anymore!"	14.9% (n = 28)	14.4% (n = 24)	14.7% (n = 52)	1.000
q5 "A positive test result (TST/IGRA) has no significance to me!"	19.4% (n = 36)	14.3% (n = 24)	16.9% (n = 60)	0.256
q6 Physicians have no insight into the efficacy of preventive treatment	50.0% (n = 94)	30.5% (n = 50)	40.9% (n = 144)	0.0002*
q7 Physicians avoid to administer preventive treatment for the risks of side effects	61.9% (n = 117)	54.5% (n = 91)	58.4% (n = 208)	0.163
q8 Patients have no insight into the efficacy of preventive treatment	56.8% (n = 108)	54.5% (n = 91)	55.8% (n = 199)	0.671
q9 Patients hesitate to enter preventive treatment for the fear of side effects	70.2% (n = 134)	67.7% (n = 113)	69% (n = 247)	0.648

nologists. This is likely due to the better knowledge of pulmonologists on tuberculosis, compared to non-pulmonologists. Although pulmonologists are more motivated to test HIV-infected individuals and other immunocompromised hosts for LTBI compared to non-pulmonologists, and they are better aware of the gaps in TB control in Germany, stringency to provide preventive chemotherapy for individuals with positive test results is lacking in all groups of professionals.

In the absence of available data from Germany, national recommendations for TB contact tracing [7] report that people living with HIV-infection (PLWH) have a risk of developing active TB of 35–162 per 1000 person-years. However these data originate from studies conducted before the advent of modern antiretroviral therapies (ART) [15] and refer to high prevalence countries of TB, where *M. tuberculosis* exposure for PLWH is much higher than in Germany. Results from the Swiss HIV cohort reported a lower incidence of active TB of 16 per 1000 person-years in TST positive individuals in the absence of preventive therapy [16]. Furthermore, the country of origin was of substantial importance for the risk of TB in that study. In Switzerland the number of PLWH with a positive TST or IGRA test result who needed to be treated to prevent a case of TB was 4 times higher for migrants from high incidence countries of TB compared to individuals originating from low incidence countries of TB [16]. The lower risk of PLWH for developing active TB in low-prevalence settings is likely related to a decreased risk of *M. tuberculosis* transmission from individuals with active disease, while in high-incidence countries the risk of *M. tuberculosis* exposure is considerably greater.

Additionally, in a low incidence setting, ART initiation leads to a 44–56% risk reduction of active TB [16,17]. PLWH predominantly receive their care from specialized outpatient clinics or private practitioners in Germany. More than 80% of PLWH in the country have suppressed levels of viral replication on ART

[18] and active TB in these patients has become a very rare opportunistic infection [19] even in the absence of preventive therapy. Persistent viral replication was also associated with a higher risk of developing TB in a large French cohort of PLWH [20]. Another recent study reporting on the German HIV cohort describes an important decrease in TB occurrence after ART initiation. The authors also suggest that country of origin and the degree of immunosuppression are also associated with the risk of developing TB. Preventive therapy was given to only a very small fraction of the population and the authors suggest a differentiated approach in ascertaining the risk of future TB and therefore the indication LTBI screening and preventive therapy within this population [21]. It is likely that because of the personal experience of physicians caring for PLWH in Germany caretakers regularly evaluate only two thirds of PLWH for LTBI and only one third of those with a positive TST or IGRA result receives preventive therapy in the present study.

Similarly, the current recommendations for TB contact tracing in Germany describe a relative risk of 37–74 for the development of TB in solid organ transplant recipients. However, in a large retrospective cohort study of lung transplant patients from Germany totaling over 7000 person-years of follow-up, only 5 patients were diagnosed with active TB corresponding to relative risk of 7.5–10 times lower than indicated, in this population [22]. In our survey, only one third of physicians indicated that they offered preventive chemotherapy to immuno-suppressed patients, e.g. solid organ transplant recipients.

Until recently, one of the dogmas of immunodiagnostic testing by TST and IGRAs in individuals from risk groups was "intention to test is intention to treat" [23]. Healthcare workers (HCW) with a positive IGRA test result in countries of low TB incidence were thought to be at risk for the development of TB and were offered preventive chemotherapy. However, there is substantial within-subject variability on serial testing [24] and positive IGRA test

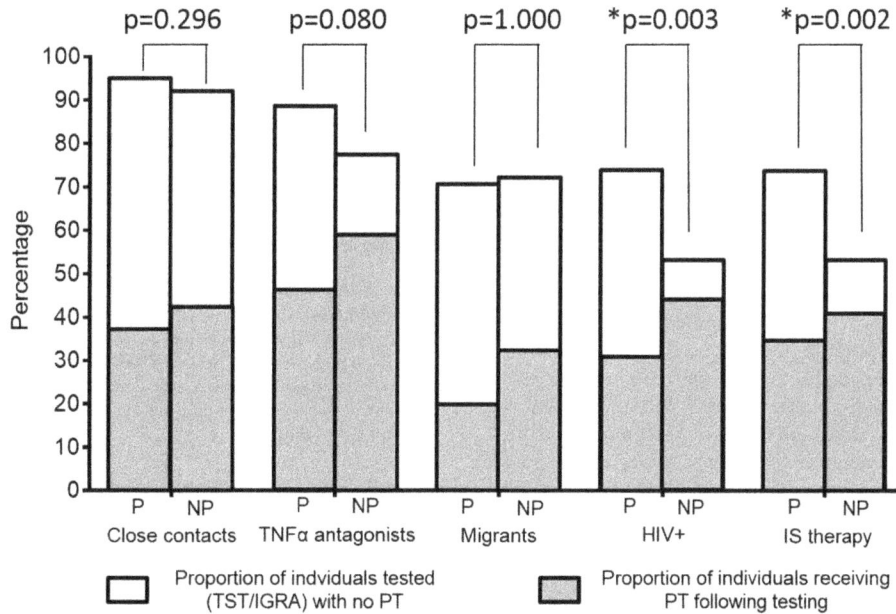

Figure 2. Rate of performed tests (IGRA/TST) and preventive treatment offered in the case of a positive test result in risk groups among pulmonologists and non-pulmonologists involved in TB prevention in Germany. P – pulmonologists; NP – non-pulmonologists; TNFα – tumor necrosis factor α; IS therapy – immunosuppressive therapy, IGRA – interferon gamma release assay; TST – tuberculin skin test, PT – preventive chemotherapy.

results revert to negative in a substantial proportion of HCW in the absence of preventive chemotherapy [25]. In a recent study from North America with more than nine thousand healthcare workers of which 1223 had positive IGRA test results, one third had reversion to a negative test result on follow-up and none of the HCW developed tuberculosis, in the absence of preventive chemotherapy [26]. Therefore the benefit of preventive therapy in HCW with positive IGRA results in the absence of a documented recent exposure to an active case or additional risk factors for TB is unclear. Preventive treatment of HCW with evidence of LTBI without evidence of recent exposure is no more recommended in Germany but can be considered in cases who had a documented contact with an index case, similar to contacts in the general population [27].

National recommendations for TB contact tracing also report that the risk of patients with silicosis to be 30 times elevated [7]. In a study on 118 retired coal miners in Germany, almost 40% with silicosis, approximately 50% had a positive IGRA test result. None of the 90 individuals who were evaluated after 2 years in follow-up developed active tuberculosis in the absence of preventive chemotherapy [28].

More than one third of close contacts of patients with contagious TB can be identified as having LTBI [29]. In the absence of preventive chemotherapy the risk of close contacts with positive TST results to progress to active disease has been estimated around 2–6% during the first 2–3 years after exposure [13,30]. However two studies report progression rates to active TB of 12–13% in close contacts with positive IGRA test results not receiving preventive chemotherapy [10,31]. It is thus possible, that close contacts are the group with the highest risk for the progression to TB in Germany. Other studies also suggest that the risk in contacts of TB patients and particularly in household contacts is underestimated [32]. Given the fact that LTBI testing of close TB contacts is mandatory in Germany according to the Infection Protection Act the low acceptance rate documented in

this survey (Fig. 2), confirming recent observations, is surprising [9,23].

In order to improve TB prevention and to achieve the goal of TB elimination in countries of low TB incidence the indication for preventive chemotherapy should be made on a risk assessment-based approach where the need to screen individuals is prioritised on the basis of the intensity of exposure and susceptibility of individuals for *M. tuberculosis* infection [3]. Additionally, due to the low positive predictive value, LTBI-testing should not be directed at individuals with a low risk of active TB in whom the risks of preventive chemotherapy may outweigh its benefits. It has been suggested that over 95% of individuals with a positive IGRA or TST do not develop active TB during follow-up further supporting targeted testing [33].

Rather surprisingly we found that physicians in Germany did not rank migrants among the groups with a high risk for TB, although it is recognized that individuals coming from high TB prevalence countries who are latently infected might have an increased risk of active TB of more than 13-fold in comparison with migrants without LTBI [34]. Other studies also report insufficient testing coverage of migrants for LTBI [35].

Even though preventive therapy is highly effective in selected populations, acceptance and adherence to a prolonged treatment are less than optimal and adverse effects, although rare, can occur in a small proportion of individuals. Mistrust against preventive strategies might explain the suboptimal acceptance rates for preventive therapy among both patients and prescribing physicians with even lower acceptance rates being recorded among HCW. On the other hand, the long duration of therapy might lead to poor adherence with fewer than half of the individuals started on preventive therapy completing the entire course according to one study [36]. Consequently in the low-prevalence setting, the decision for preventive treatment should be based on an individualized risk-benefit assessment [37,38].

This study has several limitations. Physicians' behavior was not directly analyzed but attitude of behavior was evaluated. It is possible, that actual behavior differs from the stated attitudes. Although the survey was distributed among a large group of decision makers and caretakers of TB patients in Germany from the public health care sector and different clinical areas and 510 physicians completed the online survey, the response rate of the electronic questionnaire was only approximately 20%. Due to the anonymous nature of this web-based survey, no information was available on the physicians who responded or did not respond to the invitation to participate in the study. Consequently, sampling bias cannot be excluded and generalization of the results has to be made with caution. Despite these limitations, this is the largest survey of physicians' attitude towards TB prevention in Germany to date and the results from this survey reflect actual data on acceptance of preventive chemotherapy in this country.

In conclusion, we found great uncertainty about risk factors for tuberculosis among physicians in Germany likely leading to non-stringent behavior in TB prevention. TB prevention could be improved if the definition of TB "risk groups" for LTBI screening and preventive chemotherapy will be re-classified according to data applying to local situations. Immunodiagnostic testing should be limited to risk groups in which a positive test result is associated with a significantly increased risk for developing TB in the future

and significant risk reduction can be achieved by preventive chemotherapies. This will require regional and national surveys rather than applying information from high TB prevalence countries to countries of low TB prevalence and vice versa. This approach could lead to more consequent initiation of preventive therapy following a positive test and avoid unnecessary testing and treatment.

Acknowledgments

The authors are grateful to colleague physicians from the German Society for Pulmonology (DGP e.V.), from the German working group of private physicians caring for HIV-infected patients (DAGNÄ e.V.), from the network for rheumatic diseases (DGRh), from the German network of occupational medicine physicians (ArbMedNet) and to TB officers at municipal or regional health care departments in Germany who participated in the survey.

Author Contributions

Analyzed the data: CG IDO OV CL. Contributed to the writing of the manuscript: CG IDO CL. Contributed to the idea of the manuscript: CG CL. Conceived the manuscript: CG CL. Contributed to the design of the manuscript: CG IDO CL. Contributed to the interpretation of data: CG IDO OV CL. Revised the manuscript and approved the final version of the draft for publication: CG IDO OV CL.

References

1. World Health Organization (2013) Global tuberculosis report 2013. Geneva, Switzerland.
2. Robert Koch Institute (2013) Bericht zur Epidemiologie der Tuberkulose in Deutschland für 2011 Robert Koch-Institut, Berlin 2013. 99–103.
3. Erkens CG, Kamphorst M, Abubakar I, Bothamley GH, Chemtob D, et al. (2010) Tuberculosis contact investigation in low prevalence countries: a European consensus. Eur Respir J 36: 925–949.
4. Mack U, Migliori GB, Sester M, Rieder HL, Ehlers S, et al. (2009) LTBI: latent tuberculosis infection or lasting immune responses to M. tuberculosis? A TBNET consensus statement. Eur Respir J 33: 956–973.
5. Infectious Diseases Protection Law (Gesetz zur Verhütung und Bekämpfung von Infektionskrankheiten beim Menschen, Infektionsschutzgesetz IFSG). §25 1–3 II, July 2000. Available: www.rki.de. Accessed 2014 May.
6. Schaberg T, Bauer T, Castell S, Dalhoff K, Detjen A, et al. (2012) [Recommendations for therapy, chemoprevention and chemoprophylaxis of tuberculosis in adults and children. German Central Committee against Tuberculosis (DZK), German Respiratory Society (DGP)]. Pneumologie 66: 133–171.
7. Diel R, Loytved G, Nienhaus A, Castell S, Detjen A, et al. (2011) [New recommendations for contact tracing in tuberculosis]. Gesundheitswesen 73: 369–388.
8. Fallab-Stubi CL, Zellweger JP, Sauty A, Uldry C, Iorillo D, et al. (1998) Electronic monitoring of adherence to treatment in the preventive chemotherapy of tuberculosis. Int J Tuberc Lung Dis 2: 525–530.
9. Robert Koch-Institute (2013) Anwendung und Akzeptanz der präventiven Behandlung bei Kindern mit Kontakt zu Tuberkulose-Erkrankte. Epidemiologisches Bulletin Nr 12.
10. Diel R, Loddenkemper R, Niemann S, Meywald-Walter K, Nienhaus A (2011) Negative and positive predictive value of a whole-blood interferon-gamma release assay for developing active tuberculosis: an update. Am J Respir Crit Care Med 183: 88–95.
11. European Centre for Disease Prevention and Control (2010) Progressing towards TB elimination. Stockholm: ECDC.
12. World Health Organization Media Center. New action plan lays the foundation for tuberculosis elimination. Issued on October 10th 2010. Available: http://www.who.int/mediacentre/news/releases/2010/tb_20101013/en/, Accessed 2014 Sep 5.
13. Chee CB, Sester M, Zhang W, Lange C (2013) Diagnosis and treatment of latent infection with Mycobacterium tuberculosis. Respirology 18: 205–216.
14. Chegou NN, Heyckendorf J, Walzl G, Lange C, Ruhwald M (2013) Beyond the IFN-gamma horizon: Biomarkers for immunodiagnosis of infection with M. tuberculosis. Eur Respir J 43: 1472–1486.
15. Cohn DL, El-Sadr WM (2006) Treatment of latent tuberculosis infection. In M.C. Raviglione, editor. Reichman and Hershfield's Tuberculosis: A Comprehensive International Approach, 3rd ed. Informa Healthcare, New York. 265–305.
16. Elzi L, Schlegel M, Weber R, Hirschel B, Cavassini M, et al. (2007) Reducing tuberculosis incidence by tuberculin skin testing, preventive treatment, and antiretroviral therapy in an area of low tuberculosis transmission. Clin Infect Dis 44: 94–102.
17. HIV-Causal Collaboration (2012) Impact of antiretroviral therapy on tuberculosis incidence among HIV-positive patients in high-income countries. Clin Infect Dis 54: 1364–1372.
18. Kollan C, Bartmeyer B, Bergmann F, Bogner J, Fritzsche C, et al. Antiretroviral treatment (ART) outcome in a large prospective German HIV cohort study - how much virus is still out there?, 5. Deutsch-Österreichischer AIDS-Kongress, Hannover, June 15–18, 2011; PW 49, Abstact volume 61–62.
19. Sester M, van Leth F, Bruchfeld J, Bumbacea D, Cirillo DM, et al. (2014) Risk Assessment of Tuberculosis in Immunocompromised Patients - A TBNET Study. Am J Respir Crit Care Med.
20. Abgrall S, Del Giudice P, Melica G, Costagliola D, Fhdh-Anrs CO (2010) HIV-associated tuberculosis and immigration in a high-income country: incidence trends and risk factors in recent years. AIDS 24: 763–771.
21. Karo B, Haas W, Kollan C, Gunsenheimer-Bartmeyer B, Hamouda O, et al. (2014) Tuberculosis among people living with HIV/AIDS in the German ClinSurv HIV Cohort: long-term incidence and risk factors. BMC Infect Dis 14: 148.
22. Ringshausen FC, Suhling H, Bange FC, Welte T, Gottlieb J (2013) Tuberculosis after lung transplantation, Germany, 1993–2012. Poster number 4689, European Respiratory Conference, Barcelona, 7–11 September 2013.
23. Lange C, Rieder HL (2011) Intention to test is intention to treat. Am J Respir Crit Care Med 183: 3–4.
24. Ringshausen FC, Nienhaus A, Torres Costa J, Knoop H, Schlosser S, et al. (2011) Within-subject variability of Mycobacterium tuberculosis-specific gamma interferon responses in German health care workers. Clin Vaccine Immunol 18: 1176–1182.
25. Dorman SE, Belknap R, Graviss EA, Reves R, Schluger N, et al. (2014) Interferon-gamma release assays and tuberculin skin testing for diagnosis of latent tuberculosis infection in healthcare workers in the United States. Am J Respir Crit Care Med 189: 77–87.
26. Slater ML, Welland G, Pai M, Parsonnet J, Banaei N (2013) Challenges with QuantiFERON-TB Gold assay for large-scale, routine screening of U.S. healthcare workers. Am J Respir Crit Care Med 188: 1005–1010.
27. Nienhaus A, Schablon A, Preisser AM, Ringshausen FC, Diel R (2014) Tuberculosis in healthcare workers - a narrative review from a German perspective. J Occup Med Toxicol 9: 9.
28. Ringshausen FC, Nienhaus A, Schablon A, Torres Costa J, Knoop H, et al. (2013) Frequent detection of latent tuberculosis infection among aged underground hard coal miners in the absence of recent tuberculosis exposure. PLoS One 8: e82005.
29. Marks SM, Taylor Z, Qualls NL, Shrestha-Kuwahara RJ, Wilce MA, et al. (2000) Outcomes of contact investigations of infectious tuberculosis patients. Am J Respir Crit Care Med 162: 2033–2038.
30. Ferebee SH (1970) Controlled chemoprophylaxis trials in tuberculosis. A general review. Bibl Tuberc 26: 28–106.

31. Haldar P, Thuraisingam H, Patel H, Pereira N, Free RC, et al. (2013) Single-step QuantiFERON screening of adult contacts: a prospective cohort study of tuberculosis risk. Thorax 68: 240–246.

32. Moran-Mendoza O, Marion SA, Elwood K, Patrick D, FitzGerald JM (2010) Risk factors for developing tuberculosis: a 12-year follow-up of contacts of tuberculosis cases. Int J Tuberc Lung Dis 14: 1112–1119.

33. Pai M, Denkinger CM, Kik SV, Rangaka MX, Zwerling A, et al. (2014) Gamma interferon release assays for detection of Mycobacterium tuberculosis infection. Clin Microbiol Rev 27: 3–20.

34. Mulder C, van Deutekom H, Huisman EM, Toumanian S, Koster BF, et al. (2012) Role of the QuantiFERON(R)-TB Gold In-Tube assay in screening new immigrants for tuberculosis infection. Eur Respir J 40: 1443–1449.

35. Pareek M, Abubakar I, White PJ, Garnett GP, Lalvani A (2011) Tuberculosis screening of migrants to low-burden nations: insights from evaluation of UK practice. Eur Respir J 37: 1175–1182.

36. Horsburgh CR Jr, Goldberg S, Bethel J, Chen S, Colson PW, et al. (2010) Latent TB infection treatment acceptance and completion in the United States and Canada. Chest 137: 401–409.

37. Landry J, Menzies D (2008) Preventive chemotherapy. Where has it got us? Where to go next? Int J Tuberc Lung Dis 12: 1352–1364.

38. Leung CC, Rieder HL, Lange C, Yew WW (2011) Treatment of latent infection with Mycobacterium tuberculosis: update 2010. Eur Respir J 37: 690–711.

39. Valin N, Antoun F, Chouaid C, Renard M, Dautzenberg B, et al. (2005) Outbreak of tuberculosis in a migrants' shelter, Paris, France, 2002. Int J Tuberc Lung Dis 9: 528–533.

40. Liu Y, Painter JA, Posey DL, Cain KP, Weinberg MS, et al. (2012) Estimating the impact of newly arrived foreign-born persons on tuberculosis in the United States. PLoS One 7: e32158.

41. Gomez-Reino JJ, Carmona L, Valverde VR, Mola EM, Montero MD, et al. (2003) Treatment of rheumatoid arthritis with tumor necrosis factor inhibitors may predispose to significant increase in tuberculosis risk: a multicenter active-surveillance report. Arthritis Rheum 48: 2122–2127.

42. Brassard P, Kezouh A, Suissa S (2006) Antirheumatic drugs and the risk of tuberculosis. Clin Infect Dis 43: 717–722.

43. Korner MM, Hirata N, Tenderich G, Minami K, Mannebach H, et al. (1997) Tuberculosis in heart transplant recipients. Chest 111: 365–369.

44. Torre-Cisneros J, Doblas A, Aguado JM, San Juan R, Blanes M, et al. (2009) Tuberculosis after solid-organ transplant: incidence, risk factors, and clinical characteristics in the RESITRA (Spanish Network of Infection in Transplantation) cohort. Clin Infect Dis 48: 1657–1665.

45. Bruce RM, Wise L (1977) Tuberculosis after jejunoileal bypass for obesity. Ann Intern Med 87: 574–576.

46. Pickleman JR, Evans LS, Kane JM, Freeark RJ (1975) Tuberculosis after jejunoileal bypass for obesity. JAMA 234: 744.

47. World Health Organization. Global tuberculosis control : epidemiology, strategy, financing : WHO Report 2009, Geneva, Switzerland; 2009.

48. Van den Broek J, Borgdorff MW, Pakker NG, Chum HJ, Klokke AH, et al. (1993) HIV-1 infection as a risk factor for the development of tuberculosis: a case-control study in Tanzania. Int J Epidemiol 22: 1159–1165.

49. Calvert GM, Rice FL, Boiano JM, Sheehy JW, Sanderson WT (2003) Occupational silica exposure and risk of various diseases: an analysis using death certificates from 27 states of the United States. Occup Environ Med 60: 122–129.

50. Cowie RL (1994) The epidemiology of tuberculosis in gold miners with silicosis. Am J Respir Crit Care Med 150: 1460–1462.

51. McAdam JM, Bucher SJ, Brickner PW, Vincent RL, Lascher S (2009) Latent tuberculosis and active tuberculosis disease rates among the homeless, New York, New York, USA, 1992–2006. Emerg Infect Dis 15: 1109–1111.

52. Tan de Bibiana J, Rossi C, Rivest P, Zwerling A, Thibert L, et al. (2011) Tuberculosis and homelessness in Montreal: a retrospective cohort study. BMC Public Health 11: 833.

53. Chia S, Karim M, Elwood RK, FitzGerald JM (1998) Risk of tuberculosis in dialysis patients: a population-based study. Int J Tuberc Lung Dis 2: 989–991.

54. Lundin AP, Adler AJ, Berlyne GM, Friedman EA (1979) Tuberculosis in patients undergoing maintenance hemodialysis. Am J Med 67: 597–602.

55. Baussano I, Williams BG, Nunn P, Beggiato M, Fedeli U, et al. (2010) Tuberculosis incidence in prisons: a systematic review. PLoS Med 7: e1000381.

56. Castaneda-Hernandez DM, Martinez-Ramirez JE, Bolivar-Mejia A, Rodriguez-Morales AJ (2013) Differences in TB incidence between prison and general populations, Pereira, Colombia, 2010–2011. Tuberculosis (Edinb) 93: 275–276.

57. Friedman LN, Williams MT, Singh TP, Frieden TR (1996) Tuberculosis, AIDS, and death among substance abusers on welfare in New York City. N Engl J Med 334: 828–833.

58. Girardi E, Sabin CA, d'Arminio Monforte A, Hogg B, Phillips AN, et al. (2005) Incidence of Tuberculosis among HIV-infected patients receiving highly active antiretroviral therapy in Europe and North America. Clin Infect Dis 41: 1772–1782.

59. Ku SC, Tang JL, Hsueh PR, Luh KT, Yu CJ, et al. (2001) Pulmonary tuberculosis in allogeneic hematopoietic stem cell transplantation. Bone Marrow Transplant 27: 1293–1297.

60. de la Camara R, Martino R, Granados E, Rodriguez-Salvanes FJ, Rovira M, et al. (2000) Tuberculosis after hematopoietic stem cell transplantation: incidence, clinical characteristics and outcome. Spanish Group on Infectious Complications in Hematopoietic Transplantation. Bone Marrow Transplant 26: 291–298.

61. Veening GJ (1968) Long term isoniazid prophylaxis. Controlled trial on INH prophylaxis after recent tuberculin conversion in young adults. Bull Int Union Tuberc 41: 169–171.

62. Bush OB Jr, Sugimoto M, Fujii Y, Brown FA Jr (1965) Isoniazid prophylaxis in contacts of persons with known tuberculosis. Second report. Am Rev Respir Dis 92: 732–740.

63. Coker R, McKee M, Atun R, Dimitrova B, Dodonova E, et al. (2006) Risk factors for pulmonary tuberculosis in Russia: case-control study. BMJ 332: 85–87.

64. Pablos-Mendez A, Blustein J, Knirsch CA (1997) The role of diabetes mellitus in the higher prevalence of tuberculosis among Hispanics. Am J Public Health 87: 574–579.

65. Kim CH, Im KH, Yoo SS, Lee SY, Cha SI, et al. (2014) Comparison of the incidence between tuberculosis and nontuberculous mycobacterial disease after gastrectomy. Infection.

66. Steiger Z, Nickel WO, Shannon GJ, Nedwicki EG, Higgins RF (1976) Pulmonary tuberculosis after gastric resection. Am J Surg 131: 668–671.

67. Kim HA, Yoo CD, Baek HJ, Lee EB, Ahn C, et al. (1998) Mycobacterium tuberculosis infection in a corticosteroid-treated rheumatic disease patient population. Clin Exp Rheumatol 16: 9–13.

68. Yamada T, Nakajima A, Inoue E, Tanaka E, Hara M, et al. (2006) Increased risk of tuberculosis in patients with rheumatoid arthritis in Japan. Ann Rheum Dis 65: 1661–1663.

69. Ferebee SH, Mount FW (1962) Tuberculosis morbidity in a controlled trial of the prophylactic use of isoniazid among household contacts. Am Rev Respir Dis 85: 490–510.

70. Katz J, Kunofsky S, Damijonaitis V, Lafleur A, Caron T (1965) Effect of Isoniazid Upon the Reactivation of Inactive Tuberculosis; Final Report. Am Rev Respir Dis 91: 345–350.

17

Inhibition of Platelet Activation and Thrombus Formation by Adenosine and Inosine: Studies on Their Relative Contribution and Molecular Modeling

Eduardo Fuentes[1,2]*, **Jaime Pereira**[3], **Diego Mezzano**[3], **Marcelo Alarcón**[1,2], **Julio Caballero**[4], **Iván Palomo**[1,2]*

1 Department of Clinical Biochemistry and Immunohematology, Faculty of Health Sciences, Interdisciplinary Excellence Research Program on Healthy Aging (PIEI-ES), Universidad de Talca, Talca, Chile, **2** Centro de Estudios en Alimentos Procesados (CEAP), CONICYT-Regional, Gore Maule, Talca, Chile, **3** Department of Hematology-Oncology, School of Medicine, Pontificia Universidad Católica de Chile, Santiago, Chile, **4** Center for Bioinformatics and Molecular Simulations, Faculty of Engineering in Bioinformatics, Universidad de Talca, Talca, Chile

Abstract

Background: The inhibitory effect of adenosine on platelet aggregation is abrogated after the addition of adenosine-deaminase. Inosine is a naturally occurring nucleoside degraded from adenosine.

Objectives: The mechanisms of antiplatelet action of adenosine and inosine *in vitro* and *in vivo*, and their differential biological effects by molecular modeling were investigated.

Results: Adenosine (0.5, 1 and 2 mmol/L) inhibited phosphatidylserine exposure from $52\pm4\%$ in the control group to 44 ± 4 ($p<0.05$), 29 ± 2 ($p<0.01$) and $20\pm3\%$ ($p<0.001$). P-selectin expression in the presence of adenosine 0.5, 1 and 2 mmol/L was inhibited from 32 ± 4 to 27 ± 2 ($p<0.05$), 14 ± 3 ($p<0.01$) and $9\pm3\%$ ($p<0.001$), respectively. At the concentrations tested, only inosine to 4 mmol/L had effect on platelet P-selectin expression ($p<0.05$). Adenosine and inosine inhibited platelet aggregation and ATP release stimulated by ADP and collagen. Adenosine and inosine reduced collagen-induced platelet adhesion and aggregate formation under flow. At the same concentrations adenosine inhibited platelet aggregation, decreased the levels of sCD40L and increased intraplatelet cAMP. In addition, SQ22536 (an adenylate cyclase inhibitor) and ZM241385 (a potent adenosine receptor A_{2A} antagonist) attenuated the effect of adenosine on platelet aggregation induced by ADP and intraplatelet level of cAMP. Adenosine and inosine significantly inhibited thrombosis formation *in vivo* ($62\pm2\%$ occlusion at 60 min [$n=6$, $p<0.01$] and $72\pm1.9\%$ occlusion at 60 min, [$n=6$, $p<0.05$], respectively) compared with the control ($98\pm2\%$ occlusion at 60 min, $n=6$). A_{2A} is the adenosine receptor present in platelets; it is known that inosine is not an A_{2A} ligand. Docking of adenosine and inosine inside A_{2A} showed that the main difference is the formation by adenosine of an additional hydrogen bond between the NH_2 of the adenine group and the residues Asn253 in H6 and Glu169 in EL2 of the A_{2A} receptor.

Conclusion: Therefore, adenosine and inosine may represent novel agents lowering the risk of arterial thrombosis.

Editor: James P. Brody, Irvine, United States of America

Funding: This work was funded by the CONICYT REGIONAL / GORE MAULE / CEAP / R09I2001, Interdisciplinary Excellence Research Program on Healthy Aging (PIEI-ES), and supported by grant no. 1130216 (I. P., M. G., R. M., M. A., J. C.) from Fondecyt, Chile. The funders had no role in study design, data collection and analysis, decision to publish, or preparation of the manuscript.

Competing Interests: The authors have declared that no competing interests exist.

* Email: ipalomo@utalca.cl (IP); edfuentes@utalca.cl (EF)

Introduction

Cardiovascular diseases (CVD) (i.e., acute myocardial infarction, cerebrovascular disease and peripheral arterial thrombosis) have increased significantly in recent years [1,2]. The major and independent risk factors for CVD are cigarette smoking, elevated blood pressure, elevated serum total cholesterol and diabetes, among others [3,4]. Platelet hyper-aggregability is associated with risk factors for CVD [5]. Thus platelets from patients with type 1 and type 2 diabetes exhibit enhanced platelet aggregation activity early [6,7].

Platelet accumulation at vascular injury sites is the primary event in arterial thrombosis and its activation is a critical component of atherothrombosis [8]. Patients with unstable complex lesions had a fivefold higher expression of platelet activation than patients with stable angina, indicating an intense thrombogenic potential [9]. Also platelets could be directly involved in the unstable plaque through the production and release of pro-inflammatory molecules, including a variety of cytokines, such as TGF-β, IL-1β and sCD40L, among others [10,11].

Antiplatelet therapy has been used for a long time in an effort to prevent, as well as to treat, thrombotic diseases [12–14]. The multiple pathways of platelet activation limit the effect of specific receptor/pathway inhibitors, resulting in limited clinical efficacy [15,16]. In this way, the best-known inhibitor and turn off signaling in platelet activation is cyclic adenosine monophosphate (cAMP) [17,18].

Adenosine is a key endogenous molecule that regulates tissue function by activating four G-protein-coupled adenosine receptors: A_1, A_{2A}, A_{2B} and A_3. Both A_2 adenosine receptors, A_{2A} and A_{2B}, are coupled to G_s, leading to stimulation of adenylyl cyclase and consequent elevation of cAMP [19]. Adenosine is also recognized as one of the most important endogenous molecules able to prevent tissue injury in ischemia-reperfusion [20]. Inosine is another purine nucleoside, which is formed during the breakdown of adenosine by adenosine deaminase [21]. Inosine potently inhibited the production of the proinflammatory cytokines (TNF-α, IL-1 and IL-12) and its effect was partially reversed by blockade of adenosine A_1 and A_2 receptors [22].

Given the high structural similitude between adenosine and inosine, the main aim of this work was to investigate the relative contribution of these two molecules on platelet activation and thrombus formation. Furthermore, we performed docking experiments on the adenosine receptor A_{2A} in order to explain their differential biological effects at a molecular level.

Materials and Methods

Animal research

This study was carried out under recommendations according to the Guide for the Care and Use of Laboratory Animals of the National Institutes of Health. The protocol was approved by the Committee on the Ethics of Animal Experiments of the Universidad de Talca. All efforts were made to minimize suffering.

Reagents and antibodies

The agonist adenosine 5′- diphosphate bis (ADP), acetylsalicylic acid (ASA), rose bengal, adenosine, inosine and prostaglandin E_1 (PGE$_1$) were from Sigma-Aldrich (St. Louis, Missouri/MO, U.S.A), while the collagen was obtained from Hormon-Chemie (Munich, Germany). Calcein-AM, bovine serum albumin (BSA), SQ22536 (adenylate cyclase inhibitor) and ZM241385 (adenosine receptor A_{2A} antagonist) were obtained from Sigma-Aldrich (St. Louis, Missouri/MO, USA), whereas Luciferase luciferin reagent was obtained from Chrono-Log corp (Havertown, PA) and microfluidic chambers were from Bioflux (Fluxion, San Francisco, California, USA). Annexin V FITC Apoptosis KIT and antibodies (anti-CD62P-PE and anti-CD61-FITC) were obtained from BD Pharmingen (BD Biosciences, San Diego, CA, USA).

Preparation of human platelet suspensions

After receiving written informed consent from all volunteers, venous blood samples (blood volume of 30 mL was extracted from each volunteer) were taken from six young healthy volunteers (range 20–30 years). The samples were placed in 3.2% citrate tubes (9:1 v/v) by phlebotomy with vacuum tube system (Becton Dickinson Vacutainer Systems, Franklin Lakes, NJ, USA). The protocol was authorized by the ethics committee of the Universidad de Talca in accordance with the Declaration of Helsinki (approved by the 18th World Medical Assembly in Helsinki, Finland, 1964). Samples obtained from each volunteer were processed independently for each assay and centrifuged at 240 g for 10 min to obtain platelet-rich plasma (PRP). Following this, two-thirds of PRP was removed and centrifuged (10 min at 650 g).

The pellet was then washed with HEPES-Tyrode's buffer containing PGE$_1$ (120 nmol/L). Washed platelets were prepared in HEPES-Tyrode's buffer at a concentration of 200×10^9 platelets/L (Bayer Advia 60 Hematology System, Tarrytown, NY, USA). Platelets were kept at 4°C during all the isolation steps after blood samples were taken.

Flow cytometry analysis for phosphatidylserine externalization and P-selectin exposure

Loss of platelet membrane phopholipid asymmetry with externalization of phosphatidylserine (PS) and P-selectin expression on platelets were determined by flow cytometry [23]. To 480 μL of citrated whole blood, collagen 1.5 μg/mL and ADP 8 μmol/L (final concentrations) were added for 10 min at 37°C, with stirring at 240 g. In each experiment, previous to the addition of platelet agonists, the sample was incubated with saline, adenosine (0.5 to 2 mmol/L) or inosine (1 to 4 mmol/L) for 10 min at room temperature. To determine phosphatidylserine externalization, 50 μL of PRP obtained of sample was diluted with 150 μL of binding buffer (10 mmol/L Hepes, 150 mmol/L NaCl, 5.0 mmol/L KCl, 1.0 mmol/L MgCl$_2$, 2.0 mmol/L CaCl$_2$, pH 7.4) and incubated for 25 min in the dark with 0.6 μg/mL (final concentration) of annexin V-FITC and anti-CD61-PE. To determine platelet P-selectin expression, 50 μL of sample was mixed with saturated concentrations of anti-CD62P-PE and anti-CD61-FITC and incubated for 25 min in the dark. Then, red cells were lysed using FACS lysing solution for 15 min. Samples were then centrifuged and washed for analysis. The samples were acquired and analyzed in Accuri C6 flow cytometer (BD, Biosciences, USA).

Platelet populations were gated on cell size using forward scatter (FSC) vs side scatter (SSC) and CD61 positivity to distinguish them from electronic noise. The light scatter and fluorescence channels were set at logarithmic gain and 5,000 events per sample analyzed. Fluorescence intensities of differentially stained populations were expressed as mean channel value using the cSampler Software (BD Biosciences, USA). All measurements were performed from six separate platelet donors.

Measurement of platelet secretion and aggregation

Platelet ATP secretion and aggregation were monitored by light transmission according to Born and Cross [24], using a lumi-aggregometer (Chrono-Log, Havertown, PA, USA). Briefly, 480 μL of PRP in the reaction vessel was pre-incubated with 20 μL of saline, PGE$_1$ (0.02 mmol/L), adenosine (0.5 to 2 mmol/L) or inosine (1 to 4 mmol/L). After 3 min of incubation, 20 μL of agonist (ADP 8 μmol/L or collagen 1.5 μg/mL) was added to initiate platelet aggregation, which was measured for 6 min. To determine platelet ATP secretion 50 μL of luciferin/luciferase was added within 2 min before stimulation. Platelet ATP secretion and aggregation (maximal amplitude [%]) were determined by software AGGRO/LINK (Chrono-Log, Havertown, PA, USA). Inhibition of the maximal platelet secretion and aggregation was expressed as a percentage with respect to control (saline). The concentration required to inhibit platelet secretion and aggregation by 50% (IC$_{50}$) was calculated from the dose-response curves. All measurements were performed from six separate platelet donors.

Platelet adhesion and aggregation under controlled flow

Experiments under flow were performed in a BioFlux 200 flow system (Fluxion, San Francisco, California, USA) with high shear plates (48 wells, 0–20 dyne/cm^2). Using manual mode in the

BioFlux software, the microfluidic chambers were coated for 1 hour with 20 µL of collagen 200 µg/mL at a wall shear rate of $200\ s^{-1}$.

The plaque coating was allowed to dry at room temperature for one hour. The channels were perfused with phosphate-buffered saline (PBS) for 10 min at room temperature at wall shear rate of $200\ s^{-1}$ to remove the interface. Then, the channels were blocked with BSA 5% for 10 min at room temperature at wall shear rate of $200\ s^{-1}$. Whole blood anticoagulated with sodium citrate was labeled with calcein-AM (4 µmol/L) and incubated at room temperature with saline, PGE_1 (0.02 mmol/L), adenosine (0.5 to 2 mmol/L) or inosine (1 to 4 mmol/L). After one hour of incubation, the blood was added to the inlet of the well and chambers were perfused for 10 min at room temperature a wall shear rate of $1000\ s^{-1}$. The plates were mounted on the stage of an inverted fluorescence microscope (TE200, NIKON, Japan) [25].

Platelet deposition was observed and recorded in real-time (30 frames per min) with a CCD camera (QICAM, QIMaging, Surrey, BC, Canada). Bright field and fluorescence microscopy for real-time visualization of platelet adhesion and aggregation in flowing blood was used. For each flow experiment, fluorescence images were analyzed off-stage by quantifying the area covered by platelets with the ImageJ software (version 1.26t, NIH, USA). In each field, the area covered by platelets was quantified. All measurements were performed from six separate platelet donors.

Effect of ZM241385 and SQ22536 on antiplatelet activity

To investigate whether platelet antiaggregant activity of adenosine and inosine was mediated by stimulation of adenosine receptor A_{2A}/adenylyl cyclase pathway, PRP (480 µL at 200×10^9 platelets/L) was pretreated with SQ22536 (250 µmol/L) or ZM241385 (30 µmol/L) for 3 min. Then, the same PRP was preincubated with 20 µL of adenosine (2 mmol/L) or inosine (4 mmol/L) for 3 min prior to the addition of ADP 8 µmol/L. Platelets were first exposed to ZM241385 or SQ22536 and then ADP was used as controls. All measurements were performed from six separate platelet donors.

Measurement of cAMP levels in platelets

The effect of adenosine (0.5 to 2 mmol/L) or inosine (1 to 4 mmol/L) on platelet levels of cAMP was evaluated in PRP samples (500 µL) following 5 min incubation without stirring. Reactions were stopped with 150 µL of ice-cold 10% trichloroacetic acid. Precipitated proteins were removed by centrifugation at 2.000 g for 15 min at 4°C. Following addition of 150 µL of HCl 1 mol/L, the supernatant was submitted to 6 ether extractions v/v and lyophilized. Samples were stored at −70°C until assay. Before determination, the powder was dissolved in 200 µL of PBS, pH 6.2. cAMP Direct Immunoassay Kit (BioVision Research Products, Mountain View, CA, USA) was employed. All measurements were performed from six separate platelet donors.

Molecular Docking

Docking was performed using Glide [26], which is contained in Maestro software (Maestro, Version 9.0, Schrödinger, LLC, New York, NY, 2007). Glide docking uses a series of hierarchical filters to find the best possible ligand binding locations in a previously built receptor grid space. The filters include a systematic search approach, which samples the positional, conformational, and orientational space of the ligand before evaluating the energy interactions between the ligand and the protein.

The coordinates of the adenosine receptor A_{2A} were extracted from the X-ray crystal structure of human $A_{2A}R$ with adenosine bound (accession code in Protein Data Bank (PDB): 2YDO). The structures of adenosine and inosine were sketched with Maestro software. The extra-precision (XP) module of Glide was used. A grid box of 30Å × 30Å × 30Å was first centered on the center of mass of the adenosine in PDB 2YDO. Default docking parameters were used [27]. The docking hierarchy began with the systematic conformational expansion of the ligand followed by placement in the receptor site. Then minimization of the ligand in the field of the receptor was carried out using the OPLS-AA [28] force field with a distance-dependent dielectric of 2.0. Afterward, the lowest energy poses were subjected to a Monte Carlo procedure that samples the nearby torsional minima. The best pose for a given ligand was determined by the Emodel score, while different compounds were ranked using GlideScore [29]. The docking poses for both ligands were analyzed by examining their relative total energy score. The more energetically favorable conformations were selected as the best poses.

Thrombus formation in murine model

All studies were approved by the committee on animal care and conform to the Guide for the care and use of Laboratory Animals of Universidad de Talca. The Thrombosis in mice was performed by photochemical injury using a modification of the model described by Przyklenk and Whittaker [30]. For murine model we used the same mice species (C57BL/6) and gender (male) for both in control and experimental groups. Briefly, mice (12–16 weeks old) were anesthetized with a combination of tribromoethanol (270 mg/kg) and xylazine (13 mg/kg), before anesthetizing the animals; the mice were carefully handled to minimize stress and quickly anesthetized. Twenty-four hours prior to surgery, systolic blood pressure was measured using a noninvasive blood pressure meter (BP-98A, Softron Co. Ltd., Tokyo, Japan) in awake mice and during thrombosis. Throughout the procedure, animals were kept on a heating pad maintained at 37°C. After the administration of anesthesia, the mice were placed in the supine position and the mesentery was exposed by central incision in the abdomen, permitting visualization of thrombus development in mesenteric artery. The mice were injected with rose bengal through tail vein injection in a volume of 0.1 mL at a concentration of 50 mg/kg. Just after injection, a 1.5-mW green light laser (532 nm) was applied to the desired site of mesenteric artery and blood flow was monitored for 60 min. Stable occlusion was defined as a blood flow of 0 mL/min for 3 min. Saline (control group, n = 6), ASA (200 mg/kg, n = 6), adenosine (200 mg/kg, n = 6) or inosine (200 mg/kg, n = 6) was administered intraperitoneally 30 min before experiment. After laser exposure, the image of the injury generated of the injured vessel was recorded with a charge-coupled device camera (Optronics, Goleta, CA). The recorded video image was digitized and then analyzed with ImageJ software (version 1.26t, NIH, USA) [31]. In control experiments, neither injection of rose bengal without green laser or without rose bengal with green laser, resulted in any alterations in blood flow (data not shown).

Measurement of sCD40L levels

Soluble CD40 ligand (sCD40L) was determined using a Human sCD40-Ligand Quantikine kit (R & D systems, Minneapolis, MN). Briefly, washed platelets (200×10^9 platelets/L) were pretreated with saline, ASA (0.3 mmol/L), adenosine (0.5 to 2 mmol/L) or inosine (1 to 4 mmol/L) for 15 min at 37°C and then stimulated by thrombin (2 U/mL) for 45 min at 37°C. Finally, the supernatants were collected following centrifugation at 11.000 g for 10 min at 4°C and stored at −70°C prior to sCD40L measurements by ELISA as described earlier [32]. All measurements were performed from six separate platelet donors.

Statistical analysis

Data were analyzed using SPSS version 17.0 (SPSS, Inc., Chicago, Illinois. and expressed as mean ± standard error of mean (SEM). Six or more independent experiments were performed for the different assays. Results were expressed as percent inhibition or as percentage of control (as 100%). Fifty-percent inhibitory concentration (IC_{50}) of adenosine or inosine against agonist-induced platelet function was calculated from the dose-response curves. Differences between groups were analyzed by Student's t-test or one-way analysis of variance (ANOVA) using Tukey's post-hoc test. P values <0.05 were considered significant.

Results

In vitro findings antiplatelet effects

Effects of adenosine and inosine on platelet activation events. The antiplatelet effects of adenosine and inosine were explored by testing their activity on different activation-dependent events in human platelets. Activated platelets expose PS, which is a key phenomenon for generating a burst of thrombin essential for thrombus growth. Collagen/ADP-induced externalization of PS assessed by annexin-V binding in the presence of adenosine 0.5, 1 and 2 mmol/L was inhibited from 52±4% in the control group to 44±4% (p<0.05), 29±2 (p<0.01), and 20±3% (p<0.001), respectively. Whereas collagen/ADP-induced externalization of PS assessed by annexin-V binding was only slightly inhibited by 4 mmol/L of inosine (p<0.05) (Figure 1A). The influence of adenosine (0.5 to 2 mmol/L) and inosine (1 to 4 mmol/L) on P-selectin expression by human platelet after stimulation of ADP/collagen in citrated whole blood was measured by flow cytometry. P-selectin expression in the presence of adenosine 0.5, 1 and 2 mmol/L was inhibited from 32±4 to 27±2 (p<0.05), 14±3 (p<0.01) and 9±3% (p<0.001), respectively. At the concentrations tested, inosine only to 4 mmol/L has effect on platelet P-selectin expression (p<0.05) (Figure 1B).

Effects of adenosine and inosine on platelet ATP secretion and aggregation. The effects of adenosine and inosine on platelet ATP secretion induced by ADP and collagen are shown in Figure 2A. Adenosine inhibited ADP-induced ATP secretion with

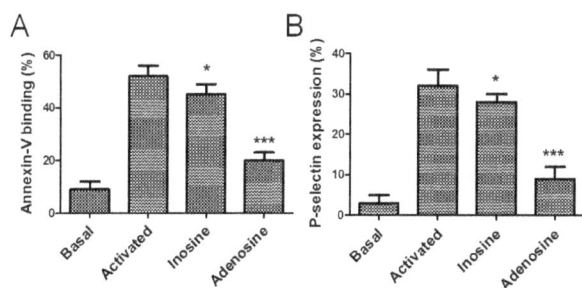

Figure 2. Effects of adenosine and inosine on ADP (8 μmol/L), collagen (1.5 μg/mL), induced platelet ATP secretion (A) and aggregation (B). PRP was pre-incubated with saline (control), adenosine (0.5 to 2 mmol/L) or inosine (1 to 4 mmol/L). After 3 min of incubation, 20 μL of agonist (ADP 8 μmol/L or collagen 1.5 μg/mL) was added to initiate platelet aggregation, which was measured for 6 min. The inhibition of the maximal platelet ATP secretion and aggregation were expressed as a percentage with respect to control (mean ± SEM; n=6). The results presented are from 6 separate volunteers (each donors performed as single triplicates).

a 50% inhibitory concentration (IC_{50}) of 0.96 mmol/L. Similarly, the IC_{50} concentration for adenosine on collagen-induced platelet ATP-secretion was about 0.78 mmol/L. Moreover, inosine effectively inhibited the collagen-induced platelet ATP secretion with an IC_{50} of 2.3 mmol/L.

The effects of adenosine and inosine on ADP- and collagen-induced platelet aggregation are shown in Figure 2B. Adenosine effectively reduced ADP-induced platelet aggregation with an IC_{50} of 0.53 mmol/L. Similarly; adenosine suppressed collagen-induced platelet aggregation with an IC_{50} of 0.87 mmol/L. Moreover, inosine effectively inhibited collagen-induced platelet aggregation with an IC_{50} of 2.38 mmol/L. In addition, inosine showed only a mild inhibitory effect (46±5%, p<0.05) over ADP-induced platelet aggregation at a concentration of 4 mmol/L.

Adenosine and inosine impair platelet adhesion on immobilized collagen under flow conditions. The effects of adenosine and inosine on platelet adhesion/aggregation to immobilized collagen under arterial flow conditions are shown in Figure 3. After perfusion of citrate-anticoagulated blood over collagen coated plaque surfaces at 37°C with a wall shear rate of 1000 s^{-1} for 10 min, rapid platelet adhesion and aggregate formation were observed (Figure 3A). Adenosine (0.5 to 2 mmol/L) and inosine (1 to 4 mmol/L) concentration-dependently reduced collagen-induced platelet adhesion and aggregate formation under controlled flow. As shown in Figure 3B, platelet adhesion and aggregate formation under controlled flow in presence of adenosine 0.5, 1 and 2 mmol/L was inhibited from 60±8 to 24±4 (p<0.001), 17±6 (p<0.001) and 3±2% (p<0.001), respectively. Similarly, in presence of inosine 1, 2 and 4 mmol/L platelet adhesion and aggregate formation under controlled flow was inhibited from 60±8 to 42±5 (p<0.01), 24±4 (p<0.001) and 12±4% (p<0.001), respectively.

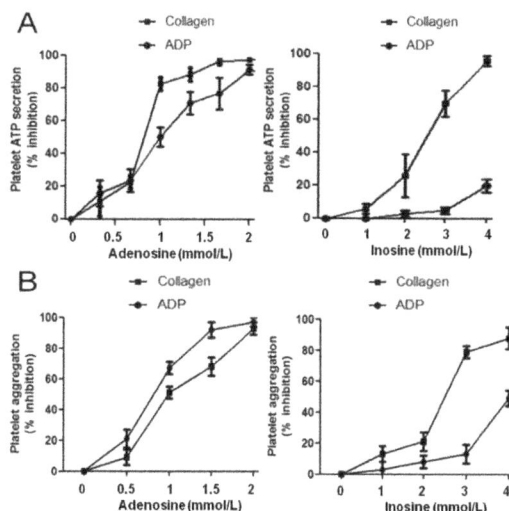

Figure 1. Effects of adenosine and inosine on platelet activation. Blood sample was incubated with saline, adenosine (2 mmol/L) or inosine (4 mmol/L) for 10 min, prior to measuring human platelet activation induced by agonists (collagen/ADP). Phosphatidylserine externalization (n=9 experiments, panel A) and P-selectin expression (n=6 experiments, panel B) were determined by flow cytometry. The basal bar represents the fluorescence in unstimulated sample. The graph depicts the mean ± SEM, *p<0.05 and ***p<0.001. The results presented are from 6 separate volunteers (each donors performed as single triplicates).

A

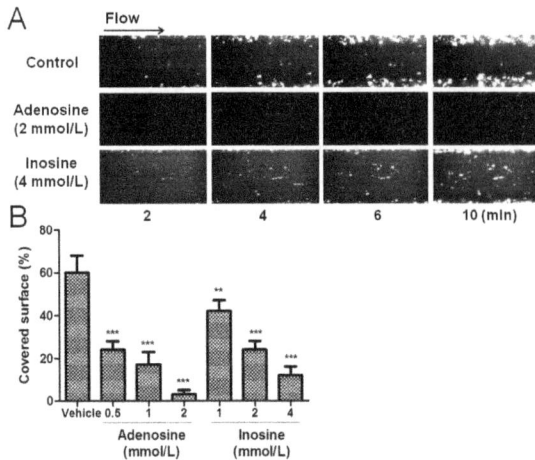

Figure 3. Effects of adenosine and inosine on collagen-induced platelet adhesion and aggregation under arterial flow conditions. Panel A shows the time-lapse of 10 min at 10 dyne/cm^2. Panel B shows the surface covered by platelets expressed as the percentage of the total surface observed, values are mean $\pm$ SEM; n = 6. **p<0.01 and ***p<0.001. The results presented are from 6 separate volunteers (each donors performed as single triplicates).

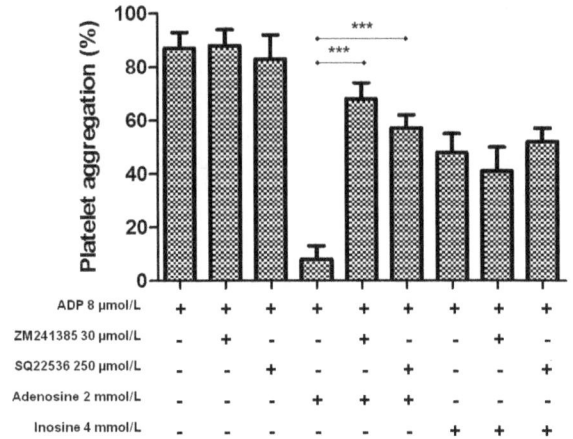

Figure 4. Effect of adenosine receptor A$_{2A}$ antagonist (ZM241385) and adenylyl cyclase inhibitor (SQ22536) on ADP-induced platelet aggregation. PRP suspension was incubated with ADP, adenosine or inosine plus ADP or pretreated with SQ22536 or ZM241385 for 3 min, followed by addition of adenosine or inosine and ADP. The graph depicts the mean $\pm$ SEM of n = 6 experiments. ***p<0.001. The results presented are from 6 separate volunteers (each donors performed as single triplicates).

Mechanisms involved

Effect of ZM241385 and SQ22536 on ADP-induced platelet aggregation. We tested whether ZM241385 and SQ22536 could reverse the inhibitory effect of adenosine and inosine on platelet aggregation induced by ADP. As shown in Figure 4, ZM241385 (30 µmol/L) and SQ22536 (250 µmol/L) attenuated the inhibitory effect of adenosine against ADP-induced platelet aggregation from 8±5 to 68±6 and 57±5%, respectively (p< 0.001). In addition, we found that SQ22536 attenuated an increase of intraplatelet levels of cAMP by adenosine from 29±2 to 9±1 pmol/10^8 platelets (p<0.05). On the contrary, ZM241385 and SQ22536 did not have any effect on the platelet antiaggregant activity of inosine (1 to 4 mmol/L). ZM241385 and SQ22536 alone did not exert any effect on ADP-induced platelet aggregation and with no statistical differences between them.

Effects of adenosine and inosine on intraplatelet levels of cAMP. We investigated whether the effects of adenosine and inosine on platelet function were mediated by changes in platelet cAMP levels. As shown in Figure 5, levels of cAMP in resting platelets were significantly lower compared with PGE$_1$ (0.02 mmol/L)-treated platelets (p<0.001). At the same concentrations adenosine significantly inhibits platelet aggregation and concentration-dependently (0.5 to 2 mmol/L) increased the intraplatelet levels of cAMP (p<0.001). On the other hand, inosine (1 to 4 mmol/L) did not show any effect on intraplatelet levels of cAMP.

Molecular docking. Figure 6 shows the alignment of the cocrystallized adenosine structure versus the docked structures for adenosine and inosine. According to this figure, the docked adenosine structure fitted in an optimal way with the adenosine in the crystal structure, and the inosine had the same orientation inside the adenosine receptor A$_{2A}$ binding pocket. Both compounds contain a ribose group that extends deep into the ligand-binding pocket where it has hydrogen bond (HB) interactions with the residues Ser277 and His278 in H7. In addition, both compounds have a π-stacking interaction with Phe168 in extracellular loop 2 (EL2).

Adenosine forms an additional HB between the NH$_2$ of the adenine group and the residues Asn253 in H6 and Glu169 in EL2

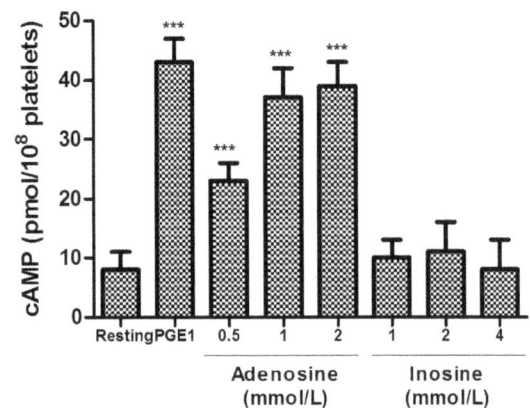

Figure 5. Effects of adenosine and inosine on intraplatelet levels of cAMP. Platelets were incubated with PGE$_1$ (0.02 mmol/L, positive control), adenosine (0.5 to 2 mmol/L) or inosine (1 to 4 mmol/L) for measurement of cAMP formations as described in *Materials and methods*. ***p<0.001 as compared with resting platelets (n = 6). The results presented are from 6 separate volunteers (each donors performed as single triplicates).

of the adenosine receptor A$_{2A}$, whereas the hypoxanthine group of inosine cannot establish these interactions. The role of Glu169 in ligand binding has been identified previously in the literature [33], suggesting that it is either directly or indirectly involved in the molecular recognition of both adenosine agonists and antagonists [33].

In vivo assessment of the antithrombotic potential

Effect on arterial thrombus formation *in vivo*. To study arterial thrombus development in mesenteric artery, anesthetized animals received saline, ASA, adenosine or inosine at a dose of

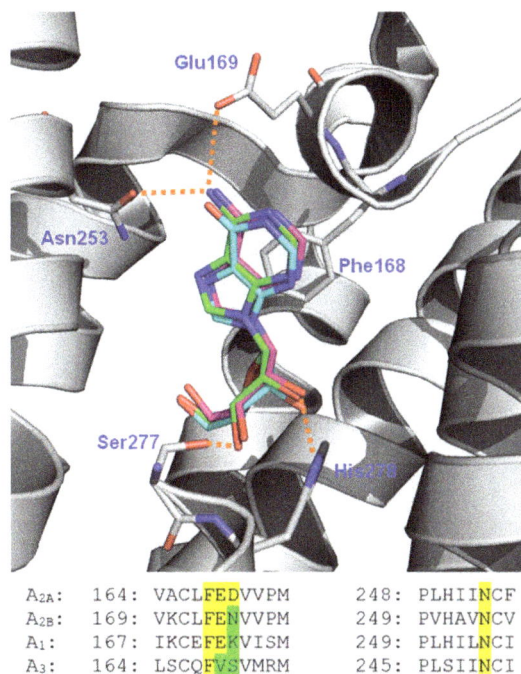

A2A:	164: VACL**FED**VVPM	248: PLHI**I**NCF
A2B:	169: VKCL**FEN**VVPM	249: PVHAV**N**CV
A1:	167: IKCE**FEK**VISM	249: PLHIL**N**CI
A3:	164: LSCQ**FVS**VMRM	245: PLSI**I**NCI

Figure 6. Molecular modeling of adenosine and inosine on adenosine receptor A2A. (top) Molecular conformations of adenosine (green) and inosine (cyan) obtained using docking inside adenosine receptor A2A binding pocket are represented. The X-ray reference structure of adenosine is represented in purple (PDB code: 2YDO). A comparison between the conformations reflects that inosine and adenosine adopt the same binding orientation inside adenosine receptor A2A (bottom). Alignment of the A2A motifs that contain residues Glu169 and Asn253 with A2B, A1, and A3.

200 mg/kg body weight by intraperitoneal injection. The effect of adenosine and inosine on arterial thrombus formation was examined and is shown in Figure 7A. Both adenosine and inosine showed a different kinetic inhibition on arterial thrombus formation (Figure 7B). The thrombotic vessel occlusion at 60 min was inhibited from 98 ± 2 to $30\pm1.8\%$ (n = 6, p<0.001) by pretreatment with ASA. Similarly, adenosine and inosine significantly inhibited arterial occlusion. Administration of adenosine showed a significant reduction in occlusion extent compared with the negative control at 60 min (62 ± 2 vs $98\pm2\%$, respectively, n = 6) (p<0.01). On the other hand, inosine exhibited a minor effect on occlusion size reduction from 98 ± 2 to $72\pm1.9\%$ (n = 6, p<0.05) (Figure 7C).

Additional anti-inflammatory properties

Effect on the levels of sCD40L. As platelets are considered the major source of sCD40L in blood, we examined the effect of adenosine and inosine on the release of sCD40L. As observed in Figure 8, we found that adenosine (0.5 to 2 mmol/L) concentration-dependently reduced thrombin-induced sCD40L released from platelets (p<0.001). Adenosine exhibited a similar effect as ASA on sCD40L release. Moreover, inosine has a residual effect only at 4 mmol/L over sCD40L released from platelet (p<0.05).

Discussion

In this study, we have demonstrated that adenosine and inosine display *in vitro* and *in vivo* antiplatelet activities and reduce platelet release of atherosclerotic-related inflammatory mediator

(sCD40L). This inhibitory effect of adenosine and inosine was demonstrated with the use of different agonists (ADP and collagen) and this inhibition was directly proportional to the concentrations used.

Adenosine is a natural product and endogenous nucleoside with antiplatelet activity [34–36]. Adenosine through G-protein linked receptors activate adenylate cyclase and increase cellular cAMP levels, showing inhibition of platelet function [37,38]. Studies have established that the inhibitory effect of adenosine on platelet aggregation disappears after the addition of adenosine-deaminase [39,40], and converts the purine nucleoside into inosine [41]. However, our results show that inosine possesses antiplatelet activity *in vitro* by significantly inhibiting platelet function (activation, secretion, aggregation and adhesion), releasing sCD40L and for the first time we have demonstrated prevention of thrombus growth *in vivo*. In addition, another study has established that inosine markedly inhibited platelet activation *in vitro* and *in vivo*, as well as cerebral ischemia [42].

Platelet-derived P-selectin seems to contribute to atherosclerotic lesion development and arterial thrombogenesis by forming large stable platelet-leukocyte aggregates [43]. Our results show that adenosine and inosine inhibited P-selectin expression on human platelets induced by ADP/collagen. In this sense, adenosine and inosine could inhibit platelet-leukocyte conjugate formation [44]. It has been shown that the increase of cAMP levels regulates P-selectin expression via activation of PKA [38,45]. In fact, we have recently demonstrated that an increase in intraplatelet cAMP by adenosine markedly increases the phosphorylation of PKA in human platelets [46].

When platelets adhere to collagen, a ligand-binding–induced signal is generated, leading to platelet spreading that render adherent platelets resistant to shear forces at the site of vascular damage [47]. Interestingly, we found that under conditions of arterial shear, adenosine and inosine significantly reduced platelet adhesion and aggregation to collagen as compared with the negative control.

In the last decade several lines of evidence have supported the notion that the secretion of platelet pro-inflammatory molecules (sCD40L, RANTES, sP-selectin, among others) plays a pathogenic role in both the onset and progression of the atherosclerotic process as well as in thrombotic occlusion of the vessels [48,49]. Platelets interact with monocytes via a CD40-CD40L-mediated pathway that causes their adherence to the inflamed endothelial layer [50]. Thus, high levels of sCD40L have been associated with platelet activation, suggesting a prognostic marker in patients with advanced atherosclerosis [51]. This study demonstrates for the first time that adenosine and inosine, among its antiplatelet activities, decreases the inflammatory component of activated platelets, by reducing the release of sCD40L.

In this study, ZM241385 (adenosine receptor A2A antagonist) and SQ22536 (adenylyl cyclase inhibitor) were able to attenuate the effect of adenosine on ADP-induced platelet aggregation, but failed to affect the platelet aggregation induced by ADP [52]. These findings suggest that inhibition of platelet aggregation by adenosine is mediated by the stimulation of adenosine receptor A2A/adenylate cyclase with increased intraplatelet cAMP concentrations. Adenosine increased cAMP levels and significantly inhibited platelet aggregation stimulated by ADP and collagen. Two recent observations may explain these findings showing that intraplatelet cAMP levels downregulate P2Y1R expression [53] and contribute to maintaining GPVI in a monomeric form on resting platelets [54]. Thus, adenosine through elevation of cAMP suppresses the sCD40L release due to the inhibition of adenylyl cyclase inhibition [46,55]. However, ZM241385 and SQ22536

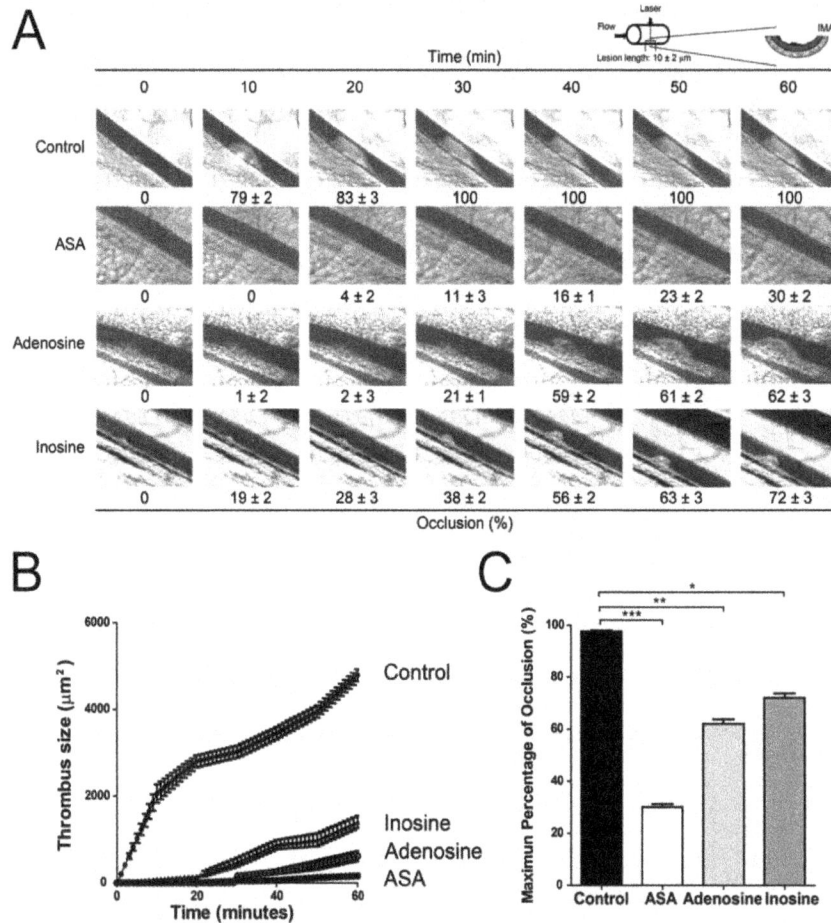

Figure 7. Adenosine and inosine inhibited arterial thrombosis formation. Panel A shows thrombus formation after laser irradiation in the saline control group (n = 6); ASA (acetylsalicylic acid) (200 mg/kg, n = 6); adenosine (200 mg/kg, n = 6) and inosine (200 mg/kg, n = 6). The figures below each photograph represent the percentages of occlusions caused by thrombus formation. Panel B shows the time course changes of thrombus size (μm^2). Panel C shows maximum percentage of occlusion at 60 min after laser irradiation. For panels A and C the percentages of occlusions were calculated using the percentage of a certain area where the occlusion is greater. The graph depicts the mean ± SEM of n = 6 experiments. *p < 0.05, **p < 0.01 and ***p < 0.001.

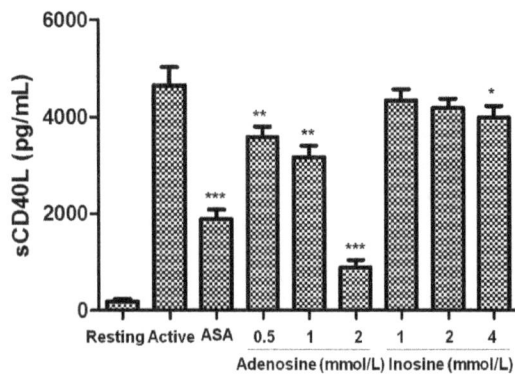

Figure 8. Effect of adenosine and inosine on release of sCD40L from platelets. Washed platelets were incubated with saline, adenosine, inosine or ASA (acetylsalicylic acid) and then stimulated with thrombin. The graph depicts the mean ± SEM of n = 6 experiments. *p < 0.05, **p < 0.01 and ***p < 0.001 as compared with the active (saline and then stimulated with thrombin). The results presented are from 6 separate volunteers (each donors performed as single triplicates).

were not able to attenuate the effect of inosine on ADP-induced platelet aggregation. Thus inosine by intraplatelet signaling pathways inhibits platelet function (phospholipase C activation rather than PKC) [42]. In this sense, different mechanisms may underlie the antiplatelet activity of adenosine and inosine. In fact, different biological functions of both nucleosides have also been demonstrated [56].

Previously, it has been suggested that adenosine is a natural ligand for the four receptors of the family (A_1, A_{2A}, A_{2B} and A_3), while inosine is only a weak agonist for the A_1 and A_3 adenosine receptors [57]. In addition, A_{2A} and A_{2B} receptors are naturally expressed in platelets [58,59]. The adenosine receptor A_{2A} has a structure consisting of seven transmembrane helices (H1–H7). The binding modes of adenosine and other adenosine receptor A_{2A} agonists have been reported recently [60]. Despite the high structural similitude and antiplatelet activity between adenosine and inosine, the latter is ineffective at adenosine receptor A_{2A} [60]. We performed docking experiments in order to explain this paradigm at a molecular level. The main difference is that adenosine forms an additional HB between the NH_2 of the adenine group and the residues Asn253 in H6 and Glu169 in EL2 of the adenosine receptor A_{2A}, whereas the hypoxanthine group of inosine cannot create these interactions, therefore losing its activity on the receptor and without an effect on cAMP levels.

In Figure 6 we have also included the alignment of the adenosine receptor A$_{2A}$ sequence motifs that include the A$_{2A}$R residues Glu169 and Asn253 to explain why inosine is not an adenosine receptor A2A ligand, but it is at least a weak agonist for A$_1$ and A$_3$ adenosine receptors. We can see that Asn253 is conserved in all the adenosine receptors. However, the FED motif in adenosine receptor A2A that contains Glu169 is different in other adenosine receptors. The FED motif is optimal for including adenine, but not optimal for including hypoxanthine. The phenylalanine forms the pi-pi stacking with the purine ring, glutamate forms the HB interaction with NH$_2$ of adenine, and aspartate is at the entrance of the pocket (it could be involved in the attraction of the ligand). The phenylalanine is conserved in all the adenosine receptors. However, the glutamate is not conserved in the A$_3$ receptor. Since there is no glutamate in the A$_3$ receptor, the negative density of the carbonyl oxygens in the hypoxanthine does not perceive a negative charge that prevents its binding. On the other hand, the aspartate at the entrance is mutated by asparagine in the A$_{2B}$ receptor (a neutral amino acid), and by a lysine in the A$_1$ receptor (positively charged amino acid). The lysine could contribute to the attraction of the hypoxanthine ring (due to the negative density of hypoxanthine). Summarizing, the changes in FED motif in A$_1$ and A$_3$ receptors could explain why inosine is at least a weak agonist for these receptors, but there is no evidence that A$_1$ and A$_3$ receptors are in platelets.

Platelet aggregation plays a key role in the pathogenesis of arterial thrombosis [61]. Therefore, inhibition of platelet aggregation by drugs has been used extensively for the prevention of thromboembolic events especially in patients with acute coronary syndromes. In this study, using a murine model of real-time thrombus formation [62], we demonstrated that adenosine and inosine significantly reduced thrombus growth *in vivo* although to a lesser extent than the effect observed with aspirin.

Conclusion

Our data supports the notion that the mechanisms underlying antiplatelet activity resulting from the interaction adenosine-adenosine receptor A$_{2A}$ seem to be related to a substantial increase in platelet cAMP levels with inhibition of P-selectin expression, sCD40L release and downregulated downstream signaling pathways of ADP and collagen receptors. On the other hand, although inosine does not seem to interact with platelet receptors it was capable of significantly inhibiting platelet adhesion and aggregation under flow and thrombus growth *in vivo*.

Author Contributions

Conceived and designed the experiments: EF MA JC JP IP. Performed the experiments: EF MA JC. Analyzed the data: JP DM IP. Contributed reagents/materials/analysis tools: IP JP. Contributed to the writing of the manuscript: EF JP IP.

References

1. Palomo GI, Icaza NG, Mujica EV, Nunez FL, Leiva ME, et al. (2007) Prevalence of cardiovascular risk factors in adult from Talca, Chile. Rev Med Chil 135: 904–912.
2. Bautista LE, Orostegui M, Vera LM, Prada GE, Orozco LC, et al. (2006) Prevalence and impact of cardiovascular risk factors in Bucaramanga, Colombia: results from the Countrywide Integrated Noncommunicable Disease Intervention Programme (CINDI/CARMEN) baseline survey. Eur J Cardiovasc Prev Rehabil 13: 769–775.
3. Grundy SM, Pasternak R, Greenland P, Smith S Jr, Fuster V (1999) Assessment of cardiovascular risk by use of multiple-risk-factor assessment equations: a statement for healthcare professionals from the American Heart Association and the American College of Cardiology. Circulation 100: 1481–1492.
4. Mujica V, Urzua A, Leiva E, Diaz N, Moore-Carrasco R, et al. (2010) Intervention with education and exercise reverses the metabolic syndrome in adults. J Am Soc Hypertens 4: 148–153.
5. Willoughby S, Holmes A, Loscalzo J (2002) Platelets and cardiovascular disease. Eur J Cardiovasc Nurs 1: 273–288.
6. Sagel J, Colwell JA, Crook L, Laimins M (1975) Increased platelet aggregation in early diabetus mellitus. Ann Intern Med 82: 733–738.
7. Palomo I, Moore-Carrasco R, Alarcon M, Rojas A, Espana F, et al. (2010) Pathophysiology of the proatherothrombotic state in the metabolic syndrome. Front Biosci (Schol Ed) 2: 194–208.
8. Ruggeri ZM (1997) Mechanisms initiating platelet thrombus formation. Thromb Haemost 78: 611–616.
9. Chakhtoura EY, Shamoon FE, Haft JI, Obiedzinski GR, Cohen AJ, et al. (2000) Comparison of platelet activation in unstable and stable angina pectoris and correlation with coronary angiographic findings. Am J Cardiol 86: 835–839.
10. Galliera E, Corsi MM, Banfi G (2012) Platelet rich plasma therapy: inflammatory molecules involved in tissue healing. J Biol Regul Homeost Agents 26: 35S–42S.
11. Fuentes QE, Fuentes QF, Andres V, Pello OM, de Mora JF, et al. (2013) Role of platelets as mediators that link inflammation and thrombosis in atherosclerosis. Platelets 24: 255–262.
12. Collins B, Hollidge C (2003) Antithrombotic drug market. Nat Rev Drug Discov 2: 11–12.
13. Palomo I, Toro C, Alarcon M (2008) The role of platelets in the pathophysiology of atherosclerosis (Review). Mol Med Rep 1: 179–184.
14. Ji X and Hou M (2011) Novel agents for anti-platelet therapy. J Hematol Oncol 4: 44.
15. Patrono C, Baigent C, Hirsh J, Roth G (2008) Antiplatelet drugs: American College of Chest Physicians Evidence-Based Clinical Practice Guidelines (8th Edition). Chest 133: 199S–233S.
16. Tantry US, Etherington A, Bliden KP, Gurbel PA (2006) Antiplatelet therapy: current strategies and future trends. Future Cardiol 2: 343–366.
17. Lerea KM, Glomset JA, Krebs EG (1987) Agents that elevate cAMP levels in platelets decrease thrombin binding. J Biol Chem 262: 282–288.
18. Lerea KM, Glomset JA (1987) Agents that elevate the concentration of cAMP in platelets inhibit the formation of a NaDodSO4-resistant complex between thrombin and a 40-kDa protein. Proc Natl Acad Sci U S A 84: 5620–5624.
19. Fredholm BB, AP IJ, Jacobson KA, Klotz KN, Linden J (2001) International Union of Pharmacology. XXV. Nomenclature and classification of adenosine receptors. Pharmacol Rev 53: 527–552.
20. Hasko G, Linden J, Cronstein B, Pacher P (2008) Adenosine receptors: therapeutic aspects for inflammatory and immune diseases. Nat Rev Drug Discov 7: 759–770.
21. Cristalli G, Costanzi S, Lambertucci C, Lupidi G, Vittori S, et al. (2001) Adenosine deaminase: functional implications and different classes of inhibitors. Med Res Rev 21: 105–128.
22. Hasko G, Kuhel DG, Nemeth ZH, Mabley JG, Stachlewitz RF, et al. (2000) Inosine inhibits inflammatory cytokine production by a posttranscriptional mechanism and protects against endotoxin-induced shock. J Immunol 164: 1013–1019.
23. Ritchie JL, Alexander HD, Rea IM (2000) Flow cytometry analysis of platelet P-selectin expression in whole blood–methodological considerations. Clin Lab Haematol 22: 359–363.
24. Born GV, Cross MJ (1963) The Aggregation of Blood Platelets. J Physiol 168: 178–195.
25. Conant CG, Schwartz MA, Nevill T, Ionescu-Zanetti C (2009) Platelet adhesion and aggregation under flow using microfluidic flow cells. J Vis Exp.
26. Friesner R, Banks J, Murphy R, Halgren T, Klicic J, et al. (2004) Glide: a new approach for rapid, accurate docking and scoring. 1. Method and assessment of docking accuracy. Journal of Medicinal Chemistry 47: 1739–1749.
27. Munoz C, Adasme F, Alzate-Morales JH, Vergara-Jaque A, Kniess T, et al. (2012) Study of differences in the VEGFR2 inhibitory activities between semaxanib and SU5205 using 3D-QSAR, docking, and molecular dynamics simulations. J Mol Graph Model 32: 39–48.
28. Jorgensen W, Maxwell D, Tirado-Rives J (1996) Development and testing of the OPLS all-atom force field on conformational energetics and properties of organic liquids. Journal of the American Chemical Society 118: 11225–11236.
29. Eldridge MD, Murray CW, Auton TR, Paolini GV, Mee RP (1997) Empirical scoring functions: I. The development of a fast empirical scoring function to estimate the binding affinity of ligands in receptor complexes. J Comput Aided Mol Des 11: 425–445.
30. Przyklenk K, Whittaker P (2007) Adaptation of a photochemical method to initiate recurrent platelet-mediated thrombosis in small animals. Lasers Med Sci 22: 42–45.
31. Abramoff MD, Magalhaes PJ, Ram SJ (2004) Image Processing with ImageJ. Biophotonics International 11: 36–42.

32. Antczak AJ, Singh N, Gay SR, Worth RG (2010) IgG-complex stimulated platelets: a source of sCD40L and RANTES in initiation of inflammatory cascade. Cell Immunol 263: 129–133.

33. Kim J, Jiang Q, Glashofer M, Yehle S, Wess J, et al. (1996) Glutamate residues in the second extracellular loop of the human A2a adenosine receptor are required for ligand recognition. Mol Pharmacol 49: 683–691.

34. Fuentes E, Castro R, Astudillo L, Carrasco G, Alarcón M, et al. (2012) Bioassay-Guided Isolation and HPLC Determination of Bioactive Compound That Relate to the Antiplatelet Activity (Adhesion, Secretion, and Aggregation) from Solanum lycopersicum. Evidence-Based Complementary and Alternative Medicine: 1–10.

35. Wang J, Huang ZG, Cao H, Wang YT, Hui P, et al. (2008) Screening of anti-platelet aggregation agents from Panax notoginseng using human platelet extraction and HPLC-DAD-ESI-MS/MS. J Sep Sci 31: 1173–1180.

36. Fuentes E, Castro R, Astudillo L, Carrasco G, Alarcon M, et al. (2012) Bioassay-Guided Isolation and HPLC Determination of Bioactive Compound That Relate to the Antiplatelet Activity (Adhesion, Secretion, and Aggregation) from Solanum lycopersicum. Evid Based Complement Alternat Med 2012: 147031.

37. Anfossi G, Russo I, Massucco P, Mattiello L, Cavalot F, et al. (2002) Adenosine increases human platelet levels of cGMP through nitric oxide: possible role in its antiaggregating effect. Thromb Res 105: 71–78.

38. Minamino T, Kitakaze M, Asanuma H, Tomiyama Y, Shiraga M, et al. (1998) Endogenous adenosine inhibits P-selectin-dependent formation of coronary thromboemboli during hypoperfusion in dogs. J Clin Invest 101: 1643–1653.

39. Altman R, Rouvier J, Weisenberger H (1985) Identification of platelet inhibitor present in the melon (Cucurbitacea cucumis melo). Thromb Haemost 53: 312–313.

40. Dutta-Roy AK, Crosbie L, Gordon MJ (2001) Effects of tomato extract on human platelet aggregation in vitro. Platelets 12: 218–227.

41. Hasko G, Sitkovsky MV, Szabo C (2004) Immunomodulatory and neuroprotective effects of inosine. Trends Pharmacol Sci 25: 152–157.

42. Hsiao G, Lin KH, Chang Y, Chen TL, Tzu NH, et al. (2005) Protective mechanisms of inosine in platelet activation and cerebral ischemic damage. Arterioscler Thromb Vasc Biol 25: 1998–2004.

43. Burger PC, Wagner DD (2003) Platelet P-selectin facilitates atherosclerotic lesion development. Blood 101: 2661–2666.

44. Storey RF, Judge HM, Wilcox RG, Heptinstall S (2002) Inhibition of ADP-induced P-selectin expression and platelet-leukocyte conjugate formation by clopidogrel and the P2Y12 receptor antagonist AR-C69931MX but not aspirin. Thromb Haemost 88: 488–494.

45. Libersan D, Rousseau G, Merhi Y (2003) Differential regulation of P-selectin expression by protein kinase A and protein kinase G in thrombin-stimulated human platelets. Thromb Haemost 89: 310–317.

46. Fuentes E, Badimon L, Caballero J, Padro T, Vilahur G, et al. (2013) Protective mechanisms of adenosine 5′-monophosphate in platelet activation and thrombus formation. Thromb Haemost 111.

47. Inoue O, Suzuki-Inoue K, Dean WL, Frampton J, Watson SP (2003) Integrin alpha2beta1 mediates outside-in regulation of platelet spreading on collagen through activation of Src kinases and PLCgamma2. J Cell Biol 160: 769–780.

48. Aukrust P, Muller F, Ueland T, Berget T, Aaser E, et al. (1999) Enhanced levels of soluble and membrane-bound CD40 ligand in patients with unstable angina. Possible reflection of T lymphocyte and platelet involvement in the pathogenesis of acute coronary syndromes. Circulation 100: 614–620.

49. Wagner DD, Burger PC (2003) Platelets in inflammation and thrombosis. Arterioscler Thromb Vasc Biol 23: 2131–2137.

50. Harding SA, Sommerfield AJ, Sarma J, Twomey PJ, Newby DE, et al. (2004) Increased CD40 ligand and platelet-monocyte aggregates in patients with type 1 diabetes mellitus. Atherosclerosis 176: 321–325.

51. Setianto BY, Hartopo AB, Gharini PP, Anggrahini DW, Irawan B (2010) Circulating soluble CD40 ligand mediates the interaction between neutrophils and platelets in acute coronary syndrome. Heart Vessels 25: 282–287.

52. Daniel JL, Dangelmaier C, Jin J, Kim YB, Kunapuli SP (1999) Role of intracellular signaling events in ADP-induced platelet aggregation. Thromb Haemost 82: 1322–1326.

53. Yang D, Chen H, Koupenova M, Carroll SH, Eliades A, et al. (2010) A new role for the A2b adenosine receptor in regulating platelet function. J Thromb Haemost 8: 817–827.

54. Loyau S, Dumont B, Ollivier V, Boulaftali Y, Feldman L, et al. (2012) Platelet glycoprotein VI dimerization, an active process inducing receptor competence, is an indicator of platelet reactivity. Arterioscler Thromb Vasc Biol 32: 778–785.

55. Enomoto Y, Adachi S, Doi T, Natsume H, Kato K, et al. (2011) cAMP regulates ADP-induced HSP27 phosphorylation in human platelets. Int J Mol Med 27: 695–700.

56. Hoffmeister HM, Betz R, Fiechtner H, Seipel L (1987) Myocardial and circulatory effects of inosine. Cardiovasc Res 21: 65–71.

57. Fredholm BB, Irenius E, Kull B, Schulte G (2001) Comparison of the potency of adenosine as an agonist at human adenosine receptors expressed in Chinese hamster ovary cells. Biochem Pharmacol 61: 443–448.

58. Zhao Z, Makaritsis K, Francis CE, Gavras H, Ravid K (2000) A role for the A3 adenosine receptor in determining tissue levels of cAMP and blood pressure: studies in knock-out mice. Biochim Biophys Acta 1500: 280–290.

59. Johnston-Cox HA, Ravid K (2011) Adenosine and blood platelets. Purinergic Signal 7: 357–365.

60. Lebon G, Warne T, Edwards PC, Bennett K, Langmead CJ, et al. (2011) Agonist-bound adenosine A2A receptor structures reveal common features of GPCR activation. Nature 474: 521–525.

61. Barrett NE, Holbrook L, Jones S, Kaiser WJ, Moraes LA, et al. (2008) Future innovations in anti-platelet therapies. Br J Pharmacol 154: 918–939.

62. Fukuoka T, Hattori K, Maruyama H, Hirayama M, Tanahashi N (2012) Laser-induced thrombus formation in mouse brain microvasculature: effect of clopidogrel. J Thromb Thrombolysis 34: 193–198.

18

Eribulin Mesylate Targets Human Telomerase Reverse Transcriptase in Ovarian Cancer Cells

Satoko Yamaguchi[1], Yoshiko Maida[1], Mami Yasukawa[1], Tomoyasu Kato[2], Masayuki Yoshida[3], Kenkichi Masutomi[1]*

1 Division of Cancer Stem Cell, National Cancer Center Research Institute, Tokyo, Japan, 2 Department of Gynecology, National Cancer Center Hospital, Tokyo, Japan, 3 Department of Pathology and Clinical Laboratories, National Cancer Center Hospital, Tokyo, Japan

Abstract

Treatment of advanced ovarian cancer involves platinum-based chemotherapy. However, chemoresistance is a major obstacle. Cancer stem cells (CSCs) are thought to be one of the causes of chemoresistance, but the underlying mechanism remains elusive. Recently, human telomerase reverse transcriptase (hTERT) has been reported to promote CSC-like traits. In this study, we found that a mitotic inhibitor, eribulin mesylate (eribulin), effectively inhibited growth of platinum-resistant ovarian cancer cell lines. Eribulin-sensitive cells showed a higher efficiency for sphere formation, suggesting that these cells possess an enhanced CSC-like phenotype. Moreover, these cells expressed a higher level of hTERT, and suppression of hTERT expression by siRNA resulted in decreased sensitivity to eribulin, suggesting that hTERT may be a target for eribulin. Indeed, we found that eribulin directly inhibited RNA-dependent RNA polymerase (RdRP) activity, but not telomerase activity of hTERT *in vitro*. We propose that eribulin targets the RdRP activity of hTERT and may be an effective therapeutic option for CSCs. Furthermore, hTERT may be a useful biomarker to predict clinical responses to eribulin.

Editor: Taro Yamashita, Kanazawa University, Japan

Funding: This work was supported by Grant in Aid for Scientific Research (26462544) (to SY) from Japan Society for the Promotion of Science (http://www.jsps.go.jp/english/e-grants/), Funding program for the Next Generation World-Leading Researchers (NEXT program) (to KM) from Japan Society for the Promotion of Science (http://www.jsps.go.jp/english/e-jisedai/), the Mitsubishi Foundation (to KM) (http://www.mitsubishi-zaidan.jp/en/), the Uehara Memorial Foundation (to KM) (http://www.ueharazaidan.or.jp/), and National Cancer Center Research and Development Funds (26-A-5) (to KM) (http://www.ncc.go.jp/jp/about/rinri/kaihatsu/). The funders had no role in study design, data collection and analysis, decision to publish, or preparation of the manuscript.

Competing Interests: The authors have declared that no competing interests exist.

* Email: kmasutom@ncc.go.jp

Introduction

Ovarian cancer is the most lethal of all gynecological malignancies, claiming around 150,000 lives annually worldwide. The majority of ovarian cancers are diagnosed at an advanced stage, and platinum-based chemotherapy is the standard first-line treatment for advanced ovarian cancer patients. However, chemoresistance is a major obstacle in treating ovarian cancer.

Serous adenocarcinoma (SAC), the most common type of ovarian cancer, usually responds well to initial platinum-based chemotherapy, although it will recur and ultimately develop drug resistance. Clear cell carcinoma (CCC), the second most common type in Japan, is often resistant to initial platinum-based chemotherapy [1]. Regardless of whether the resistance is acquired or primary, more promising therapeutic strategies are necessary to overcome chemoresistance and improve the prognosis of ovarian cancer patients.

Recent studies have suggested that cancer stem cells (CSCs) are, at least in part, responsible for chemoresistance in many types of cancers including ovarian cancer [reviewed in [2]]. CSCs are a subpopulation of tumor cells, which are characterized by a self-renewal capacity and ability to differentiate into distinct cell types. The emergence of CSCs occurs at least partly as a result of epithelial-mesenchymal transition (EMT), a process essential for embryonic development, which is induced during cancer progression and crucial for cancer metastasis. CSCs possess the self-renewal feature of normal stem cells, and similar signaling pathways regulate self-renewal of CSCs and normal stem cells [3]. One such pathway involves telomerase reverse transcriptase (TERT), the rate-limiting catalytic subunit of telomerase, which is expressed in the majority of cancers. Recent evidence indicates that TERT regulates stem cell traits in a telomere length-independent manner. For example, TERT activates quiescent epidermal stem cells *in vivo* in a manner independent of the intrinsic RNA component of the telomerase enzyme TERC [4]. In addition, together with the SWItch-Sucrose NonFermentable (SWI-SNF) complex protein brahma-related gene 1 (BRG1), TERT acts as a transcriptional modulator of the Wnt/β-catenin signaling pathway, contributing to self-renewal and proliferation during development [5]. More recently, accumulating evidence indicates that TERT also operates in CSCs and promotes EMT and CSC-like traits. Specifically, overexpression of human TERT (hTERT) results in an enhanced sphere-forming capacity, increased expression of EMT/CSC markers, and increased *in vivo* tumorigenesis caused by hTERT interacting with β-catenin and enhancing its transcriptional activity [6]. Conversely, suppression of hTERT expression results in a decreased sphere-forming capacity and decreased expression of the CSC marker

CD44 [7]. This function of hTERT in promotion of EMT and CSC-like traits appears to be independent of its telomerase activity [6]. Indeed, we have reported that hTERT in a complex with BRG1 and the nucleolar GTP-binding protein nucleostemin (NS) (TBN complex) participates in maintenance of CSCs. Moreover, we found that overexpression of the TBN complex enhances tumorigenicity and expression of EMT/CSC markers in an hTERT-dependent manner but in a telomere length-independent manner [8]. The exact telomerase-independent mechanisms by which the TBN complex regulates CSCs remain elusive. One possible mechanism is via the RNA-dependent RNA polymerase (RdRP) activity of hTERT [9]. RdRP induces RNA interference through production of double-stranded RNAs from single-stranded template RNAs and regulates the assembly of heterochromatin and mitotic progression [10]. Similar to RdRPs in model organisms, we found that the RdRP activities of the TBN complex are high in mitotic cells, and suppression of the TBN complex results in mitotic arrest [11].

To address chemoresistance, therapeutic strategies targeting EMT and CSCs are increasingly attracting attention. Recently, because eribulin mesylate (eribulin) was reported to inhibit metastasis by reversing EMT [12], we speculated that eribulin might target CSCs. Eribulin is a non-taxane inhibitor of microtubule dynamics [13], which induces irreversible mitotic blockade, leading to persistent inactivation of Bcl-2 and subsequent apoptosis [14]. In the United States, eribulin has been approved for treatment of metastatic breast cancer after at least two treatment regimens including an anthracycline and a taxane. Furthermore, eribulin is approved for treatment of inoperable or recurrent breast cancer in Japan.

In this study, we found that eribulin effectively inhibited growth of platinum-resistant ovarian cancer cells. Eribulin-sensitive cells showed enhanced CSC-like characteristics and high hTERT expression. Suppression of hTERT expression resulted in decreased sensitivity to eribulin. Moreover, eribulin inhibited the RdRP activity of hTERT *in vitro*, demonstrating that hTERT is a direct target of eribulin.

Results

Eribulin inhibits growth of cisplatin-resistant ovarian adenocarcinoma cell lines

Fourteen ovarian adenocarcinoma cell lines were investigated for sensitivity to cisplatin [cis-diamminedichloroplatinum(II)], including six SAC cell lines (PEO1, PEO4, PEO14, PEO23, OVKATE, and OVSAHO), six CCC cell lines (RMG-I, ES-2, OVISE, OVMANA, OVTOKO, and TOV21G), and two undifferentiated/unclassified adenocarcinoma cell lines (OV-CAR-3 and A2780) (Table S1). As shown in Figure 1A, OVKATE, RMG-I, PEO4, and PEO23 cells were particularly resistant to cisplatin, presumably via different mechanisms. OVKATE cells have been previously reported as resistant to platinum agents with elevated expression of glutathione-S-transferase, a drug-resistance marker [15]. RMG-I cells are also resistant to cisplatin, which involves the extracellular signal-regulated kinase (ERK) pathway [16]. PEO4 and PEO23 cells were derived from the same patients as PEO1 and PEO14 cells, respectively, after development of clinical chemoresistance, and are therefore platinum resistant [17]. BRCA2 mutation has been found to contribute to platinum resistance in PEO4 cells [18].

We screened a series of known anti-cancer compounds for growth inhibition of platinum-resistant ovarian cancer cell lines. We found that eribulin, a mitotic inhibitor that suppresses microtubule dynamics [13], inhibited growth of RMG-I,

PEO23, and PEO4 cells (Figure 1B). Strikingly, eribulin was not as effective in some of the cisplatin-sensitive cell lines such as OVTOKO, PEO14, and TOV21G (Figure 1A and 1B). For further characterization, we defined eight cell lines with an IC_{50} of <100 nM for eribulin as "eribulin-sensitive" (Eribulin S) and six cell lines with an IC_{50} of >100 nM for eribulin as "eribulin-resistant" (Eribulin R).

Eribulin-sensitive cell lines show a higher sphere-forming capacity

CSCs are thought to be responsible for chemoresistance, and CSCs have been reported to contribute to cisplatin resistance in several types of cancer [19]. Moreover, it was recently reported that eribulin reverses EMT [12], a phenotype that is highly related to CSCs. Therefore, we investigated whether eribulin-sensitive cells possess an enhanced CSC-like phenotype. Because a sphere-forming capacity is a CSC-like characteristic, we performed sphere formation assays under serum-free conditions, and found that eribulin-sensitive cell lines showed high sphere formation efficiency (Figure 2A and 2B). The sphere formation efficiency of Eribulin S cell lines was significantly higher than that of Eribulin R cell lines (Figure 2C, p = 0.0013), suggesting that eribulin-sensitive cell lines possess enhanced CSC-like characteristics.

Since we have recently demonstrated that NS together with hTERT and BRG1 maintains CSCs [8] and we and others have also demonstrated that NS is a useful CSC marker [20–22], we investigated the expression of BRG1 and NS in Eribulin S and Eribulin R cell lines. The protein expression level of BRG1 was significantly higher in Eribulin S cell lines (Figure 2D and 2E, p = 0.0189), while only a modest tendency of higher level of NS in Eribulin S cell lines was observed (Figure 2D and 2E, p = 0.1216). We did not detect a difference in the expression level of CD133 or CD44 (Figure S1), the cell surface markers implied in some CSCs [23].

Eribulin S cells express higher levels of hTERT protein

Overexpression of hTERT results in an enhanced sphere-forming capacity in gastric cancer cells [6]. Conversely, suppression of hTERT expression results in a decreased sphere-forming capacity in breast cancer cells [7]. Therefore, we determined whether the ovarian cancer cells with a higher sphere-forming capacity express a higher level of hTERT. We observed a tendency in cell lines with high sphere-forming efficiency, such as RMG-I, PEO23, and A2780, to express relatively high levels of hTERT protein, while cell lines with low sphere-forming efficiency, such as TOV21G, OVTOKO, and OVMANA, expressed low levels of hTERT protein, as demonstrated by enzyme-linked immunosorbent assay (ELISA) (Figure 3A). The high level of hTERT expression in RMG-I cells can be accounted for by a gain-of-function mutation (-124 G>A) in the hTERT promoter region (Table S1 and Figure S2). This cancer-specific mutation was recently reported in melanoma and several other types of cancer [24–27], which creates new binding motifs for E-twenty six/ternary complex factors (ETS/TCF) and thus contributes to upregulated hTERT transcription [24,25].

We found that Eribulin S cell lines expressed higher levels of hTERT protein than those in Eribulin R cell lines (Figure 3B, p = 0.008).

Suppression of hTERT expression results in decreased sensitivity to eribulin

The correlation between hTERT expression and eribulin sensitivity led us to postulate that eribulin inhibits growth of

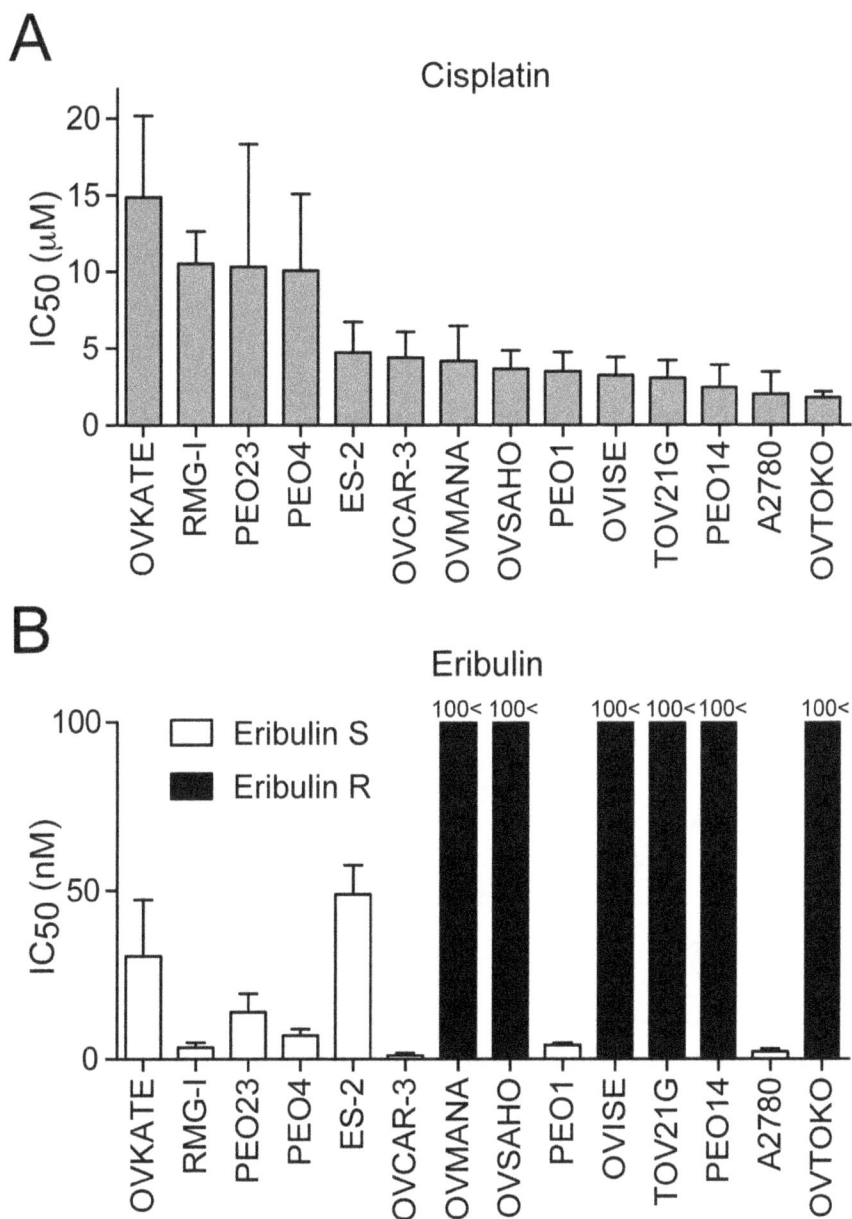

Figure 1. Eribulin inhibits growth of cisplatin-resistant ovarian cancer cells. Cells were treated with cisplatin or eribulin for 72 h, and then cell viability was determined by MTT assays. (A) Mean IC_{50} values for cisplatin (μM). (B) Mean IC_{50} values for eribulin (nM). Eribulin-sensitive (Eribulin S) cell lines are shown as open bars, and eribulin-resistant (Eribulin R) cell lines are shown as closed bars. Error bars represent the SD of at least three independent experiments.

ovarian cancer cells via inhibition of hTERT. To test this hypothesis, we examined whether suppression of hTERT expression in ovarian cancer cells leads to decreased sensitivity to eribulin. Two independent hTERT-specific siRNAs were introduced into A2780 cells, and sensitivity to eribulin was compared with cells expressing control siRNA. As expected, cells expressing hTERT siRNAs showed decreased sensitivity to eribulin (Figure 4A). TERT siRNA1 showed a tendency of stronger suppression of hTERT expression than TERT siRNA2 as demonstrated by ELISA (Figure 4B). This finding may explain why cells expressing TERT siRNA1 tended to be less sensitive to eribulin than those expressing TERT siRNA2 (Figure 4A). Similar results were obtained in ES-2 cells (Figure 4C and 4D). These results suggest that hTERT might be a direct target for eribulin.

Eribulin inhibits RdRP activity of hTERT *in vitro*

It is widely believed that any effect of hTERT suppression is mediated by telomere shortening. However, because we observed decreased sensitivity to eribulin in a relatively short period (Figure 4, 96 h after transfection of siRNA against hTERT), we speculated that this effect is independent of the telomere maintenance function of hTERT. Moreover, the function of hTERT in promotion of EMT and CSC-like traits is independent of its telomerase activity [6]. Together with our recent report showing that hTERT has an RdRP activity independent of telomere maintenance [9], we investigated whether eribulin directly targets hTERT-RdRP activity. We monitored the inhibitory effect of eribulin on hTERT-RdRP activity using an

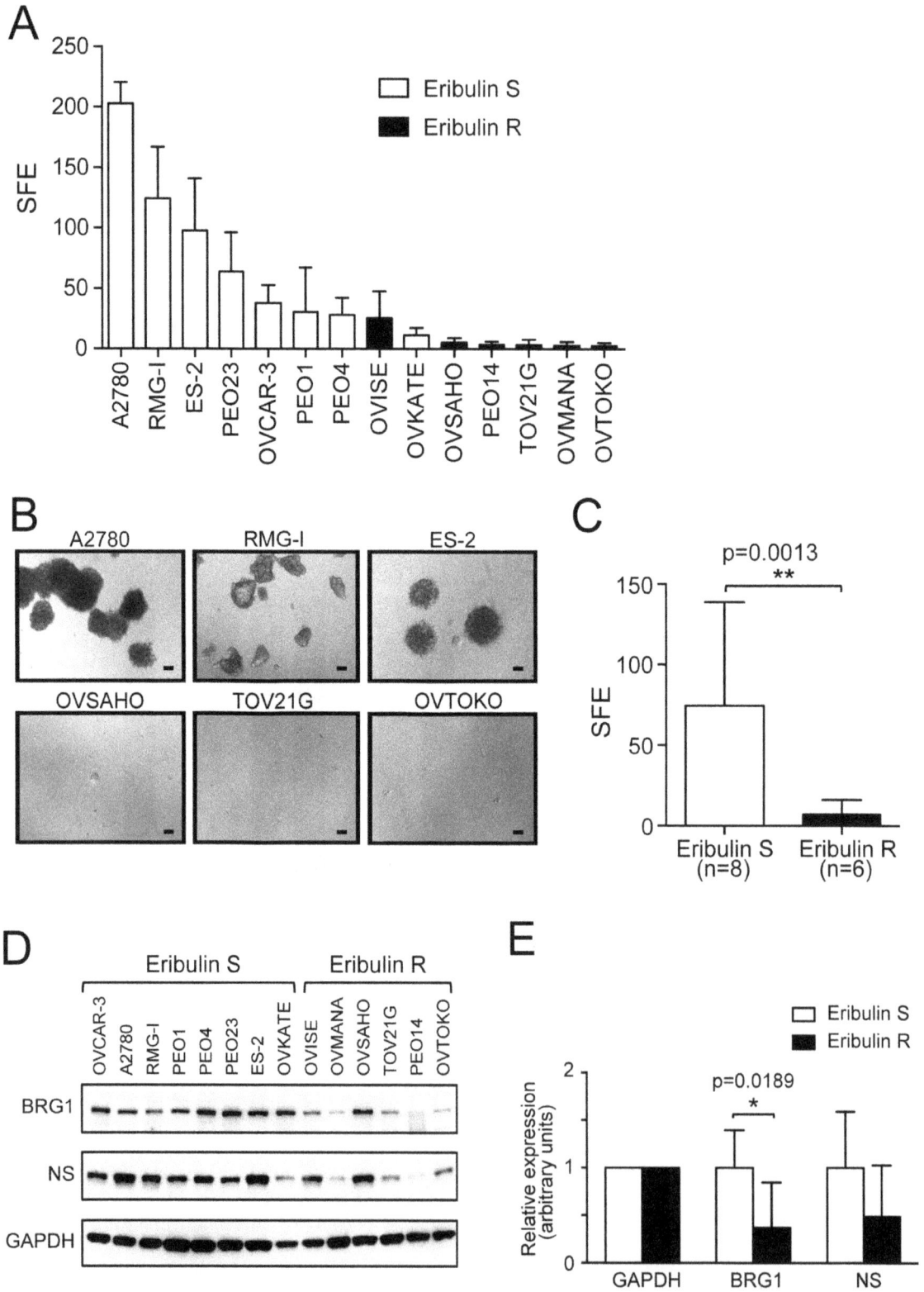

Figure 2. Eribulin-sensitive ovarian cancer cells show high sphere formation efficiency and higher BRG1 expression. (A) Sphere formation efficiency (SFE) of each cell line was indicated per 1,000 cells. Eribulin S cell lines are shown as open bars, and Eribulin R cells are shown as closed bars. Each experiment was performed at least three times, and mean values ± SD are indicated. (B) Morphology of tumorspheres under serum-free conditions. Representative images of spheres formed by A2780, RMG-I, ES-2, OVSAHO, TOV21G, and OVTOKO cells are shown. Scale bar = 50 μm. (C) The mean SFE of Eribulin S cell lines (n = 8) and Eribulin R cell lines (n = 6) shown in (A). Error bars indicate SD. (D) The level of BRG1 and NS protein expression was detected by immunoblotting. GAPDH expression was shown as loading control. (E) Signals in (D) were quantified with ImageJ software and normalized to GAPDH signal. The mean values of relative expression level ± SD are indicated.

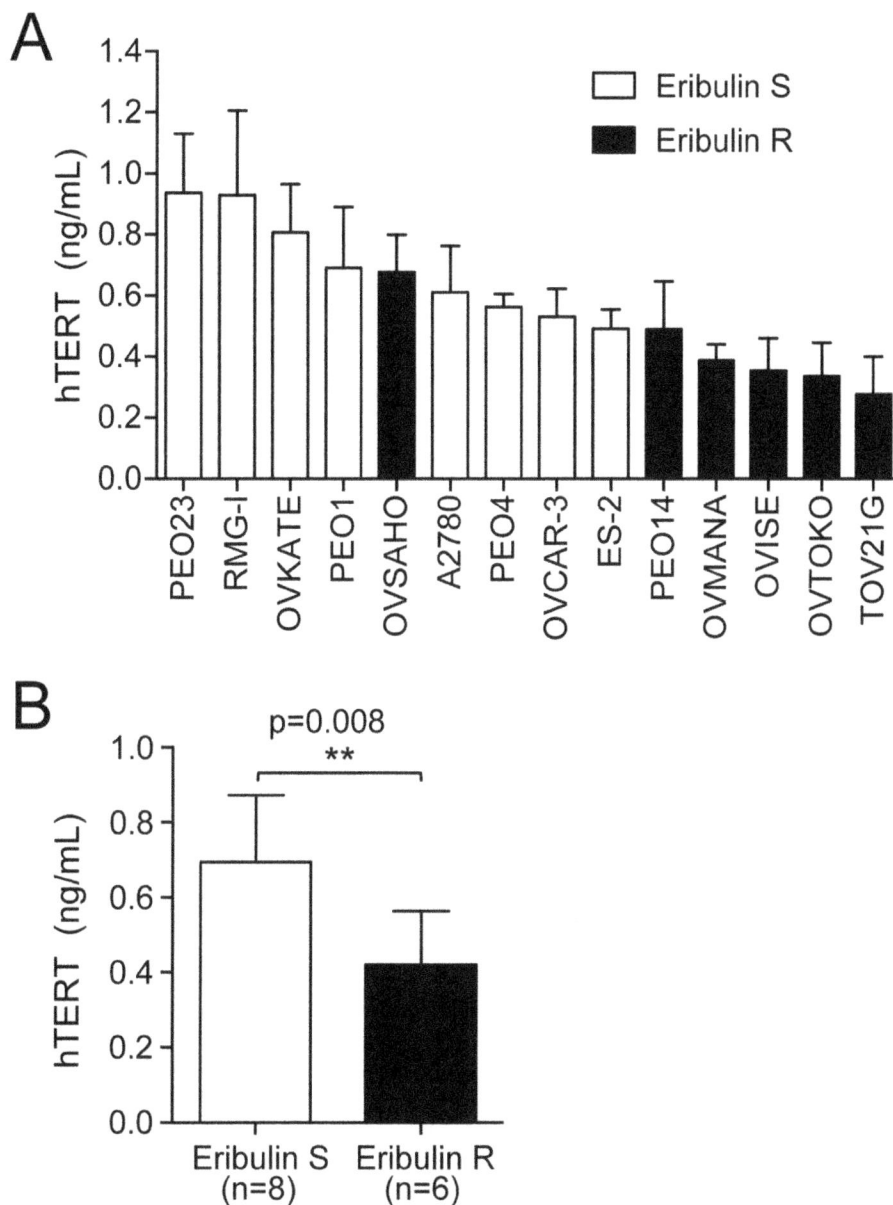

Figure 3. Eribulin-sensitive ovarian cancer cells express higher levels of hTERT protein. (A) The level of hTERT protein expression was determined by ELISA (indicated as ng/ml). Eribulin S cell lines are shown as open bars, and Eribulin R cells are shown as closed bars. Each experiment was performed at least three times, and mean values ± SD are indicated. (B) The mean hTERT level of Eribulin S cell lines (n = 8) and Eribulin R cell lines (n = 6) shown in (A). Error bars indicate SD.

in vitro RdRP assay [11], and found that eribulin inhibited hTERT-RdRP activity *in vitro* at a concentration of 50 μM (Figure 5A). The same concentration of eribulin did not inhibit the telomerase activity of hTERT as shown by telomeric repeat amplification protocol (TRAP) assay (Figure 5B). These results suggest that the effects of eribulin on hTERT are not mediated via telomerase activity, but via RdRP activity. Interestingly, another mitotic inhibitor, paclitaxel, a representative taxane, did not inhibit RdRP activity (Figure 5C), suggesting that eribulin has a specific inhibitory effect on hTERT-RdRP activity.

Discussion

Among gynecological cancers, ovarian cancer is the leading cause of death. In particular, resistance to conventional platinum-based chemotherapy has been a barrier in the improvement of prognoses for ovarian cancer patients, and new therapeutic strategies are urgently required. Here, we found that eribulin was effective to inhibit growth of platinum-resistant ovarian cancer cells. Effects of eribulin were correlated with hTERT expression levels (Figure 3), and suppression of hTERT expression resulted in decreased sensitivity to eribulin (Figure 4), suggesting that hTERT could be a target of eribulin in these cells. Indeed, eribulin inhibited the RdRP activity but not the reverse transcriptase activity of hTERT *in vitro* (Figure 5).

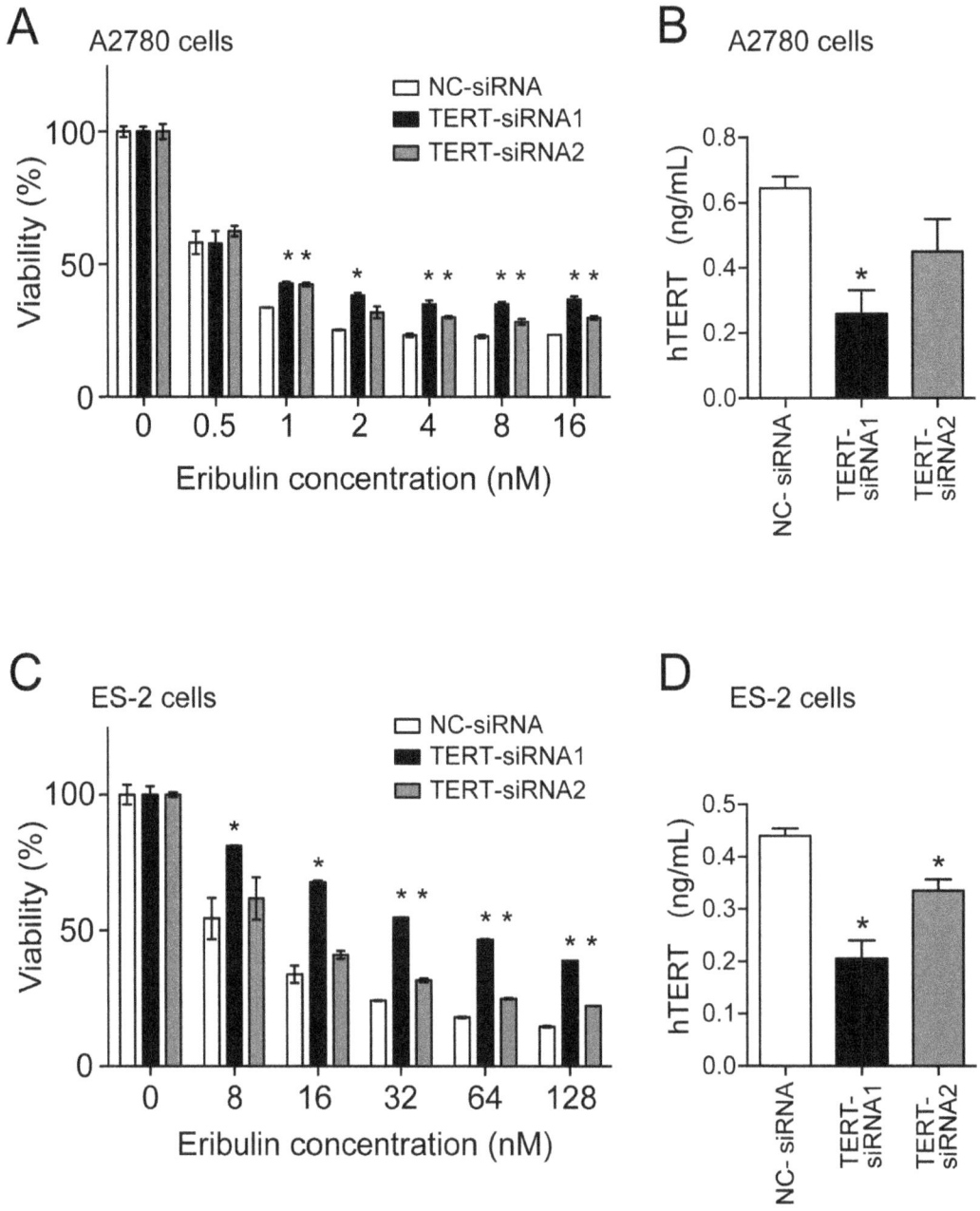

Figure 4. Suppression of hTERT expression by siRNA results in decreased sensitivity to eribulin. (A) A2780 cells expressing control siRNA (open bars), TERT siRNA1 (closed bars), or TERT siRNA2 (shaded bars) were treated with eribulin for 72 h, and then cell viability was determined by MTT assays. *$p < 0.05$ vs. cells expressing control siRNA. (B) The level of hTERT protein expression in A2780 cells expressing control siRNA (open bars), TERT siRNA1 (closed bars), or TERT siRNA2 (shaded bars) was determined by ELISA (indicated as ng/ml). (C and D) The experiments described in (A and B) were performed in the same manner using ES-2 cells expressing control siRNA (open bars), TERT siRNA1 (closed bars), or TERT siRNA2 (shaded bars). *$p < 0.05$ vs. cells expressing control siRNA.

CSCs and hTERT

CSCs are thought to be involved in chemoresistance, and several pathways have been found to contribute to the promotion or maintenance of CSCs. We and others have shown that hTERT plays an important role in promotion and maintenance of CSCs in telomere maintenance-independent manners [6–8]. Eribulin effectively inhibited growth of platinum-resistant cells (Figure 1). Eribulin-sensitive cells exhibited higher hTERT expression (Figure 3) and a higher sphere-forming capacity (Figure 2), suggesting that these cells have enhanced CSC-like characteristics,

possibly due to the high levels of hTERT protein. Consistently, eribulin-sensitive cells exhibited higher BRG1 expression (Figure 2), another component of the TBN complex that maintains CSCs. We did not detect a significant difference in the expression of CD133 or CD44 (Figure S1). Although CD133 and CD44 are thought to be indicative of CSCs in some types of cancer, it remains to be elucidated what markers are appropriate for CSCs in ovarian cancers [23].

Because telomere maintenance by telomerase is indispensable for infinite proliferation of malignant cells, efforts have been made

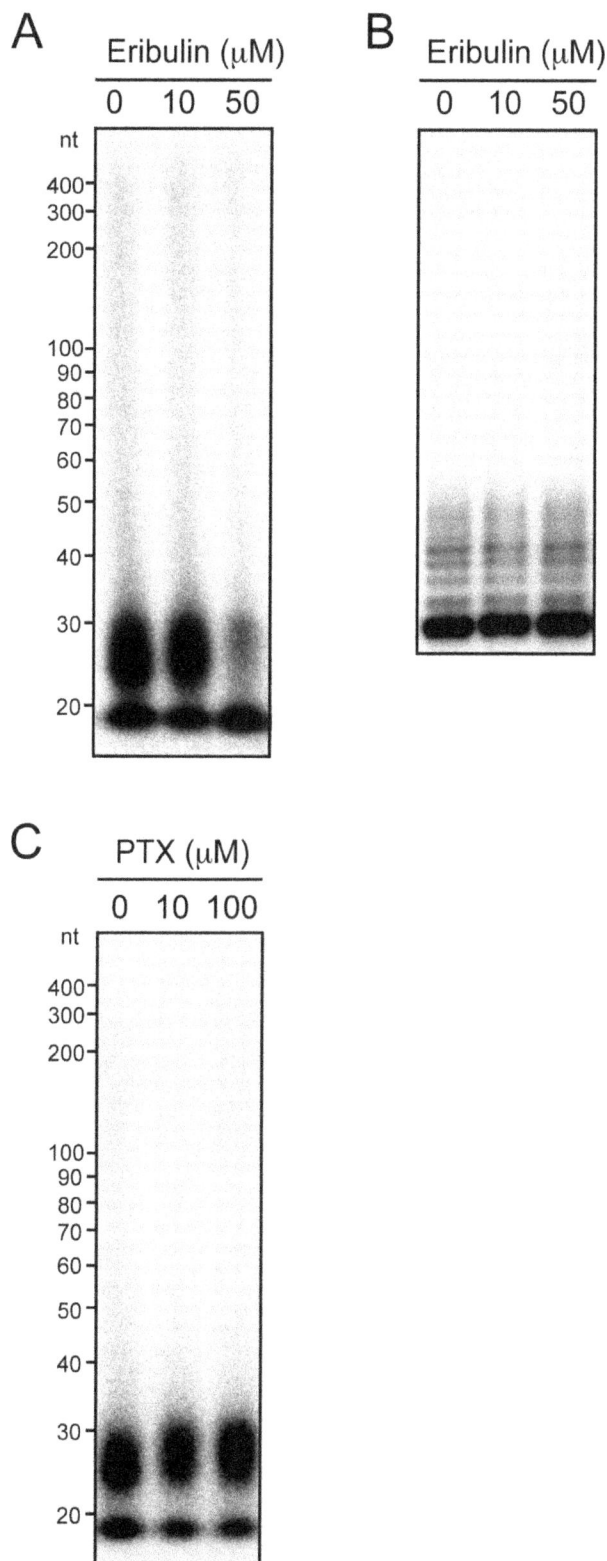

Figure 5. Eribulin inhibits RdRP activity but not telomerase activity of hTERT. (A) RdRP activity of hTERT immune complexes prepared from HeLa cells arrested in the mitotic phase was assayed without or with 10 and 50 μM eribulin. (B) Telomerase activity in HeLa cell extracts was assayed without or with 10 and 50 μM eribulin. (C) RdRP activity of hTERT immune complexes was assayed without or with 10 and 100 μM paclitaxel (PTX).

to develop anticancer therapeutics targeting telomerase. Recent studies indicate that TERT plays functional roles beyond telomere maintenance. Indeed, the function of TERT to activate normal quiescent stem cells or CSC-like traits has been shown to be independent of its telomerase activity [4,6,28]. We have also found that the TBN complex maintains CSCs in a telomere length-independent manner [8]. It is possible that this telomerase-independent mechanism is mediated by the RdRP activity of TERT, because the TBN complex itself is responsible for the RdRP activity and is involved in heterochromatin regulation and mitotic progression [11]. We speculate that the RdRP activity of hTERT is involved in gene expression through heterochromatin regulation in cancer cells, and it could be a novel anticancer therapeutic target. Whether RdRP activity is prerequisite for hTERT function in the promotion of CSCs remains to be determined.

Eribulin and hTERT

Eribulin binds to microtubule plus ends and inhibits the growth phase of microtubule dynamics [29]. Recently, eribulin was shown to reverse EMT by downregulating transforming growth factor-β (TGF-β)-induced Smad phosphorylation [12]. Smad proteins bind to microtubules in the absence of TGF-β and TGF-β triggers dissociation from microtubules and phosphorylation of Smad proteins [30]. Yoshida *et al.* speculated that eribulin inhibits Smad phosphorylation possibly by suppressing Smad dissociation from microtubules [12]. Because we have recently demonstrated that hTERT localizes to mitotic spindles and centromeres during mitosis [11], it is also possible that eribulin inhibits hTERT functions by interfering with the interaction between hTERT and microtubules. Eribulin improves overall survival of patients with metastatic breast cancer, who had prior anthracycline- and taxane-based chemotherapy [31]. A taxane drug, paclitaxel, did not inhibit the RdRP activity of hTERT (Figure 5C), providing one of the potential molecular bases for the different clinical outcomes of taxanes and eribulin. The exact mechanism by which eribulin inhibits hTERT function is yet to be understood.

hTERT as a biomarker

It is important to identify biomarkers to predict responses to anticancer therapies. By determination of hTERT levels in clinical specimens, patients who are likely to respond well to eribulin may be identified before they receive chemotherapy. In particular, an ELISA would be able to measure hTERT levels in clinical practice.

In summary, we found that eribulin inhibits RdRP activity of hTERT, which may contribute to chemoresistance in ovarian cancer by maintaining CSCs. Eribulin inhibited the growth of ovarian cancer cells with high hTERT expression and strong platinum resistance, suggesting it may be a promising therapeutic agent for chemoresistant ovarian cancer. Moreover, hTERT may be a useful biomarker to predict clinical responses to eribulin.

Materials and Methods

Cell lines

RMG-I [32], OVMANA [33], OVTOKO [34], OVISE [34], OVSAHO [33], and OVKATE [33] cells were obtained from the Japanese Collection of Research Bioresources Cell Bank. OV-CAR-3 cells [35] were obtained from the RIKEN BioResource Center. PEO1, PEO4, PEO14, PEO23 [17], and A2780 [36] cells were purchased from the European Collection of Cell Cultures, and TOV21G [37] and ES-2 [38] cells were purchased from the American Type Culture Collection. RMG-I cells were cultured in

Ham's F12 medium supplemented with 10% fetal bovine serum, ES-2 cells in McCoy's 5a medium supplemented with 10% fetal bovine serum, TOV21G cells in MCDB105/Medium 199 (1:1) supplemented with 10% fetal bovine serum, and HeLa cells in Dulbecco's modified Eagle's medium (DMEM) supplemented with 10% fetal bovine serum. All other cell lines (A2780, OVCAR-3, OVMANA, OVTOKO, OVISE, OVSAHO, OVKATE, PEO1, PEO4, PEO14, and PEO23) were cultured in RPMI-1640 medium supplemented with 10% fetal bovine serum and 1 mM sodium pyruvate (Gibco, Grand Island, NY, USA).

Compounds

Cisplatin was purchased from Sigma-Aldrich (St Louis, MO, USA), paclitaxel was purchased from Wako (Osaka, Japan), and eribulin (Halaven) was purchased from Eisai Co., Ltd (Tsukuba, Japan).

MTT assay

Cells (5,000–10,000 per well) were seeded in 96-well plates and then treated with cisplatin or eribulin after 24 h. At 72 h of treatment, an MTT proliferation assay (Cell Proliferation Kit I MTT, Roche Diagnostics, Mannheim, Germany) was performed according to the manufacturer's protocol. Briefly, 10 μl MTT labeling reagent was added to each well, followed by 4 h of incubation. Then, 100 μl solubilization solution was added to each well, followed by overnight incubation. The reaction product was quantified by measuring the absorbance at 570 and 690 nm using a microplate reader (Viento 808, BioTek, Winooski, VT, USA). Cell viability was determined by comparisons to untreated cells.

Sphere formation assay

Single cells were seeded in 96-well ultra low attachment plates (Corning Inc, Corning, NY, USA) at 100–1,000 cells/100 μl medium in each well. Cells were grown in serum-free DMEM/F12 medium (Gibco) supplemented with 20 ng/ml basic fibroblast growth factor (Wako), 20 ng/ml epidermal growth factor (Wako), and B27 supplement (Gibco). Cultures were supplemented with 25 μl of fresh medium every 3–4 days, and the number of spheres was counted on days 7 and 14. Microscopic images were obtained with a CKX41 inverted microscope and DP21 digital camera (Olympus, Tokyo, Japan).

Immunoblotting

Cells were lysed in radioimmunoprecipitation assay (RIPA) buffer containing 1% NP-40, 1 mM EDTA, 50 mM Tris-HCl (pH 7.4) and 150 mM NaCl. After sonication and centrifugation of the lysates, proteins (20 μg) were subjected to SDS-PAGE in 7.5% poly-acrylamide gels, followed by immunoblot analysis. The following antibodies were used: anti-BRG1 (a gift from Dr. Tsutomu Ohta, National Cancer Center, Japan), anti-NS (A300–600A; Bethyl Laboratories, Montgomery, TX, USA), anti-GAPDH (3H12; Medical & Biological Laboratories (MBL), Nagoya, Japan), anti-CD133 (W6B3C1; Miltenyi Biotec, Bergisch Gladbach, Germany) and anti-CD44 (2C5; R&D Systems, Minneapolis, MN, USA). Signals were detected by LAS-3000 (Fujifilm, Tokyo, Japan), quantified with ImageJ software (National Institutes of Health, USA) and normalized using GAPDH loading control.

hTERT ELISA

The hTERT ELISA employed a rabbit anti-hTERT polyclonal antibody as the capture antibody (MBL), and a mouse anti-hTERT monoclonal antibody (mAb) (clone 2E4-5) as the detection antibody (MBL code no. 5340, Ab-Match Assembly Human TERT Kit). The 2E4-5 antibody was generated against recombinant hTERT as an immunogen as described previously [11]. Cells were lysed in RIPA buffer. After sonication and centrifugation of the lysates, 100 μg total protein (100 μl in volume) was added to each well of a 96-well plate (MBL code no. 5310, Ab-Match Universal Kit). The ELISA was performed according to the manufacturer's instructions. Absorbances at 450 and 630 nm were measured by a microplate reader. Each experiment was performed at least three times, and mean values were calculated.

TERT promoter mutation analysis

Genomic DNA was extracted from ovarian cancer cell lines using a Blood and Cell Culture DNA Kit (Qiagen, Hilden, Germany) according to the manufacturer's protocol. The TERT promoter region (-146 to -124-bp upstream from the start codon) was amplified by PCR using KOD FX (Toyobo, Osaka, Japan) and the following primers: 5′-GTCCTGCCCCTTCACCTT-3′ and 5′-CAGCGCTGCCT-GAAACTC-3′ [25]. PCR was performed under the following conditions: 40 cycles of 98°C for 10 s, 55°C for 30 s, and 68°C for 60 s. Purified PCR products were sequenced by Sanger sequencing.

Transfection of siRNA

Cells were transfected with siRNA by Lipofectamine RNAi-MAX (Invitrogen) and then seeded at 5,000–10,000 cells per well in 96-well plates. At 24 h after transfection, the cells were treated with eribulin, and an MTT assay was performed after 72 h of treatment. For the ELISA, $2–5.0 \times 10^6$ cells transfected with siRNA were plated in a 10-cm petri dish, and then collected after 48 h of incubation. hTERT siRNA1 and hTERT siRNA2 have been described previously [8]. The negative control siRNA (MISSION siRNA Universal Negative Control; Sigma-Aldrich) was also used.

IP-RdRP assay

In order to detect RdRP activity in vitro, the hTERT immune complex was isolated by mAb against hTERT. An IP-RdRP assay has been established in mitotically arrested HeLa cells [11]. Therefore, HeLa cells were used for this assay. To synchronize HeLa cells undergoing mitosis, the cells were cultured in medium containing 2.5 mM thymidine (Nacalai Tesque, Kyoto, Japan) for 24 h. At 6 h after release, the cells were incubated in medium containing 0.1 μg/ml nocodazole (Sigma-Aldrich) for 14 h. After shaking gently, mitotic cells were retrieved. The IP-RdRP assay was performed as described previously [11].

TRAP assay

A TRAP assay was used to detect telomere specific reverse transcriptase activity as described previously [39].

Statistical analysis

Statistical analyses were performed with GraphPad Prism 6 (GraphPad Software, La Jolla, CA, USA). The Student's t-test or Mann Whitney test was used. Two-sided p-values of <0.05 were considered statistically significant.

Supporting Information

Figure S1 CD133 and CD44 expression in Eribulin S and Eribulin R ovarian cancer cells. (A) The level of CD133 and CD44 protein expression was detected by immunoblotting.

Since the data was obtained in the same experiment as Figure 2 panel D, GAPDH gel was identical with Figure 2 panel D. (B) Signals in (A) were quantified with ImageJ software and normalized to GAPDH signal. The mean values of relative expression level ± SD are indicated.

Figure S2 ES-2 and RMG-I cells possess hTERT promoter mutations. The hTERT promoter was sequenced in each cell line. ES-2 cells harbor a -138/-139 GG>AA mutation as described previously [27], and RMG-I cells harbor a -124 G>A mutation. The wild-type sequences of the corresponding regions from OVKATE and OVSAHO cells are shown as controls.

References

Acknowledgments

We thank Dr. Tsutomu Ohta for the gift of anti-BRG1 antibody, Dr. Koichi Ichimura for technical assistance with promoter mutation analysis, and MBL for their assistance in establishing the ELISA kit for hTERT detection.

Author Contributions

Conceived and designed the experiments: SY KM. Performed the experiments: SY YM M. Yasukawa. Analyzed the data: SY YM. Contributed reagents/materials/analysis tools: TK M. Yoshida. Contributed to the writing of the manuscript: SY YM KM.

1. Takano M, Tsuda H, Sugiyama T (2012) Clear cell carcinoma of the ovary: is there a role of histology-specific treatment? J Exp Clin Cancer Res 31: 53.
2. Singh A, Settleman J (2010) EMT, cancer stem cells and drug resistance: an emerging axis of evil in the war on cancer. Oncogene 29: 4741–4751.
3. Pardal R, Clarke MF, Morrison SJ (2003) Applying the principles of stem-cell biology to cancer. Nat Rev Cancer 3: 895–902.
4. Sarin KY, Cheung P, Gilison D, Lee E, Tennen RI, et al. (2005) Conditional telomerase induction causes proliferation of hair follicle stem cells. Nature 436: 1048–1052.
5. Park JI, Venteicher AS, Hong JY, Choi J, Jun S, et al. (2009) Telomerase modulates Wnt signalling by association with target gene chromatin. Nature 460: 66–72.
6. Liu Z, Li Q, Li K, Chen L, Li W, et al. (2013) Telomerase reverse transcriptase promotes epithelial-mesenchymal transition and stem cell-like traits in cancer cells. Oncogene 32: 4203–4213.
7. Chung SS, Aroh C, Vadgama JV (2013) Constitutive Activation of STAT3 Signaling Regulates hTERT and Promotes Stem Cell-Like Traits in Human Breast Cancer Cells. PLoS One 8: e83971.
8. Okamoto N, Yasukawa M, Nguyen C, Kasim V, Maida Y, et al. (2011) Maintenance of tumor initiating cells of defined genetic composition by nucleostemin. Proc Natl Acad Sci U S A 108: 20388–20393.
9. Maida Y, Yasukawa M, Furuuchi M, Lassmann T, Possemato R, et al. (2009) An RNA-dependent RNA polymerase formed by TERT and the RMRP RNA. Nature 461: 230–235.
10. Martienssen RA, Zaratiegui M, Goto DB (2005) RNA interference and heterochromatin in the fission yeast Schizosaccharomyces pombe. Trends Genet 21: 450–456.
11. Maida Y, Yasukawa M, Okamoto N, Ohka S, Kinoshita K, et al. (2014) Involvement of telomerase reverse transcriptase in heterochromatin maintenance. Mol Cell Biol 34: 1576–1593.
12. Yoshida T, Ozawa Y, Kimura T, Sato Y, Kuznetsov G, et al. (2014) Eribulin mesilate suppresses experimental metastasis of breast cancer cells by reversing phenotype from epithelial-mesenchymal transition (EMT) to mesenchymal-epithelial transition (MET) states. Br J Cancer 110: 1497–1505.
13. Towle MJ, Salvato KA, Budrow J, Wels BF, Kuznetsov G, et al. (2001) In vitro and in vivo anticancer activities of synthetic macrocyclic ketone analogues of halichondrin B. Cancer Res 61: 1013–1021.
14. Towle MJ, Salvato KA, Wels BF, Aalfs KK, Zheng W, et al. (2011) Eribulin induces irreversible mitotic blockade: implications of cell-based pharmacodynamics for in vivo efficacy under intermittent dosing conditions. Cancer Res 71: 496–505.
15. Ohta I, Gorai I, Miyamoto Y, Yang J, Zheng JH, et al. (2001) Cyclophosphamide and 5-fluorouracil act synergistically in ovarian clear cell adenocarcinoma cells. Cancer Lett 162: 39–48.
16. Wang J, Zhou JY, Wu GS (2011) Bim protein degradation contributes to cisplatin resistance. J Biol Chem 286: 22384–22392.
17. Langdon SP, Lawrie SS, Hay FG, Hawkes MM, McDonald A, et al. (1988) Characterization and properties of nine human ovarian adenocarcinoma cell lines. Cancer Res 48: 6166–6172.
18. Sakai W, Swisher EM, Jacquemont C, Chandramohan KV, Couch FJ, et al. (2009) Functional restoration of BRCA2 protein by secondary BRCA2 mutations in BRCA2-mutated ovarian carcinoma. Cancer Res 69: 6381–6386.
19. Vidal SJ, Rodriguez-Bravo V, Galsky M, Cordon-Cardo C, Domingo-Domenech J (2014) Targeting cancer stem cells to suppress acquired chemotherapy resistance. Oncogene 33: 4451–4463.
20. Tamase A, Muraguchi T, Naka K, Tanaka S, Kinoshita M, et al. (2009) Identification of tumor-initiating cells in a highly aggressive brain tumor using promoter activity of nucleostemin. Proc Natl Acad Sci U S A 106: 17163–17168.
21. Kobayashi T, Masutomi K, Tamura K, Moriya T, Yamasaki T, et al. (2014) Nucleostemin expression in invasive breast cancer. BMC Cancer 14: 215.
22. Lin T, Meng L, Li Y, Tsai RY (2010) Tumor-initiating function of nucleostemin-enriched mammary tumor cells. Cancer Res 70: 9444–9452.
23. Medema JP (2013) Cancer stem cells: the challenges ahead. Nat Cell Biol 15: 338–344.
24. Huang FW, Hodis E, Xu MJ, Kryukov GV, Chin L, et al. (2013) Highly recurrent TERT promoter mutations in human melanoma. Science 339: 957–959.
25. Horn S, Figl A, Rachakonda PS, Fischer C, Sucker A, et al. (2013) TERT promoter mutations in familial and sporadic melanoma. Science 339: 959–961.
26. Killela PJ, Reitman ZJ, Jiao Y, Bettegowda C, Agrawal N, et al. (2013) TERT promoter mutations occur frequently in gliomas and a subset of tumors derived from cells with low rates of self-renewal. Proc Natl Acad Sci U S A 110: 6021–6026.
27. Wu RC, Ayhan A, Maeda D, Kim KR, Clarke BA, et al. (2013) Frequent somatic mutations of the telomerase reverse transcriptase promoter in ovarian clear cell carcinoma but not in other major types of gynecologic malignancies. J Pathol 232: 473–481.
28. Choi J, Southworth LK, Sarin KY, Venteicher AS, Ma W, et al. (2008) TERT promotes epithelial proliferation through transcriptional control of a Myc- and Wnt-related developmental program. PLoS Genet 4: e10.
29. Smith JA, Wilson L, Azarenko O, Zhu X, Lewis BM, et al. (2010) Eribulin binds at microtubule ends to a single site on tubulin to suppress dynamic instability. Biochemistry 49: 1331–1337.
30. Dong C, Li Z, Alvarez R Jr, Feng XH, Goldschmidt-Clermont PJ (2000) Microtubule binding to Smads may regulate TGF beta activity. Mol Cell 5: 27–34.
31. Cortes J, O'Shaughnessy J, Loesch D, Blum JL, Vahdat LT, et al. (2011) Eribulin monotherapy versus treatment of physician's choice in patients with metastatic breast cancer (EMBRACE): a phase 3 open-label randomised study. Lancet 377: 914–923.
32. Nozawa S, Tsukazaki K, Sakayori M, Jeng CH, Iizuka R (1988) Establishment of a human ovarian clear cell carcinoma cell line (RMG-I) and its single cell cloning–with special reference to the stem cell of the tumor. Hum Cell 1: 426–435.
33. Yanagibashi T, Gorai I, Nakazawa T, Miyagi E, Hirahara F, et al. (1997) Complexity of expression of the intermediate filaments of six new human ovarian carcinoma cell lines: new expression of cytokeratin 20. Br J Cancer 76: 829–835.
34. Gorai I, Nakazawa T, Miyagi E, Hirahara F, Nagashima Y, et al. (1995) Establishment and characterization of two human ovarian clear cell adenocarcinoma lines from metastatic lesions with different properties. Gynecol Oncol 57: 33–46.
35. Hamilton TC, Young RC, McKoy WM, Grotzinger KR, Green JA, et al. (1983) Characterization of a human ovarian carcinoma cell line (NIH:OVCAR-3) with androgen and estrogen receptors. Cancer Res 43: 5379–5389.
36. Hamilton TC, Young RC, Ozols RF (1984) Experimental model systems of ovarian cancer: applications to the design and evaluation of new treatment approaches. Semin Oncol 11: 285–298.
37. Provencher DM, Lounis H, Champoux L, Tetrault M, Manderson EN, et al. (2000) Characterization of four novel epithelial ovarian cancer cell lines. In Vitro Cell Dev Biol Anim 36: 357–361.
38. Lau DH, Lewis AD, Ehsan MN, Sikic BI (1991) Multifactorial mechanisms associated with broad cross-resistance of ovarian carcinoma cells selected by cyanomorpholino doxorubicin. Cancer Res 51: 5181–5187.
39. Kim NW, Piatyszek MA, Prowse KR, Harley CB, West MD, et al. (1994) Specific association of human telomerase activity with immortal cells and cancer. Science 266: 2011–2015.

19

A CLDN1-Negative Phenotype Predicts Poor Prognosis in Triple-Negative Breast Cancer

Fei Ma[1][⅁][¶], Xiaoyan Ding[2][⅁][¶], Ying Fan[1], Jianming Ying[3], Shan Zheng[3], Ning Lu[3]*, Binghe Xu[1]*

1 Department of Medical Oncology, Cancer Hospital, Chinese Academy of Medical Sciences and Peking Union Medical College, Beijing, China, **2** Department of Medical Oncology, Beijing DiTan Hospital, Capital Medical University, Beijing, China, **3** Department of Pathology, Cancer Hospital, Chinese Academy of Medical Sciences and Peking Union Medical College, Beijing, China

Abstract

Introduction: Triple-negative breast cancer (TNBC) is a heterogeneous disease with no definitive prognostic markers. As a major component of tight junctions, claudins (CLDNs) presumably play an important role in carcinogenesis and progression of breast cancer. This study was aimed at determining the relationship between the expression of CLDNs and the clinical outcomes of TNBCs.

Materials and Methods: The surgical specimens of primary breast tumors from a consecutive cohort of 173 TNBC patients were retrospectively collected. The membranous expression of CLDN1, CLDN2, CLDN4, and CLDN7 was measured by immunohistochemistry. Then, the associations between CLDN expression, clinicopathological features, and clinical outcomes were assessed.

Results: Positive CLDN1, CLDN2, CLDN4, and CLDN7 membrane expression was detected in 44.5%, 54.9%, 76.9%, and 73.4% of the cohort specimens, respectively. A lack of CLDN1 expression was related to only lymph node metastasis ($P = 0.014$). The rate of CLDN4-positive tumors was significantly increased in tumors of a higher grade ($P = 0.003$). Importantly, negative CLDN1 expression was associated with worse relapse-free survival (RFS) in both lymph node positive (LN+) and negative (LN−) cases (both $P < 0.001$). Similarly it was also associated with shorter overall survival (OS)($P = 0.003$ in LN+ cases; $P = 0.018$ in LN− cases). In the LN+ subgroup, CLDN2-negative cases had a significantly higher risk of recurrence ($P = 0.008$). Multivariate analysis revealed that negative CLDN1 expression was an independent prognostic factor for high risk of both recurrence and death (HR 5.529, 95% CI 2.664–11.475, $P < 0.001$; HR 3.459, 95% CI 1.555–7.696, $P = 0.002$). However, neither CLDN4 nor CLDN7 expression was associated with survival.

Conclusion: In TNBC, the CLDN1-negative phenotype predicts a high risk of recurrence and death. The absence of CLDN1 expression is strongly suggested to be an independent adverse prognostic factor in this heterogeneous subtype of breast cancer.

Editor: Ruby John Anto, Rajiv Gandhi Centre for Biotechnology, India

Funding: The present study was supported by Beijing Medicine Research and Development Fund (2011-4002-02) and Beijing Hope Run Special Fund (LC2012A51). The funders had no role in study design, data collection and analysis, decision to publish, or preparation of the manuscript.

Competing Interests: The authors have declared that no competing interests exist.

* Email: binghxu@126.com (BX); nlu03@126.com (NL)

⅁ These authors contributed equally to this work.

¶ These authors are first authors on this work

Introduction

Triple-negative breast cancer (TNBC) is a therapeutically relevant definition of a subgroup of breast cancers (BCs) characterized by the absence of staining for the estrogen receptor (ER), the progesterone receptor (PR), and human epidermal factor receptor 2 (HER2). TNBC has proven to be remarkably heterogeneous with various prognoses stratified by clinical, pathological, genetic factors, and treatment modalities [1–5]. For example, stage II TNBC cases treated with adjuvant chemotherapy would have a better prognosis than those receiving no chemotherapy [5]. Certain histological types, such as metaplastic carcinomas, have been shown to have a very poor outcome, but medullary carcinomas have been shown to have a particularly good prognosis [6]. In addition, the "basal-like" type (with CK5/6 and EGFR expression) of TNBC generally has a worse prognosis than non-basal-like TNBC [7,8]. Due to a lack of specific targets for treatment, standard chemotherapy regimens for TNBC have not been established and dose-dense chemotherapy regimens tend to be effective in improving survival [9,10]. Thus far, data on definitive predictive markers of TNBC are insufficient. Therefore, it is urgent that we elucidate novel predictive biomarkers of TNBC to assist in selecting patients with high-risk tumors before initiating dose-dense chemotherapy to avoid overtreatment-related complications and to identify potential molecular targets.

Claudins (CLDNs), a family comprising 27 members, are the primary family of proteins that make up tight junctions between neighboring cells [11]. As major trans-membrane proteins, CLDNs play crucial roles in the formation and maintenance of tight junctions [12]. It is generally accepted that the disruption of tight junctions leads to the loss of intercellular cohesion, which contributes to the invasiveness and lack of differentiation of cancer cells and thus promotes metastasis. Earlier studies have suggested that mRNA or membrane protein expression levels of CLDNs were strongly correlated with carcinogenesis in BC and especially CLDN1 [13–19]. However, clinical studies are still relatively limited. Two reports have suggested a correlation between CLDN1 down-regulation and BC recurrence [16,17]. One study reported that down-regulation of CLDN2 was associated with advanced BC [18]. Of the few publications on CLDN7 expression in BC, researchers have reported that positive CLDN7 expression was significantly associated with an increased risk of recurrence and nodal involvement but with lower histological grade in a small sample of invasive ductal carcinoma (IDC) tumors [19,20]. The roles of the four CLDNs listed above are not well understood with respect to the various subtypes of TNBC.

Recently, a claudin-low phenotype of BC was described as a new subtype by gene microarray. It is typically triple negative by immunohistochemistry (IHC) and accounts for 25–39% of TNBCs. Defined by low mRNA expression of CLDN3, CLDN4, and CLDN7 [21], this subtype was reported to be a frequent phenomenon in metaplastic and basal-like BCs and has been shown to have a poor prognosis similar to that of basal-like BCs [21–23]. However, the expression profiles of CLDNs in TNBC have not yet been well analyzed.

Taken together, we hypothesize that the expression of CLDNs, including CLDN1, CLDN2, CLDN4, and CLDN7, associates with prognostic heterogeneity of TNBC. Therefore, we associated clinicopathological parameters with protein expression of CLDN1, CLDN2, CLDN4, and CLDN7 to uncover prognostic biomarkers for TNBC.

Materials and Methods

Ethics statement

This study was a retrospective study. All of the specimens were retrieved from the Biological Specimen Bank. The study was approved by the Independent Ethics Committee of the Cancer Hospital, Chinese Academy of Medical Sciences (CH-BC-018). The informed consent was also remitted by the Ethics Committee.

Study population

Between June 1, 2004 and January 1, 2007, a total of 2835 operable BC patients at the Cancer Hospital, Chinese Academy of Medical Sciences (CAMS) were retrospectively collected for this study. Of these, 292 patients were identified as TNBC cases. Triple-negative breast cancer was defined as estrogen receptor/progesterone receptor $<1\%$ [24] and HER2 0, 1+ or 2+ (with negative fluorescence by in situ hybridization) on immunohistochemistry. A gene copy/CEP-17 ratio <2.0 was considered to indicate negative amplification [25]. A total of 119 patients were excluded from the analysis because they had synchronous or metachronous bilateral BCs (n = 4), pure ductal carcinoma in situ (n = 4), other malignant tumors (n = 8), their tumor specimens were not archived properly (n = 71), or they missed a follow-up (n = 32). In total, 173 cases were included, and the surgical specimens of the primary breast tumors prior to adjuvant chemotherapy were retrieved from the Biological Specimen Bank of the Cancer Hospital, CAMS. Data on the patients' medical history, tumor features, demographic characteristics, and treatment modalities were recorded. Staging of tumors was performed according to the American Joint Committee on Cancer

Staging Group's Cancer Staging Manual [26]. Grading and histologic classification of the tumors were based upon the WHO's criteria [27]. All of the patients undergoing breast-conserving surgery received post-operative radiotherapy. Adjuvant chemotherapy was administered depending on the risk of recurrence in accordance with the National Comprehensive Cancer Network guidelines [28].

Immunohistochemistry (IHC)

To measure CLDN expression, polyclonal antibodies against claudin-1 (1:50) and monoclonal antibodies against claudin-2 (12H12, 1:100), claudin-4 (3E2C1, 1:50), and claudin-7 (5D10F3, 1:50) were used. The four CLDN antibodies were purchased from Zymed (CA, USA). The primary antibodies were detected using a secondary antibody conjugated to HRP (Cytomation Envision System HRP, DAKO, Carpinteria, CA). Diaminobenzidine was used as a chromogen. Sections were counterstained with hematoxylin. Normal breast skin served as a positive control for CLDN1 and CLDN2, and normal colon tissue served as a positive control for CLDN4 and CLDN7. In negative control slides, the same method was employed and the primary antibody was substituted with 1% TBS.

Interpretation of IHC sections

Based on previous studies, CLDN1, CLDN2, CLDN4 and CLDN7 IHC staining was interpreted according to the extent of membrane staining [16,22,29]. Two independent pathologists observed the immunostaining under a light microscope at a $200\times$ magnification, and positive cells, negative cells and total cells from five different visual fields were counted for each specimen. For pathological results with discrepancies, a third pathologist was asked to independently examine the slides to reach a unanimous decision. Scoring was performed as follows: negative (−), $<10\%$ positive tumor cells; positive (+), $\geq 10\%$ positive tumor cells [16]. Only membranous staining was considered positive staining [29]. Furthermore, interstitial lymphocyte infiltration (ILI) was defined as the number of lymphocytes in the tumor interstitium in five different visual fields.

Statistical analysis

Statistical analysis was performed using SPSS 16.0 statistical software (SPSS Inc, Chicago, IL, USA). Relapse-free survival (RFS) was measured from the date of curative surgery to the first day of documented recurrence. Overall survival (OS) was measured from the date of curative surgery to the date of death or final follow-up.

Independent sample t-tests and chi-square tests were used to compare continuous and categorical variables. The Kaplan-Meier product limit method was used to estimate the survival outcomes; groups were compared using the log-rank test. Cox proportional hazards models were fit to determine the association between clinicopathological characteristics, especially CLDN expression, and patient survival. $P<0.05$ was considered to be statistically significant.

Results

Baseline clinicopathological characteristics by lymph node status

The study cohort had a median age of 54 years (range: 24–78 years). The median follow-up time for the cohort was 64.6 months (range: 8.1–95.8 months). Table 1 lists the demographics, characteristics, treatment, and metastatic patterns of the cohort according to nodal status. According to the status of lymph node metastasis, patients were stratified into two subgroups: node positive (LN+, n = 97) and node negative (LN−, n = 76). Patients in the LN+ subgroup tended to have a more advanced stage of disease and a larger tumor size with more vascular involvement (P<0.001) than those in the LN− group. Among all patients, 161 (93.1%) received adjuvant chemotherapy, consisting of primarily anthracycline-and/or taxane-based regimens. At the end of follow-up, 67 patients had relapsed and 47 patients had died from metastatic BC. Although a significantly larger number of patients in the LN+ group received radiotherapy, more patients relapsed in the LN+ group than in the LN− group (P<0.001). The sites of metastasis were similar between the LN+ and LN− subgroups.

Expression of CLDN1, CLDN2, CLDN4, and CLDN7

Membrane expression of CLDN1, CLDN2, CLDN4, and CLDN7 was detected in 44.5% (77), 54.9% (95), 76.9% (133), and 73.4% (127) of the patients, respectively. Only one patient was positive for CLDN1, CLDN2, and CLDN7 expression, and two of three patients with medullary carcinomas were positive for

CLDN4 expression. For three cases with metaplastic tumors, positive expression of CLDN1, CLDN2, CLDN4, and CLDN7 was detected in 0, 1, 3, and 2 cases, respectively. Both CLDN2 and CLDN4 expression associated with positive expression of CLDN1 with p values <0.001 and = 0.014, respectively. Similarly, CLDN7 expression was associated with CLDN4 expression (P = 0.001) (Table S1).

Expression of the four CLDNs was predominantly localized to the membrane, but CLDN2 was also expressed in the cytoplasm of some TNBC specimens (Fig. 1). CLDN1 and CLDN2 stained positive in 10–50% of tumor cells, while CLDN4 and CLDN7 stained positive in ≥50% of tumor cells.

Association between CLDN expression and clinical parameters

Chi-square tests were used to compare CLDNs expression in the LN− and LN+ groups. CLDN1 expression was significantly

Table 1. Demographics and characteristics of patients by nodal status.

Clinical characteristics	Nodal positive (n = 97) n (%)	Nodal negative (n = 76) n (%)	P value
Age (mean±SD)	50.1±11.9	52.4±11.1	0.197[a]
Body weight index (mean±SD)	25.0±3.6	25.0±3.6	0.948 [a]
Family history	17 (17.5)	16 (21.1)	0.565
Histologic type			0.389
IDC	92 (94.9)	73 (96.1)	
Metaplastic	3 (3.1)	0 (0)	
Medullary	1 (1.0)	2 (2.6)	
ILC	1 (1.0)	1 (1.3)	
Tumor grade			0.541
Grade 2	47 (48.5)	33 (43.4)	
Grade 3	50 (51.5)	43 (56.6)	
Tumor size (>2 cm)			0.01
T1	24 (24.7)	34 (44.7)	
T2/T3/T4	73 (75.3)	42 (55.3)	
Stage			<0.001
I	0 (0)	33 (43.4)	
II	39 (40.2)	43 (56.6)	
III	58 (59.8)	0(0)	
Vascular involvement	27 (27.8)	4 (52.6)	<0.001
Surgery Mode			0.153
Modified Radical Mastectomy	89 (91.7)	64 (88.2)	
Breast conservation	8 (8.3)	12 (11.2)	
Adjuvant radiotherapy	59 (60.8)	16 (21.1)	<0.001
Adjuvant chemotherapy	93 (95.9)	68 (89.5)	0.133
Adjuvant Taxane	68(73.1)	32(47.1)	0.001
Adjuvant Anthracycline	92(98.9)	66(97.1)	0.574
Recurrence	51 (52.6)	16 (21.1)	<0.001
Site of recurrence before death			
Local-regional	10 (19.6)	7 (43.8)	0.096
Non-visceral	36 (70.6)	11 (68.8)	1.0
Visceral	43 (84.3)	13 (81.3)	0.716

%: positive numbers/total numbers of the subgroup according to nodal status; IDC: infiltrating ductal carcinoma; ILC: infiltrating lobular carcinoma; [a] by t test; other data were evaluated by X^2 test;"recurrence" was defined before the last follow-up.

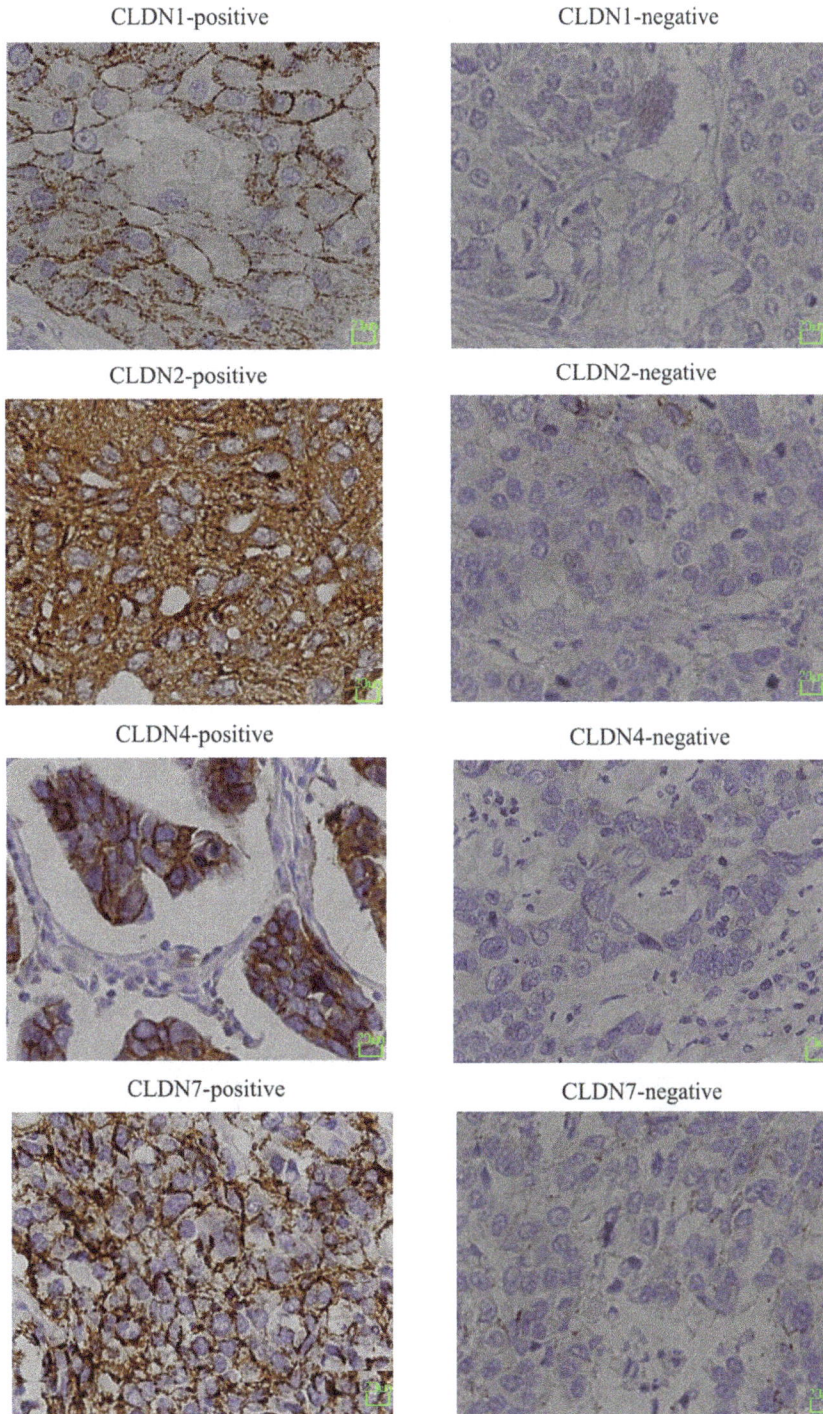

Figure 1. Membrane protein expression was assessed in 173 TNBC specimens using our optimized CLDNs IHC protocol. Representative CLDN-positive and CLDN-negative sections are shown. CLDN expression was primarily localized to the membrane (≥10% tumor cells), and CLDN2 was also expressed in the cytoplasm. (Original magnification: ×200.) Cells nuclei were counterstained with hematoxylin.

higher in the LN− group, 55.3% (42/76) compared to 36.1% (35/97) in the LN+ group, suggesting that the absence of CLDN1 expression is related to lymph node metastasis (P = 0.014) (Table 2). CLDN1 expression was also associated with interstitial lymphocyte infiltration (P = 0.017) (Table 2). No significant differences were observed between the subgroups stratified by other clinicopathological parameters (age, histology grade, vascular involvement, and tumor size) and CLDNs expression, except CLDN4 expression was found to be significantly higher in TNBC patients ≤50 years old with a tumor grade 3 compared to TNBC

Table 2. Comparison of CLDN expression and clinical parameters.

Clinical parameters	CDLN1+ % (n)	CLDN2+ % (n)	CLDN4+ % (n)	CLDN7+ % (n)
Nodal status				
Negative (n = 76)	55.3%(42)[a]	60.5% (46)	76.3% (58)	77.6% (59)
Positive (n = 97)	36.1% (35)[a]	50.5% (49)	77.3% (75)	70.1% (68)
Age				
≤50 years (n = 87)	42.5% (37)	55.2% (48)	85.1% (74)[b]	67.8% (59)
>50 years (n = 86)	46.5% (40)	54.7% (47)	68.6% (59)[b]	79.1% (68)
Vascular involvement				
Yes (n = 31)	35.5% (11)	61.3% (19)	80.6% (25)	74.2%(23)
No (n = 142)	46.5% (66)	53.5% (76)	76.1% (108)	73.2% (104)
Tumor size				
≤2 cm (n = 59)	47.5% (28)	54.2% (32)	78.0% (46)	72.9% (43)
>2 cm (n = 114)	43.0% (49)	55.3% (63)	76.3% (87)	73.7% (84)
Histology				
IDC (n = 167)	45.5% (76)	55.7% (93)	76.6% (128)	74.3% (124)
MC (n = 6)	16.7% (1)	33.3% (2)	83.3% (5)	50.0% (3)
ILI				
Yes (n = 31)	64.5% (20)[c]	64.5% (20)	80.6% (25)	74.2% (23)
No (n = 142)	40.1% (57)[c]	52.8% (75)	76.1% (108)	73.2% (104)
Tumor grade				
Grade 2 (n = 72)	38.9% (28)	55.6% (40)	65.3% (47)[d]	77.8% (56)
Grade 3 (n = 93)	50.5% (47)	55.9% (52)	86.0% (80) [d]	69.9% (65)

%: number of positivity/total number of the subgroup; MC, included 3 medullary carcinomas and 3 metaplastic carcinomas; IDC: invasive ductal carcinoma; ILI: interstitial lymphocyte infiltration. [a] P = 0.014, [b]P = 0.012, [c]P = 0.017, [d]P = 0.003.

patients >50 years old or having a tumor grade 2 (P = 0.012 and P = 0.003, respectively) (Table 2).

Significance of CLDN expression in TNBC

The 5-year RFS and OS rates of 173 TNBC were 61.4% and 73.5%, respectively. All clinical factors were investigated by univariate analysis to determine whether there was a significant difference in RFS (Table 3). Among all TNBC patients, negative CLDN1 or CLDN2 expression was associated with significantly worse RFS (P<0.001 and P = 0.001, respectively) (Fig. 2A, 2C). Other factors such as node positive, vascular invasion, and with adjuvant radiotherapy were also related to a high risk of recurrence(P<0.001, 0.027 and 0.014, respectively) (Table 3). Similar associations were noted between CLDN1, CLDN2 expression and OS (P<0.001 and P = 0.038, respectively) (Fig. 2B, 2D).

Further analysis revealed that cases with both CLDN1- and CLDN2-positive expression had a similar survival rate as cases with only positive CLDN1 expression (P = 0.576 for RFS and P = 0.427 for OS), but these cases had significantly longer RFS and OS than those cases that were positive for only CLDN2 expression or those cases that were negative for CLDN1 and CLDN2 expression (P<0.001 for each comparison) (Fig. 2E, 2F). Importantly, negative CLDN1 expression was associated with worse relapse-free survival (RFS) in both lymph node positive (LN+) and negative (LN−) cases (both P<0.001). Similarly it was also associated with shorter overall survival (OS)(P = 0.003 in LN+ cases; P = 0.018 in LN− cases). However, negative CLDN2

expression was associated with worse RFS in only LN+ cases, P = 0.008 (Fig. S1).

Similar results were observed for the 161 patients who received surgery plus adjuvant chemotherapy as for the whole cohort of TNBC cases. Both negative CLDN1 and CLDN2 expression were associated with significantly worse survival in terms of RFS and OS (RFS, P<0.001 and P = 0.001, respectively; OS, P<0.001 and P = 0.035, respectively) (Fig. S2).

Multivariate Cox regression analysis for RFS identified negative CLDN1 expression to be an independent adverse factor for tumor recurrence and death (HR 5.529, 95% CI 2.664–11.475, P< 0.001; HR 3.459, 95% CI 1.555–7.696, P = 0.002) (Table 4, 5). Lymph node metastasis was also associated with RFS and OS in the multivariate analysis (P = 0.005 and P = 0.004, respectively). No other clinical factors were associated with a significantly higher risk of recurrence or death in the multivariate analysis (Table 4, 5).

Discussion

TNBC has already been widely acknowledged as a distinct subtype of BC associated with a poor prognosis [2,3]. Increasing evidence has shown that TNBC is a heterogeneous group of diseases with different biological characteristics and clinical outcomes [2,3]. Claudins (CLDNs), major components of tight junctions, presumably play an important role in carcinogenesis and progression of BC, but little is known about the impact of these molecules on tumor recurrence. Furthermore, "claudin-low" is a special subtype of BC identified by gene microarray that is associated with a poor prognosis. Most patients with "claudin-low"

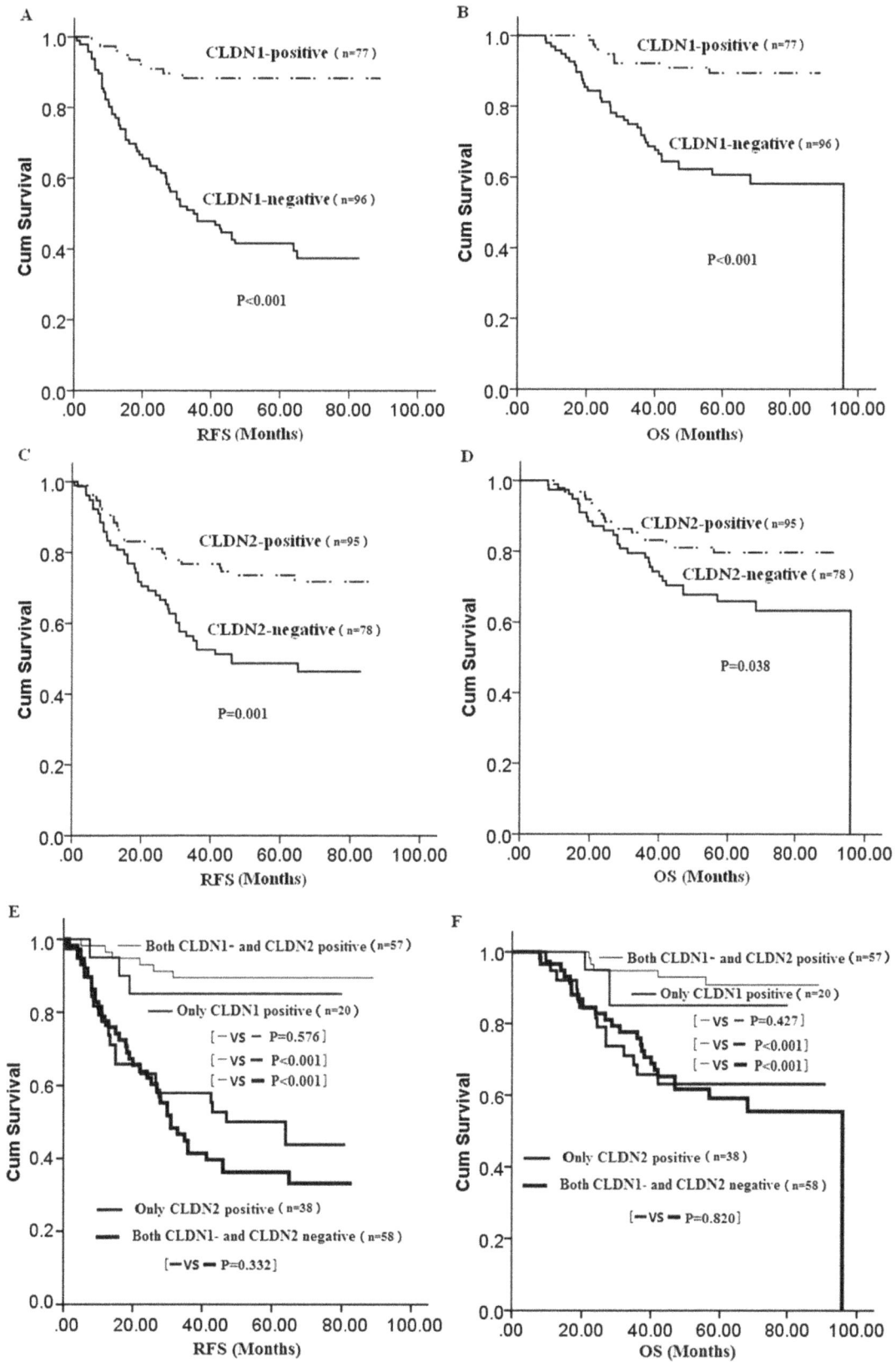

Figure 2. Kaplan-Meier survival curves of RFS and OS based on CLDN1- and CLDN2–membrane expression (CLDN1: A for RFS, B for OS; CLDN2: C for RFS, D for OS); (combination of CLDN1 and CD LN−2: E for RFS, F for OS).

Table 3. Univariate analyses of RFS by clinical factors.

Clinical factors	Events (n, %)	HR (95% CI)	P value
CLDN1 expression		0.139 (0.069–0.281)	<0.001
Negative	58 (60.4%)		
Positive	9 (11.7%)		
CLDN2 expression		0.450 (0.275–0.737)	0.001
Negative	41 (52.6%)		
Positive	26 (27.4%)		
CLDN4 expression		1.362 (0.743–2.496)	0.317
Negative	13 (32.5%)		
Positive	54 (40.6%)		
CLDN7 expression		0.764 (0.453–1.289)	0.313
Negative	20 (43.5%)		
Positive	47 (37.0%)		
Age		0.786 (0.486–1.271)	0.327
≤50 years	36 (41.4%)		
>50 years	31 (36.0%)		
BMI (Kg/m^2)		1.170 (0.725–1.889)	0.520
≤25	33 (36.3%)		
>25	34 (41.5%)		
Nodal status		3.276 (1.866–5.752)	<0.001
Negative	16 (21.1%)		
Positive	51 (52.6%)		
Tumor size		1.600 (0.932–2.747)	0.088
<2 cm	18 (30.5%)		
>2 cm	49 (43.0%)		
Tumor Grade		0.717(0.439–1.170)	0.183
Grade 2	33 (45.8%)		
Grade 3	31 (33.3%)		
With vascular invasion		1.864 (1.074–3.235)	0.027
No	50 (35.2%)		
Yes	17 (54.8%)		
Adjuvant radiotherapy		1.822 (1.127–2.948)	0.014
No	31 (31.6%)		
Yes	36 (48.0%)		
(Neo) adjuvant chemotherapy		0.739 (0.319–1.710)	0.480
No	6 (50.0%)		
Yes	61 (37.9%)		
Chemo with taxanes		0.903 (0.542–1.505)	0.696
No	25 (41.0%)		
Yes	36 (36.0%)		

%: number of events/total number of the subgroup.

are triple negative. But the associations between the CLDNs-negative phenotypes, defined by immunohistochemical methods, and the "claudin-low" subtype were unclear. Before this study, it was not sure whether the CLDNs-negative phenotypes associated with the poor prognosis in TNBC.

In accordance with previous studies, positive CLDN expression was defined as ≥10% membrane expression for four CLDNs in this study [12,16]. Positive CLDN1 and CLDN2 expression was

detected in 44.5% and 55.9% of cases, respectively. And the extent of immunostaining in most cases was 10–50%. Consistent with our results, Marohashi's study showed that CLDN1 was expressed in 61.4% of 83 BCs (cut-off value 10%) [16]. Because a different criterion for positive expression was used, the rate of CLDN1-high expression was much lower in Gerhard's study, with only 12.6% in 103 TNBC tumors having high levels of CLDN1 expression [23]. In addition, the majority of TNBC patients showed positive

Table 4. Multivariate Cox regression analysis of RFS.

Factors	HR (95% CI)	P value
CLDN1 negativity	5.529 (2.664–11.475)	<0.001
Lymph node metastasis	2.339 (1.292–4.233)	0.005
CLDN2 negativity	1.424 (0.854–2.373)	0.175
Adjuvant radiotherapy	1.150 (0.670–1.974)	0.613
With vascular invasion	1.289 (0.698–2.381)	0.417
Tumor size >2 cm	1.293 (0.739–2.264)	0.368

membrane staining of CLDN4 (76.9%) and CLDN7 (73.4%). Similar to our results, increased protein expression of CLDN4 was found in ER-negative BC, especially in basal-like BC (in which subtype tumors were mainly TNBC) [22,30,31]. However, a study conducted by Blanchard et al. found contradictory results in 152 breast tumors. No significant difference in CLDN4 expression was observed between basal-like BC and non-basal-like BC (P = 0.18) [32]. Therefore, further investigations in CLDN4 expression levels and TNBC subtypes should be performed.

In this study, positive CLDN1 expression was associated with interstitial lymphocyte infiltration. These lymphocytes may down-regulate cytokines to induce the expression of CLDN1. For instance, loss of keratin 8 and 18 expression could increase CLDN1 expression in epithelial cancer cells [33]. However, negative CLDN1 expression was significantly more frequent in the LN+ TNBC subgroup compared to the LN− subgroup (55.3% vs. 36.1%, P = 0.014). These finding were consistent with one study that demonstrated that CLDN1-negative expression was associated with node metastasis in 83 BCs [16]. Thus, loss of CLDN1 may lead to lack of intercellular cohesion between cancer cells, promote invasiveness, and contribute to lymph node metastasis [15]. This finding suggests that CLDN1 may play a pivotal role in the invasion of TNBC. In addition, positive CLDN4 expression was associated with higher tumor grade (P = 0.003). In addition, a study conducted by Szasz et al. with 97 cases of IDC and invasive lobular carcinomas reported a similar result [29]. In agreement with previous studies of TNBCs [2,3], patients with node metastasis had a significantly worse prognosis in terms of RFS (P<0.001).

More importantly, this study consisted of the largest series of TNBCs to clarify the relationship between CLDN1 expression and survival outcomes. We demonstrated that a lack of CLDN1 expression on the membrane was associated with worse RFS and OS in both LN+ and LN− cases. One mechanism to explain this phenomenon could be that, as in the case of E-cadherin, the transcription factors slug and snail, which are key markers of EMT, could bind to the *CLDN1* promoter to repress its activation and promote the activation of *MMP-2* and *MMP-9*, resulting in TNBC invasion [34,35]. In line with our observations, studies conducted by Morohashi et al. and Szasz et al. with a smaller sample of BCs reported that CLDN1-negative or -low expression was associated with tumor recurrence in different subtypes of BC (P<0.001 and P = 0.038) [16,29]. In contrast, research conducted by Kolokytha et al. with 76 TNBC tumors showed that CLDN1 expression was not related to survival [36]. In the 161 TNBC cases that received adjuvant chemotherapy, negative CLDN1 expression was also associated with a worse outcome (P<0.001). Additionally, CLDN1-negative expression was identified as an adverse prognostic factor by multivariate Cox regression analysis. These results suggest that negative CLDN1 expression may be an adverse prognostic factor in TNBC.

In the current study, in subgroups analysis by lymph node status, we also observed that CLDN2-negative expression was only associated with worse RFS in LN+ TNBC cases (P = 0.008). In a previous study, Kim reported that down-regulation of CLDN2 in breast carcinomas was related to advanced disease and lymph node metastasis [18]. Tabariès et al. identified that only decreased expression of CLDN2 promoted breast cancer liver metastases by reducing adhesion between tumor cells [37]. Our results further supported previous studies that imply that CLDN2 is implicated in the development of metastatic potential within TNBC.

Finally, neither CLDN4 nor CLDN7 expression was signifi-cantly associated with survival of patients with TNBC, which contradicts the previously reported association between CLDN4 expression and BC tumor recurrence [29,36]. A Japanese group demonstrated that there was no association between CLDN4

Table 5. Multivariate Cox regression analysis of OS.

Factors	HR (95% CI)	P value
CLDN1 negativity	3.459 (1.555–7.696)	0.002
Lymph node metastasis	3.496 (1.500–8.150)	0.004
CLDN2 negativity	1.310 (0.708–1.425)	0.390
Adjuvant radiotherapy	1.557 (0.795–3.050)	0.196
With vascular invasion	1.394 (0.695–2.795)	0.350
Tumor size >2 cm	1.495 (0.726–3.078)	0.275

expression and BC tumor recurrence [16]. However, IHC analysis performed on tissue microarray samples from 97 BC patients by Szasz et al. demonstrated that higher expression of CLDN4 was significantly associated with increased risk of recurrence (P = 0.045) [29]. Conversely, Kolokytha et al. analyzed 76 TNBC tumors and found that positive CLDN4 expression was associated with a favorable prognosis [36]. Further investigation of a larger sample of TNBCs is needed.

Because this was a retrospective study, a few limitations were expected. First, the sample size determination was not previously planned, and the detrimental effects of a possibly underpowered study on some significant associations between CLDNs and clinical outcomes could be unavoidable. Second, no validation cohort was used to confirm the positive or negative findings.

Acknowledgments

The authors are grateful to every patient and their relatives for their cooperation during the follow-up. We are also thankful to our colleagues in the Department of Pathology for their technical assistance.

Author Contributions

Conceived and designed the experiments: FM XD JY NL BX. Performed the experiments: FM XD SZ. Analyzed the data: FM XD YF BX. Contributed reagents/materials/analysis tools: FM XD YF JY SZ. Wrote the paper: FM XD YF BX.

References

1. Kennecke H, Yerushalmi R, Woods R, Cheang MC, Voduc D, et al. (2010) Metastatic behavior of breast cancer subtypes. J Clin Oncol 28: 3271–3277.
2. Dent R, Trudeau M, Pritchard KI, Hanna WM, Kahn HK, et al. (2007) Triple-negative breast cancer: clinical features and patterns of recurrence. Clin Cancer Res 13: 4429–4434.
3. Hernandez-Aya LF, Chavez-Macgregor M, Lei X, Meric-Bernstam F, Buchholz TA, et al. (2011) Nodal status and clinical outcomes in a large cohort of patients with triple-negative breast cancer. J Clin Oncol 29: 2628–2634.
4. Nielsen TO, Hsu FD, Jensen K, Cheang M, Karaca G, et al. (2004) Immunohistochemical and clinical characterization of the basal-like subtype of invasive breast carcinoma. Clin Cancer Res 10: 5367–5374.
5. Kashiwagi S, Yashiro M, Takashima T, Aomatsu N, Ikeda K, et al. (2011) Advantages of adjuvant chemotherapy for patients with triple-negative breast cancer at Stage II: usefulness of prognostic markers E-cadherin and Ki67. Breast Cancer Res 13: R122.
6. Eichhorn JH (2004) Medullary carcinoma, provocative now as then. Semin Diagn Pathol 21: 65–73.
7. De Brot M, Soares FA, Stiepcich MM, Cúrcio VS, Gobbi H (2009) Basal-like breast cancers: clinicopathological features and outcome. Rev Assoc Med Bras 55: 529–534.
8. Rakha EA, El-Sayed ME, Green AR, Lee AH, Robertson JF, et al. (2007) Prognostic markers in triple-negative breast cancer. Cancer 109: 25–32.
9. Gluz O, Liedtke C, Gottschalk N, Pusztai L, Nitz U, Harbeck N (2009) Triple negative breast cancer-current status and future directions. Ann Oncol 20: 1913–1927.
10. Fountzilas G, Dafni U, Bobos M, Batistatou A, Kotoula V, et al. (2012) Differential Response of Immuno- histochemically Defined Breast Cancer Subtypes to Anthracycline-Based Adjuvant Chemotherapy with or without Paclitaxel. PLoS One 7: e37946.
11. Mineta K, Yamamoto Y, Yamazaki Y, Tanaka H, Tada Y, et al. (2011) Predicted expansion of the claudin multigene family. FEBS Lett 585(4): 606–612.
12. Hewitt KJ, Agarwal R, Morin PJ (2006) The claudin gene family: expression in normal and neoplastic tissues. BMC Cancer 6: 186.
13. Tökés AM, Kulka J, Paku S, Szik A, Páska C, et al. (2005) Claudin-1, −3 and −4 proteins and mRNA expression in benign and malignant breast lesions: a research study. Breast Cancer Res 7: R296–305.
14. Hoevel T, Macek R, Mundigl O, Swisshelm K, Kubbies M (2004) Re-expression of the TJ protein CLDN1 induces apoptosis in breast tumor spheroids. International Journal of Cancer 108: 374–383.
15. Myal Y, Leygue E, Blanchard AA (2010) Claudin 1 in breast tumorigenesis: revelation of a possible novel"claudin high" subset of breast cancers. J Biomed Biotechnol 2010: 956897.
16. Morohashi S, Kusumi T, Sato F, Odagiri H, Chiba H, et al. (2007) Decreased expression of claudin-1 correlates with recurrence status in breast cancer. Int J Mol Med 20: 139–143.
17. Charpin C, Tavassoli F, Secq V, Giusiano S, Villeret J, et al. (2012) Validation of an immunohistochemical signature predictive of 8-year outcome for patients with breast carcinoma. Int J Cancer 131: E236–243.
18. Kim TH, Huh JH, Lee S, Kang H, Kim GI, An HJ (2008) Down-regulation of claudin-2 in breast carcinomas is associated with advanced disease. Histopathology 53: 48–55.
19. Kominsky SL, Argani P, Korz D, Evron E, Raman V, et al. (2003) Loss of the tight junction protein claudin-7 correlates with histological grade in both ductal carcinoma in situ and invasive ductal carcinoma of the breast. Oncogene 22: 2021–2033.
20. Sauer T, Pedersen MK, Ebeltoft K, Naess O (2005) Reduced expression of Claudin-7 in fine needle aspirates from breast carcinomas correlate with grading and metastatic disease. Cytopathology 16: 193–198.
21. Prat A, Parker JS, Karginova O, Fan C, Livasy C, et al. (2010) Phenotypic and molecular characterization of the claudin-low intrinsic subtype of breast cancer. Breast Cancer Res 12: R68.
22. Lu S, Singh K, Mangray S, Tavares R, Noble L, et al. (2013) Claudin expression in high-grade invasive ductal carcinoma of the breast: correlation with the molecular subtype. Mod Pathol 26(4): 485–495.
23. Gerhard R, Ricardo S, Albergaria A, Gomes M, Silva AR, et al. (2012) Immunohistochemical features of claudin-low intrinsic subtype in metaplastic breast carcinomas. Breast 21: 354–360.
24. Hammond ME, Hayes DF, Wolff AC, Mangu PB, Temin S (2010) American Society of Clinical Oncology/College of American Pathologists guideline recommendations for immunohistochemical testing of estrogen and progesterone receptors in breast cancer. J Oncol Pract 6: 195–197.
25. Wolff AC, Hammond ME, Schwartz JN, Hagerty KL, Allred DC, et al. (2007) American Society of Clinical Oncology/College of American Pathologists guideline recommendations for human epidermal growth factor receptor 2 testing in breast cancer. J Clin Oncol 25: 118–145.
26. Singletary SE, Allred C, Ashley P, Bassett LW, Berry D, et al. (2003) Staging system for breast cancer: Revisions for the 6th edition of the AJCC cancer staging manual. Surg Clin North Am 83: 803–819.
27. (1982) The World Health Organization Histological Typing of Breast Tumors: Second Edition –The World Organization. Am J ClinPathol 78: 806–816.
28. Bevers TB, Anderson BO, Bonaccio E, Buys S, Daly MB, et al. (2009) National Comprehensive Cancer Network: NCCN clinical practice guidelines in oncology: breast cancer screening and diagnosis. J Natl Compr Canc Netw 7: 1060–1096.
29. Szasz AM, Tokes AM, Micsinai M, Krenacs T, Jakab C, et al. (2011) Prognostic significance of claudin expression changes in breast cancer with regional lymph node metastasis. Clin Exp Metastasis 28: 55–63.
30. Blanchard AA, Skliris GP, Watson PH, Murphy LC, Penner C, et al. (2009) Claudins 1, 3, and 4 protein expression in ER negative breast cancer correlates with markers of the basal phenotype. Virchows Archiv 454: 647–656.
31. Blanchard AA, Ma X, Dueck KJ, Penner C, Cooper SC, et al. (2013) Claudin 1 expression in basal-like breast cancer is related to patient age. BMC Cancer 30;13: 268.
32. Kulka J, Szász AM, Németh Z, Madaras L, Schaff Z, et al. (2009) Expression of tight junction protein claudin-4 in basal-like breast carcinomas. Pathol Oncol Res 15: 59–64.
33. Fortier AM, Asselin E, Cadrin M (2013) Keratin 8 and 18 loss in epithelial cancer cells increases collective cell migration and cisplatin sensitivity through claudin1 up-regulation. J Biol Chem 288(16): 11555–11571.
34. Martínez-Estrada OM, Cullerés A, Soriano FX, Peinado H, Bolós V, et al. (2006) The transcription factors Slug and Snail act as repressors of claudin-1 expression in epithelial cells. Biochemical Journal 394: 449–457.

35. Gorcsan J 3rd, Deswal A, Mankad S, Mandarino WA, Mahler CM, et al. (2008) Reduction of E-cadherin expression is associated with non-lobular breast carcinomas of basal-like and triple negative phenotype. J Clin Pathol 61: 615–620.

36. Kolokytha P, Yiannou P, Keramopoulos D, Kolokythas A, Nonni A, et al. (2014) Claudin-3 and claudin-4: distinct prognostic significance in triple-negative and luminal breast cancer. Appl Immunohistochem Mol Morphol 22(2): 125–131.

37. Tabariès S, Dupuy F, Dong Z, Monast A, Annis MG, et al. (2012) Claudin-2 promotes breast cancer liver metastasis by facilitating tumor cell interactions with hepatocytes. Mol Cell Biol 32: 2979–2991.

20

Prevalence of NRT Use and Associated Nicotine Intake in Smokers, Recent Ex-Smokers and Longer-Term Ex-Smokers

Lion Shahab[1]*, Emma Beard[1], Jamie Brown[1,2], Robert West[1]

1 Department of Epidemiology and Public Health, University College London, London, United Kingdom, **2** Department of Clinical, Educational and Health Psychology, University College London, London, United Kingdom

Abstract

Background: Nicotine replacement therapy (NRT) is used by smokers wanting to reduce their smoking and to quit. However, there are very little data on nicotine intake associated with NRT use in representative population samples. This study aimed to provide estimates for NRT use and associated nicotine exposure among smokers, recent and longer-term ex-smokers in England, a country with a permissive regulatory regime for nicotine substitution.

Methods: In the Smoking Toolkit Study, a monthly series of representative household surveys of adults aged 16+ in England, current and recent ex-smokers who agreed to be re-contacted were followed up 6 months later and standard socio-demographic and smoking characteristics assessed (N = 5,467, response rate 25.1%). A random sub-sample (N = 1,614; 29.5%) also provided saliva, analysed for cotinine.

Results: The sample followed up was broadly representative of the original sample. At follow-up, 11.8% (95%CI 10.9–12.8, N = 565) of current smokers, 34.8% (95%CI 28.9–41.3, N = 77) of recent (≤3 months) ex-smokers, and 7.8% (95%CI 5.6–10.6, N = 36) of longer-term (>3 months) ex-smokers reported using NRT. Smokers who used NRT had similar saliva cotinine concentrations to smokers who did not use NRT (mean ± sd = 356.0±198.6 ng/ml vs. 313.1±178.4 ng/ml). Recent ex-smokers who used NRT had levels that were somewhat lower, but not significantly so, than current smokers (216.7±179.3 ng/ml). Longer-term ex-smokers using NRT had still lower levels (157.3±227.1 ng/ml), which differed significantly from smokers using NRT (p = 0.024).

Conclusions: Concurrent use of nicotine replacement therapy while smoking is relatively uncommon and is not associated with higher levels of nicotine intake. Among ex-smokers, NRT use is common in the short but not longer-term and among longer-term users is associated with lower nicotine intake than in smokers.

Editor: Anil Kumar, University of Missouri-Kansas City, United States of America

Funding: This study was funded by the Department of Health, Cancer Research UK, Pfizer, GlaxoSmithKline and Johnson and Johnson. The funders had no role in study design, data collection and analysis, decision to publish, or preparation of the manuscript.

Competing Interests: EB has received conference funding from Pfizer. JB has no further competing interests. RW undertakes research and consultancy for developers and manufacturers of smoking cessation treatments such as nicotine replacement products.

* Email: lion.shahab@ucl.ac.uk

Introduction

Harm reduction may be defined as reducing psychological or physiological harm from substance use without complete cessation [1]. In the case of tobacco use, harm reduction can involve the partial substitution of cigarettes with non-combustible forms such as nicotine replacement therapy (NRT) to reduce cigarette consumption or for temporary abstinence. Harm reduction may also constitute the complete and permanent substitution of cigarettes with less harmful products, switching smokers from combustible to non-combustible nicotine delivery devices, including NRT [2].

The rationale for harm reduction with NRT is based on the knowledge that most harm is caused by the burning of tobacco and not nicotine *per se* [3]. There is evidence from both population studies and clinical trials that the use of NRT among current smokers can result in reduced cigarette consumption [4]. Moreover, it is associated with both increased motivation to stop and improved quit rates [1,5] and does not increase overall nicotine intake [6]. Permanent replacement of cigarettes with NRT among ex-smokers has been shown to result in 40% of baseline levels of nicotine being substituted by nicotine replacement products in clinical trials [7,8]. Trials have also shown that extended use of NRT by ex-smokers may result in better long-term abstinence rates [9,10].

For this reason, NRT licensing is being changed to allow its use for harm reduction purposes among current and ex-smokers [11,12]. Yet, little real world data exist on the impact of NRT use for harm reduction. Most data come from clinical trials which are limited by the fact that trial samples tend to differ from general population samples [13] and that NRT is provided free together with behavioural support which may influence usage patterns. By contrast, most NRT is used without advice and bought over the counter [14] and given the recent proliferation of available products [15], up-to-date information is needed. In the UK, NICE therefore has called for further research in the area of harm reduction [16] as investigating this issue will allow more precise quantification of the likely benefits or harms of substituting cigarettes with NRT among current and ex-smokers.

As a first step in this direction, this report describes the prevalence of NRT use and associated exposure to nicotine in three conditions that it might be used in a general population sample: among current smokers for temporary abstinence or smoking reduction, during a quit attempt by recent ex-smokers or for subsequent maintenance of quitting by longer-term ex-smokers. Although it is unlikely that a substantially increased nicotine intake from NRT would be harmful [17,18], it clearly is a concern for some people and a potential barrier to effective use of nicotine products [19]. Moreover, the question has been raised whether NRT use perpetuates nicotine dependence [20] and this issue can be addressed by looking at relative exposure to nicotine among ex-smokers using and not using NRT as compared with current smokers. Lastly, given that NRT is mainly used over the counter, focusing on real-life general population data provides the best insight into this topic from a public health perspective.

Specifically, this study aimed to answer the following research questions:

1) What is the prevalence of NRT use among current smokers, recent ($\leq$3 months) and longer-term ($>$3 months) ex-smokers?
2) What is the nicotine intake associated with NRT use among current smokers, recent ($\leq$3 months) and longer-term ($>$3 months) ex-smokers?

Methods

Study design and sampling

The data come from follow-up waves of the Smoking Toolkit Study (www.smokinginengland.info), which is an ongoing series of cross-sectional household surveys in England designed to provide information about smoking prevalence and behaviour. Each month a new sample of approximately 1,800 adults aged 16 and over completes a face to face computer-assisted survey with a trained interviewer. Current smokers and ex-smokers who have quit within the last year are asked at baseline whether they agree to be followed up and those consenting are re-contacted via a postal questionnaire at 6 months. Half of those who are followed up are randomised to receive also a saliva kit and asked to provide a sample. The survey methodology has been described in detail elsewhere and has been shown to result in a baseline sample that is nationally representative in its socio-demographic composition and proportion of smokers [21]. Participants provided verbal consent. As this was an omnibus household survey conducted every week by the survey company and data were anonymised, written consent was not required. Verbal consent was noted by the interviewer and ethics approval for this study and the consent procedure was granted by the University College London ethics committee.

Participants

Between November 2006 (the survey start) and July 2011 (when follow-up saliva collection was paused), 21,821 current smokers and recent ex-smokers at baseline agreed to be followed up. Of these, 5,539 responded at 6 months follow-up. Seventy-two participants (1.3%) were excluded due to missing information on NRT use or smoking status which resulted in a response rate of 25.1% and a total analytic sample of N = 5,467, of whom 29.5% (N = 1,614) also provided saliva.

Measures

At baseline, standard socio-demographic characteristics including age, gender and social-grade (AB = higher and intermediate professional/managerial, C1 = supervisory, clerical, junior managerial/administrative/professional, C2 = skilled manual workers, D = semi-skilled and unskilled manual workers, E = on state benefit, unemployed, lowest grade workers) were assessed. Participants were asked if they (a) smoked cigarettes (including hand-rolled) every day; (b) smoked cigarettes (including hand-rolled) but not every day; (c) did not smoke cigarettes at all but did smoke tobacco of some kind (e.g. pipe or cigar); (d) had stopped smoking completely in the last year; (e) had stopped smoking completely more than a year ago; or (f) had never been a smoker (i.e. smoked for a year or more). Current smokers, classified as answering 'yes' to (a) or (b), and recent ex-smokers, classified as answering 'yes' to (d), were eligible for follow-up. Those answering 'yes' to (c), (e) or (f) were excluded from analysis. Additionally, current smokers were asked questions to determine nicotine dependence (measured by heaviness of smoking index, HSI [22], and strength of urges to smoke, SUTS [23]) as well as motivation to quit (measured by the motivation to stop scale, MTSS [24]).

At 6-months follow-up, all participants were asked whether they smoked cigarettes at all nowadays, including hand-rolled cigarettes (Yes/No). Those who self-classified as smokers were asked whether they were trying to reduce how much they smoked and, if so, whether they used NRT for cutting down and/or temporary abstinence (Yes/No). Those who had stopped smoking were asked how long ago they had stopped smoking, categorised into ex-smokers who had stopped up to three months ago or more than three months ago, whether they had used NRT to help them stop, and if so, whether they still used NRT (Yes/No). We chose this cut-off to distinguish standard from longer-term NRT use because three months is the standard recommendation for treatment length. As postal collection of saliva for cotinine analysis, a reliable marker of nicotine intake, has been shown to be practical and reliable [25], saliva was collected with a postal saliva sample kit at follow-up. The kit contained a salivette cotton roll and instructions on how to collect the sample. Participants then returned the kit by post directly to the laboratory where it was assayed for cotinine using rapid liquid-gas chromatography [26].

Analysis

Data were analysed with IBM SPSS Statistics 20.0.0. Comparisons were made between those who were and were not followed up and among those who were followed-up, between those who did and did not provide a saliva sample. Differences were assessed with χ^2-tests and independent t-tests for categorical and continuous variables, respectively. Due to the positively skewed distribution of cotinine values, generalised linear models with a gamma distribution and log link were used to determine the impact of NRT use and smoking status on cotinine values. In sensitivity analysis, findings were re-examined with a general linear model using log-transformed cotinine values (all zero values being replaced with 0.001). Given unequal group sizes and non-normality of cotinine values, post-hoc analyses of group differences were assessed with Kruskal-Wallis pairwise comparison. All analyses were unweighted, statistical significance was set at the standard level ($p<0.05$), and the Bonferroni correction was applied in post-hoc analyses.

Results

1. Prevalence of NRT use among current smokers, recent and longer-term ex-smokers

Participants followed-up at 6 months who constituted the analytic sample were somewhat older and more likely to be female than those lost to follow-up (Table 1). The majority of the analytic sample, 87.5% (95%CI 86.6–88.3, N = 4,783/5,467), were smoking, 4.0% (95%CI 3.6–4.6, N = 221/5,467) had stopped smoking up to three months ago and 8.5% (95%CI 7.8–9.2, N = 463/5,467) more than three months ago. NRT use was most common among recent ($\leq$3 months) ex-smokers, a third of whom (34.8%, 95%CI 28.9–41.3, N = 77/221) were still using NRT. A significantly smaller proportion of current smokers (11.8%; 95%CI 10.9–12.8, N = 565/4,783; $\chi^2(1)$ = 100.2, $p<0.001$) or longer-term (>3 months) ex-smokers (7.8%; 95%CI 5.6–10.6, N = 36/463; $\chi^2(1)$ = 79.5, $p<0.001$), were currently using NRT.

2. Nicotine intake associated with NRT use among current smokers, recent and longer-term ex-smokers

A subsample of the analytic sample provided a saliva sample, analysed for cotinine to estimate exposure to nicotine. Socio-demographic and smoking characteristics did not differ as a function of whether participants did or did not have cotinine results (all $p>0.05$, Table 1). In addition, the prevalence of NRT use among either current or ex-smokers did not differ as a function of cotinine availability (all $p>0.05$). In the presence of a significant interaction between NRT use and smoking status (Wald $\chi^2(2)$ = 55.7, $p<0.001$), main effects were not considered. As Figure 1 shows, cotinine levels were greatest among current smokers and lowest among longer-term ex-smokers but also differed as a function of NRT use.

Among participants not using NRT, cotinine levels were significantly higher in smokers (arithmetic mean ($\tilde{x}_a$) $\pm$ sd = 313.1 $\pm$ 178.4 ng/ml, geometric mean ($\tilde{x}_g$) = 226.0 ng/ml, N = 1,263) than ex-smokers. This was the case for both recent ex-smokers ($\tilde{x}_a$ = 16.1 $\pm$ 51.1 ng/ml, $\tilde{x}_g$ = 1.8 ng/nl, N = 47; Kruskal-Wallis pairwise comparison = 729.7, $p<0.001$) and longer-term ex-smokers ($\tilde{x}_a$ = 3.8 $\pm$ 18.8 ng/ml, $\tilde{x}_g$ = 0.6 ng/ml, N = 120; Kruskal-Wallis pairwise comparison = 789.6, $p<0.001$). Yet, even among ex-smokers there was some variation and some 7.2% (N = 12) had cotinine values above standard cut-off levels for smoking abstinence ($\geq$15 ng/ml), most likely due to misreporting.

Among participants using NRT, cotinine levels of current smokers ($\tilde{x}_a$ = 356.0 $\pm$ 198.6 ng/ml, $\tilde{x}_g$ = 283.6 ng/ml; N = 155) were significantly higher only compared with longer-term ex-smokers ($\tilde{x}_a$ = 157.3 $\pm$ 227.1 ng/ml, $\tilde{x}_g$ = 34.2 ng/ml, N = 9; Kruskal-Wallis pairwise comparison = 504.5; p = 0.024). Cotinine levels of recent ex-smokers using NRT ($\tilde{x}_a$ = 216.7 $\pm$ 179.3 ng/ml, $\tilde{x}_g$ = 113.3 ng/nl, N = 20) did not differ from current smokers using NRT (Kruskal-Wallis pairwise comparison = 317.0; p = 0.063). Excluding recent ex-smokers who had stopped within the last week (N = 32) did not change results.

Further pairwise comparisons revealed that recent ex-smokers using NRT had significantly higher cotinine levels than recent ex-smokers not using NRT (Kruskal-Wallis pairwise comparison = 503.0, $p<0.001$). Longer-term ex-smokers using NRT also appeared to have higher cotinine levels than long-term ex-smokers not using NRT but this difference did not reach significance (Kruskal-Wallis pairwise comparison = 375.4; p = 0.297). Lastly, smokers with concurrent NRT use had similar cotinine values to those not using NRT (Kruskal-Wallis pairwise comparison = 90.2; p = 0.344) and this remained the case when controlling for cigarette consumption in sensitivity analysis. Excluding participants who had indicated ever using electronic cigarettes at baseline (N = 9) did not alter results.

Table 1. Baseline characteristics by follow-up status and cotinine availability.

	Total sample (N = 21821)	Not followed-up (N = 16354)	Followed-up (N = 5467)	Cotinine analysed	
				Yes (N = 1614)	No (N = 3853)
Socio-demographic characteristics					
Mean (SD) Age	41.6 (16.3)	39.8 (16.1)	47.0 (15.6)***	46.8 (15.8)	47.1 (15.5)
% (N) Women	53.1 (11589)	51.9 (8493)	56.6 (3096)***	55.5 (895)	57.1 (2201)
% (N) C2DE[1]	67.8 (14788)	68.1 (11132)	66.9 (3656)	66.7 (1076)	67.0 (2580)
Smoking characteristics					
% (N) Current Smokers	93.7 (20445)	94.3 (15426)	91.8 (5019)***	91.5 (1477)	91.9 (3542)
Mean (SD) Heaviness of smoking index^	2.25 (1.5)	2.22 (1.5)	2.35 (1.5)***	2.41 (1.5)	2.33 (1.5)
Mean (SD) Strength of urges^[2]	2.29 (0.9)	2.28 (0.9)	2.32 (0.9)**	2.32 (0.9)	2.30 (0.9)
Mean (SD) Motivation to stop^[3]	3.85 (2.0)	3.92 (2.0)	3.64 (2.0)***	3.67 (2.0)	3.62 (2.0)

[1]In socio-economic group C2 (Skilled manual worker), D (Semi-skilled and unskilled manual worker), or E (On state benefit, unemployed, lowest grade workers);
[2]From 1 'slight' to 5 'extremely strong';
[3]From 1 'Don't want to stop' to 7 'Really want to and intend to stop in next month',
^Only current smokers included;
*p<.05;
**p<.01;
***p<.001.

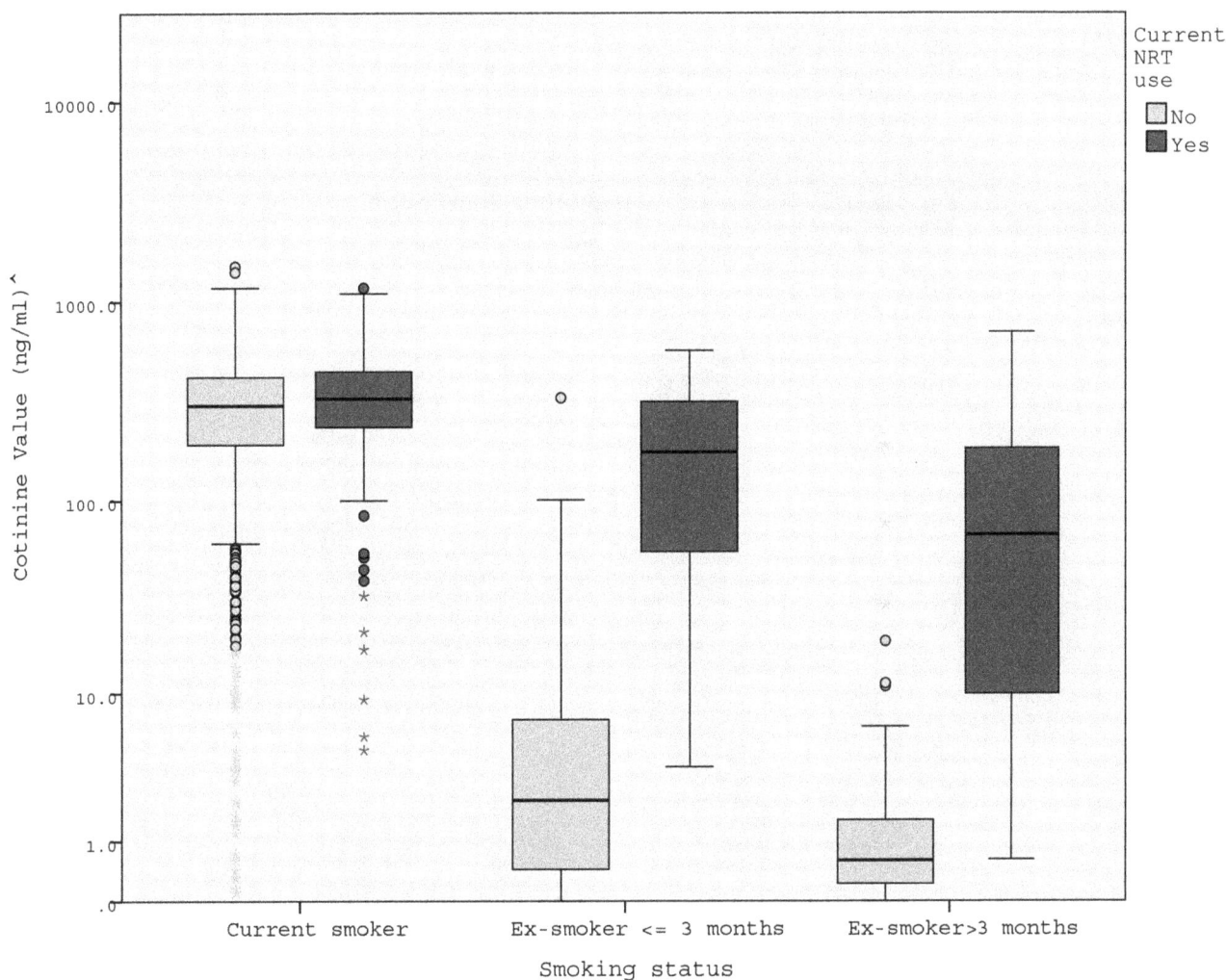

Figure 1. Box-plot of cotinine levels by NRT use and smoking status. Box provides interquartile range and median value is indicated by black line; whiskers represent normal range (up to 1.5 times of interquartile range); circle indicates outliers 1.5–3 times of the interquartile range and asterisks extreme outliers more than 3 times of the interquartile range; ^Plotted on logarithmic scale.

Discussion

Whilst a third of ex-smokers in England use nicotine replacement therapy for smoking cessation in the short-term, its use for harm reduction is relatively uncommon. Only around one in ten smokers uses NRT concurrently and a similar proportion of ex-smokers uses NRT beyond the standard length of three months. Despite recent policy and licensing changes, long-term NRT use does not appear to have increased materially since 2002, when one year usage rates were estimated at around 5% [27]. Similarly, concurrent NRT use among smokers, either for temporary abstinence or cutting down, has remained relatively stable since 2002 [28] and mostly reflects short-term use [29]. These findings are in agreement with a similar lack of change in general NRT usage pattern following an earlier relaxation of NRT licensing in 2005 [30].

Notwithstanding concerns among potential users and stop smoking advisors (e.g. [19]), what little research exists suggests that long-term NRT use is safe and any associated health risks small [17,31,32], certainly compared with continued smoking [33]. This study adds further evidence, suggesting that longer-term NRT use is associated with significantly lower exposure to nicotine than among current smokers. By contrast, recent ex-smokers using NRT had concentrations not greatly dissimilar to those of smokers. This finding is consistent with previous clinical studies which show that nicotine substitution from NRT tapers off over time [7]. In line with other work from the Smoking Toolkit Study, NRT use among current smokers was not associated with greater cotinine levels [6,34], suggesting that smokers are relatively adept at titrating nicotine levels, with some nicotine otherwise obtained from cigarettes being replaced by nicotine from NRT. While this study cannot provide exact estimates of substitution rates as no NRT usage data were available, some substitution is likely given previous findings of smokers maintaining nicotine levels when using acute forms of NRT whilst dramatically reducing cigarette consumption [4]. The fact that longer-term use among ex-smokers was associated with lower cotinine levels suggests that NRT is unlikely to maintain nicotine dependence in the long run. These results should allay the fears of potential NRT users that it will lead to an increase in nicotine exposure.

This study has a number of limitations. Despite an initial large sample size, there were few ex-smokers who used NRT which reduced power to detect differences between groups. In addition, the baseline sample differed somewhat from the sample followed up. However, differences were modest and unlikely to substantially influence the findings. Lastly, due to the cross-sectional design we cannot make causal attributions about the direction of the observed effects. This study's strengths include the use of a general population sample enabling us to look at actual use of NRT and assessment with established, ecologically valid measures. Further research would benefit from measuring a wider array of biomarkers of smoking-related harm such as lung function tests or carcinogen metabolites to complement these results and provide a more complete assessment of the potential harm of long-term NRT use.

In conclusion, use of NRT while smoking is not associated with higher overall nicotine levels; its use for more than 3 months after stopping is uncommon and is associated with significantly lower cotinine levels compared with current smokers.

Author Contributions

Conceived and designed the experiments: RW. Analyzed the data: LS. Wrote the paper: LS EB JB RW.

References

1. Beard E, McNeill A, Aveyard P, Fidler J, Michie S, et al. (2011) Association between use of nicotine replacement therapy for harm reduction and smoking cessation: a prospective study of English smokers. Tob Control 22: 118–122. tobaccocontrol-2011-050007 [pii];10.1136/tobaccocontrol-2011-050007 [doi].

2. Le Houezec J, McNeill A, Britton J (2011) Tobacco, nicotine and harm reduction. Drug Alcohol Rev 30: 119–123. 10.1111/j.1465-3362.2010.00264.x [doi].

3. Stratton S, Shetty P, Wallace R, Bondurant S (2001) Clearing the smoke: addressing the science base for tobacco harm reduction. Washington, DC: National Academy Press.

4. Fagerstrom KO, Hughes JR (2002) Nicotine concentrations with concurrent use of cigarettes and nicotine replacement: a review. Nicotine Tob Res 4 Suppl 2: S73–S79. 10.1080/1462220021000032753 [doi].

5. Wang D, Connock M, Barton P, Fry-Smith A, Aveyard P, et al. (2008) 'Cut down to quit' with nicotine replacement therapies in smoking cessation: a systematic review of effectiveness and economic analysis. Health Technol Assess 12: iii–xi.

6. Beard E, Fidler J, West R (2011) Is use of nicotine replacement therapy while continuing to smoke associated with increased nicotine intake? Evidence from a population sample. Psychopharmacology (Berl) 218: 609–610. 10.1007/s00213-011-2359-4 [doi].

7. Tonnesen P, Paoletti P, Gustavsson G, Russell MA, Saracci R, et al. (1999) Higher dosage nicotine patches increase one-year smoking cessation rates: results from the European CEASE trial. Collaborative European Anti-Smoking Evaluation. European Respiratory Society. Eur Respir J 13: 238–246.

8. Wennike P, Danielsson T, Landfeldt B, Westin A, Tonnesen P (2003) Smoking reduction promotes smoking cessation: results from a double blind, randomized, placebo-controlled trial of nicotine gum with 2-year follow-up. Addiction 98: 1395–1402.

9. Schnoll RA, Patterson F, Wileyto EP, Heitjan DF, Shields AE, et al. (2010) Effectiveness of extended-duration transdermal nicotine therapy: a randomized trial. Ann Intern Med 152: 144–151. 152/3/144 [pii]; 10.7326/0003-4819-152-3-201002020-00005 [doi].

10. Joseph AM, Fu SS, Lindgren B, Rothman AJ, Kodl M, et al. (2011) Chronic disease management for tobacco dependence: a randomized, controlled trial. Arch Intern Med 171: 1894–1900. 171/21/1894 [pii]; 10.1001/archinternmed.2011.500 [doi].

11. MHRA (2009) MHRA Public Assessment Report: The use of nicotine replacement therapy to reduce harm in smokers. London: Medicine and Healthcare Products Regulatory Agency (MHRA).

12. Fucito LM, Bars MP, Forray A, Rojewski AM, Shiffman S, et al. (2014) Addressing the evidence for FDA nicotine replacement therapy label changes: a policy statement of the Association for the Treatment of Tobacco use and Dependence and the Society for Research on Nicotine and Tobacco. Nicotine Tob Res 16: 909–914. ntu087 [pii];10.1093/ntr/ntu087 [doi].

13. Le Strat Y, Rehm J, Le FB (2011) How generalisable to community samples are clinical trial results for treatment of nicotine dependence: a comparison of common eligibility criteria with respondents of a large representative general population survey. Tob Control 20: 338–343. tc.2010.038703 [pii];10.1136/tc.2010.038703 [doi].

14. Shiffman S, Sweeney CT (2008) Ten years after the Rx-to-OTC switch of nicotine replacement therapy: what have we learned about the benefits and risks of non-prescription availability? Health Policy 86: 17–26. S0168-8510(07)00197-2 [pii];10.1016/j.healthpol.2007.08.006 [doi].

15. Shahab L, Brose LS, West R (2013) Novel Delivery Systems for Nicotine Replacement Therapy as an Aid to Smoking Cessation and for Harm Reduction: Rationale, and Evidence for Advantages over Existing Systems. CNS Drugs 27: 1007–1019. 10.1007/s40263-013-0116-4 [doi].

16. NICE (2013) Tobacco - Harm reduction. Available: http://publications.nice.org.uk/tobacco-harm-reduction-approaches-to-smoking-ph45.

17. Benowitz NL, Gourlay SG (1997) Cardiovascular toxicity of nicotine: implications for nicotine replacement therapy. J Am Coll Cardiol 29: 1422–1431. S073510979700079X [pii].

18. Benowitz NL, Jacob P III, Jones RT, Rosenberg J (1982) Interindividual variability in the metabolism and cardiovascular effects of nicotine in man. J Pharmacol Exp Ther 221: 368–372.

19. Black A, Beard E, Brown J, Fidler J, West R (2012) Beliefs about the harms of long-term use of nicotine replacement therapy: perceptions of smokers in England. Addiction 107: 2037–2042. 10.1111/j.1360-0443.2012.03955.x [doi].

20. Etter JF (2009) Dependence on the nicotine gum in former smokers. Addict Behav 34: 246–251. S0306-4603(08)00300-6 [pii]; 10.1016/j.addbeh.2008.10.018 [doi].

21. Fidler JA, Shahab L, West O, Jarvis MJ, McEwen A, et al. (2011) 'The Smoking Toolkit Study': A national study of smoking and smoking cessation in England. BMC Public Health 11: 479.

22. Heatherton TF, Kozlowski LT, Frecker RC, Rickert W, Robinson J (1989) Measuring the heaviness of smoking: using self-reported time to the first cigarette of the day and number of cigarettes smoked per day. Br J Addict 84: 791–799.

23. Fidler JA, Shahab L, West R (2011) Strength of urges to smoke as a measure of severity of cigarette dependence: comparison with the Fagerstrom Test for Nicotine Dependence and its components. Addiction 106: 631–638.

24. Kotz D, Brown J, West R (2013) Predictive validity of the Motivation To Stop Scale (MTSS): A single-item measure of motivation to stop smoking. Drug Alcohol Depend 128: 15–19. S0376-8716(12)00286-4 [pii]; 10.1016/j.drugalcdep.2012.07.012 [doi].

25. Foulds J, Bryant A, Stapleton J, Jarvis MJ, Russell MAH (1994) The Stability of Cotinine in Unfrozen Saliva Mailed to the Laboratory. American Journal of Public Health 84: 1182–1183.

26. Feyerabend C, Russell MA (1990) A rapid gas-liquid chromatographic method for the determination of cotinine and nicotine in biological fluids. J Pharm Pharmacol 42: 450–452.

27. Hajek P, McRobbie H, Gillison F (2007) Dependence potential of nicotine replacement treatments: effects of product type, patient characteristics, and cost to user. Prev Med 44: 230–234.

28. West R, DiMarino ME, Gitchell J, McNeill A (2005) Impact of UK policy initiatives on use of medicines to aid smoking cessation. Tob Control 14: 166–171.

29. Silla K, Beard E, Shahab L (2014) Characterization of long-term users of nicotine replacement therapy: evidence from a national survey. Nicotine Tob Res 16: 1050–1055. ntu019 [pii]; 10.1093/ntr/ntu019 [doi].

30. Shahab L, Cummings KM, Hammond D, Borland R, West R, et al. (2009) The impact of changing nicotine replacement therapy licensing laws in the United Kingdom: findings from the International Tobacco Control Four Country Survey. Addiction 104: 1420–1427.

31. Hubbard R, Lewis S, Smith C, Godfrey C, Smeeth L, et al. (2005) Use of nicotine replacement therapy and the risk of acute myocardial infarction, stroke, and death. Tob Control 14: 416–421. 14/6/416 [pii]; 10.1136/tc.2005.011387 [doi].

32. Eliasson B, Taskinen MR, Smith U (1996) Long-term use of nicotine gum is associated with hyperinsulinemia and insulin resistance. Circulation 94: 878–881.

33. Sims TH, Fiore MC (2002) Pharmacotherapy for treating tobacco dependence: what is the ideal duration of therapy? CNS Drugs 16: 653–662. 161001 [pii].

34. Fidler JA, Stapleton JA, West R (2011) Variation in saliva cotinine as a function of self-reported attempts to reduce cigarette consumption. Psychopharmacology (Berl) 217: 587–593. 10.1007/s00213-011-2317-1 [doi].

21

The Glasgow Prognostic Score Predicts Poor Survival in Cisplatin-Based Treated Patients with Metastatic Nasopharyngeal Carcinoma

Cui Chen[1][9], **Peng Sun**[2,3][9], **Qiang-sheng Dai**[1][9], **Hui-wen Weng**[1], **He-ping Li**[1], **Sheng Ye**[1]*

1 Department of Oncology, The First Affiliated Hospital, Sun Yat-Sen University, Guangzhou, China, **2** Department of Medical Oncology, Sun Yat-sen University Cancer Center, Guangzhou, China, **3** Collaborative Innovation Center for Cancer Medicine, State Key Laboratory of Oncology in South China, Guangzhou, China

Abstract

Background: Several inflammation-based prognostic scoring systems, including Glasgow Prognostic Score (GPS), neutrophil to lymphocyte ratio (NLR) and platelet to lymphocyte ratio (PLR) have been reported to predict survival in many malignancies, whereas their role in metastatic nasopharyngeal carcinoma (NPC) remains unclear. The aim of this study is to evaluate the clinical value of these prognostic scoring systems in a cohort of cisplatin-based treated patients with metastatic NPC.

Methods: Two hundred and eleven patients with histologically proven metastatic NPC treated with first-line cisplatin-based chemotherapy were retrospectively evaluated. Demographics, disease-related characteristics and relevant laboratory data before treatment were recorded. GPS, NLR and PLR were calculated as described previously. Response to first-line therapy and survival data were also collected. Survival was analyzed in Cox regressions and stability of the models was examined by bootstrap resampling. The area under the receiver operating characteristics curve (AUC) was calculated to compare the discriminatory ability of each scoring system.

Results: Among the above three inflammation-based prognostic scoring systems, GPS ($P<0.001$) and NLR ($P=0.019$) were independently associated with overall survival, which showed to be stable in a bootstrap resampling study. The GPS consistently showed a higher AUC value at 6-month (0.805), 12-month (0.705), and 24-month (0.705) in comparison with NLR and PLR. Further analysis of the association of GPS with progression-free survival showed GPS was also associated independently with progression-free survival ($P<0.001$).

Conclusions: Our study demonstrated that the GPS may be of prognostic value in metastatic NPC patients treated with cisplatin-based palliative chemotherapy and facilitate individualized treatment. However a prospective study to validate this prognostic model is still needed.

Editor: Konradin Metze, University of Campinas, Brazil

Funding: The authors received no specific funding for this work.

Competing Interests: The authors have declared that no competing interests exist.

* Email: yes20111212@163.com

[9] These authors contributed equally to this work.

Introduction

Nasopharyngeal carcinoma (NPC) is a distinct disease with unique ethnic and geographic characteristics, whose incidence varies from 0.5–3/100 000/year in North Africa to 20–30 in some areas of southern China. [1,2] Although the cure rate has been significantly improved owing to advances in diagnostic imaging, radiotherapeutic techniques and chemotherapy regimens recently, distant metastases remain the main reason for failure of treatment. [3] In these cases, palliative systemic therapy remains the primary therapeutic option and cisplatin-based combination chemotherapy is considered the standard front-line regimen for decades, offering response rates in the range of 50–80% and a significant prolongation of overall survival (OS). [4] However, there are still wide individual differences in clinical response and outcomes. Some reports indicate that overall survival may exceed ten years for specific subgroups of patients. It is therefore of paramount interest to find an easily available model to help evaluate individual prognosis which will greatly improve the ability of clinical decision-making.

Currently, clinical characteristics are dominating indexes for judging prognosis of metastatic NPC patients, such as performance status and disease-free interval. [5] The prognostic value of circulating Epstein–Barr virus (EBV) DNA load has also been well established in various reports. [6,7] Besides aforementioned prognostic factors representing tumor status and clinical characteristics, it is now recognized that the host inflammatory response, in particular the systemic inflammatory response, plays an important role in disease development and progression by inhibition of apoptosis, promotion of angiogenesis, and damage of DNA. [8,9,10] Several inflammation-based prognostic scoring systems have been devised and found to be strongly correlated with prognosis in patients with a variety of neoplasms. These include a combination of neutrophil and lymphocyte counts as the neutrophil to lymphocyte ratio (NLR) and a combination of platelet and lymphocyte counts as the platelet to lymphocyte ratio (PLR), both of which reflect full blood count derangements induced by the acute phase reaction, while the Glasgow Prognostic Score (GPS) incorporates raised circulating C-reactive protein (CRP) and hypoalbuminemia. [11,12,13,14,15] Recently some researches have also shown that markers of systemic inflammatory response represent reliable prognostic factors in patients with early nasopharyngeal carcinoma. [16] However, to the best of our knowledge, there is no data regarding the prognostic impact of systemic inflammation-based scoring systems in metastatic NPC. In the present study, we therefore evaluated the clinical value of several inflammation-based prognostic scoring systems including GPS, NLR and PLR in a cohort of cisplatin-based treated patients with metastatic NPC.

Patients and Methods

Patient selection

From October 2005 to October 2011, 211 patients with histologically proven metastatic NPC treated with first-line cisplatin-based chemotherapy were included in the study at Sun Yat-Sen University Cancer Center. Entry criteria consisted of: (1) radiologically measurable disease; (2) treated with at least two cycles of first-line cisplatin-based palliative chemotherapy; (3) Karnofsky Performance Scores (KPS) ≥60; (4) normal hepatic and renal function. Exclusion criteria included: (1) patients with other types of malignancy; (2) patients with brain metastases; (3) patients with clinical evidence of infection or other inflammatory conditions. This study was approved by the institutional review board and ethics committee of Sun Yat-Sen University Cancer Center. All patients provided written informed consent to

participate in this study. Parental written consent was obtained for minors in current study.

Treatment

All eligible patients received 1 of the following cisplatin-based chemotherapy regimens as the first-line treatment: (1) cisplatin (25 mg/m^2 intravenously [IV] on Days 1–3 of a 21-day cycle) plus 5-fluorouracil (500 mg/m^2 IV on Days 1–5 of a 21-day cycle), (2) paclitaxel (175 mg/m^2 IV over 3 hours with standard premedication on Day 1 of a 21-day cycle) plus cisplatin (25 mg/m^2 IV on Days 1–3 of a 21-day cycle), (3) paclitaxel (135 mg/m^2 IV over 3 hours with standard premedication on Day 1 of a 21-day cycle) plus cisplatin (25 mg/m^2 IV on Days 1–3 of a 21-day cycle) plus 5-fluorouracil (800 mg/m^2, continuous IV infusion for 24 hours, on Days 1–5 of a 21-day cycle). Of the 211 eligible patients, 78 (37.0%) patients were given the PF regimen, 24 (11.4%) patients were given the TP regimen, and 109 (51.6%) patients received the TPF regimen.

Relevant Evaluation

Basic demographics, baseline characteristics, detailed medical history as well as relevant laboratory data before treatment (C-reactive protein (CRP), Serum lactate dehydrogenase (LDH), albumin, neutrophil, lymphocyte, platelet (Plt) count and plasma EBV DNA level) were recorded. The GPS, NLR and PLR were constructed as described previously. In GPS, patients with both an elevated CRP level (>1.0 mg/dl) and hypoalbuminemia (<3.5 g/dl) were allocated a score of 2, patients with only one of these biochemical abnormalities were allocated a score of 1, and patients with neither of these abnormalities were allocated a score of 0. NLR was divided into two groups (<5 and ≥5) while PLR was categorized into three groups (<150, 150–300 and >300).

Progression-free survival (PFS) and overall survival (OS) were defined as the time from the first diagnosis of metastasis to the date of documented progression and to the date of death, respectively. Tumor response was evaluated according to the Response Evaluation Criteria in Solid Tumors (RECISTs) 1.0.

Table 1. Demographic and Baseline Characteristics of Patients.

Patient characteristics	Number (%)
Total evaluated	211 (100)
Age, years (median/range)	46/14–72
Gender (male/female)	181/30 (85.8/14.2)
KPS (median/range)	90/60–100
Number of involved sites (median/range)	2/1–6
Synchronous metastasis (yes/no)	53/158 (25.1/74.9)
Liver metastasis (yes/no)	73/138 (34.6/65.4)
Lung metastasis (yes/no)	97/114 (45.9/54.1)
Bone metastasis (yes/no)	88/123 (41.7/58.3)
Disease-free interval, months (median/range)	6/0–65
Chemotherapy regimen (PF/TP/TPF)	78/24/109 (37.0/11.4/51.6)
Serum LDH, U/L (median/range)	247/81–632
Pre-treatment EBV DNA, copies/mL (median/range)	4.93×10^4/0–9.73×10^7
GPS (0/1/2)	125/66/20 (59.2/31.3/9.5)
NLR (median/range)	3.12/0.81–11.03
PLR (median/range)	71.2/31.3–422.5

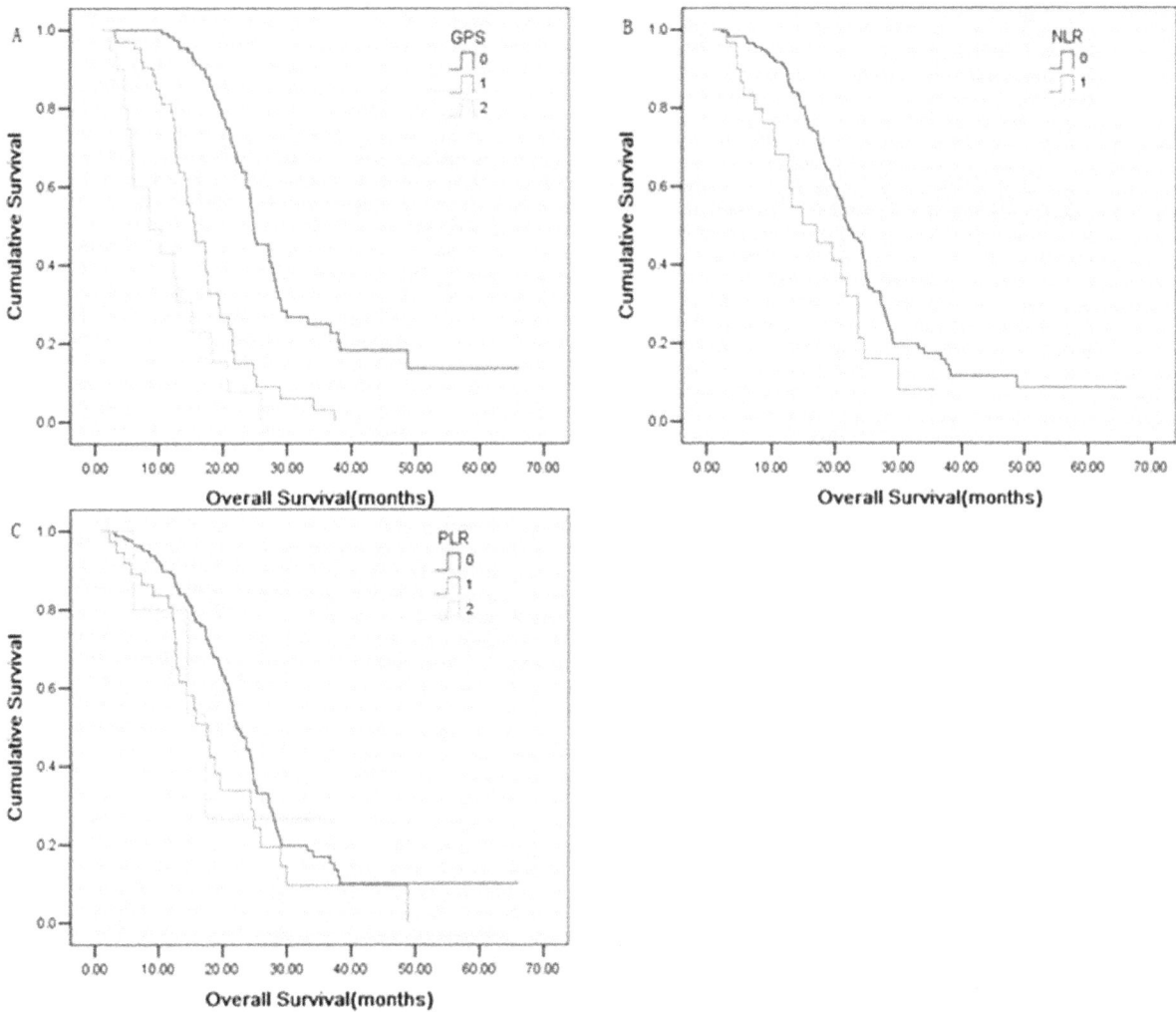

Figure 1. Comparison of overall survival according to scoring systems, GPS (A), NLR (B) and PLR (C).

Follow up

Patients were regularly followed up after chemotherapy until death or their last follow-up appointment. Physical examination and imaging studies of the relevant region(s) were performed every 3 months after the completion of the chemotherapy or when clinical indications dictated for follow-up. The start date of follow-up period was the date of initial metastatic NPC diagnosis. The time of last follow-up was 31st December 2013 or death.

Statistical analysis

All statistical analysis was performed using SPSS version 13.0 software or WinStat software. PFS and OS were obtained by using the Kaplan–Meier method and differences between the groups were compared by the log-rank test. A univariate analysis was performed for the potential prognostic factors. Age, karnofsky performance score before treatment, number of involved sites, disease-free interval, serum LDH, pre-treatment EBV DNA entered the calculations in a continuous way. NLR and PLR were also tested at first as continuous variables in order to avoid the bias induced by binarization of continuous data. And we tested the GPS and the other variables entering the analysis as categorical variables. Multivariable analysis including variables that proved to be significant in the univariate analysis was

performed subsequently using the Cox model to analyse factors related to prognosis (P<0.05 was used as the cut-off value of statistical significance). The stability of the COX model was tested by bootstrap resampling. New data sets of equal size were created by random sampling of the original data with replacement. In each new bootstrap data set, a patient may be represented once, multiple times or not at all. Cox regressions with the same conditions as in the original data set were then calculated for the new data sets in order to obtain the bootstrap parameter estimates. Descriptive statistics for the patient groups are reported as mean, median, and range. Categorical variables were presented numbers and percentages. Non-parametric test was applied for comparison of data among groups. A receiver operating characteristics (ROC) curve was also generated and the area under the curve (AUC) was calculated to evaluate the discriminatory ability of each scoring systems. A two-tailed P value less than 0.05 was considered to be statistically significant.

Results

Patient characteristics and Outcomes

A total of 211 patients with metastatic NPC were included in the present study. All of the patients were from epidemic areas in

Table 2. Univariate and Multivariate Analysis of Prognostic Factors of Overall Survival.

Variable	Univariate analysis		Multivariate analysis	
	P	HR (95% CI)	P	HR (95% CI)
Age	0.444	1.006 (0.990–1.023)		
Gender (male/female)	0.631	1.147 (0.655–2.008)		
KPS	0.934	1.020 (0.637–1.633)		
Liver metastasis (yes/no)	0.989	1.003 (0.694–1.449)		
Lung metastasis (yes/no)	0.848	1.035 (0.726–1.476)		
Number of involved sites	0.020	1.282 (1.040–1.580)	0.560	1.064 (0.864–1.310)
Synchronous metastasis (yes/no)	0.696	0.920 (0.604–1.400)		
Disease-free interval	0.278	1.218 (0.853–1.739)		
Chemotherapy regimen (PF/TP/TPF)	0.358	0.767 (0.435–1.351)		
Serum LDH	0.014	1.210 (1.040–1.409)	0.911	1.011 (0.835–1.225)
Pre-treatment EBVDNA	0.024	1.234 (1.028–1.481)	0.037	1.239 (1.013–1.515)
GPS (0/1/2)	<0.001	3.078 (2.393–3.959)	<0.001	2.520 (1.977–3.212)
NLR	0.025	1.732 (1.071–2.800)	0.019	1.800 (1.103–2.940)
PLR	0.125	1.311 (0.928–1.853)		

China, with a male predominance (85.8%). The mean age of diagnosis of metastatic NPC was 46 (range 14–72) years. About half of the patients had more than one metastatic site with lung being the most common site (45.9%). The pretreatment plasma EBV DNA ranged from 0 to 9.73×10^7 copies/mL, with a median of 4.93×10^4 copies/mL. One hundred and fifty (71.1%) patients showed an elevated pretreatment EBV DNA level ($>1 \times 10^3$ copies/mL). One hundred and twenty-five (59.2%) patients were allocated to GPS 0, 66 (31.3%) patients were allocated to GPS 1, and 20 (9.5%) patients were allocated to GPS 2, respectively. The median NLR level was 3.12 (range 0.81~11.03). Thirty patients (14.2%) had an NLR≥5 and the rest had an NLR<5. The PLR ranged from 31.3 to 422.5, with a median of 71.2. A PLR greater than 300 was seen in 5 patients (2.4%), 168 patients (79.6%) had PLR<150, and the rest had a PLR in between. Other patient characteristics are summarized in Table 1.

At the time of analysis, 124 (58.8%) patients had died, and the median PFS and OS were 7.9 and 21.6 months, respectively. The overall clinical response rate was 70.1% for all 211 patients.

Prognostic factor analysis for overall survival

Various potential prognostic factors including age, gender, karnofsky performance score before treatment, metastasis sites (liver and lung), number of involved sites, synchronous metastasis, disease-free interval, chemotherapy regimen, serum LDH, pre-treatment EBV DNA, GPS status, NLR and PLR were analyzed. Univariate analysis revealed that a larger number of involved sites ($P = 0.020$), higher baseline serum LDH level ($P = 0.014$), higher pretreatment EBV DNA level ($P = 0.024$), higher score of GPS ($P<0.001$) and higher value of NLR ($P = 0.025$) were considered adverse factors for overall survival (Table 2, Fig. 1). Age, gender, PLR and the other variables in the analysis had no prognostic relevance. In multivariate analysis, pre-treatment EBV DNA ($P = 0.037$), GPS ($P<0.001$) and NLR ($P = 0.019$) were independent prognostic factors (Table 2). The stability of this model was confirmed in a bootstrap resampling procedure. Among 1000 new

models, pre-treatment EBV DNA was present in 69%, GPS appeared in 89% and NLR in 71%.

Moreover, the two inflammation-based prognostic scoring systems constructed by categorizing the continuous variables of NLR and PLR as described before were compared with the GPS. Receiver operating characteristic curves were constructed for survival status at 6-month, 12-month, and 24-month of follow-up, and the area under the ROC curve (AUC) was compared (Fig. 2) to assess the discrimination ability of each scoring system. The GPS consistently show a higher AUC value at 6-month (0.805), 12-month (0.705), and 24-month (0.705) in comparison with other inflammation-based prognostic scores.

Association of GPS with clinicopathologic characteristics

Baseline patient and disease-related characteristics for each GPS group and comparisons between groups are depicted in Table 3. Although the difference was not statistically significant, a trend towards an association of GPS with BMI was observed. Of note, an elevated GPS was significantly associated with higher serum LDH and higher pretreatment EBV DNA.

Association of GPS with progression-free survival

GPS was further associated with PFS. Kaplan–Meier curves for PFS for the total cohort according to GPS was shown in Fig. 3. Median PFS (95% CI) was 8.73 (7.64–9.82), 5.27 (4.51–6.02) and 3.40 (1.21–5.59) months for patients with GPS 0, 1 and 2, respectively. As shown in Table 4, multivariate analysis including the aforementioned parameters and GPS revealed that GPS was also the independent predictor for PFS ($P<0.001$). The stability of this model was also confirmed in a bootstrap resampling procedure. In the bootstrap resampling, GPS entered in 100% and pre-treatment EBV DNA appeared in 25%.

Discussion

Markers of systemic inflammatory response represent reliable prognostic factors in patients with advanced cancer.

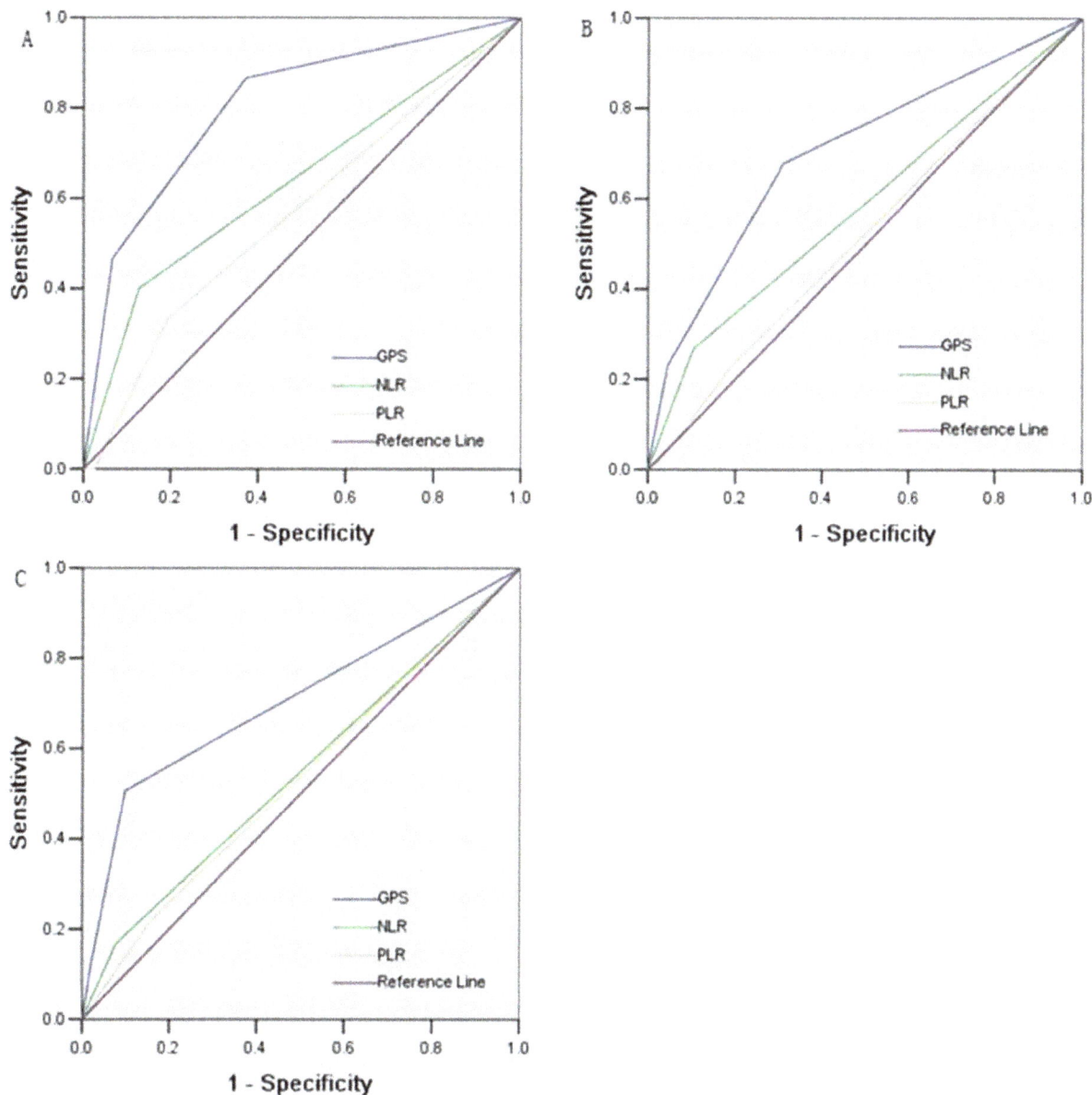

Figure 2. Comparisons of the area under the receiver operating curve for survival status between scoring systems at 6 month (A), 12 month (B) and 24 month (C).

[8,11,12,13,14,16] To the best of our knowledge, this study has firstly demonstrated that the GPS, an inflammation-based prognostic score, is an independent marker of poor prognosis in patients with metastatic NPC and is superior to the NLR in terms of prognostic ability. Furthermore, our data demonstrated a significant, independent association between GPS and PFS.

Accumulating evidence indicates the prognostic importance of GPS in various solid cancers, such as colorectal cancer, [17,18] esophageal cancer, [19] lung cancer, [13] pancreatic cancer, [12] and gastric cancer. [14] A similar result was achieved in our study. The biological basis for the correlation between the GPS and survival are not completely understood. Below are some supposed mechanisms. First, cachexia, which often manifests as nutritional depletion (weight loss, elevated resting energy expenditure and loss of lean tissue) and functional decline, is common in patients with advanced cancer and has been recognized to be associated with

poorer outcome. [20,21,22] CRP has been reported to be associated with the nutrition status and development of cachexia while albumin represents a negative acute phase protein and also represents a marker of nutritional status. [8] As we know, lower serum albumin correlates to nutritional depletion closely. Our study also shows a trend towards an association of GPS with BMI. Based on these reports, GPS, incorporating CRP and serum albumin levels, may reflect both presence of the nutritional depletion and functional decline, resulting in poor survival outcome. Second, a strong association was found between EBV infection and NPC in previous studies. [23] Plasma EBV DNA has been identified to be prognostic in metastatic NPC patients. [6,7] EBV infection stimulated the release of pro-inflammatory cytokine including IL-1, IL-6, and TNF-α from the tumor microenvironment, which results in the induction of CRP synthesis from the liver and the reduction of albumin by hepatocytes. [24,25] In

Table 3. Association of GPS with characteristics of patients.

characteristics	GPS = 0	GPS = 1	GPS = 2	P
Age (≤45/>45)	65/60	30/36	12/8	0.472
Gender (male/female)	103/22	60/6	18/2	0.236
KPS (≤80/>80)	24/101	12/54	4/16	0.978
BMI (≤18.5/>18.5)	21/104	20/46	6/14	0.070
Number of involved sites (1/≥2)	61/64	36/30	8/12	0.493
Synchronous metastasis (yes/no)	26/99	22/44	5/15	0.165
Liver metastasis (yes/no)	43/82	21/45	9/11	0.553
Lung metastasis (yes/no)	53/72	35/31	9/11	0.373
Bone metastasis (yes/no)	50/75	28/38	10/10	0.694
Serum LDH, U/L (<245/≥245)	83/42	27/39	8/12	0.001
Pre-treatment EBV DNA, copies/mL (<median/≥median)	99/26	5/61	2/18	0.0001

other words, GPS level may be a marker of inflammation from EBV infection and may indicate the magnitude of inflammation and the prognosis of patients as EBV DNA load. Previous studies have also indicated that inflammation in the tumor microenvironment play an important role in promoting tumor growth, invasion, and metastasis. [9,10] Our data shows that an elevated GPS is significantly associated with higher EBV-DNA level, which will, to certain extent, add further support to the proposal. In addition to these explanations, because our data find an elevated GPS is also significantly associated with elevated LDH, which has been reported to be an indicator of high tumor burden, an

elevated GPS score may indirectly reflect a high tumor burden. [26] In general, these explanations suggest that it is reasonable that GPS is a significant and independent predictor of survival outcome.

Recently a study by Wei-xiong Xia et al also showed that elevated CRP and CRP kinetics correlated with poor prognosis in patients with metastatic NPC. This study had similar aims and results compared with our study. However there are still some differences between the two studies. Firstly, the GPS incorporates CRP and hypoalbuminemia and may be more suitable to reflect systemic inflammatory response than CRP alone. Secondly, the

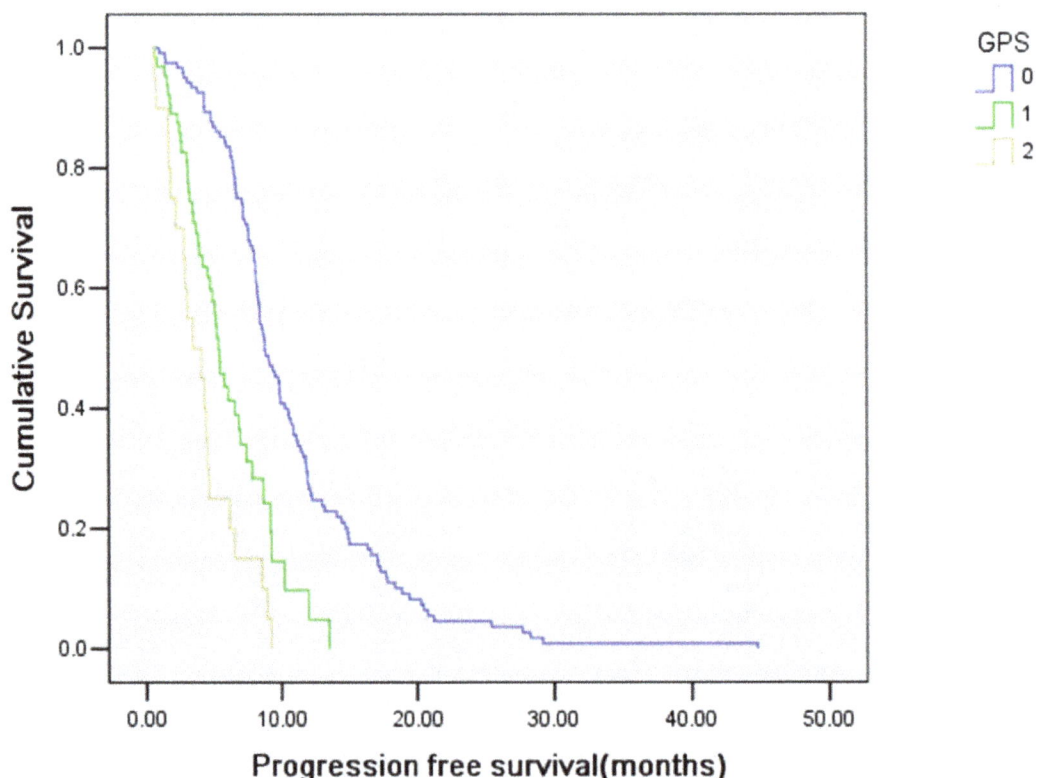

Figure 3. Kaplan–Meier estimates for progression-free survival according to GPS.

Table 4. Univariate and Multivariate Analysis of Prognostic Factors of Progression-free Survival.

Variable	Univariate analysis		Multivariate analysis	
	P	HR (95% CI)	P	HR (95% CI)
Age	0.613	0.996 (0.981–1.011)		
Gender (male/female)	0.489	1.162 (0.760–1.776)		
KPS	0.372	0.998 (0.994–1.002)		
Liver metastasis (yes/no)	0.477	0.893 (0.655–1.219)		
Lung metastasis (yes/no)	0.127	1.261 (0.936–1.698)		
Number of involved sites	0.043	1.201 (1.0066–1.435)	0.493	1.063 (0.893–1.266)
Synchronous metastasis (yes/no)	0.933	1.015 (0.719–1.434)		
Disease-free interval	0.238	1.198 (0.887–1.617)		
Chemotherapy regimen (PF/TP/TPF)	0.609	0.884 (0.552–1.417)		
Serum LDH	0.340	1.072 (0.93–1.235)		
Pre-treatment EBVDNA	<0.001	1.426 (1.170–1.739)	0.133	1.206 (0.945–1.539)
GPS (0/1/2)	<0.001	2.417 (1.916–3.050)	<0.001	2.248 (1.753–2.833)
NLR	0.054	1.400 (0.995–1.971)		
PLR	0.611	1.061 (0.844–1.334)		

eligibility criteria are different. All patients enrolled in current study received first-line cisplatin-based regimens. Thus, it is helpful to exclude the potential confounding effect of different regimens.

The GPS test is simple and based on standardized, wildly available protein assays. Therefore assessment of the GPS can be routinely in most clinical centers. Based on the present results, the significant value of GPS test is that it can identify patients at high risk of disease progression and death as a clinically convenient and useful biomarker. Thus it not only provides guidance of follow-up care at clinic but also has the potential to be a stratification factor or a selection criterion in randomized clinical trials for metastatic NPC. Moreover, in our study, most of the patients evaluated as disease progression at the end of second cycle of chemotherapy were allocated a score of 2. Patients in the good GPS group (GPS 0) had a more prolonged progression-free survival. As a consequence we believe that the presence of a systemic inflammatory response should be evaluated in the pretreatment period and might become the promising new targets of anti-tumor therapy. Nowadays there was an amount of ongoing research into the effect of non-steroidal anti-inflammatory drugs on anti-tumor treatment, including colon cancer, [27] lung cancer, [28] esophagus cancer [29] and so on. Accordingly, it is also interesting and significant to study the modification of the systemic inflammatory response in patients with metastatic nasopharyngeal carcinoma. And the GPS which is inexpensive, reliable, and widely available may have a certain guiding significance for selecting patients who might be candidates for modulation of systemic inflammatory response and provide a well defined therapeutic target for future clinical trials. Further evaluation is required to confirm this hypothesis.

In addition, the NLR and PLR have been reported to be important prognostic models in patients with a variety of solid cancers, such as colorectal cancer, esophageal cancer, gastric cancer, pancreatic cancer, and lung cancer. Several studies have also shown that an elevated NLR is associated with poor prognosis in patients with NPC. [12,14,30,31] In accord with the study of Jian-rong He et al. who tested the prognostic value of NLR in 1410 patients with various stages of NPC [32] and the study of Xin An et al. who tested the prognostic value of NLR in 363 patients with non-disseminated NPC, [16] we also found a significant association between NLR and OS. However, the COX model and the AUC analysis have shown that the GPS was superior to NLR in terms of discriminating ability and prognostic accuracy. For PLR, it was not independently associated with overall survival. In general, this study is the first to show the superior prognostic ability of the GPS over the NLR and PLR in patients with metastatic NPC.

In conclusion, our study demonstrated that the GPS may be useful to predict the prognosis of metastatic NPC patients treated with cisplatin-based palliative chemotherapy and facilitate individualized treatment. A prospective study to validate this prognostic model is needed. The mechanisms underlying the relationship between high GPS and poor prognosis in NPC still need further study.

Author Contributions

Conceived and designed the experiments: SY. Performed the experiments: CC PS HPL. Analyzed the data: CC PS QSD. Contributed reagents/materials/analysis tools: PS SY HWW. Contributed to the writing of the manuscript: CC PS.

References

1. Yu MC, Yuan JM (2002) Epidemiology of nasopharyngeal carcinoma. Semin Cancer Biol 12: 421–429.
2. Chang ET, Adami HO (2006) The enigmatic epidemiology of nasopharyngeal carcinoma. Cancer Epidemiol Biomarkers Prev 15: 1765–1777.
3. Chiesa F, De Paoli F (2001) Distant metastases from nasopharyngeal cancer. ORL J Otorhinolaryngol Relat Spec 63: 214–216.
4. Bensouda Y, Kaikani W, Ahbeddou N, Rahhali R, Jabri M, et al. (2011) Treatment for metastatic nasopharyngeal carcinoma. Eur Ann Otorhinolaryngol Head Neck Dis 128: 79–85.
5. Liu MT, Hsieh CY, Chang TH, Lin JP, Huang CC, et al. (2003) Prognostic factors affecting the outcome of nasopharyngeal carcinoma. Jpn J Clin Oncol 33: 501–508.

6. Twu CW, Wang WY, Liang WM, Jan JS, Jiang RS, et al. (2007) Comparison of the prognostic impact of serum anti-EBV antibody and plasma EBV DNA assays in nasopharyngeal carcinoma. Int J Radiat Oncol Biol Phys 67: 130–137.
7. An X, Wang FH, Ding PR, Deng L, Jiang WQ, et al. (2011) Plasma Epstein-Barr virus DNA level strongly predicts survival in metastatic/recurrent nasopharyngeal carcinoma treated with palliative chemotherapy. Cancer 117: 3750–3757.
8. McMillan DC (2009) Systemic inflammation, nutritional status and survival in patients with cancer. Curr Opin Clin Nutr Metab Care 12: 223–226.
9. Grivennikov SI, Greten FR, Karin M (2010) Immunity, inflammation, and cancer. Cell 140: 883–899.
10. Chiang AC, Massague J (2008) Molecular basis of metastasis. N Engl J Med 359: 2814–2823.
11. Kinoshita A, Onoda H, Imai N, Iwaku A, Oishi M, et al. (2013) The Glasgow Prognostic Score, an inflammation based prognostic score, predicts survival in patients with hepatocellular carcinoma. BMC Cancer 13: 52.
12. Wang DS, Luo HY, Qiu MZ, Wang ZQ, Zhang DS, et al. (2012) Comparison of the prognostic values of various inflammation based factors in patients with pancreatic cancer. Med Oncol 29: 3092–3100.
13. Gioulbasanis I, Pallis A, Vlachostergios PJ, Xyrafas A, Giannousi Z, et al. (2012) The Glasgow Prognostic Score (GPS) predicts toxicity and efficacy in platinum-based treated patients with metastatic lung cancer. Lung Cancer 77: 383–388.
14. Wang DS, Ren C, Qiu MZ, Luo HY, Wang ZQ, et al. (2012) Comparison of the prognostic value of various preoperative inflammation-based factors in patients with stage III gastric cancer. Tumour Biol 33: 749–756.
15. McMillan DC (2013) The systemic inflammation-based Glasgow Prognostic Score: a decade of experience in patients with cancer. Cancer Treat Rev 39: 534–540.
16. An X, Ding PR, Wang FH, Jiang WQ, Li YH (2011) Elevated neutrophil to lymphocyte ratio predicts poor prognosis in nasopharyngeal carcinoma. Tumour Biol 32: 317–324.
17. Maeda K, Shibutani M, Otani H, Nagahara H, Sugano K, et al. (2013) Prognostic value of preoperative inflammation-based prognostic scores in patients with stage IV colorectal cancer who undergo palliative resection of asymptomatic primary tumors. Anticancer Res 33: 5567–5573.
18. Ishizuka M, Nagata H, Takagi K, Iwasaki Y, Kubota K (2013) Inflammation-based prognostic system predicts survival after surgery for stage IV colorectal cancer. Am J Surg 205: 22–28.
19. Vashist YK, Loos J, Dedow J, Tachezy M, Uzunoglu G, et al. (2011) Glasgow Prognostic Score is a predictor of perioperative and long-term outcome in

patients with only surgically treated esophageal cancer. Ann Surg Oncol 18: 1130–1138.
20. Laviano A, Meguid MM, Inui A, Muscaritoli M, Rossi-Fanelli F (2005) Therapy insight: Cancer anorexia-cachexia syndrome–when all you can eat is yourself. Nat Clin Pract Oncol 2: 158–165.
21. Donohoe CL, Ryan AM, Reynolds JV (2011) Cancer cachexia: mechanisms and clinical implications. Gastroenterol Res Pract 2011: 601434.
22. Fearon KC, Voss AC, Hustead DS (2006) Definition of cancer cachexia: effect of weight loss, reduced food intake, and systemic inflammation on functional status and prognosis. Am J Clin Nutr 83: 1345–1350.
23. Senba M, Zhong XY, Senba MI, Itakura H (1994) EBV and nasopharyngeal carcinoma. Lancet 343: 1104.
24. Eliopoulos AG, Stack M, Dawson CW, Kaye KM, Hodgkin L, et al. (1997) Epstein-Barr virus-encoded LMP1 and CD40 mediate IL-6 production in epithelial cells via an NF-kappaB pathway involving TNF receptor-associated factors. Oncogene 14: 2899–2916.
25. Pepys MB, Hirschfield GM (2003) C-reactive protein: a critical update. J Clin Invest 111: 1805–1812.
26. Liaw CC, Wang CH, Huang JS, Kiu MC, Chen JS, et al. (1997) Serum lactate dehydrogenase level in patients with nasopharyngeal carcinoma. Acta Oncol 36: 159–164.
27. Fuchs CS, Ogino S (2013) Aspirin therapy for colorectal cancer with PIK3CA mutation: simply complex!. J Clin Oncol 31: 4358–4361.
28. Gridelli C, Gallo C, Ceribelli A, Gebbia V, Gamucci T, et al. (2007) Factorial phase III randomised trial of rofecoxib and prolonged constant infusion of gemcitabine in advanced non-small-cell lung cancer: the GEmcitabine-COxib in NSCLC (GECO) study. Lancet Oncol 8: 500–512.
29. Szumilo J, Burdan F, Szumilo M, Lewkowicz D, Kedzierawska-Kurylcio A (2009) Cyclooxygenase inhibitors in chemoprevention and treatment of esophageal squamous cell carcinoma. Pol Merkur Lekarski 27: 408–412.
30. Kwon HC, Kim SH, Oh SY, Lee S, Lee JH, et al. (2012) Clinical significance of preoperative neutrophil-lymphocyte versus platelet-lymphocyte ratio in patients with operable colorectal cancer. Biomarkers 17: 216–222.
31. Feng JF, Huang Y, Chen QX (2014) Preoperative platelet lymphocyte ratio (PLR) is superior to neutrophil lymphocyte ratio (NLR) as a predictive factor in patients with esophageal squamous cell carcinoma. World J Surg Oncol 12: 58.
32. He JR, Shen GP, Ren ZF, Qin H, Cui C, et al. (2012) Pretreatment levels of peripheral neutrophils and lymphocytes as independent prognostic factors in patients with nasopharyngeal carcinoma. Head Neck 34: 1769–1776.

22

The Impact of Antiretroviral Therapy on Mortality in HIV Positive People during Tuberculosis Treatment

Anna Odone[1,2,3]*, **Silvia Amadasi[4]**, **Richard G. White[1,5]**, **Theodore Cohen[6,7]**, **Alison D. Grant[5,8]**, **Rein M. G. J. Houben[1,5]**

1 TB Modelling Group, Centre for the Mathematical Modelling of Infectious Diseases, London School of Hygiene and Tropical Medicine, London, United Kingdom, **2** Department of Global Health and Social Medicine, Harvard Medical School, Boston, Massachusetts, United States of America, **3** University of Parma, School of Medicine, Parma, Italy, **4** University Division of Infectious and Tropical Diseases, University of Brescia and Spedali Civili General Hospital, Brescia, Italy, **5** TB Centre, London School of Hygiene and Tropical Medicine, London, United Kingdom, **6** Center for Communicable Disease Dynamics, Department of Epidemiology, Harvard School of Public Health, Boston, Massachusetts, United States of America, **7** Division of Global Health Equity, Brigham and Women's Hospital, Boston, Massachusetts, United States of America, **8** Department of Clinical Research, London School of Hygiene and Tropical Medicine, London, United Kingdom

Abstract

Objective: To quantify the impact of antiretroviral therapy (ART) on mortality in HIV-positive people during tuberculosis (TB) treatment.

Design: We conducted a systematic literature review and meta-analysis. Studies published from 1996 through February 15, 2013, were identified by searching electronic resources (Pubmed and Embase) and conference books, manual searches of references, and expert consultation. Pooled estimates for the outcome of interest were acquired using random effects meta-analysis.

Subjects: The study population included individuals receiving ART before or during TB treatment.

Main Outcome Measures: Main outcome measures were: (i) TB-case fatality ratio (CFR), defined as the proportion of individuals dying during TB treatment and, if mortality in HIV-positive people not on ART was also reported, (ii) the relative risk of death during TB treatment by ART status.

Results: Twenty-one studies were included in the systematic review. Random effects pooled meta-analysis estimated the CFR between 8% and 14% (pooled estimate 11%). Among HIV-positive TB cases, those receiving ART had a reduction in mortality during TB treatment of between 44% and 71% (RR = 0.42, 95%CI: 0.29–0.56).

Conclusion: Starting ART before or during TB therapy reduces the risk of death during TB treatment by around three-fifths in clinical settings. National programmes should continue to expand coverage of ART for HIV positive in order to control the dual epidemic.

Editor: Katharina Kranzer, London School of Hygiene and Tropical Medicine, United Kingdom

Funding: This work was funded through a UNAIDS direct commission (AIEP1201338/3.4.58680). AO is funded through a residency fellowship in Hygiene and Preventive Medicine. RGW, TC, and RMGJH are funded by the TB Modelling and Analysis Consortium (TB MAC) grant (OPP1084276) from the Bill and Melinda Gates Foundation. RGW is also funded by the Medical Research Council (UK) (Methodology Research Fellowship: G0802414 and grant MR/J005088/1) and CDC/ PEPFAR via the Aurum Institute (U2GPS0008111). AG is funded by Global Health Trials (G1100689) and the Bill and Melinda Gates Foundation (OPP1083118). The funders had no role in study design, data collection and analysis, decision to publish, or preparation of the manuscript.

Competing Interests: The authors have declared that no competing interests exist.

* Email: anna.odone@mail.harvard.edu

Introduction

Infection with HIV dramatically increases individuals' risk of developing active tuberculosis (TB) disease, as well as the risk of death during TB treatment [1]. While 13% of all people with TB are estimated to be HIV positive, they account for approximately a quarter of TB deaths [2]. The African region, where 250,000 deaths occurred among HIV-positive TB cases in 2012, accounts for 75% of HIV-positive TB cases [2].

Globally, in 2012, 46% of notified TB cases had a documented HIV test result and the coverage of Antiretroviral therapy (ART) among TB patients known to be HIV-positive was estimated to be 57% [2]. ART reduces the impact of HIV on incident TB, as illustrated by Suthar *et al.* who showed that the risk of TB is reduced by 65% [3]. Also, results from various trials and observational studies have consistently shown a benefit of ART on TB outcomes, and indicated that ART should be initiated as early as possible in the course of a TB episode [4,5,6,7,8,9,10,11]. However, to date, there has been no systematic overview of the magnitude of benefit of ART on TB mortality. A recent systemic review by Straetemans *et al.* on TB mortality stratified subjects by HIV status but did not explore the effect of ART [12].

TB mortality in HIV-positive people is a key parameter to describe current state and progress in TB care and control [2]. Ideally, TB mortality is estimated through direct measurements using vital registration systems or mortality surveys, but these are often unavailable in resource limited settings, where TB incidence is highest [2]. Alternatively, TB mortality can be estimated indirectly by calculating the case fatality ratio (CFR), which is defined as the proportion of people with incident TB that die as a result of this episode of disease [13]. TB-CFR has been defined by Maher *et al.* as the proportion of TB cases that die within a specified time [14]. In particular, Mukadi *et al.* defined TB-CFR as the proportion of tuberculosis patients that die during TB treatment [15], which is the definition applied by Straetemans *et al.* in their review [12].

In this paper we systematically review the literature to estimate the mortality during TB treatment among HIV-positive TB patients receiving ART as well as its value relative to HIV-positive TB patients not receiving ART.

Methods

The review's methods were defined in advance following the Prepared Items for Systematic Reviews and Meta-Analysis (PRISMA) guidelines [16].

Criteria for considering studies

Study population. We included studies that described mortality among HIV positive patients receiving TB treatment who initiated combination ART before or during TB treatment. All sex and age groups were included.

Our focus was on estimating the effect of ART as it applied to TB patients from the general population, and we excluded cohorts that were limited to recurrent, extra-pulmonary or known drug-resistant TB patients only. We also excluded studies focusing on populations of patients not representative of the general population such as miners [17], prisoners [18], healthcare workers [19] or injecting drug users [20].

Study design and sample size. Eligible study designs included clinical trials, prospective cohort, retrospective cohort and case-control studies. Literature reviews were screened to retrieve relevant primary data. Studies which reported mortality results on fewer than 50 TB patients receiving ART were also excluded.

Outcome measures. We focused on deaths occurring *during* TB treatment, the main operational parameter used in the field by most TB control programmes. This outcome has the benefit of a clearly defined at-risk period which facilitates between-study comparisons as well as programmme monitoring and evaluation. Papers were therefore excluded if they did not report mortality within six to eight months after start of TB treatment or otherwise restrict patient follow-up to the end of treatment.

We considered two primary outcome measures. Firstly, the TB-CFR defined as percentage of deaths among the study population occurring during TB treatment. Secondly, if the paper also reported TB mortality in HIV-positive individuals not on ART, we recorded the estimated relative risk (odds ratio (OR), relative risk (RR) or hazard ratio (HR)) of death during TB treatment by ART status.

Search methods for identification of studies

Studies were identified by searching the electronic databases Medline and Embase. The strategy was first developed in Medline and then adapted for use in the other databases (Appendix A). Studies published in English from 1996 (when combination ART first became available) through July2014 were included. In addition, the abstract books of the world conferences on lung health of the International Union against Tuberculosis and Lung Diseases (IUATLD) were manually scanned for the period 2004–2013 and further studies were retrieved from reference lists of relevant articles and consultation with experts in the field.

Data collection and analysis

Data extraction. Identified studies were independently reviewed for eligibility by two authors in a two-step process; a first screen was performed based on title and abstract while full texts were retrieved for the second screen. At both stages disagreements between reviewers were resolved by discussion.

Data were extracted by one author supervised by a second author using a standardised data extraction spreadsheet. The data extraction spreadsheet was piloted on 10 randomly selected papers and modified accordingly. Data extraction included: authors' names, year and country of publication, study design, study setting, study period, age of study participants, information on TB type, TB diagnosis and drug resistance, information on time of ART initiation, follow-up time, information on analysis performed and outcomes of interest. We defined TB treatment to be standardized (following the definition used by Straetemans [12]) if it was described to be: i) in line with WHO recommendations, ii) following national or governmental guidelines, iii) direct observed treatment strategy (DOTS) or iv) defined as 'standard' [12].

Analysis. We performed descriptive analysis to report the characteristics of the included studies. Midpoint values for the age of the included cohorts was based on the reported mean or median and were pooled as weighted averages. With regard to the pre-specified outcomes, we would expect variability between studies, e.g. based on average CD4 count in the study population or general quality of local health systems. We therefore applied random effects analyses to acquire an estimate of the average effect of ART on TB mortality, rather than assuming a single true value in a fixed effects approach [21]. With regard to the pre-specified outcomes, heterogeneity was assessed using the I^2 statistic and visual inspection of forest plots [21]. Depending on data availability, we planned to conduct sub-group analyses (where relevant and possible) by WHO region, age-group, time interval between TB treatment start and ART start, laboratory-confirmed TB diagnosis and median CD4 count at start of study. If unadjusted and adjusted outcomes were available, we recorded the adjusted estimate to reduce the risk of confounding.

Quality assessment. The same two authors who performed data extraction independently assessed the quality of the included studies using the Newcastle-Ottawa Assessment Scale (NOS) [22]. Level of quality was not set as a criterion for exclusion. Disagreements by reviewers were resolved by consensus.

Results

Identified studies

We identified 2,129 records by searching the selected databases and listing references of relevant articles. After removing duplicates, 1,825 articles were retrieved. Papers were screened

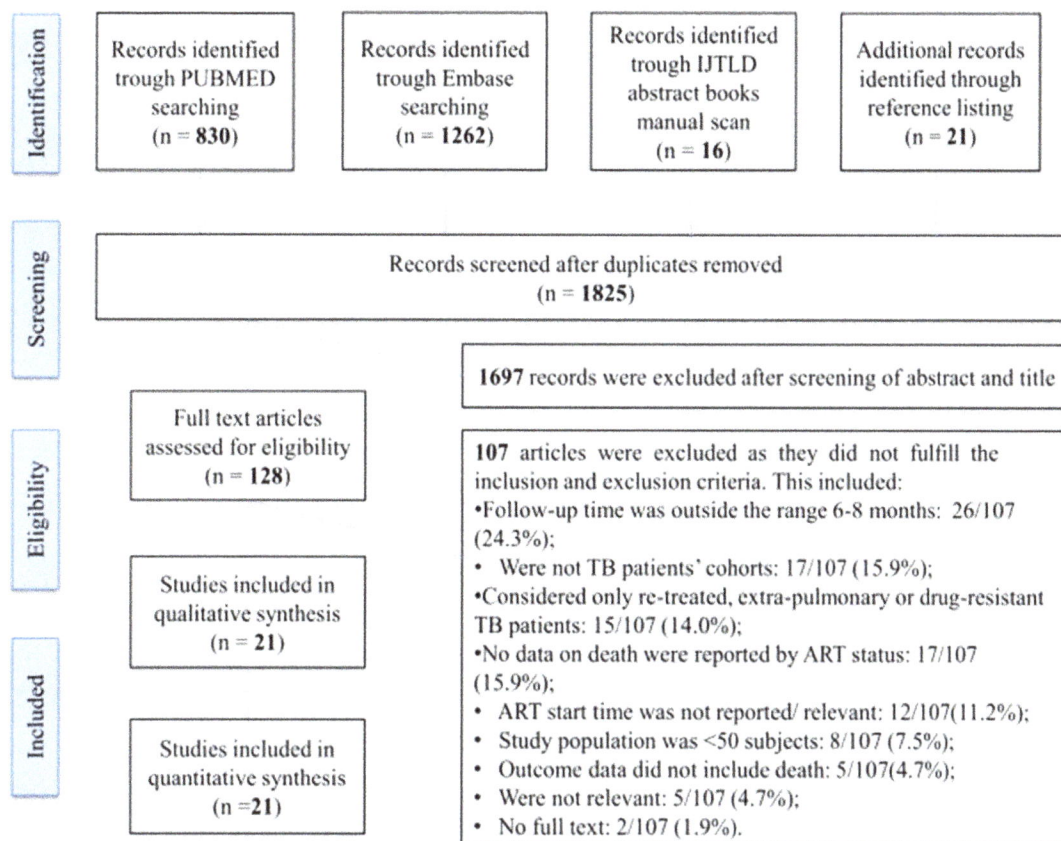

Figure 1. PRISMA flow diagram of papers selected.

and selected as illustrated in Figure 1, resulting in 21 studies that were included in the systematic review and meta-analysis.

Characteristics of included studies

The characteristics of the included studies are reported in Table 1. The majority of the studies were conducted in the African (n = 11, 52%) [14,23,24,25,26,27,28,29,30,31,32] and South-East Asian (n = 7, 33%) [33,34,35,36,37,38,39] regions; two studies were conducted in South America [40,41] and one in Europe [42]. Four out of seven studies in the South-East Asian region were conducted in Thailand [33,35,37,38] while one used data from eighteen sites in the Asia-Pacific region [39]. Both South American studies were conducted in Brazil.

More than half of included studies (n = 13, 62%) described a retrospective cohort [23,24,25,27,34,37,40,42], seven (33.3%) described prospective cohort studies [14,26,33,35,38,41] and one was a clinical trial [36]. We excluded seven papers [5,6,7,8,9,43,44] reporting results from large trials that focused on time of ART initiation during TB treatment as TB mortality data was only reported at time points that lay beyond our pre-specified 'during treatment' period [6,7,43,44], the outcome was death combined with AIDS-defining illness and mortality data could not be extrapolated [7] or focused only on tuberculous meningitis [9]. Study enrollment periods ranged from 4 months [30] to 8 years [40]. The majority of the studies were conducted predominantly in urban settings (n = 14, 66.7%) [12,23,24,25,26,29,30,31,32,36,40,41,42]. Table 2 shows the levels of quality assigned to each study. We determined that the majority of the studies were susceptible to mild cohort selection

bias because of their retrospective study design [23,24,25,27,34,37,40,42]. We did not assess ten eligible studies for comparability as they were descriptive studies not reporting effect estimates [14,23,25,27,28,31,36,37,39,42]. Among the rest, we judged that five had moderate comparability, because confounding factors were not fully adjusted or they were not specified [24,29,30,34,35]. For most studies, the assessment of outcomes was done by medical record review which we regarded as susceptible to mild outcome bias (Table 2).

Characteristics of the study populations

86% (n = 18) studies reported on source of data and method of data collection; of these, data were mostly collected from medical records (n = 10, 56%) and TB registers (n = 5, 28%). Three studies explicitly reported on how death was ascertained or confirmed (Table 2) [38,39,45].

For most studies (n = 19, 90.5%) only a fraction of the total patient population included TB cases that started ART before or during TB treatment. For example, in Agodokpessi et al., of the total patient population, 259/1086 (24%) were HIV positive and of these 259, 85 (33%) initiated ART before or during TB treatment [23]. On average, 50% of the studies' study population (range: 12–100%) fitted our criteria (Table 1). The number of included patients per study ranged from 75 [33] to 21,851 [29], with a median of 191 subjects. Studies included predominantly young adults (age midpoint: 34. years, SD: ±1.9).

All but two [14,25] studies reported on TB type: among them, the percentage of individuals with pulmonary TB ranged between 19.4% and 100% (median: 66%). Where reported, most subjects

Table 1. Characteristics of included studies.

Reference	Country	WHO Region	Study Design	Study Period	Patient Source	Population Main Study	Population For Review (%)	Age b (Years)	PTB (%)	New TB Cases (%)	MDR-TB (%)	Standardized TB Treatment	Follow-Up Period	ART Start Time Before TB (%)	ART Start Time During TB Treatment c (Midpoint (Range))
Agodokpessi 2012 [23]	Benin	AFRO	Cohort (Ret)	Jan–Dec 2009	1 Urban Hospital	259	85 (33)^A	36 (15–72)^$	88^$	Na	Na	Yes	TB Treatment	0	Na
Akksilp 2007 [33]	Thailand	SEARO	Cohort (Pros)	Feb2003–Jan 2004	25 Health Clinics	329	75 (23)	32 (1–68)^$	69^$	93^$	1^$	Yes	TB Treatment	40	93 (0–170)
Dean 2002 [42]	UK	EURO	Cohort (Ret)	Jan1996–Jun 1999	12 Urban Hospitals	188	85 (45)	34 (21–70)^$	51^$	Na	7^$	Not All	TB Treatment	18	60 (0–14)
Dos Santos 2013 [40]	Brazil	AMRO	Cohort (Ret)	Jan1995–Dec 2003	2 Urban Hospitals	347	191 (55)	Na	63^$	Na	0	Yes	TB Treatment	0	Na
Ferrousier 2013 [28]	Benin	AFRO	Cohort (Ret)	Jan 2006–Jan 2008	20 Health Clinics	1255	462 (37)	83% aged 16–45^$	91^$	67^$	0.1^$	Na	TB Treatment	44	60 (TB treatment intensive phase)
Gandhi 2012 [14]	South Africa	AFRO	Cohort (Pros)	Oct 2003–Jan 2006	1 Rural Hospital	119	119 (100)	34 (±7)	Na	Na	Na	Yes	TB Treatment	0	67 (60–83)
Henegar 2012 f [24]	DRC	AFRO	Cohort (Ret)	Jan 2006–May 2007	14 Health Clinics	933	129 (14)	38 (±10)^$	66^$	80^$	Na	Yes	TB Treatment	36	Na
Kaplan 2013 [29]	South Africa	AFRO	Cohort (Ret)	Jan 009–Dec 2011	100 Health Clinics	77499	21851 (28)	34 (28–40)^$	76^$	69^$	0	Yes	TB Treatment	24	Na
Kayigamba 2013 [30]	South Africa	AFRO	Cohort (Ret)	Jan–Apr2007	48 Health Clinics	581	110 (19)	31 (25–41)^$	72	100	Na	Yes	TB Treatment	66	179^1
Kendon 2012 [25]	South Africa	AFRO	Cohort (Ret)	Jan 2008–Dec 2010	1 Urban Hospital	468	388 (83)	35 (31–42)	Na	Na	Na	Na	6 Months From ART Start	0	(0–56)
Nansera 2012 [26]	Uganda	AFRO	Cohort (Pros)	Feb 2007–Mar 2010	1 Urban Hospital	386	228 (59)	33 (18–69)^$	83^$	90^$	Na	Yes	TB Treatment	30	49 (4–18)
Raizada 2009 [34]	India	SEARO	Cohort (Ret)	Mar 2007–Aug 2007	154 Health Clinics	734	380 (52)	34 (8–89)^$	75^$	87^$	Na	Yes	TB Treatment	35	Na
Sanguanwongse 2008 [35]	Thailand	SEARO	Cohort (Pros)	Oct 2004–Mar 2006	1 Urban Hospital + Several Healthcare Clinics	1269	626 (49)	34 (1–71)	48	100	1^$	Not All	TB Treatment	0	Na
Schmaltz 2009 [41]	Brazil	AMRO	Cohort (Pros)	Apr 2000–Jul 2005	1 Urban Hospital	106	83 (78)	Na	49^$	Na	7^$	Yes	TB Treatment	41	43 (28–74)
Sileshi 2013 [31]	Ethiopia	AFRO	Cohort (Ret)	Apr 2009–Jan 2012	1 Urban Hospital + 3 Health Clinics	422	272 (64)	30 (27–37.5)	44^$	78	Na	Na	TB Treatment	Na	Na

Table 1. Cont.

Reference	Country	WHO Region	Study Design	Study Period	Patient Source	Population Main Study	Population For Review (%)	Age[b] (Years)	PTB (%)	New TB Cases (%)	MDR-TB (%)	Standardized TB Treatment	Follow-Up Period	ART Start Time Before TB (%)	ART Start Time During TB Treatment[c] (Midpoint (Range))
Sinha 2012 [36]	India	SEARO	RCT	May 2006–Mar 2011	1 Urban Hospital	150	150 (100)	35 (±8)	23	Na	0	Yes	6 months/TB Treatment Completion	0	41 (14–84)
Tansuphasawadikul 2007 [37]	Thailand	SEARO	Cohort (Ret)	Jan 2004–Jun 2005	1 Urban Hospital	101	82 (81)	33 (20–58)	19	86	6	Na	TB Treatment	0	68 (0–381)
Tweya 2013 [32]	Malawi	AFRO	Cohort (Ret)	Jan 2008–Dec 2010	1 Urban Hospital	2478	492 (20)	31 (26–38) $	100	100	Na	Yes	TB Treatment	0	60
Varma 2009 [38]	Thailand	SEARO	Cohort (Pros)	May 2005–Sept 2006	1 Urban Hospital + 32 Health Clinics	667	273 (41)	34 (18–77)$	58$	100	2$	Not All	TB Treatment	27	62 (0–386)
Zachariah 2007 [27]	Malawi	AFRO	Cohort (Ret)	Jan–Dec 2004	1 Rural Hospital	983	180 (18)	32 (2–74)	79	100	Na	Yes	TB Treatment	0	88 (66–125)
Zhao 2014 [39]	Asia	SEARO WPRO	Cohort (Pros)	Sep 2003–May 2004	18 sites	768	429 (56)	34 (29–39) $	42$	Na	Na	Na	TB Treatment	191	42 (17–64)

RCT: Randomized Controlled Trial; Pros: prospective; Ret: retrospective PTB: pulmonary tuberculosis; DS: drug-sensitive; DR: drug-resistant; Na: not available; IQR: interquartile range.

$Values refer to the total population of main study (in absence of detailed data available on TB cases receiving ART).

[a]Total study population included also 827 HIV-negative subjects. Data in the table refer to the HIV positive subset.

[b]reported estimated midpoint + range or SD; [c] (in days), relative to TB treatment start/TB diagnosis date, range either complete range or IQR depending on data availability.

[c]refers to subjects included in the meta-analysis. Detailed information on CD4 count for the whole study population for each study is reported in Table S1.

[d1]subjects already on ART by the start of TB treatment,

[d2]subjects that started ART within 90 days from TB treatment start.

[e]range.

[1]21% (n = 37) of them started within 3 months of TB treatment start.

Table 2. Source of data, method of death ascertainment or confirmation and quality assessment of the included studies.

Reference	Source of data and method of data collection	Method of death ascertainment/confirmation	The Newcastle-Ottawa Scale		
			Selection	Comparability	Outcome
Agodokpessi 2012 [23]	Data were extracted from medical records	Na	***		**
Akksilp 2007 [33]	Surveillance and monitoring data from public health program	Na	***	**	**
Dean 2002 [42]	Data were extracted from medical records	Na	**		**
Dos Santos 2013 [40]	Data were extracted from medical records by trained health care workers	Na	***	**	**
Ferroussier 2013 [28]	Data were extracted from TB registers	Na	***		**
Gandhi 2012 [14]	Na	Na	**		**
Henegar 2012 [24]	Na (we assume Data were extracted from medical records)	Na	**		*
Kaplan 2013[29]	Data were extracted from the national electronic TB register	Na	***	*	**
Kayigamba 2013 [30]	Data were extracted from TB registers and TB treatment charts	Na	**		**
Kendon 2012 [25]	Data were extracted from medical records	Na	**		**
Nansera 2012 [26]	Na	Na	**	**	*
Raizada 2009 [34]	Data were extracted from medical records	Na	***	*	**
Sanguanwongse 2008 [35]	Data were extracted from medical records	Na	***	*	**
Schmaltz 2009 [41]	Data were extracted from medical records	Na	**	*	**
Sileshi 2013 [31]	Data were extracted from medical records (Pre-ART registers, lab requests, follow-up forms, anti TB record forms, ART intake forms, and patient cards).	The patients' date of death was extracted from TB registration log books	*		**
Sinha 2012 [36]	Clinical and laboratory data actively collected and reported on an *ad hoc* electronic data base.	Na	_a	_a	_a
Tansuphasawadikul 2007 [37]	Data were extracted from medical records	Na	*		**
Tweya 2013 [32]	Data were extracted from TB registers and TB treatment cards. Deaths were ascertained mainly through active follow-up.	Na	***	**	**
Varma 2009 [38]	Data were extracted from medical records and the Thailand TB Active Surveillance Network.	To determine if patients died after defaulting notification data were linked to the Thai government's vital status registry.	***	**	**
Zachariah 2007 [27]	Data were extracted from TB registers (counselling registers, district TB registers, TB patient cards, ART Patient Master Cards and ART Registers)	Na	**		**
Zhao 2014 [39]	TREAT Asia HIV Observational Database (TAHOD)	Death was confirmed by local medical staff and reported using standardized Cause of Death (CoDe) forms	**		**

-ᵃNewcastle-Ottawa Quality assessment scale not applicable (study design: randomized trial, higher level of evidence as compared to observational studies [60].

were new TB cases (median percentage: 90%, range: 67%–100%). Drug susceptibility profiles were reported by nine studies. Three studies only included drug-sensitive TB cases and in the remaining studies, the proportion with multi-drug resistance was low and ranged from 0.1%–7% (median: 1.5%; included in the review). Three studies reported that some TB patients did not receive standardized therapy [35,38,42]. Details on TB treatment regimens are available in Table S3. Descriptions of TB type, TB category and drug susceptibility in the majority of studies referred to the original studies' entire cohorts and not to the subsets of the study population selected for this analysis.

Eleven studies reported that a proportion of their patients initiated ART before TB treatment (between 18 and 66%, Table 1), but the actual ART start dates were not reported [24,26,28,29,30,33,34,38,39,41,42]. Where all patients were initiated on ART during TB treatment, the median start times occurred in month 2 or 3 after starting TB treatment [14,25,27,32,36,37]. The variability in reporting between studies

Table 3. Outcomes considered in the included studies.

Reference	Subgroups	Sample size	N. Deaths	TB-CFR (%)	Effect estimate type	Effect estimate value (95% CI)	Univariable/Multivariable (adjusted for)
Agodokpessi 2012 [23]		85	9	11			
Akksilp 2007 [33]		75	5	7	RR	0.2 (0.1–0.4)	Multivariable (CD4, smear status, co-trimoxazole use, treatment facility)
Dean 2002 [42]		85	3	4*			
Dos Santos 2013 [40]		191			HR	0.1 (0.03–0.29)	Multivariable (age, sex, marital status and total lymphocyte count)
Ferroussier 2013 [28]		462	65	14			
Gandhi 2012 [14]		119	11	9			
Henegar 2012 [24]		129			IRR	0.63 (0.36–1.10)	Univariable
Kaplan 2013 [29]	On ART at start of TB	21851			OR	0.53 (0.46–0.60)	Multivariable (na)
	Started ART during TB				OR	0.42 (0.39–0.47)	Multivariable (na)
Kayigamba 2013 [30]		72	15	21	OR	1.43 (1.28–1.61)	Univariable
Kendon 2012 [25]		388	54	14			
Nansera 2012 [26]		228			HR	0.13 (0.07–0.25)^S	Multivariable (sex and disease category)
Raizada 2009 [34]		380	43	11	HR	0.41 (0.28–0.6)	Multivariable[a]
Sanguanwongse 2008 [35]	All	626	68	11	RR	0.18 (0.13–0.25)	Multivariable[b]
	Only bact. confirmed	583^£			RR	0.15 (0.09–0.24)	Multivariable[b]
	CD4 <10 cell/mm³	56	12	21	RR	0.26 (0.16–0.44)	Multivariable[b]
Schmaltz 2009 [41]		83	11	13	HR	0.55 (0.52–0.59)*	Multivariable[b]
Sileshi 2013 [31]		272	49	18			
Sinha 2012 [36]		150	10	7			
Tansuphasawadikul 2007 [37]		82	5	6			
Tweya 2013 [32]		492			OR	0.46 (0.26–0.83)	Multivariable (sex, age, HIV status, registration year)
Varma 2009 [38]	All	273	24	9	HR	0.16 (0.07–0.36)	Multivariable (CD4, TB severity)
	Only bact. confirmed	na			HR	0.06 (0.02–0.23)	Multivariable (CD4, TB severity)
Zachariah 2007 [27]		180	56	31			
Zhao 2014 [39]		429	13	3			

*Calculated with the available data.
^S Assumed to be a coding error in the original article (reciprocal HR reported).
^ Deaths occurred during TB treatment's initial phase.
^£ Assuming all 110 culture positive patients were not included in 473 smear positive patients.
[a] Variables to include in the model were chosen based on the literature.
[b] Variables to include in the model were chosen for inclusion in the multivariate analyses based on one or more of the following: p<0.20 in bivariate analysis, biologic plausibility, or previously published evidence.

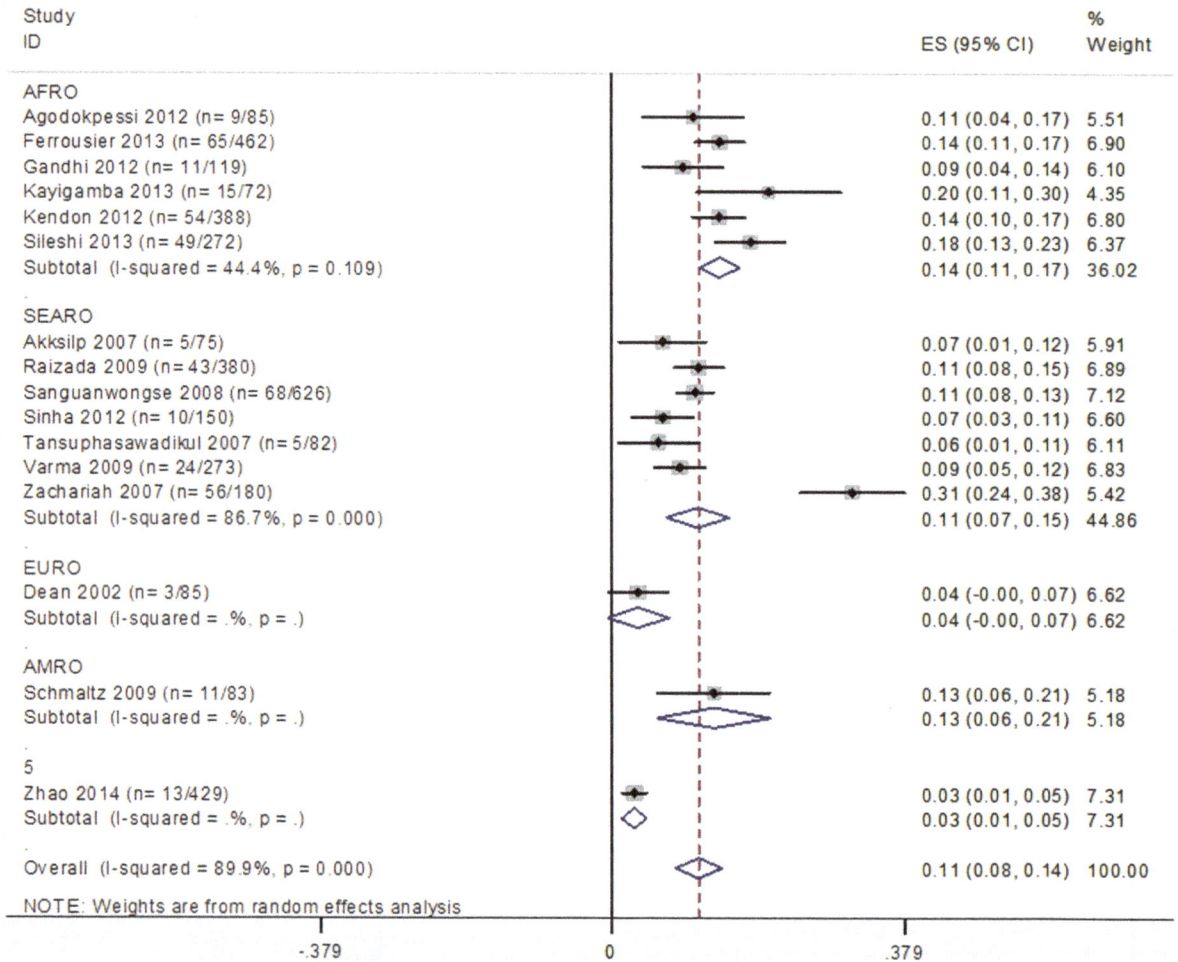

Figure 2. Forest plot of 16 studies reporting TB-CFR for HIV positive patients receiving ART (by Region).

limited our ability to examine the mortality impact of different ART initiation times with respect to the start of TB treatment.

Data on CD4 count were very heterogeneous and incomplete and did not allow quantitative assessment of effect modification (Table S2). In six (29%) studies, data on CD4 count were not reported at all [24,27,30,32,34,40]; in four (19%) studies they were not available for the subgroup of the study population included in the meta-analysis [14,33,38,41]; and in five (24%) studies the percentage of the study population included in the meta-analysis for which some measures of CD4 count were available did not exceed 55% [23,26,28,37,42]. Median CD4 count was available for >98% of subjects included in the meta-analysis in four (19%) studies [31,35,36,39] and ranged from 48 to 152 cells/mm^3.

Follow-up time corresponded to TB treatment duration in 18 (75%) studies. In Sinha et al., follow-up time was set at six months after TB treatment start or at TB treatment completion, and in Kendon et al., it was set at six months from ART start (ART was started within 56 days from TB treatment start) [36].

One study reported outcomes which were limited to bacterio-logically-confirmed (positive sputum smear or culture result) TB

cases [27,35] and one study included only culture-confirmed TB cases [35].

Outcome measures

Sixteen studies reported data on CFR (Table 3) [14,23,25,27,28,30,31,33,34,35,36,37,38,39,41,42]. Meta-analysis of the CFR showed high heterogeneity (I-squared = 89.9%, p< 0.001, Figure 2). The random-effects analysis suggested the CFR lay between 8% and 14% (point value = 11%; Figure 2). The pooled CFR appeared slightly higher in the African region (11%–17%), and lower in the South-East Asian (7%–15%) region. The CFR was 4% (95%CI: 0%–7%) and 13% (95%CI: 6%–21%) in single studies set in the UK and Brazil respectively (Figure 2). Sanguanwongse et al. considered a subgroup of patients with very low CD4 counts at the start of TB treatment (CD4 <10 cells/mm3), which experienced a CFR of 21% (95%CI: 1%–32%) [35]. When restricted to the four studies where all patients were initiated on ART after starting TB treatment, the CFR was 12% (95% CI 8%–17%).

Eleven out of 21 studies reported data on estimated relative risk of mortality comparing people taking vs. not taking ART

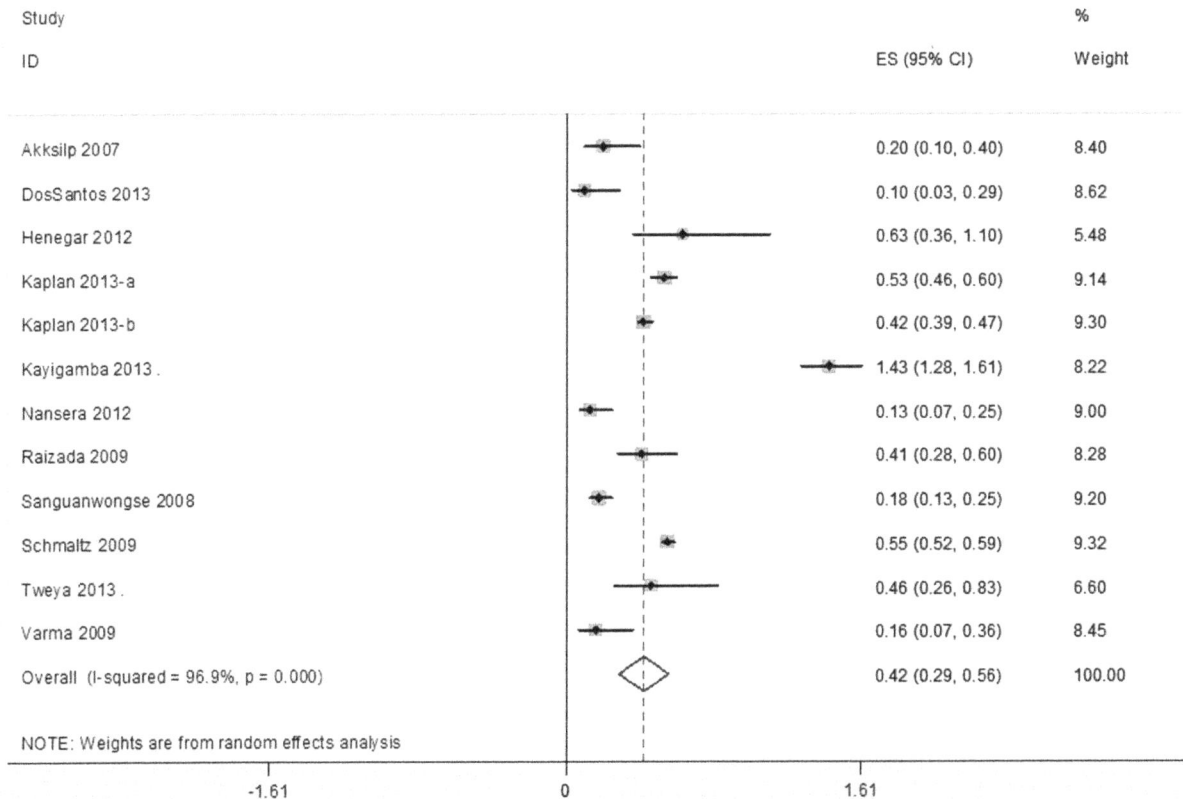

Figure 3. Forest plot studies reporting the relative risk of death during TB treatment by ART status.

[24,26,29,30,32,33,34,35,38,40,41]. Adjusted relative risks were available for all but one study [26]. A random effects meta-analysis showed that the relative risk of death during TB treatment by ART status was 0.42 with a 95%CI: 0.29–0.56; (I-squared = 96.9%, p<0.001, Figure 3), which corresponds to a 44% to 71% reduction in mortality. When we restricted the analysis to studies considering only patients with smear positive TB (n = 2) the random effects relative risk was 0.11 (95%CI: 0.03–0.20) [35,38].

Discussion

We estimate that mortality during TB treatment in HIV-positive individuals receiving ART under routine programmatic conditions lies between 8% and 14% and that ART reduces the mortality during TB treatment for HIV-positive TB cases by between 44 to 71%.

This is the first systematic assessment to quantify the impact of ART on TB mortality during TB treatment. In addition, we report not only pooled absolute mortality figures as done elsewhere [12] but also estimate the relative effect of ART on mortality, which has the advantage of being a less setting-specific and a more easily interpretable and generalizable parameter.

Our focus on deaths *during* TB treatment allowed us to make optimal use of the limited data, while providing a clear conceptual parameter that is widely used and reported by National TB Programmes, and which allows comparison between studies and

other reviews. Mortality estimates over longer follow-up periods have been reported in recent trials [6,7,8,43], but are not usually reported in surveillance systems, operational research and clinical settings. Previous reviews and reports have discussed the difficulties in trying to determine which deaths are directly attributable to TB, especially in low-resource settings [2,12]. Different studies classified TB as either the primary or a contributory cause of death [12,46]. In addition, according to the 10th revision of the International classification of diseases (ICD-10), deaths in HIV-positive TB patients are classified as HIV deaths [1]. In light of these considerations, we systematically assessed the effect of ART on death *during* TB treatment rather than deaths *due* to TB.

While the exclusion of several large RCTs reduced the number of studies and patients included, it was necessary to ensure between-study comparability regarding the time at risk of death. When reported, we note that these RCTs found relatively comparable TB-CFRs to our review [7]. We note that in the CAMELIA trial, the CFR was substantially higher than our estimate (18% and 27% for those initiating ART two or eight weeks into TB treatment), but this is likely to be due to the very low baseline CD4 count of patients included in that study (median = 25 cells/mm^3) and the longer follow-up time (median = 25 months) [6]. As expected, other observational studies that considered follow-up periods greater than 3.5 years also find higher absolute mortality estimates [47].

The estimated range for CFR estimate of 8–14% in TB patients receiving ART is also below than the 19% point value reported by Straetemans *et al.* amongst all HIV-positive TB cases, which included some individuals receiving ART. This is consistent with expected effect of ART to reduce TB mortality [12,27].

Sub-group analyses by geographical region suggested that the CFR was higher in the African region (14%, estimates based on 7 studies) and lower in the one study from a Western European setting (4%, in the UK), which mirror global TB mortality patterns [2]. The reported differences in CFR between regions might also be attributable to differences in immunosuppression at the time of clinical presentation which could affect the estimated benefits of ART. The protective effect of ART appeared stronger in people with smear-positive TB, reflecting the better treatment outcomes in this population across HIV/ART groups compared to patients without smear or culture confirmation. This could be due to some people who do not genuinely have TB being erroneously included in the smear negative group. However, given the small number of studies with bacteriological confirmation (n = 2), this result should be interpreted with caution.

A limitation of our work is that – due to a lack of data - we could not explore the effect of ART by CD4 count. The lack of data is due to the fact that the majority of the included studies reported data from TB registers, and surveillance systems in high HIV-TB burden and resource-limited settings where CD4 measurements are often unavailable [48]. Recent data from large RCTs have provided solid evidence that ART reduces mortality across a wide range of CD4 counts [5,6,7]. In addition, the 2013 WHO guidelines for antiretroviral therapy provide the evidence-based recommendation that in subjects with active tuberculosis ART should be initiated as soon as possible, irrespective of CD4 count [49]. However, we found that on average patients were started two to three months post TB treatment initiation, suggesting this may not have been policy or practice in the majority of observational studies included. If ART were provided to all HIV positive TB patients as per current guidelines, we would expect the CFR to decrease [8,43], and to see an even greater reduction in relative mortality. The question of when to start ART in HIV-positive TB patients has been addressed by the above-cited RCTs [5,6,7,8,50] and - based on their findings - HIV and TB guidelines recommend that among HIV-positive TB patients with CD4 less than 50 cells/mm^3, ART should be initiated within 2 weeks from TB treatment start and if CD4 above 50 cell/mm^3, within 8 weeks [51,52,53,54,55]. Nonetheless, the issue remains controversial as results from a recent trial reported no difference in mortality between early and delayed ART for HIV-positive TB patients with CD4 counts of 220 cells/mm^3 or more with authors arguing WHO guidelines should be updated accordingly [44] while, on the other hand, some researchers question the need of investing resources in other randomized, controlled trials on the same topic [56].

Nearly all data came from observational studies, which are more vulnerable to bias. For example, sicker patients might be more likely to be selected to start ART, thus introducing selection bias that would under-estimate the effect of ART. However, observational studies may better represent the patient population and clinical care provided in most settings. The majority of the studies considered single hospitals, local or district-level data and this might limit the ability to generalize results to national or regional level. Patients seen at referral hospitals may be sicker and

may experience higher mortality, while at the same time, those treated in urban centres might have lower mortality than those treated in rural settings. Last but not least, most studies relied on TB notification registers and medical records whose degree of completeness and quality of reporting might be different in different settings, potentially introducing bias to pooled estimates. Similar to other reviews, we did not consider mortality amongst people lost to follow-up in our CFR estimates. Given that studies have suggested mortality among patients lost to follow up and transferred out averages 21% [57], our CFR is probably similarly underestimated [12]. As we did not consider studies focusing on special populations, our findings might not be generalizable to subpopulations with additional risk factors for mortality.

We found a high degree of heterogeneity between studies, which could be due to differences in clinical (e.g. CD4 count) or health system variables. We did not apply meta-regression because of the low number of studies, and the lack of information such as duration on ART and CD4 at start of TB treatment. By reporting results from random effects estimates, we acknowledge this heterogeneity. Due to the low number of studies contributing to the analysis, stratification by study quality was not possible. In addition, 95% of studies included in our systematic assessment have an observational study design which is subject to some risk of bias. However, since our aim was to describe the risk of death among HIV-infected TB patients under routine programmatic conditions, observational studies likely provide the most relevant data for this analysis.

In conclusion, we quantified the substantial impact of ART on reducing mortality during TB treatment. Collaborative tuberculosis-HIV activities are key components of the new Post-2015 Global Tuberculosis Strategy, approved by the World Health Assembly in May 2014 [58]. They include expanded collaboration between TB and HIV programmes and integrated tuberculosis and HIV service delivery in the field. For individuals newly diagnosed with TB, this means increased on-site HIV testing, and prompt referral for HIV care for all found to be HIV positive [59]. Improved harmonization relies on more sharing of clinical space and integration of medical records, staff, and training. These interventions promise to reduce delays to HIV diagnosis, facilitate early implementation of effective ART and reduce TB-related mortality in HIV positive patients.

Supporting Information

Table S1   MEDLINE search strategy.

Table S2   CD4 count at baseline and during follow up in the included studies.

Table S3   TB treatment regimen in the included studies.

Author Contributions

Conceived and designed the experiments: AO RMGJH. Performed the experiments: AO SA RMGJH. Analyzed the data: AO SA RMGJH. Wrote the paper: AO SA RMGJH RGW TC ADG.

References

1. Corbett EL, Watt CJ, Walker N, Maher D, Williams BG, et al. (2003) The growing burden of tuberculosis: global trends and interactions with the HIV epidemic. Arch Intern Med 163: 1009–1021.
2. WHO (2013) Global Tuberculosis Report 2013. Geneva: World Health Organisation.
3. Suthar AB, Lawn SD, del Amo J, Getahun H, Dye C, et al. (2012) Antiretroviral therapy for prevention of tuberculosis in adults with HIV: a systematic review and meta-analysis. PLoS Med 9: e1001270.
4. Curran A, Falco V, Pahissa A, Ribera E (2012) Management of tuberculosis in HIV-infected patients. AIDS Rev 14: 231–246.
5. Abdool Karim SS, Naidoo K, Grobler A, Padayatchi N, Baxter C, et al. (2010) Timing of initiation of antiretroviral drugs during tuberculosis therapy. New England Journal of Medicine 362: 697–706.
6. Blanc FX, Sok T, Laureillard D, Borand L, Rekacewicz C, et al. (2011) Earlier versus later start of antiretroviral therapy in HIV-infected adults with tuberculosis. New England Journal of Medicine 365: 1471–1481.
7. Havlir DV, Kendall MA, Ive P, Kumwenda J, Swindells S, et al. (2011) Timing of antiretroviral therapy for HIV-1 infection and tuberculosis. N Engl J Med 365: 1482–1491.
8. Manosuthi W, Mankatitham W, Lueangniyomkul A, Thongyen S, Likanonsakul S, et al. (2012) Time to initiate antiretroviral therapy between 4 weeks and 12 weeks of tuberculosis treatment in HIV-infected patients: results from the TIME study. J Acquir Immune Defic Syndr 60: 377–383.
9. Torok ME, Yen NT, Chau TT, Mai NT, Phu NH, et al. (2011) Timing of initiation of antiretroviral therapy in human immunodeficiency virus (HIV)–associated tuberculous meningitis. Clin Infect Dis 52: 1374–1383.
10. Boulle A, Clayden P, Cohen K, Cohen T, Conradie F, et al. (2010) Prolonged deferral of antiretroviral therapy in the SAPIT trial: did we need a clinical trial to tell us that this would increase mortality? S Afr Med J 100: 566, 568, 570–561.
11. Laureillard D, Marcy O, Madec Y, Chea S, Chan S, et al. (2013) Paradoxical tuberculosis-associated immune reconstitution inflammatory syndrome after early initiation of antiretroviral therapy in a randomized clinical trial. AIDS 27: 2577–2586.
12. Straetemans M, Glaziou P, Bierrenbach AL, Sismanidis C, van der Werf MJ (2011) Assessing tuberculosis case fatality ratio: A meta-analysis. PLoS One 6.
13. Glaziou P, Floyd K, Raviglione M (2009) Global burden and epidemiology of tuberculosis. Clin Chest Med 30: 621–636, vii.
14. Gandhi NR, Moll AP, Lalloo U, Pawinski R, Zeller K, et al. (2009) Successful integration of tuberculosis and HIV treatment in rural South Africa: the Sizonq'oba study. J Acquir Immune Defic Syndr 50: 37–43.
15. Mukadi YD, Maher D, Harries A (2001) Tuberculosis case fatality rates in high HIV prevalence populations in sub-Saharan Africa. AIDS 15: 143–152.
16. Moher D, Liberati A, Tetzlaff J, Altman DG, Group P (2010) Preferred reporting items for systematic reviews and meta-analyses: the PRISMA statement. Int J Surg 8: 336–341.
17. Lim MS, Dowdeswell RJ, Murray J, Field N, Glynn JR, et al. (2012) The impact of HIV, an antiretroviral programme and tuberculosis on mortality in South African platinum miners, 1992–2010. PLoS One 7: e38598.
18. Davies NE, Karstaedt AS (2012) Antiretroviral outcomes in South African prisoners: a retrospective cohort analysis. PLoS One 7: e33309.
19. Casas EC, Decroo T, Mahoudo JA, Baltazar JM, Dores CD, et al. (2011) Burden and outcome of HIV infection and other morbidities in health care workers attending an Occupational Health Program at the Provincial Hospital of Tete, Mozambique. Trop Med Int Health 16: 1450–1456.
20. Altice FL, Kamarulzaman A, Soriano VV, Schechter M, Friedland GH (2010) Treatment of medical, psychiatric, and substance-use comorbidities in people infected with HIV who use drugs. Lancet 376: 367–387.
21. Higgins JP, Green S (2011) Cochrane Handbook for Systematic Reviews of Interventions Version 5.1.0 [updated March 2011], 5.1.0 ed. The Cochrane Collaboration.
22. Wells G (2011) The Newcastle-Ottawa Scale (NOS) for assessing the quality of nonrandomised studies in meta-analyses. Available: http://www.ohri.ca/programs/clinical_epidemiology/oxford.asp. Accessed 2014 Oct 23.
23. Agodokpessi G, Ade G, Ade S, Wachinou AP, Affolabi D, et al. (2012) Management of tuberculosis and HIV co-infection in Cotonou, Benin. Med Mal Infect 42: 561–566.
24. Henegar CE, Behets F, Vanden Driessche K, Tabala M, Bahati E, et al. (2012) Mortality among tuberculosis patients in the Democratic Republic of Congo. International Journal of Tuberculosis and Lung Disease 16: 1199–1204.
25. Kendon M, Knight SE, Ross A, Giddy J (2012) Timing of antiretroviral therapy initiation in adults with HIV-associated tuberculosis: Outcomes of therapy in an urban hospital in KwaZulu-Natal. South African Medical Journal 102: 931–935.
26. Nansera D, Bajunirwe F, Elyanu P, Asiimwe C, Amanyire G, et al. (2012) Mortality and loss to follow-up among tuberculosis and HIV co-infected patients in rural southwestern Uganda. International Journal of Tuberculosis and Lung Disease 16: 1371–1376.
27. Zachariah R, Fitzgerald M, Massaquoi M, Acabu A, Chilomo D, et al. (2007) Does antiretroviral treatment reduce case fatality among HIV-positive patients with tuberculosis in Malawi? Int J Tuberc Lung Dis 11: 848–853.
28. Ferroussier O, Dlodlo RA, Capo-Chichi D, Boillot F, Gninafon M, et al. (2013) Results of rapid and successful integration of HIV diagnosis and care into tuberculosis services in Benin. International Journal of Tuberculosis and Lung Disease 17 (11): 1405–1410.
29. Kaplan R, Caldwell J, Middelkoop K, Bekker LG, Wood R (2014) Impact of ART on TB Case Fatality Stratified by CD4 Count for HIV-Positive TB Patients in Cape Town, South Africa (2009–2011). J Acquir Immune Defic Syndr 66: 487–494.
30. Kayigamba FR, Bakker MI, Mugisha V, de Naeyer L, Gasana M, et al. (2013) Adherence to Tuberculosis Treatment, Sputum Smear Conversion and Mortality: A Retrospective Cohort Study in 48 Rwandan Clinics. PLoS ONE 8 (9).
31. Sileshi B, Deyessa N, Girma B, Melese M, Suarez P (2013) Predictors of mortality among TB-HIV Co-infected patients being treated for tuberculosis in Northwest Ethiopia: A retrospective cohort study. BMC Infectious Diseases 13 (1).
32. Tweya H, Feldacker C, Phiri S, Ben-Smith A, Fenner L, et al. (2013) Comparison of treatment outcomes of new smear-positive pulmonary tuberculosis patients by HIV and antiretroviral status in a TB/HIV clinic, Malawi. PLoS ONE 8 (2).
33. Akksilp S, Karnkawinpong O, Wattanaamornkiat W, Viriyakitja D, Monkongdee P, et al. (2007) Antiretroviral therapy during tuberculosis treatment and marked reduction in death rate of HIV-infected patients, Thailand. Emerg Infect Dis 13: 1001–1007.
34. Raizada N, Chauhan LS, Babu BS, Thakur R, Khera A, et al. (2009) Linking HIV-infected TB patients to cotrimoxazole prophylaxis and antiretroviral treatment in India. PLoS One 4.
35. Sanguanwongse N, Cain KP, Suriya P, Nateniyom S, Yamada N, et al. (2008) Antiretroviral therapy for HIV-infected tuberculosis patients saves lives but needs to be used more frequently in Thailand. J Acquir Immune Defic Syndr 48: 181–189.
36. Sinha S, Shekhar RC, Singh G, Shah N, Ahmad H, et al. (2012) Early versus delayed initiation of antiretroviral therapy for Indian HIV-Infected individuals with tuberculosis on antituberculosis treatment. BMC Infect Dis 12.
37. Tansuphasawadikul S, Saito W, Kim J, Phonrat B, Dhitavat J, et al. (2007) Outcomes in HIV-infected patients on antiretroviral therapy with tuberculosis. Southeast Asian J Trop Med Public Health 38: 1053–1060.
38. Varma JK, Nateniyom S, Akksilp S, Mankatittham W, Sirinak C, et al. (2009) HIV care and treatment factors associated with improved survival during TB treatment in Thailand: an observational study. BMC Infect Dis 9: 42.
39. Zhao H, Chen YMA, Lee C, Omar SFS, Phanuphak N, et al. (2014) Prognostic significance of the interval between the initiation of antiretroviral therapy and the initiation of anti-tuberculosis treatment in HIV/tuberculosis-coinfected patients: Results from the TREAT Asia HIV Observational Database. HIV Medicine 15 (2): 77–85.
40. Dos Santos APG, Pacheco AG, Staviack A, Golub JE, Chaisson RE, et al. (2013) Safety and effectiveness of HAART in tuberculosis-HIV co-infected patients in Brazil. International Journal of Tuberculosis and Lung Disease 17: 192–197+i.
41. Schmaltz CA, Sant'Anna FM, Neves SC, Velasque Lde S, Lourenco MC, et al. (2009) Influence of HIV infection on mortality in a cohort of patients treated for tuberculosis in the context of wide access to HAART, in Rio de Janeiro, Brazil. J Acquir Immune Defic Syndr 52: 623–628.
42. Dean GL, Edwards SG, Ives NJ, Matthews G, Fox EF, et al. (2002) Treatment of tuberculosis in HIV-infected persons in the era of highly active antiretroviral therapy. AIDS 16: 75–83.
43. Abdool Karim SS, Naidoo K, Grobler A, Padayatchi N, Baxter C, et al. (2010) Timing of initiation of antiretroviral drugs during tuberculosis therapy. N Engl J Med 362: 697–706.
44. Mfinanga SG, Kirenga BJ, Chanda DM, Mutayoba B, Mthiyane T, et al. (2014) Early versus delayed initiation of highly active antiretroviral therapy for HIV-positive adults with newly diagnosed pulmonary tuberculosis (TB-HAART): a prospective, international, randomised, placebo-controlled trial. Lancet Infect Dis 14: 563–571.
45. Sinha S, Shekhar RC, Singh G, Shah N, Ahmad H, et al. (2012) Early versus delayed initiation of antiretroviral therapy for Indian HIV-Infected individuals with tuberculosis on antituberculosis treatment. BMC Infect Dis 12: 168.
46. Walpola HC, Siskind V, Patel AM, Konstantinos A, Derhy P (2003) Tuberculosis-related deaths in Queensland, Australia, 1989-1998: characteristics and risk factors. Int J Tuberc Lung Dis 7: 742–750.
47. Dheda K, Lampe FC, Johnson MA, Lipman MC (2004) Outcome of HIV-associated tuberculosis in the era of highly active antiretroviral therapy. J Infect Dis 190: 1670–1676.
48. Lawn SD, Meintjes G, McIlleron H, Harries AD, Wood R (2013) Management of HIV-associated tuberculosis in resource-limited settings: A state-of-the-art review. BMC Medicine 11 (1).
49. Doherty M, Ford N, Vitoria M, Weiler G, Hirnschall G (2013) The 2013 WHO guidelines for antiretroviral therapy: Evidence-based recommendations to face new epidemic realities. Current Opinion in HIV and AIDS 8 (6): 528–534.
50. Abdool Karim SS, Naidoo K, Grobler A, Padayatchi N, Baxter C, et al. (2011) Integration of antiretroviral therapy with tuberculosis treatment. N Engl J Med 365: 1492–1501.

51. World Health Organization (2010) Treatment of tuberculosis: guidelines, 4th ed. 2010 (WHO/HTM/TB/2009.420) Available: http://whqlibdoc.who.int/publications/2010/9789241547833_eng.pdf?ua=1. Accessed August 14, 2014.

52. TB CARE I (2014) International Standards for Tuberculosis Care, Edition 3. TB CARE I, The Hague. Available: http://www.thoracic.org/assemblies/mtpi/resources/istc-report.pdf. Accessed August 14, 2014.

53. Panel on Antiretroviral Guidelines for Adults and Adolescents (2013) Guidelines for the use of antiretroviral agents in HIV-1-infected adults and adolescents. Department of Health and Human Services. Available: http://aidsinfo.nih.gov/ContentFiles/AdultandAdolescentGL.pdf. Accessed August 14, 2014.

54. Thompson MA, Aberg JA, Hoy JF, Telenti A, Benson C, et al. (2012) Antiretroviral treatment of adult HIV infection: 2012 recommendations of the International Antiviral Society-USA panel. JAMA 308: 387–402.

55. World Health Organization (2013) Consolidated guidelines on the use of antiretroviral drugs for treating and preventing HIV infection, 2013. Available: www.who.int/hiv/pub/guidelines/arv2013. Accessed August 14, 2014.

56. The Lancet Global Heath Blog (2013) Clinical trials and global health equity. Available: http://globalhealth.thelancet.com/2013/07/08/clinical-trials-and-global-health-equity. Accessed October 23, 2014.

57. Korenromp EL, Bierrenbach AL, Williams BG, Dye C (2009) The measurement and estimation of tuberculosis mortality. Int J Tuberc Lung Dis 13: 283–303.

58. The Stop TB Partnership (2014) WHA approves Post-2015 Global Strategy and Targets For Tuberculosis Prevention, Care and Control. Available: http://www.stoptb.org/news/stories/2014/ns14_031.asp. Accessed October 23, 2014.

59. Legido-Quigley H, Montgomery CM, Khan P, Atun R, Fakoya A, et al. (2013) Integrating tuberculosis and HIV services in low- and middle-income countries: a systematic review. Trop Med Int Health 18: 199–211.

60. Oxford Centre for Evidence-Based Medicine website. Available: http://www.cebm.net/ocebm-levels-of-evidence/. Accessed October 23, 2014.

23

Optimal Dosage of Methylprednisolone for the Treatment of Sudden Hearing Loss in Geriatric Patients: A Propensity Score-Matched Analysis

Myoung Su Choi, Ho Yun Lee*, Chin Saeng Cho

Department of Otorhinolaryngology, Department of Otorhinolaryngology, Head & Neck Surgery, School of Medicine, Eulji University Medical Center, Eulji University, Daejeon, Korea

Abstract

We aimed to compare the treatment outcomes and the occurrence rates of adverse events associated with different steroid regimens in geriatric patients (aged 65 years or older) with unilateral idiopathic sudden sensorineural hearing loss (ISSNHL). After thorough medical chart reviews of 109 patients with ISSNHL between May 2006 and December 2013, we performed a propensity score-matched analysis using previously known prognostic factors, steroid regimens, and other cointerventions. Patients were divided based on their steroid regimens into group I (which initially received 48 mg of methylprednisolone daily with a subsequently tapered dose) and group II (which initially received 24 mg of methylprednisolone daily with a subsequently tapered dose). We compared final hearing and the occurrence of adverse events between the two groups. As a result, 20 pairs of propensity score-matched patients (n = 40) were enrolled. Group I patients showed better final hearing levels compared with group II patients (42.00 ± 22.35 dB and 57.38 ± 26.40 dB, respectively), although this difference was marginally significant (p = 0.058). Based on the comparative analysis of each of the frequencies in the final audiograms, lower hearing thresholds at 2 KHz were observed in group I (p = 0.049). There was no significant difference in the occurrence of adverse effects between the two groups (p>0.05). In conclusion, conventional steroid regimens produced adverse event occurrence rates that were similar to those of low-dose treatment but may also have produced superior hearing recovery. The use of steroid dose reduction in geriatric patients with ISSNHL is not preferable to conventional steroid regimens.

Editor: Hanjun Liu, Sun Yat-sen University, China

Funding: This research was supported by EMBRI Grants 2013 EMBRI-DJ-0005 from Eulji University. The funders had no role in study design, data collection and analysis, decision to publish, and had a role in the preparation of the manuscript.

Competing Interests: The authors have declared that no competing interests exist.

* Email: hoyun1004@gmail.com

Introduction

According to recent guidelines, initial corticosteroid treatment can be administered to patients with idiopathic sudden sensori-neural hearing loss (ISSNHL) [1]. Such treatment is commonly used on the basis of the hypothesis that it may affect the inner ear and induce suppression of the immune response, changes in microcirculation, and a decrease in endolymphatic pressure [2]. However, the effects of steroids on the treatment of sudden hearing loss remain unclear [3]. Although the adverse effects that occur after a 10- to 14-day course of steroids are usually acceptable and manageable [1], various symptoms may occur, including weight gain, gastritis, hypertension, hyperglycemia, cataracts, avascular necrosis of the hip, as well as changes in appetite, mood, sleep patterns, and even death [1,4,5].

A study of 18226 patients with diabetes revealed that patients with diabetes and chronic obstructive pulmonary disease who used high-dose corticosteroids were at a greater risk of diabetes-related hospitalization and suggested that the minimally effective cortico-steroid dose should be used [6]. More than two-thirds of the geriatric population (aged 65 years or older) have hypertension and 22% to 33% have diabetes, which are associated with a high risk of major complications such as lower-extremity amputation, myocardial infarction, and visual impairment [7,8]. Therefore, the burden of complications associated with corticosteroid use may be larger in the elderly population than in younger patients.

Prednisone at a dose of 60 mg daily or methylprednisolone (MPD) at a dose of 48 mg for 7 to 14 days is frequently used as an initial medication in the treatment of ISSNHL, and the doses are subsequently tapered [1]. However, many clinicians use slightly different protocols in terms of the type of steroid, dosage, and duration in different clinical settings, and the number of comparative studies of different steroid protocols is limited [1,9].

Based on these findings, we assumed that, if treatment outcomes following low-dose steroid treatments were as effective as those following higher-dose steroid treatments, the low-dose treatments would be accompanied by a reduced risk of adverse effects and that the use of low-dose steroid treatments for ISSNHL in geriatric patients would be more rational.

In this study, we aimed to compare the treatment outcomes and the occurrence rates of adverse events according to different

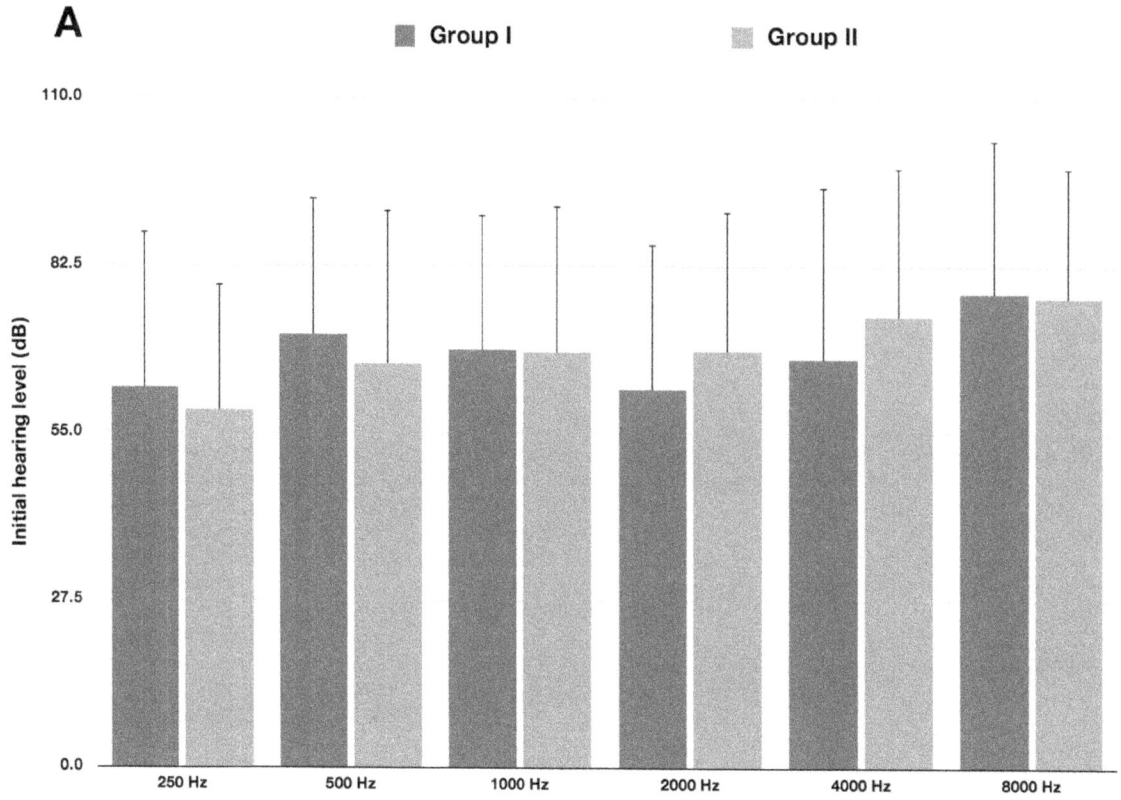

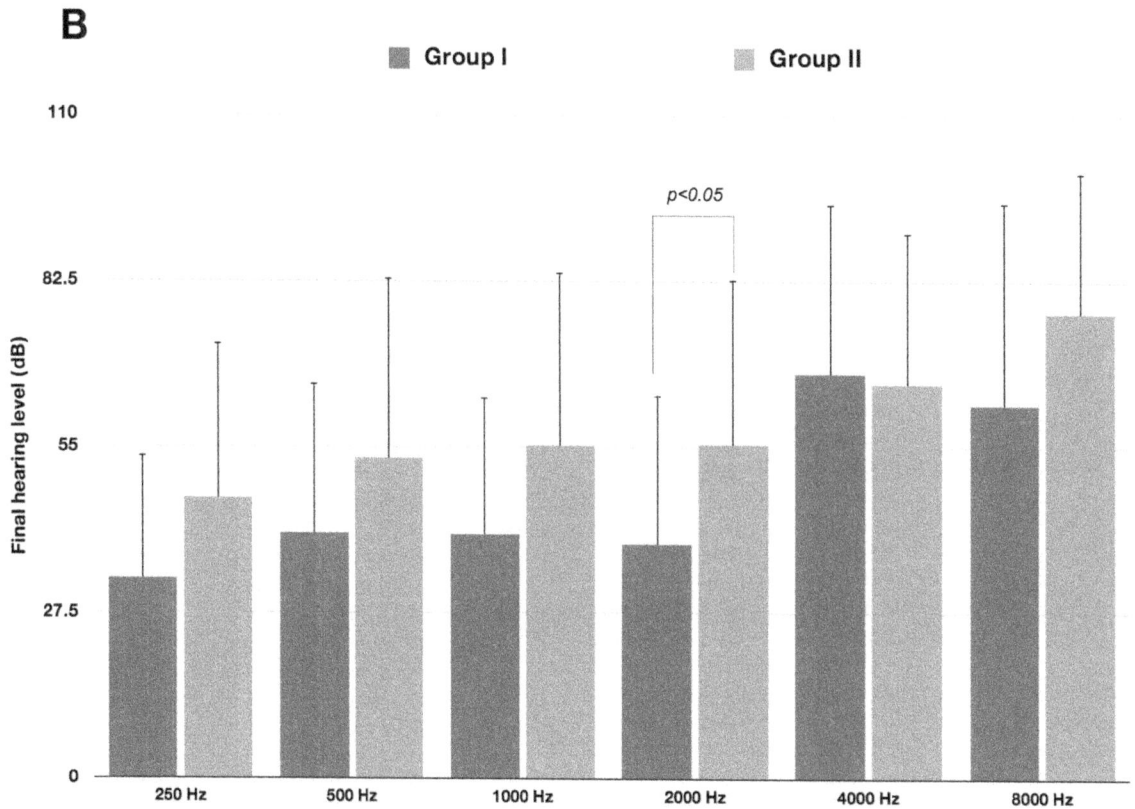

Figure 1. Changes in hearing levels at each frequency before and after treatment in propensity-score matched population. (A) Comparison of the pretreatment hearing levels at each frequency. (B) Comparison of the posttreatment hearing levels at each frequency.

steroid regimens in ISSNHL patients aged 65 years or older by using a propensity score-matched (PSM) analysis.

Materials and Methods

Ethics Statement

This study was approved by the Institutional Review Board of the Eulji University (No. 2014-02-010). The Board granted a waiver of written informed consent for this retrospective study.

Patients

Based on retrospective medical chart reviews, we enrolled patients who were aged 65 years or older and had been diagnosed with ISSNHL and admitted to the university hospital between May 2006 and December 2013. The exclusion criteria were as follows: 1) concomitant meningitis, myelitis, vasculopathy, or neuropsychiatric disease; 2) a clinical observation period less than 3 months; 3) previous histories of sudden hearing loss and/or the possibility of Meniere's disease; and 4) uncontrolled hypertension or uncontrolled diabetes mellitus.

Age, sex, comorbid diabetes and hypertension, the presence of dizziness and/or tinnitus, the period of time from onset to treatment, the initial hearing levels of both ears, and the final hearing level of the affected side 3 months after the onset of treatment were documented.

Treatment Protocols

All patients were hospitalized for 1 week, and one of two types of treatment was provided using the time-variant differential approach: either oral MPD treatment or "low-dose" oral MPD treatment. Oral MPD treatment was administered between 2006 and 2008. Subsequently, oral "low-dose" MPD treatment became

the mainstream treatment and was commonly used until 2010. From early 2011, an additional intratympanic dexamethasone injection (IT-DEX) administered as a salvage therapy following oral MPD treatment has been the main treatment for sudden deafness.

Patients who received the oral MPD treatment were treated with steroids for 10 days using the same recommended dosage protocol for MPD (48 mg/d for 4 days, followed by a taper of 8 mg every 2 days) [9]. The total cumulative dose of MPD was 432 mg (equivalent to 530 mg of prednisolone) over 14 days. These patients were classified as group I. Patients who received the oral "low-dose" MPD treatment were treated with a half-dose of oral MPD (24 mg/d for the first 4 days, followed by a taper by 8 mg every 2 days). The total cumulative dose of MPD was 144 mg (equivalent to 180 mg of prednisolone) over 8 days. These patients were classified as group II.

Moreover, for patients who required an additional cointervention, a continuous infusion of 10 μg/d of alprostadil over 7 days or daily intravenous infusions of 88 mg of zinc sulfate hydrate were provided.

Calculation of Hearing Levels and Estimation of Recoveries

Hearing levels were calculated using the arithmetic mean of the hearing levels at 500 Hz, 1 kHz, 2 kHz, and 4 kHz. Hearing improvement rates were calculated as the hearing gain divided by the initial hearing difference between the lesion side and the healthy side and then multiplied by 100 [10,11]. Complete recovery was defined by a final hearing level within 20 dB or equal to the hearing level of the unaffected ear [10,11]. Good recovery was defined as hearing gains greater than 30 dB [10,11]. Fair recovery was defined as hearing gains of 10 to 29 dB. Hearing

Table 1. Baseline clinical characteristics.

	Total population			Propensity-matched population		
	Group I (n=66)	Group II (n=43)	p-value	Group I (n=20)	Group II (n=20)	p-value
Age	72.52±5.00	70.49±5.24	0.045	71.45±5.56	71.10±5.15	0.816
Male	26 (59.1)	18 (58.1)	0.798	9 (45.0)	9 (45.0)	1.000
Body mass index (kg/m²)	25.10±3.58	24.46±3.14	0.342	25.43±3.87	24.79±3.32	0.555
Diabetes mellitus	17 (25.8)	9 (20.9)	0.563	4 (20.0)	4 (20.0)	1.000
Hypertension	29 (43.9)	27 (62.8)	0.054	10 (50.0)	7 (35.0)	0.337
Days from onset to treatment	3.98±2.73	3.86±3.24	0.829	4.00±3.04	3.40±1.96	0.333
Right side	33 (50.0)	23 (53.5)	0.722	9 (45.0)	9 (45.0)	1.000
Dizziness	12 (18.2)	4 (9.3)	0.200	3 (15.0)	2 (10.0)	0.633
Tinnitus	43 (65.2)	33 (76.7)	0.198	16 (80.0)	15 (75.0)	0.705
Intratympanic injection	5 (7.6)	4 (9.3)	0.749	0 (0.0)	0 (0.0)	–
Alprostadil injection	48 (72.7)	30 (69.8)	0.738	15 (75.0)	18 (90.0)	0.212
Zinc injection	7 (10.6)	1 (2.3)	0.144	0 (0.0)	0 (0.0)	–
Initial hearing (dB)	65.70±23.34	73.92±22.51	0.071	67.38±22.16	69.38±22.25	0.800
Initial contralateral hearing (dB)	43.22±26.89	43.66±22.08	0.928	41.38±27.55	42.63±22.19	0.890
Final hearing (dB)	46.67±26.20	56.54±26.98	0.060	42.00±22.35	57.38±26.40	0.058

Data are presented as mean±standard deviation or number (percentage).

Table 2. Comparison of the posttreatment hearing levels at each frequency.

	250 Hz	500 Hz	1000 Hz	2000 Hz	4000 Hz	8000 Hz
Group I (dB)	33.25±20.28	40.75±24.83	40.50±22.65	39.00±24.53	67.25±28.03	62.00±33.50
Group II (dB)	46.50±25.76	53.25±29.84	55.25±28.72	55.50±27.38	65.50±24.92	77.25±23.25
p-value	0.096	0.142	0.065	0.049*	0.864	0.109

Data are presented as mean±standard deviation; *: p<0.05.

gains of less than 10 dB were defined as no change or deterioration [10,11].

Adverse Events

From the medical chart reviews, insomnia, abdominal discomfort, high blood pressure that occurred more than twice per day (systolic pressure, ≥150 mmHg, and/or diastolic pressure, ≥ 90 mmHg), and hyperglycemia for which insulin had been newly prescribed or increased were documented. Additionally, major complications such as myocardial infarction, gastrointestinal bleeding, and death were also documented.

Statistical Analyses

The details of the estimation of the propensity scores were as follows: (1) age, sex, accompanying hypertension and diabetes, presence of tinnitus or dizziness, initial hearing levels of the lesion and healthy sides, IT-DEX treatment, and other cointerventions (alprostadil or zinc injection) were selected as covariates based on the results of the previous studies [12–16]; (2) treatment assignment (group I or II) was used as the outcome variable; (3) logistic regression was performed, and propensity scores were calculated. The 1:1 nearest-neighbor method was used for matching. Next, a test of the balance of the covariates was performed, and the treatment effects were finally compared using paired t-tests and McNemar's tests. All statistical analyses were performed using the SPSS software (ver. 18.0, SPSS Inc., Chicago, IL, USA), and the level of statistical significance was set at a p-value of less than 0.05.

Results

A total of 109 patients were enrolled in this study, including 44 men (40.4%) and 65 women (59.6%), with a mean age of 71.72 years (range, 65–87 years) and mean ISSNHL duration (from the onset to treatment) of 3.94±2.93 days. Diabetes was reported in 26 patients (23.9%) and hypertension in 56 (51.4%). Of accompanying symptoms, 76 patients (69.7%) had tinnitus and 16 (14.7%) had dizziness. The mean initial hearing level was 68.95±23.26 dB and the initial contralateral hearing level was 43.39±25.00 dB. The baseline characteristics revealed marginally significant differences in age (p=0.045), accompanying hypertension (p=0.054), and initial hearing levels (p=0.071) between the steroid regimen groups.

After the PSM analysis, 20 pairs of patients were allocated either to group I or II (Table 1), and the balance test revealed that there were no significant differences in any of the covariates (p>0.05). The final hearing level in group I was 42.00±22.35 dB and that in group II was 57.38±26.40 dB (p=0.058, 95% confidence interval of the difference: −31.30 dB to 0.55 dB). Comparison of the individual frequencies in the PSM population revealed that the pretreatment audiograms were not different at any of the frequencies between the two groups (Figure 1A, p>0.05); however, the posttreatment audiograms showed marginally significant differences at 1000 Hz (p=0.065) and 2000 Hz (p=0.049) (Figure 1B, Table 2).

The hearing improvement rates did not differ between groups I and II (114.69±299.56% and 123.32±392.28%, respectively; p=0.941). Regarding hearing recovery, group I showed a tendency for better recovery compared with group II, but the difference was not significant (Table 3, p>0.05).

Table 3. Treatment outcomes according to different steroid regimens.

Total population (n=109)	Total population			Propensity-matched population		
	Group I (n=66)	Group II (n=43)	p-value	Group I (n=20)	Group II (n=20)	p-value
Recovery, n (%)						
CR	7 (10.6)	1 (2.3)	0.144	2 (10.0)	1 (5.0)	0.370
CR+GR	25 (37.9)	11 (25.6)	0.182	8 (40.0)	3 (15.0)	0.109
CR+GR+FR	42 (63.6)	23 (53.5)	0.291	15 (75.0)	10 (50.0)	0.227
HIR	40.46±270.90	80.13±269.90	0.456	114.69±299.56	123.32±392.28	0.941
Adverse effects, n (%)						
Insomnia	5 (7.6)	1(2.3)	0.400	2 (10.0)	1(5.0)	1.000
Abdominal discomfort	14 (21.2)	12 (27.9)	0.493	3(15.0)	6(15.0)	0.375
High BP	17 (25.8)	15 (34.9)	0.309	7 (35.0)	6 (30.0)	1.000
Hyperglycemia	17 (25.8)	6 (14.0)	0.140	7 (35.0)	4 (20.0)	0.453

CR: complete recovery; GR: good recovery; FR: fair recovery; HIR: hearing improvement rate; BP: blood pressure.

Regarding severe adverse events during treatment, one patient in group II experienced pulmonary edema and upper gastrointestinal bleeding. However, other major complications, such as myocardial infarction and death, did not occur in any of the groups.

Regarding minor adverse events, the PSM analysis revealed that patients in group I complained of insomnia (10% of the patients), abdominal discomfort (15%), high blood pressure (35%), and hyperglycemia (35%). However, the occurrence rates of these adverse events were not significantly different between the two groups (Table 3).

Discussion

Our study showed that patients receiving conventional steroid treatment had slightly better hearing recovery than patients who received reduced steroid doses, although the difference was marginally significant. Similar trends were found when the final audiograms at all frequencies were compared, with the exception of the 4 kHz frequency. No significant differences in the occurrence rates of adverse effects were found between the two groups.

These findings may suggest that steroid dose reduction is not preferable to the conventional steroid regimen in geriatric patients with ISSNHL.

In contrast, a prospective randomized trial reported that therapeutic outcomes did not differ between 7-day prednisolone and 300 mg dexamethasone pulse therapies [17]. The colleagues of those authors also reported newly developed myocardial infarctions in patients following the pulse therapy and urged clinicians to consider the severe risks of steroid treatment [18]. These findings suggest that the potential benefits of high-dose pulse therapy may not exceed the risks of severe complications. In addition, the duration of steroid use as well as the dosage may be important variables, both of which determine the cumulative steroid dose that may affect the hearing outcome or occurrence of adverse events. The relatively short-term duration of treatment in group II (8 days) compared with that in group I (14 days) might have affected the treatment outcome in our study. A recent survey conducted in the United States reported that 32.2% of the physicians preferred a 14-day steroid treatment, 33.2%, 10-day treatment, and 16.1%, 7-day treatment [19]. This may be attributed to the fact that the optimal dosage and duration of steroid treatment, particularly in elderly population with comorbidities, have not been determined.

With aging, liver function, which is primarily responsible for the metabolism of steroids, is mostly maintained, but phase I metabolism catalyzed by cytochrome P450 tends to decrease, and an increase in interindividual variability is distinctive [20]. Moreover, the affinities of the receptor protein for dexamethasone and corticosterone tend to decrease [21]. Therefore, the use of higher steroid doses might be more rational than lower-dose

steroid treatment; however, excessively high-dose steroid treatments have failed to show additional benefits [17]. Based on these findings, we suggest that further studies comparing a greater range of steroid regimens for the treatment of ISSNHL should be performed to identify the optimal dose because we still do not have many options other than steroid treatment [9].

Apart from systemic steroid treatment, intratympanic steroid injection is currently recommended after the failure of the initial treatment [1]. Other possible treatment options include hyperbaric oxygen therapy, and a significant improvement in hearing was reported in the acute stage of ISSNHL following this therapy [22]. The mechanism of action in this therapy is now thought to be the control of cochlear ischemia by increasing oxygen partial pressure. However, in most hospitals, this therapy is not available because it requires a specific sealed chamber. Moreover, it is an expensive and time-consuming treatment method. Other possible options include medications such as antiviral agents [23], vasodilators (such as carbogen, alprostadil, naftidrofuryl, and low-molecular-weight dextran) [24], high-dose vitamins [25,26], and zinc supplementation [27]. However, the effects of these agents have not been sufficiently studied and there is no evidence to support their use.

To reduce the confounding effects between diverse treatment options and the observed baseline characteristics, we performed the PSM analysis [28,29]. Selection bias was decreased as far as possible by controlling for the diverse prognostic factors and cointerventions that may have influenced the treatment outcomes. As a result, we were able to compare the intervention effects of the examined steroid regimens by the PSM analysis in order to overcome the limitations of the retrospective, observational study design [29].

Our study has several limitations. It seems unnatural to include covariates such as IT-DEX, alprostadil, and zinc, which may act as confounding factors to the outcome, in the PSM analysis. However, the exclusion of all patients who were treated with cointerventions could result in insignificant conclusions owing to a small sample size. Therefore, we controlled cointerventions as covariates to be able to evaluate the sole effect of steroid dose by minimizing the between-group difference.

In conclusion, conventional steroid regimens produced the occurrence rates of adverse events that were similar to those of low-dose treatment but may also have produced better recoveries. The use of steroid dose reduction in geriatric patients with ISSNHL is not preferable to conventional steroid regimen.

Author Contributions

Conceived and designed the experiments: HYL CSC. Performed the experiments: MSC HYL. Analyzed the data: MSC HYL. Contributed reagents/materials/analysis tools: MSC HYL. Wrote the paper: MSC HYL.

References

1. Stachler RJ, Chandrasekhar SS, Archer SM, Rosenfeld RM, Schwartz SR, et al. (2012) Clinical practice guideline: sudden hearing loss. Otolaryngol Head Neck Surg 146(3 Suppl): S1-35.

2. Schreiber BE, Agrup C, Haskard DO, Luxon LM (2010) Sudden sensorineural hearing loss. Lancet 375: 1203–1211.

3. Wei BP, Stathopoulos D, O'Leary S (2013) Steroids for idiopathic sudden sensorineural hearing loss. Cochrane Database Syst Rev 7: CD003998.

4. Rauch SD, Halpin CF, Antonelli PJ, Babu S, Carey JP, et al. (2011) Oral vs intratympanic corticosteroid therapy for idiopathic sudden sensorineural hearing loss: a randomized trial. JAMA 305: 2071–2079.

5. Ogino-Nishimura E, Nakagawa T, Tateya I, Hiraumi H, Ito J (2013) Systemic steroid application caused sudden death of a patient with sudden deafness. Case Rep Otolaryngol 3: 734131–7341312. doi:10.1155/2013/734131

6. Caughey GE, Preiss AK, Vitry AI, Gilbert AL, Roughead EE (2013) Comorbid diabetes and COPD: impact of corticosteroid use on diabetes complications. Diabetes Care 36: 3009–3014. doi:10.2337/dc12-2197

7. Lionakis N, Mendrinos D, Sanidas E, Favatas G, Georgopoulou M (2012) Hypertension in the elderly. World J Cardiol 4: 135–147.

8. Kirkman MS, Briscoe VJ, Clark N, Florez H, Haas LB, et al. (2012) Diabetes in older adults. Diabetes Care 35: 2650–2664.

9. Rauch SD (2008) Clinical practice. Idiopathic sudden sensorineural hearing loss. N Engl J Med 359: 833–840.

10. Kanzaki J, Taiji H, Ogawa K (1988) Evaluation of hearing recovery and efficacy of steroid treatment in sudden deafness. Acta Otolaryngol Suppl 456: 31–36.

11. Suzuki H, Hashida K, Nguyen KH, Hohchi N, Katoh A, et al. (2012) Efficacy of intratympanic steroid administration on idiopathic sudden sensorineural hearing

loss in comparison with hyperbaric oxygen therapy. Laryngoscope 122: 1154–1157.

12. Xenellis J, Karapatsas I, Papadimitriou N, Nikolopoulos T, Maragoudakis P, et al. (2006) Idiopathic sudden sensorineural hearing loss: prognostic factors. J Laryngol Otol 120: 718–724.

13. Cvorović L, Deric D, Probst R, Hegemann S (2008) Prognostic model for predicting hearing recovery in idiopathic sudden sensorineural hearing loss. Otol Neurotol 29: 464–469.

14. Hikita-Watanabe N, Kitahara T, Horii A, Kawashima T, Doi K, et al. (2010) Tinnitus as a prognostic factor of sudden deafness. Acta Otolaryngol 130: 79–83.

15. Yang CH, Ko MT, Peng JP, Hwang CF (2011) Zinc in the treatment of idiopathic sudden sensorineural hearing loss. Laryngoscope 121: 617–621. doi:10.1002/lary.21291 Epub 2010 Oct 6.

16. Kim MG, Jung YG, Eun YG (2011) Effect of steroid, carbogen inhalation, and lipoprostaglandin E1 combination therapy for sudden sensorineural hearing loss. Am J Otolaryngol 32: 91–95. doi:10.1016/j.amjoto.2009

17. Westerlaken BO, de Kleine E, van der Laan B, Albers F (2007) The treatment of idiopathic sudden sensorineural hearing loss using pulse therapy: a prospective, randomized, double-blind clinical trial. Laryngoscope 117: 684–690.

18. Free RH, Smale ND, de Kleine E, van der Laan BF (2009) Side effects of oral dexamethasone pulse therapy for idiopathic sudden sensorineural hearing loss. Otol Neurotol 30: 691.

19. Coelho DH, Thacker LR, Hsu DW (2011) Variability in the management of idiopathic sudden sensorineural hearing loss. Otolaryngol Head Neck Surg 145: 813–817.

20. Schmucker DL (2001) Liver function and phase I drug metabolism in the elderly: a paradox. Drugs Aging 18: 837–851.

21. Bolla R (1980) Age-dependent changes in rat liver steroid hormone receptor proteins. Mech Ageing Dev 12: 249–259.

22. Bennett MH, Kertesz T, Perleth M, Yeung P, Lehm JP (2012) Hyperbaric oxygen for idiopathic sudden sensorineural hearing loss and tinnitus. Cochrane Database Syst Rev 17: CD004739.

23. Awad Z, Huins C, Pothier DD (2012) Antivirals for idiopathic sudden sensorineural hearing loss. Cochrane Database Syst Rev 15: CD006987.

24. Agarwal L, Pothier DD (2009) Vasodilators and vasoactive substances for idiopathic sudden sensorineural hearing loss. Cochrane Database Syst Rev 7: CD003422.

25. Kaya H, Koç AK, Sayın I, Güneş S, Altıntaş A, et al. (2014) Vitamins A, C, and E and selenium in the treatment of idiopathic sudden sensorineural hearing loss. Eur Arch Otorhinolaryngol. doi:10.1007/s00405-014-2922-9 Epub ahead of print.

26. Kang HS, Park JJ, Ahn SK, Hur DG, Kim HY (2013) Effect of high dose intravenous vitamin C on idiopathic sudden sensorineural hearing loss: a prospective single-blind randomized controlled trial. Eur Arch Otorhinolaryngol 270: 2631–2636.

27. Yang CH, Ko MT, Peng JP, Hwang CF (2011) Zinc in the treatment of idiopathic sudden sensorineural hearing loss. Laryngoscope 121: 617–621.

28. Stuart EA (2010) Matching methods for causal inference: A review and a look forward. Stat Sci 25: 1–21.

29. Austin PC, Laupacis A (2011) A tutorial on methods to estimating clinically and policy-meaningful measures of treatment effects in prospective observational studies: a review. Int J Biostat 7: 6. doi:10.2202/1557-4679.1285

Permissions

The contributors of this book come from diverse backgrounds, making this book a truly international effort. This book will bring forth new frontiers with its revolutionizing research information and detailed analysis of the nascent developments around the world.

We would like to thank all the contributing authors for lending their expertise to make the book truly unique. They have played a crucial role in the development of this book. Without their invaluable contributions this book wouldn't have been possible. They have made vital efforts to compile up to date information on the varied aspects of this subject to make this book a valuable addition to the collection of many professionals and students.

This book was conceptualized with the vision of imparting up-to-date information and advanced data in this field. To ensure the same, a matchless editorial board was set up. Every individual on the board went through rigorous rounds of assessment to prove their worth. After which they invested a large part of their time researching and compiling the most relevant data for our readers.

The editorial board has been involved in producing this book since its inception. They have spent rigorous hours researching and exploring the diverse topics which have resulted in the successful publishing of this book. They have passed on their knowledge of decades through this book. To expedite this challenging task, the publisher supported the team at every step. A small team of assistant editors was also appointed to further simplify the editing procedure and attain best results for the readers.

Apart from the editorial board, the designing team has also invested a significant amount of their time in understanding the subject and creating the most relevant covers. They scrutinized every image to scout for the most suitable representation of the subject and create an appropriate cover for the book.

The publishing team has been an ardent support to the editorial, designing and production team. Their endless efforts to recruit the best for this project, has resulted in the accomplishment of this book. They are a veteran in the field of academics and their pool of knowledge is as vast as their experience in printing. Their expertise and guidance has proved useful at every step. Their uncompromising quality standards have made this book an exceptional effort. Their encouragement from time to time has been an inspiration for everyone.

The publisher and the editorial board hope that this book will prove to be a valuable piece of knowledge for researchers, students, practitioners and scholars across the globe.

List of Contributors

Isabella Monia Montagner and Anna Merlo
Veneto Institute of Oncology IOV - IRCCS, Padua, Italy

Gaia Zuccolotto
Department of Medicine, University of Padua, Padua, Italy

Davide Renier and Monica Campisi
Fidia Farmaceutici S.p.A., Abano Terme, Italy

Gianfranco Pasut
Department of Pharmaceutical and Pharmacological Sciences, University of Padua, Padua, Italy

Paola Zanovello and Antonio Rosato
Department of Surgery, Oncology and Gastroenterology, University of Padua, Padua, Italy

Paul E. Sax
Division of Infectious Diseases, Brigham and Women's Hospital, Boston, Massachusetts, United States of America
Harvard University Center for AIDS Research, Harvard University, Boston, Massachusetts, United States of America

Alexis Sypek, Bethany K. Berkowitz, Bethany L. Morris and Kathleen A. Kelly
Division of General Medicine, Department of Medicine, Massachusetts General Hospital, Boston, Massachusetts, United States of America
Medical Practice Evaluation Center, Department of Medicine, Massachusetts General Hospital, Boston, Massachusetts, United States of America

Elena Losina
Department of Orthopedic Surgery, Brigham and Women's Hospital, Boston, Massachusetts, United States of America
Harvard University Center for AIDS Research, Harvard University, Boston, Massachusetts, United States of America
Division of General Medicine, Department of Medicine, Massachusetts General Hospital, Boston, Massachusetts, United States of America
Medical Practice Evaluation Center, Department of Medicine, Massachusetts General Hospital, Boston, Massachusetts, United States of America

Department of Biostatistics, Boston University School of Public Health, Boston, Massachusetts, United States of America

A.David Paltiel
Yale School of Public Health, New Haven, Connecticut, United states of America

George R. Seage III and Milton C. Weinstein
Harvard School of Public Health, Harvard University, Boston, Massachusetts, United States of America

Rochelle P. Walensky
Division of Infectious Diseases, Brigham and Women's Hospital, Boston, Massachusetts, United States of America
Harvard University Center for AIDS Research, Harvard University, Boston, Massachusetts, United States of America
Division of Infectious Diseases, Department of Medicine, Massachusetts General Hospital, Boston, Massachusetts, United States of America
Medical Practice Evaluation Center, Department of Medicine, Massachusetts General Hospital, Boston, Massachusetts, United States of America

Joseph Eron
Division of Infectious Disease, School of Medicine, University of North Carolina at Chapel Hill, Chapel Hill, North Carolina, United States of America

Kenneth A. Freedberg
Harvard University Center for AIDS Research, Harvard University, Boston, Massachusetts, United States of America
Harvard School of Public Health, Harvard University, Boston, Massachusetts, United States of America
Division of General Medicine, Department of Medicine, Massachusetts General Hospital, Boston, Massachusetts, United States of America
Division of Infectious Diseases, Department of Medicine, Massachusetts General Hospital, Boston, Massachusetts, United States of America
Medical Practice Evaluation Center, Department of Medicine, Massachusetts General Hospital, Boston, Massachusetts, United States of America

Department of Epidemiology, Boston University School of Public Health, Boston, Massachusetts, United States of America

Luca Massacesi
Dipartimento di Neuroscienze, Psicologia, Farmaco e Salute del Bambino Universita` di Firenze, Firenze, Italy Neurologia , Azienda Ospedaliero-Universitaria Careggi, Firenze, Italy

Irene Tramacere, Clara Milanese, Graziella Filippini and Alessandra Solari
Fondazione IRCCS Istituto Neurologico Carlo Besta, Milano, Italy

Salvatore Amoroso
Dipartimento di Neuroscienze, Sezione di Farmacologia, Universita` Politecnica delle Marche, Ancona, Italy

Mario A. Battaglia
Associazione Italiana Sclerosi Multipla (AISM), Fondazione Italiana Sclerosi Multipla (FISM), Genova, Italy

Maria Donata Benedetti
Dipartimento Universitario di Neurologia, Azienda Ospedaliera Universitaria Integrata di Verona, Verona, Italy

Loredana La Mantia
Unitá di Neurologia - Multiple Sclerosis Center, I.R.C.C.S. Santa Maria Nascente Fondazione Don Gnocchi, Milano, Italy

Anna Repice
Neurologia, Azienda Ospedaliero-Universitaria Careggi, Firenze, Italy

Gioacchino Tedeschi
Clinica Neurologica, Universitá di Napoli, Napoli, Italy

Min Wang, Jun-Xia Cao, Yi-Shan Liu, Bei-Lei Xu, Duo Li, Xiao-Yan Zhang, Jun-Li Li, Jin-Long Liu, Hai-Bo Wang and Zheng-Xu Wang
Biotherapy Center, General Hospital of Beijing Military Command, Beijing, China

Jian-Hong Pan
Department of Biostatistics, Peking University Clinical Research Institute, Peking University Health Science Center, Beijing, China

Shing Chan, Godfrey Chi-fung Chan, Yiu-fai Cheung and Mei-pian Chen
Department of Pediatrics and Adolescent Medicine, The University of Hong Kong, Hong Kong, China

Z. Ioav Cabantchik
Department of Biological Chemistry, Alexander Silberman Institute of Life Sciences, Hebrew University of Jerusalem, Safra Campus at Givat Ram, Jerusalem, Israel

Reginald M. Gorczynski
University Health Network, Toronto General Hospital, Toronto, Canada
Department of Immunology, Faculty of Medicine, University of Toronto, and Institute of Medical Science, University of Toronto, Toronto, Ontario, Canada

Zhiqi Chen, Ismat Khatri and Anna Podnos
University Health Network, Toronto General Hospital, Toronto, Canada

Nuray Erin
Department of Medical Pharmacology, Akdeniz University, School of Medicine, Antalya, Turkey

Man Li, Zhen Liang, Xun Sun, Tao Gong and Zhirong Zhang
Key Laboratory of Drug Targeting and Drug Delivery Systems, Ministry of Education, West China School of Pharmacy, Sichuan University, Chengdu, Sichuan, PR China

Rong Lin, Yiyi Tao, Yibing Yu, Zhendong Xu, Jing Su and Zhiqiang Liu
Department of Anaesthesiology, Shanghai First Maternity and Infant Hospital, Tongji University School of Medicine, Shanghai, China

Diana Amorim, Ana David-Pereira, Patrícia Marques, Sónia Puga, Patrícia Rebelo, Patrício Costa, Armando Almeida and Filipa Pinto-Ribeiro
Life and Health Sciences Research Institute (ICVS), School of Health Sciences (ECS), University of Minho, Braga, Portugal, 2 ICVS/3B's - PT Government Associate Laboratory, Braga/Guimarães, Portugal

Antti Pertovaara
Institute of Biomedicine/Physiology, University of Helsinki, Helsinki, Finland

Anders W. Jørgensen
The Nordic Cochrane Centre, Dept 7811, Rigshospitalet, Copenhagen, Denmark

Lars H. Lundstrøm and Jørn Wetterslev
Copenhagen Trial Unit, Copenhagen Centre of Clinical Intervention Research, Dept 7812, Rigshospitalet, Copenhagen, Denmark

Arne Astrup
Department of Nutrition, Exercise and Sports, Faculty of Science, University of Copenhagen, Frederiksberg, Denmark

Peter C. Gøtzsche
Institute of Medicine and Surgery, Faculty of Health Sciences, University of Copenhagen, Copenhagen, Denmark

Skye P. Barbic and Zachary Durisko
Social Aetiology of Mental Illness (SAMI) Canadian Institute of Health Research (CIHR) Training Program, Centre for Addiction and Mental Health, Toronto, Ontario, Canada

Paul W. Andrews
Department of Psychology, Neuroscience & Behaviour, McMaster University, Hamilton, Canada

Chi T. Viet and Brian L. Schmidt
Department of Oral Maxillofacial Surgery, New York University, New York, New York, United States of America
Bluestone Center for Clinical Research, New York University, New York, New York, United States of America

Dongmin Dang, Stacy Achdjian, Yi Ye and Samuel G. Katz
Bluestone Center for Clinical Research, New York University, New York, New York, United States of America

Paola Genevini, Giulia Papiani, Annamaria Ruggiano and Francesca Navone
Institute of Neuroscience, Consiglio Nazionale delle Ricerche, and Department of Medical Biotechnology and Translational Medicine (BIOMETRA), Universitá degli Studi di Milano, Milano, Italy

Lavinia Cantoni
Department of Molecular Biochemistry and Pharmacology, Istituto di Ricerche Farmacologiche "Mario Negri", Milan, Italy

Nica Borgese
Institute of Neuroscience, Consiglio Nazionale delle Ricerche, and Department of Medical Biotechnology and Translational Medicine (BIOMETRA), Universitádegli Studi di Milano, Milano, Italy
Department of Health Science, Magna Graecia University of Catanzaro, Catanzaro, Italy

Matteo Cerri, Flavia Del Vecchio, Marco Mastrotto, Marco Luppi, Davide Martelli, Emanuele Perez, Domenico Tupone, Giovanni Zamboni and Roberto Amici
Department of Biomedical and NeuroMotor Sciences, Alma Mater Studiorum - University of Bologna, Bologna, Italy

Max Seidensticker, Ricarda Seidensticker, Robert Damm, Konrad Mohnike and Jens Ricke
Universitätsklinik Magdeburg, Klinik für Radiologie und Nuklearmedizin, Magdeburg, Germany
International School of Image-Guided Interventions, Deutsche Akademie für Mikrotherapie, Magdeburg, Germany

Maciej Pech
Universitätsklinik Magdeburg, Klinik für Radiologie und Nuklearmedizin, Magdeburg, Germany
International School of Image-Guided Interventions, Deutsche Akademie für Mikrotherapie, Magdeburg, Germany
Medical University of Gdansk, 2nd Department of Radiology, Gdansk, Poland

Bruno Sangro
Clinica Universidad de Navarra, Liver Unit, Department of Internal Medicine, Pamplona, Spain

Peter Hass and Günther Gademann
Universitätsklinik Magdeburg, Klinik für Strahlentherapie, Magdeburg, Germany

Peter Wust
Charité Universitätsmedizin Berlin, Klinik für Radioonkologie und Strahlentherapie, Berlin, Germany

Siegfried Kropf
Universitätsklinik Magdeburg, Institut für Biometrie und Medizinische Informatik, Magdeburg, Germany

Christian Gutsfeld
Division of Clinical Infectious Diseases, German Center for Infection Research Tuberculosis Unit, Research Center Borstel, Borstel, Germany

Department of Psychosomatic Medicine, Sachsenklinik, Bad Lausick, Germany

Ioana D. Olaru
Division of Clinical Infectious Diseases, German Center for Infection Research Tuberculosis Unit, Research Center Borstel, Borstel, Germany

Oliver Vollrath
Institute of Medical Informatics and Statistics, University Hospitals Schleswig-Holstein, Campus Kiel, Kiel, Germany

Christoph Lange
Division of Clinical Infectious Diseases, German Center for Infection Research Tuberculosis Unit, Research Center Borstel, Borstel, Germany
International Health/Infectious Diseases, University of Lübeck, Lübeck, Germany
Department of Internal Medicine, University of Namibia School of Medicine, Windhoek, Namibia
Department of Medicine, Karolinska Institute, Stockholm, Sweden

Eduardo Fuentes, Iván Palomo and Marcelo Alarcón
Department of Clinical Biochemistry and Immunohematology, Faculty of Health Sciences, Interdisciplinary Excellence Research Program on Healthy Aging (PIEI-ES), Universidad de Talca, Talca, Chile
Centro de Estudios en Alimentos Procesados (CEAP), CONICYT-Regional, Gore Maule, Talca, Chile

Jaime Pereira and Diego Mezzano
Department of Hematology- Oncology, School of Medicine, Pontificia Universidad Católica de Chile, Santiago, Chile

Julio Caballero
Center for Bioinformatics and Molecular Simulations, Faculty of Engineering in Bioinformatics, Universidad de Talca, Talca, Chile

Satoko Yamaguchi, Yoshiko Maida, Mami Yasukawa and Kenkichi Masutomi
Division of Cancer Stem Cell, National Cancer Center Research Institute, Tokyo, Japan

Tomoyasu Kato
Department of Gynecology, National Cancer Center Hospital, Tokyo, Japan

Masayuki Yoshida
Department of Pathology and Clinical Laboratories, National Cancer Center Hospital, Tokyo, Japan

Fei Ma Binghe Xu and Ying Fan
Department of Medical Oncology, Cancer Hospital, Chinese Academy of Medical Sciences and Peking Union Medical College, Beijing, China

Xiaoyan Ding
Department of Medical Oncology, Beijing DiTan Hospital, Capital Medical University, Beijing, China

Jianming Ying, Shan Zheng and Ning Lu
Department of Pathology, Cancer Hospital, Chinese Academy of Medical Sciences and Peking Union Medical College, Beijing, China

Christian Tudorache
Institute Biology Leiden, Leiden University, Leiden, The Netherlands

Erik Burgerhout
Institute Biology Leiden, Leiden University, Leiden, The Netherlands
NewCatch B.V., Leiden, The Netherlands

Sebastiaan Brittijn and Guido van den Thillart
NewCatch B.V., Leiden, The Netherlands

Cui Chen, Qiang-sheng Dai, Hui-wen Weng, He-ping Li and Sheng Ye
Department of Oncology, The First Affiliated Hospital, Sun Yat-Sen University, Guangzhou, China

Peng Sun
Department of Medical Oncology, Sun Yat-sen University Cancer Center, Guangzhou, China
Collaborative Innovation Center for Cancer Medicine, State Key Laboratory of Oncology in South China, Guangzhou, China

Anna Odone
TB Modelling Group, Centre for the Mathematical Modelling of Infectious Diseases, London School of Hygiene and Tropical Medicine, London, United Kingdom
Department of Global Health and Social Medicine, Harvard Medical School, Boston, Massachusetts, United States of America
University of Parma, School of Medicine, Parma, Italy

Silvia Amadasi
University Division of Infectious and Tropical Diseases, University of Brescia and Spedali Civili General Hospital, Brescia, Italy

Richard G. White and Rein M. G. J. Houben
TB Modelling Group, Centre for the Mathematical Modelling of Infectious Diseases, London School of Hygiene and Tropical Medicine, London, United Kingdom
TB Centre, London School of Hygiene and Tropical Medicine, London, United Kingdom

Theodore Cohen
Center for Communicable Disease Dynamics, Department of Epidemiology, Harvard School of Public Health, Boston, Massachusetts, United States of America
Division of Global Health Equity, Brigham and Women's Hospital, Boston, Massachusetts, United States of America

Alison D. Grant
TB Centre, London School of Hygiene and Tropical Medicine, London, United Kingdom
Department of Clinical Research, London School of Hygiene and Tropical Medicine, London, United Kingdom

Index

www.ingramcontent.com/pod-product-compliance
Lightning Source LLC
Chambersburg PA
CBHW061253190326
41458CB00011B/3659

www.ingramcontent.com/pod-product-compliance
Lightning Source LLC
Chambersburg PA
CBHW061253190326

41458CB00011B/3659